MODERN HOME
MEDICAL ADVISER

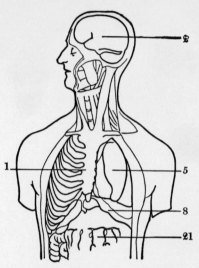

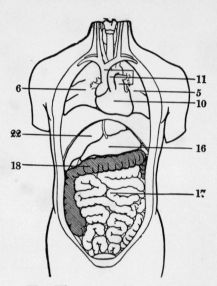

I. Head and chest. (*Explanation to color plate 1*)

II. Thoracic and abdominal cavities. External layer. (*Explanation to color plate 2*).

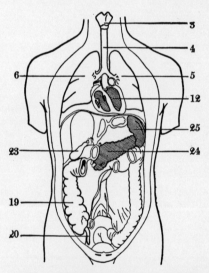

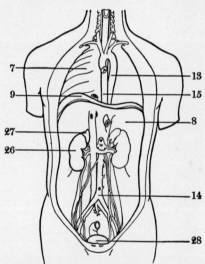

III. Thoracic and abdominal cavities. Median layer. (*Explanation to color plate 3*.)

IV. Thoracic and abdominal cavities. Posterior wall. (*Explanation to color plate 4*.)

1. Sternum. 2. Brain. 3. Larynx. 4. Trachea. 5. Left lung. 6. Right lung. 7. Right thorax. 8. Diaphragm. 9. Right dome of the diaphragm. 10. Heart. 11. Large cardiac vessels. 12. Cavities of the heart (shaded). 13. Large thoracic artery. 14. Large abdominal artery. 15. Esophagus. 16. Stomach. 17. Small intestine. 18. Large intestine (shaded). 19. Cecum. 20. Vermiform appendix of the cecum. 21. Omentum. 22. Liver. 23. Gall bladder. 24. Pancreas (shaded). 25. Spleen (shaded). 26. Right kidney. 27. Adrenal. 28. Urinary bladder.

These diagrams and the following four color plates are reproduced from *Man: Development, Nature and Function of Human Organism* (*Der Mensch: Von Werden, Wesen und Wirken des menschlichen Organismus*). Martin Vogel, Editor. Published by the German Hygiene Museum, Leipzig, 1930. Used by permission of Johann Ambrosius Barth.

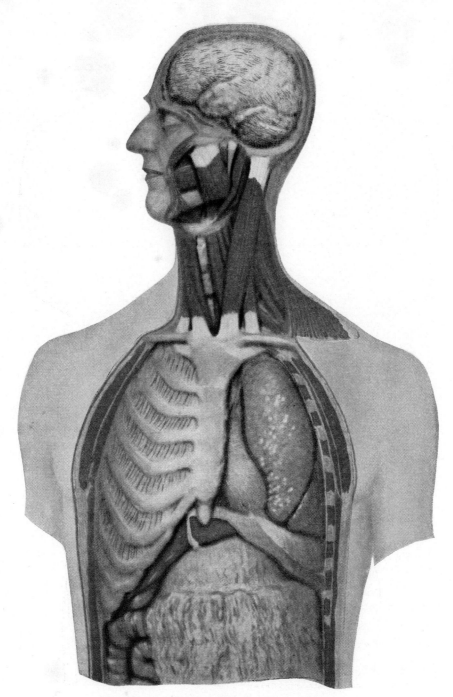

I. Cranial and thoracic cavities.

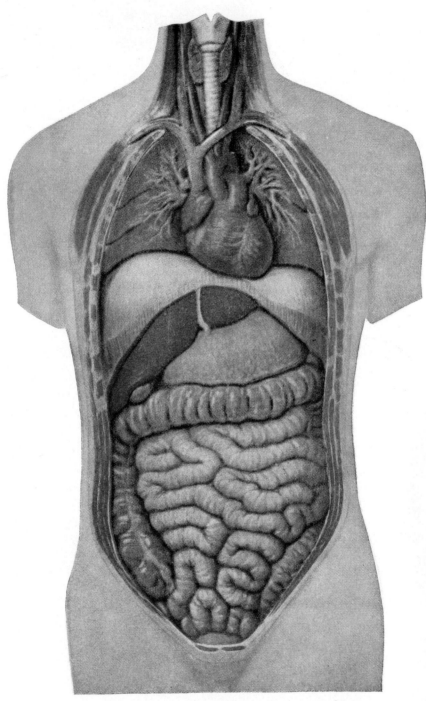

II.   Thoracic and abdominal cavities, external layer.

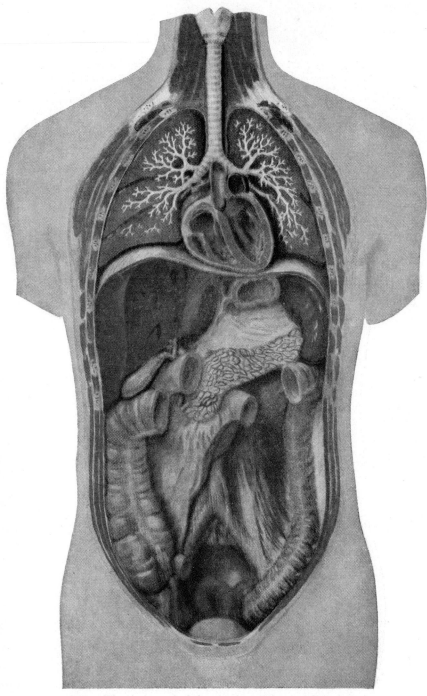

III. Thoracic and abdominal cavities, median layer.

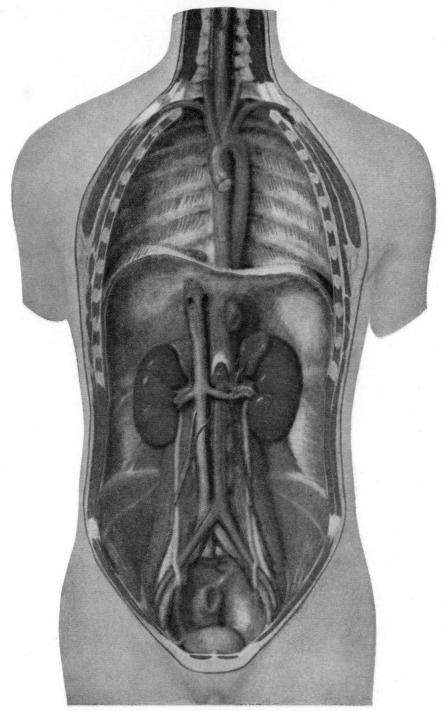

IV. Thoracic and abdominal cavities, posterior wall.

MODERN HOME
MEDICAL ADVISER

YOUR HEALTH AND HOW TO PRESERVE IT

EDITED BY
Morris Fishbein, M.D.

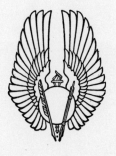

WITH MANY LINECUT AND HALFTONE ILLUSTRATIONS

New York
P. F. COLLIER & SON CORPORATION

BY SPECIAL ARRANGEMENT WITH
DOUBLEDAY, DORAN & COMPANY, INC.

NEW YORK

Preface

THIS VOLUME is planned to tell what every intelligent person ought to know about medicine and hygiene. It is in a way a modern substitute for the old-time family medicine book that used to be on the table in the sitting room along with the Bible in many a home in the United States.

The book is planned to answer questions concerning all the common, and even some of the extraordinary, illnesses that may develop in any family. Thus, all the common infectious diseases, deficiency diseases, disturbances of metabolism and digestion are discussed; also diseases due to disorders of the glands of internal secretion, to hyper-sensitivity, and to industrial causes. There are also special sections for such medical specialties as diseases of the skin, the eye, ear, nose and throat.

The book is planned also as an adequate guide to hygiene and first aid. It concerns not only prenatal care and the care of the child, but also the selection of a suitable diet, posture, mental hygiene, care of the feet, old age, the family medicine chest, and the choice of a physician.

An attempt has been made to write in a language that anyone can understand. In some conditions a knowledge of the structure and function of organs—anatomy and physiology—is necessary for understanding. Therefore such knowledge is provided and will require careful study.

In the preparation of this especially revised edition material which has been well established by use during the past five years has not been revised. However, much that is new has been developed during that time. An attempt has been made to introduce such new material in the proper places so as to enable readers to know whether or not new technics have been developed which will be helpful to them when applied by the physician in overcoming their troubles.

The editor wishes to express his sincere appreciation to all of those who have collaborated in making this book possible.

Chicago, November, 1940   MORRIS FISHBEIN, M.D.

Collaborators

WILLIAM W. DUKE, M.D.,
Visiting Physician to St. Mary's Hospital; Formerly Professor of Experimental Medicine, University of Kansas School of Medicine, Kansas City, Mo.

MORRIS FISHBEIN, M.D.,
Editor, *Journal American Medical Association*, Chicago.

NEWELL C. GILBERT, M.D.,
Associate Professor Medicine, Northwestern Univ. Med. School, Chicago.

JACOB P. GREENHILL, M.D.,
Associate Professor Gynecology, Loyola Univ. Medical School, Chicago.

PHILIP S. HENCH, M.D.,
Associate in Section in Division of Medicine, Mayo Clinic; Instructor in Medicine on Mayo Foundation for Medical Education and Research, Graduate School, University of Minnesota, Rochester, Minn.

RAPHAEL ISAACS, M.D.,
Associate Professor Internal Medicine, Univ. Mich. Med. School, Ann Arbor, Mich.

PHILIP C. JEANS, M.D.,
Professor Pediatrics, State Univ. of Iowa College of Medicine, Iowa City, Iowa.

WINGATE M. JOHNSON, M.D.,
Winston-Salem, N. C.

ELLIOTT P. JOSLIN, M.D.,
  Clinical Professor Medicine, Harvard University Medical School
  Boston, Mass.

OLIVER P. KIMBALL, M.D.,
  Cleveland, Ohio.

PHILIP LEWIN, M.D.,
  Associate Professor Orthopedic Surgery, Northwestern Univ.
  Med. School, Chicago.

CAREY P. McCORD, M.D.,
  Associate Professor Preventive Medicine, Univ. Cincinnati Coll.
  of Med., Cincinnati, Ohio.

R. TAIT McKENZIE, M.D.,
  Research Professor Physical Education, Univ. of Pa. School of
  Med., Philadelphia, Pa.

MILTON M. PORTIS, M.D.,
  Formerly Clinical Professor Medicine, Loyola Univ. Medical
  School, Chicago.

SIDNEY A. PORTIS, M.D.,
  Clinical Professor Medicine, Loyola Univ. Medical School,
  Chicago.

GEORGE K. PRATT, M.D.,
  Recently Associate Medical Officer, National Committee for
  Mental Hygiene, New York City.

THURMAN B. RICE, M.D.,
  Associate Professor Bacteriology and Public Health, Indiana
  Univ. School of Medicine, Indianapolis, Ind.

ARTHUR W. STILLIANS, M.D.,
  Professor Dermatology Northwestern Univ. Medical School,
  Chicago.

SOLOMON STROUSE, M.D.,
  Associate Clinical Professor Medicine, Rush Medical College,
  Chicago.

WALTER TIMME, M.D.,
  Professor Clinical Neurology, Columbia Univ. Coll. Phys. and
  Surgeons. New York, N. Y.

FREDERICK F. TISDALL, M.D.,
  Professor Pediatrics, University of Toronto, Toronto, Canada.

DWIGHT L. WILBUR, M.D.,
  Assistant in Section in Division of Medicine, Mayo Clinic; Fellow
  in Medicine, Mayo Foundation for Medical Education and Research, Graduate School, University of Minnesota, Rochester,
  Minn.

RUSSELL M. WILDER, M.D.,
  Head of Section in Division of Medicine, Mayo Clinic; Professor
  of Medicine, Mayo Foundation for Medical Education and Research, Graduate School, University of Minnesota, Rochester,
  Minn.

FRANCIS CARTER WOOD, M.D.,
  Editor, *American Journal of Cancer;* Professor and Director of
  Institute for Cancer Research, Columbia University, New York,
  N. Y.

Contents

                                                                    PAGE

Preface   V

CHAPTER

I. The Choice of a Physician, by Morris Fishbein, M.D.

    The Family Doctor   1
        Graduation from a Medical College. License by the State. The Doctor's Internship. Membership in the County Medical Society. Characteristics of an Ethical Doctor.

    The Scientific Advancement of Medicine   4
    Development of Specialists   6
        Consult the Family Doctor First.
    Picking a Family Doctor   7

II. The Family Medicine Chest, by Morris Fishbein, M.D.   9
    Taking Medicine   9
    Equipment of the Family Medicine Chest   16
    The Drugs and Medical Supplies   17

III. First Aid, by Morris Fishbein, M.D.   19
    Accidents   19
        Falls.
    Bleeding or Hemorrhage   20
        Nosebleed. Control of Bleeding.
    Bruises   22
    Foreign Bodies   23
    Fireworks and Toy Firearms   24
    Wounds   25
        Burns. Resuscitation. Electric Shock.

CHAPTER   PAGE
            Gas Poisoning   30
            Fainting and Unconsciousness   32
            Heat Stroke   33
            Bite Wounds   34
            Hiccups   35
            Migraine or Sick Headache   37
            Metallic and Food Poisoning   40
            Symptoms and Treatment of Acute Poisoning   41

IV. HYGIENE OF WOMEN, by Morris Fishbein, M.D.   50
            Disorders of Menstruation   52
            Exercises   53
            Painful Menstruation   54
            Absence of Menstruation   55
            The Rhythm of Menstruation and the Safe Period for
                    Prevention of Conception   60

V. SEX HYGIENE, by Thurman B. Rice, M.D.   64
            Introduction by M. F.   64
            The Ideals and Purposes of Sex Education   65
            Reproduction in the Plant and Animal Kingdoms   68
            The Anatomy and Physiology of the Reproductive
                    System   76
            The Teaching of Sex to the Young Child   82
            The School Child   90
            The Period of Adolescence   96
            The Mating Period   104
            The Honeymoon   111
            The Young Married Couple   116
            Sex in Middle and Advanced Life   121
            The Purpose of Marriage   128
            Abnormalities of Sexual Function   133
                    Masturbation. Excessive Sexuality. Sexual Frigidity.
                    Sexual Complexes.
            The Hygiene of the Reproductive System   137
                    Cleanliness. Menstruation. Diseases of the Genital
                    Organs. Sexual Intercourse in Pregnancy. Contracep-
                    tives. Abortion. Sexual Stimulation.

VI. CARE OF MOTHER BEFORE AND AFTER CHILDBIRTH, by
            J. P. Greenhill, M.D.   147
            Introduction by M. F.   147

CHAPTER   PAGE

Signs of Pregnancy   149
Visit to Physician   149
Serious Symptoms during Pregnancy   150
Estimating the Day of Birth   150
The Diet   151
   Special Diets.
Care of the Bowels   155
Care of the Kidneys in Pregnancy   156
Treatment of Kidney Complications   157
Clothing in Pregnancy   157
Exercise in Pregnancy   159
   Walking. Violent Exercise. Travel. Housework.
Bathing   162
   Kind of Bath to Take. Warm Bath Daily.
Care of the Breasts   163
Care of the Genital Organs   164
Care of the Hair   164
Care of the Teeth   164
The Mind   165
Signs of Trouble   165
Minor Ailments during Pregnancy   166
   Heartburn and Belching. Fainting and Dizziness.
   Varicose Veins. Hemorrhoids or Piles. Cramps in the
   Legs. Prevention of Goiter.
Preparations for Confinement   168
When to Call the Doctor for Confinement   170
What to Do if the Baby Is Born at Home Before the
   Patient Can Go to the Hospital   171
Postnatal Care   172
Weaning the Baby   176
Superstitions and Misconceptions about Childbirth   177

VII. CARE AND FEEDING OF THE CHILD, by Philip C. Jeans,
         M.D.   182
Introduction by M. F.   182
Development of the Infant   183
Physical Care and Hygiene   185
Crying   187
Exercise   188
Training   188

CHAPTER | PAGE

Nutrition of the Infant 189
Introductory Discussion.
Digestion 194
Stools 195
Breast Feeding 196
Technic of Nursing. Difficulties. Weaning.
Artificial Feeding 199
Sugars and Carbohydrates. Diluents. Synthetic Food
Mixtures. Formulas for Well Babies. Formulas with
Undiluted Milk. The Preparation of Formulas.
Choice and Care of Bottles and Nipples. Technic of
Feeding. Additions to the Milk Diet.
Care of the Sick Infant 205
Common Illnesses and Abnormalities 206
Jaundice in the Newborn. Hernia or "Rupture."
Common Colds. Otitis Media. Croup. Pneumonia.
Thrush. Intussusception. Rectal Prolapse. Pyelitis.
Vaginitis. Convulsions. Feeding in Acute Illness.
Vomiting. Colic. Constipation. Diarrhea. Malnu-
trition. Rickets.

VIII. INFANT HYGIENE, by Frederick F. Tisdall, M. D. 220
Exercise for Baby 220
Fresh Air for Baby 221
Exposure of Baby to Sunshine 221
Sleep for Baby 223
Diet 224
Toilet Habits 225
Bathing 226
Clothing 228
Mental Development of the Child 229

IX. THE PREVENTION AND TREATMENT OF INFECTIOUS
DISEASE, by Morris Fishbein, M.D. 230
About Germs 230
Incubation Periods 231
Resistance to Infectious Disease 232
Carriers of Disease 233
Paths by Which Germs Invade 234
Response of the Body to Germ Invasion 235
Stamping out Disease 236
Prevention of Infection 237
Personal Hygiene 238

CHAPTER   PAGE
        Incidence of Infectious Disease   238
        Cleanliness and Infection   239
        Treatment of Infectious Diseases   239

X. INFECTIOUS DISEASES OF CHILDHOOD, by Morris Fishbein, M.D.   241
        Diphtheria   241
           Treatment of Diphtheria.
        Measles   249
        German Measles   254
        Scarlet Fever   255
        Whooping Cough   259
        Chicken Pox   261
        Mumps   263
        Infantile Paralysis   265

XI. TRANSMISSIBLE DISEASES, by Morris Fishbein, M.D.   272
        Typhoid Fever   272
        Erysipelas   277
        Tetanus or Lockjaw   279
        Rabies or Hydrophobia   282
        Vincent's Angina   284
        Undulant Fever   285
        Amebiasis and Dysentery   287
        Tularemia   290
        Malaria   292
        Rat-Bite Fever   295
        Rocky Mountain Spotted Fever   296
        Glanders   297
        Psittacosis or Parrot Disease   298
        Epidemic Encephalitis   300

XII. THE RESPIRATORY DISEASES, by Morris Fishbein, M.D.   304
        The Common Cold   304
           Causes of Colds. Symptoms of Colds. Prevention of Colds. Vaccines against Colds. Treatment of Colds. General Treatment. Summer Colds.
        Pneumonia   314
        Tuberculosis   319
           Medical Treatment of Tuberculosis. Diet in Tuberculosis. Control of Tuberculous Cattle. Climate in

CHAPTER PAGE

Prevention and Treatment of Tuberculosis. Skin
Tests for Tuberculosis. Rest in Tuberculosis. Treatment of Tuberculosis. Mental Aspects in Tuberculosis. Health Hints for the Tuberculous. Conclusions.

XIII. RHEUMATISM, ARTHRITIS, AND GOUT, by Morris Fish-
bein, M.D. 337
Rheumatism and Arthritis 337
Causes of Chronic Arthritis. Symptoms of Inflam-
mation of Joints. Diets in Arthritis.
Gout 344

XIV. DISEASES OF THE HEART AND CIRCULATION, by Newell
C. Gilbert, M.D. 346
Introduction by M. F. 346
The Anatomy of the Heart 348
The Pericardium. Construction of the Heart. The
Heart Muscle.
The Function of the Heart 351
Changes in the Heart.
Congenitally Defective Hearts 355
Hearts Defective because of Disease 356
Manifestations of Rheumatic Fever in Childhood 356
Chorea 359
Rheumatic Inflammation of the Heart (Car-
ditis) 360
The Attack on Rheumatic Fever 363
Prevention.
Endocarditis 368
Syphilis of the Heart 371
Heart Changes in Hyperthyroidism 371
Angina Pectoris and Coronary Thrombosis 371
Angina Pectoris. Coronary Thrombosis.
Disordered Action of the Heart 377

XV. DIGESTION AND DIGESTIVE DISEASES, by Drs. Milton
M. and Sidney A. Portis 380
Introduction by M. F. 380
The Feces or "Stool" 384
Methods of Studying Digestion 388
Examination of Excreted Materials.

CHAPTER   PAGE

Acute Indigestion   391
Treatment of Indigestion   392
Difficulty in Swallowing   394
Dyspepsia   395
Gastroptosis   397
Ulcer of the Stomach and Duodenum   398
Disease of the Gall Bladder   401
Jaundice   403
Appendicitis   404
Ulcer, Gall-Bladder Disease, and Appendicitis   406
Cancer of the Stomach   407
Constipation   407
Colitis and Diarrhea   410
Chronic Diarrhea and Dysentery   411
Cancer of the Bowels   413
Intestinal Obstruction   414
Intestinal Parasites or "Worms"   415
Cathartics, Laxatives, and Enemas   417

XVI.   THE KIDNEY: ITS DISEASES AND DISTURBANCES, by
          Philip S. Hench, M.D.   418

Introduction by M. F.   418
Anatomy of the Kidney   421
Functions of the Kidney   424
Physiology of the Kidney: How It Carries on Its
       Functions   425
History of Kidney Disease before the Time of
       Richard Bright   428
   The Work of Richard Bright   432
   Modern Significance of Albuminuria   433
       Incidence. Types of Albuminuria. Nonrenal Albu-
       minuria. Chemical Types of Albuminuria. Conclu-
       sions Regarding Albuminuria.
   Modern Methods of Examining the Kidneys   440
   Knowledge Derived from Kidney Tests   443
   General Causes of Kidney Disease   444
   General Symptoms and Signs of Kidney Disease   445
   Uremia   446
   Aims in the Treatment of Kidney Disease and
       Kidney Failure   448

        Classification of Kidney Diseases: Synopsis of
            Chief Forms   452
            Group I. Diseases where Nephritis Becomes the
            Chief Cause of Ill Health. Group II. Nephrosis.
            Group III. Conditions in which the Urine Is Ab-
            normal but no Nephritis Is Present. Group IV.
            Disturbances of the Kidney Dependent on Malfor-
            mation.
        Conclusion   462

XVII.   THE BLOOD AND ITS DISEASES, by Raphael Isaacs,
            M.D.   464
        Introduction by M. F.   464
        The Meaning of a "Blood Count"   465
            Red Blood Cells. Red Coloring Matter. White Blood
            Cells. Blood Platelets.
        Why the Doctor Makes Certain Laboratory
            Tests and What They Tell Him   468
            The Wassermann and Kahn Tests.
        The Causes of Anemia   469
        Treatment of Anemia   472
        Blood Transfusion   473
        Symptoms of Anemia   474
        Prevention of Anemia   476
        Polycythemia, or Too Many Blood Cells   476
        Leukemia, or Too Many White Blood Cells   478
        Hemophilia, Purpura, and Abnormal Bleeding   479
        Enlargement of the Lymph Glands and the
            Spleen   481

XVIII. DEFICIENCY DISEASES, by Russell M. Wilder, M.D.,
            and Dwight L. Wilbur, M.D.   483
        Introduction by M. F.   483
        Vitamin A Deficiency and Xerophthalmia   488
            History. Effects. Source, Nature, and Action of
            Vitamin A. Prevention and Treatment.
        Beriberi: A Vitamin B Deficiency   491
            History. Symptoms. Treatment.
        Scurvy, or Vitamin C Deficiency   492
            History. Symptoms. Course. Treatment.
        Rickets: A Vitamin D Deficiency   494
            History. Incidence. Cause. Symptoms. Prevention
            and Treatment.

CHAPTER   PAGE

     Pellagra   *498*
        Cause. Incidence. Symptoms. Course. Treatment.
     Vitamin E   *501*

XIX. ALLERGY AND HYPERSENSITIVITY, INCLUDING HAY
     FEVER, ASTHMA, HIVES, HEADACHE,
     ECZEMA, STOMACH AND INTESTINAL DIS-
     ORDERS, AND OTHER FUNCTIONAL AND
     ORGANIC DISEASES, by William W.
     Duke, M.D.   *504*

     Introduction by M. F.   *504*
     Defining Allergy   *506*
     History   *507*
     Heredity   *508*
     Age of Onset   *508*
     Natural and Acquired Sensitiveness   *509*
     Effect of Environment and Climate   *509*
     Permanence of Sensitiveness   *510*
     Multiple Sensitiveness   *510*
     Specificity of Sensitiveness   *511*
     Degree of Sensitiveness   *511*
     Periodicity of Allergy   *511*
     The Nature of the Cause of Allergy   *512*
     Relationship of Allergy to General Health   *512*
     Personality of the Allergy Patient   *513*
     The Ill Effects of Careless Advice   *514*
     Agents which Tend to Sensitize   *514*
        Pollen. Foods. Animal Hair and Feathers. Cotton-
        seed, Linseed, Orris, Glue, and Corn Products. Molds
        and Fungi. Insects. Dust. Smoke. Drug Idiosyn-
        crasies. Animal Parasites. Bacteria. Therapeutic
        Serums. Sensitiveness of One Individual to Another.
     Sensitiveness to Heat and Effort, Cold, Light,
        and Scratches   *518*
     Deformities Caused by Allergy   *520*
     Symptoms of Allergy   *521*
        General Symptoms. Eye Symptoms. Nasal Symptoms.
        Mouth and Throat Symptoms. Lung Symptoms.
        Stomach and Intestinal Symptoms. Skin Symptoms.
        Headache. Nerve Manifestations. Bladder Symp-
        toms. Miscellaneous Symptoms.
     Diagnosis of Allergy   *523*

CHAPTER   PAGE

Treatment   524
Allergic Shock and General Illnesses, Removal of
Cause. Pollen Avoidance and Pollen Disease. Specific
Treatment. Nonspecific Treatment. Treatment with
Heat, Cold, Exercise, Light, and Scratches. Results
of Therapy.

XX. THE INTERNAL GLANDULAR SYSTEM   530
I. The Glands, by Walter Timme, M.D.   530
Introduction by M. F.   530
Thymus Gland   535
Pineal Gland   538
Thyroid Gland   539
Parathyroid Glands   542
Pituitary Gland   543
The Superarenal Glands   547
Addison's Disease   549
The Gonads or Sex Glands   551
Mechanism of Menstruation   552

II. Goiter: The Cause and Prevention, by Oliver
P. Kimball, M.D.   554
Endemic Goiter Districts   555
The Thyroid Gland   556
Periods When Goiter Is Most Likely to Occur   556
Chemistry of the Thyroid Secretion   557
Prevention of Goiter   557
Other Sources of Food Iodine.
The Results of Goiter   560

XXI. DIABETES, by Elliott P. Joslin, M.D.   563
Introduction by M. F.   563
Death Rate from Diabetes   565
What Is Diabetes?   567
Why Is Diabetes Increasing?   571
Prevention of Diabetes   571
Should a Diabetic Marry? The Wise Control
Their Weight. And If You Discover Diabetes in a
Relative. Louisa Drum and What She Did.
"A Little Child Shall Lead Them"   576
Diabetes Is Best Studied in Children. The Diabetic
Child's Splendid Teeth. The Diabetic Child and
Early Old Age.

CHAPTER   PAGE

      Dogs and Diabetics   579
      Treatment of Diabetes   579
          Week-end Hospital Treatment. Home Treatment.
          Plan Your Visit to Your Doctor.
      Diabetic Diets   581
          Composition of Diet.
      A Diabetic's Menu   586
      Exercise   587
      Insulin   588
          Insulin Reactions.
      The Usefulness of Diabetes   595
      Diabetics and Old Age   597
      Diabetic Gangrene   598
      Care of the Feet   599
      Infections   600
      Diabetic Coma   601
          Rules to Avoid and Prevent Diabetic Coma. Dia-
          betic Coma Needless. Dangers of Diabetic Coma.
      Diabetic Camps   604

XXII. BLOOD PRESSURE, by Wingate M. Johnson, M.D.   607
      Introduction by M. F.   607
      Measuring the Blood Pressure   608
      Normal Blood Pressure   610
      High Blood Pressure, or Hypertension   610
          Treatment of High Blood Pressure.
      Low Blood Pressure, or Hypotension   617
          Treatment of Low Blood Pressure.

XXIII. CANCER, by Francis Carter Wood, M.D.   622
      Introduction by M. F.   622
      The Causes of Cancer   624
      Distribution of Cancer   625
      Classification of Cancer   627
      The Nature of Cancer   627
      Heredity   628
      Race   629
      Sex   629
      Contagion   630
      Varieties of Cancer and Their Symptoms   630
      Cancer of the Breast   632

CHAPTER   PAGE

Cancer of the Womb 632

Cancer of the Stomach 633

Cancer of the Intestine and Rectum 633

Cancer of the Kidney, Bladder, and Prostate 633

Sarcoma of the Bone 634

The Diagnosis of Cancer 634

Treatment of Cancer 636

The Prevention of Cancer 637

XXIV. THE HAZARDS OF INDUSTRY, by Carey P. McCord, M.D. 639

Introduction: Occupational Diseases, by M. F. 639

Caisson Disease 640

Dampness 640

Dust as a Hazard 641

Infections of Industry 641

Radiant Energy Diseases 642

Poisoning from Drugs and Chemicals Used in Industry 645

XXV. THE SKIN, by Arthur W. Stillians, M.D. 661

The Functions of the Skin 664

Keeping the Skin Healthy 666
    Constipation. Bathing. Soap. Powders. Cold Cream. Antiseptics. Massage. Steaming. Electricity. Sun Baths and Artificial Substitutes for Them.

Care of the Skin at Various Periods of Life 676
    Infancy. Childhood. Adolescence. Middle Life. Age.

Inflammations and Abnormalities of the Skin 678
    Chapping. Chafing. Sunburn. Eczema. Dermatitis from External Irritants. Heat Rash. Impetigo. Seborrheic Dermatitis. Acne Vulgaris. Acne Rosacea. Excessive Sweating. Body Odor. Ringworm. Lousiness. Corns. Warts. Keloids. Vascular Birthmark. Blood Vessel Tumors of Older Skin. Chloasma. Freckles and Tanning. Senile Keratoses. Cancer of the Skin. Wrinkles. Xanthoma.

The Hair 694
    The Function of the Hair. The Care of the Hair. Combs and Brushes. Dandruff. Toxic Baldness. Alopecia Areata. Senile Alopecia. Graying of the Hair. Superfluous Hair.

CHAPTER   PAGE

Shaving — 700
Sycosis (Barber's Itch).

The Nails — 701
Hygiene of the Nails.

XXVI. EYE, EAR, TONGUE, NOSE, AND THROAT, by Morris Fishbein, M.D. — 704

Diseases of the Eye — 704
Spots or Specks in Vision. Seeing Colored Lights. Black Eye. Penetrating Injury. Sympathetic Ophthalmia. Care of Eye in Industry. Foreign Bodies in Eye. Conjuctivitis. Pink Eye. Trachoma. Styes. Tear Ducts. Ulcer on Eye. Inflammation of the Iris. Cataract. Inflammation of Retina. Detachment of Retina. Glaucoma.

The Ear and Its Disturbances — 714
Erysipelas of Ear. Tin Ear. Infection of Ear Canal. Hard Wax. Earache. Otitis Media. Mastoids.

The Tongue and Its Disorders — 718
Geographic Tongue. Inflammation of Tongue.

The Nose — 720
Hygiene of Nose. Plastic Surgery of Nose. Foreign Bodies in Nose. Polyps in Nose. Nosebleed. Sinus Disease. The Sense of Smell.

The Throat — 729
Sore Throat. Mouth Washes and Gargles. Tonsillitis.

XXVII. THE VENEREAL DISEASES, by Morris Fishbein, M.D. — 738

Syphilis — 738
Transmission of Syphilis. First Signs of Syphilis. Facts about Syphilis. Instructions for Those with Syphilis. When People with Syphilis May Marry.

Gonorrhea — 745
First Signs of Gonorrhea. Treatment of Gonorrhea. Advice to Those with Gonorrhea. Marriage after Gonorrhea.

XXVIII. THE CARE OF THE TEETH, by Morris Fishbein, M.D. — 748

The Care of Baby's Teeth — 748
Orthodontia — 750
The Care of Adults' Teeth — 751

Toothbrush. Toothpaste, Mouth Washes, and
Tooth Powders.

Pyorrhea   754
Halitosis or Bad Breath   756
False Teeth   757

XXIX.   ADVICE ON THE DIET, by Solomon Strouse, M.D.   759
.. Introduction by M. F.   759
The Development of the Normal Diet   760
Foods, Fads, and Fancies   761
Food Poisoning   764
Extraneous Factors in Diet   764
The Need for Food   765
Calories   767
Classification of Foods   768
Acid-Base Ratio   773
Vitamins   774
Digestion, Assimilation, Absorption   774
Preparation   776
Building the Diet   776
Varieties of Meat in the Diet   778
Carbohydrate and Fat   780
Milk   781
Cereals   782
Sugars   783
Fruits   784
Vegetables   785
Nuts   786
Fats   786
Condiments and Seasoning   786
Alcohol   787
Protein Yield of Various Foods   788
Caloric Yield of Various Foods   789
Distribution of Protein, Fat, and Carbohydrate   790
Essentials of a Normal Diet   791
Constipation   791
Sample Diet   792
Sample Menu   792
Bland Diet   793

CHAPTER PAGE

Diet for Hyperacidity 794
Diet for Hypo-Acidity 795

XXX. POSTURE, by Tait McKenzie, M.D. 797
Correct Sitting Posture 798
Kindergarten Training. Training in Higher Grades.
Bad Posture 799
Endurance Test 799
Physical Training 800
Posture of Students of College Age 800
Physical Education for Women 801
Games for Women.
Postural Effect of Clothing 802
Clothing and Round Shoulders 803
Exercises for Faulty Posture 804

XXXI. THE FOOT, by Philip Lewin, M.D. 806
Functions of the Feet 807
Shoes 807
Hygiene 809
Flat-Feet 810
Fallen Arches 815
Sprained Ankle 817
Painful Heels 818
Club-Foot 819
Ingrown Toenails 820
Warts 821
Bunions 822
Corns 822
Treatment of a Soft Corn.
Perspiring Feet 824

XXXII. NERVOUS AND MENTAL DISORDERS, by George K. Pratt, M.D. 825
Causes of Mental Disorders 828
Adjustment of Behavior 832
Mental Training in Childhood 834
Insanity 836
Mental Defect 837

CHAPTER   PAGE
              Feeble-Mindedness   *838*
              Prevention of Mental Disorder   *840*
              Treatment of Mental Disorder   *841*
              Psychotherapy   *843*
              Community Hospitals for Mental Disorder   *846*

XXXIII.   OLD AGE, by Morris Fishbein, M. D.   *848*
              The Span of Life   *848*
              Changes in Old Age   *850*
              Diseases of Old Age   *851*
              Exercises and Hygiene   *852*
              Cancer in Old Age   *853*

Illustrations

FRONTISPIECE

			PAGE
FIG.	1.	What periodical medical examination discloses	*5*
FIG.	2.	Effect of periodical medical examination upon mortality	*5*
FIG.	3.	Disorderly medicine chest	*10*
FIG.	4.	Never take a cathartic for abdominal pain, unless cause of pain is known	*12*
FIG.	5.	Danger of medicine chest within child's reach	*16*
FIG.	6.	Application of tourniquet	*20*
FIG.	7.	Modified Barton bandage	*20*
FIG.	8.	Four-tailed bandage in place	*20*
FIG.	9.	*Upper:* Wrong way of saving a drowning person *Lower:* Right way of saving a drowning person	*26*
FIG.	10.	Technic of artificial respiration	*29*
FIG.	11.	*Top left:* Method of carrying person with serious injury. *Top right:* Basket method of carrying injured person. *Bottom:* Method of removing injured person from contact with live wire	*32*
FIG.	12.	Black Widow spider (*Lathrodoctus mactans*)	*36*
FIG.	13.	Lateral view of female pelvic organs	*57*
FIG.	14.	Abdominal female organs	*57*
FIG.	15.	Aluminum bassinet	*184*
FIG.	16.	Taking the baby's temperature and bathing (*sponge bath*)	*184*
FIG.	17.	Washing the baby's eyes	*185*
FIG.	18.	Bathing the baby (*tub bath*)	*185*
FIG.	19.	Thumb sucking	*188*
FIG.	20.	Thumbs deformed by sucking	*188*

PAGE

FIG. 21. As soon as possible, the child should be taught to drink from a cup   204

FIG. 22. Permitting child to sleep with nursing bottle in mouth may deform face   204

FIG. 23. A weekly weighing of the child indicates state of nutrition   212

FIG. 24. Applying the square diaper   225

FIG. 25. New clothes for the baby, avoiding pins and buttons   227

FIG. 26. Patient ready for bed bath   236

FIG. 27. Bathing the patient   236

FIG. 28. Making the patient's bed   236

FIG. 29. Vaccination against smallpox   237

FIG. 30. Mortality from diphtheria and croup   243

FIG. 31. Injection of toxin-antitoxin for prevention of diphtheria   248

FIG. 32. Pool at Warm Springs Foundation for Treatment of Infantile Paralysis   268

FIG. 33. Home-constructed pool for giving treatment to children with infantile paralysis   268

FIG. 34. Physical therapy technician treating child in pool for infantile paralysis   269

FIG. 35. Typhoid is in retreat in the registration area of the United States   273

FIG. 36. A fly is the most dangerous animal known   274

FIG. 37. Life cycle of a fly   275

FIG. 38. Female malarial mosquito (*enlarged*)   293

FIG. 39. Female yellow fever mosquito (*enlarged*)   293

FIG. 40. Chest examinations of suspected tuberculous children   324

FIG. 41. Children suitably dressed for outdoor study and sleep   324

FIG. 42. Outdoor sun bath   325

FIG. 43. Indoor sun bath   325

FIG. 44. Deaths per 100,000 population United States Registration Area   347

FIG. 45. Position of the heart in the chest cavity   349

FIG. 46. Circulation of the blood   352

FIG. 47. Circulation and blood supply of the heart   373

FIGS. 48 and 49. The journey of the carbohydrate   386, 387

FIG. 50. Normal stomach   400

FIG. 51. Tube in stomach   400

PAGE

FIG. 52. Duodenal tube at outlet of stomach 400

FIG. 53. Hourglass stomach 400

FIG. 54. Normal gall bladder showing injection of dye, indicating normal filling, concentration of bile, and emptying after a meal of fat 401

FIG. 55. Gall bladder containing numerous small gallstones 401

FIG. 56. Gall bladder containing several large stones 401

FIG. 57. A little journey through the kidney 427

FIG. 58. Blood transfusion 472

FIG. 59. The large wheals indicate hypersensitivity to ragweed pollen 516

FIG. 60. *Top left:* Box elder. *Middle left:* Sycamore. *Bottom left:* Oak. *Top right:* Cottonwood. *Middle right:* Maple. *Bottom right:* Pigweed 517

FIG. 61. *Top:* Orchard grass—Redtop—Rye. *Bottom:* Bluegrass—Southern ragweed—Timothy 524

FIG. 62. Sagebrush. Pigweed. Lambs'-quarters 525

FIG. 63. Location of various important glands in the human body 533

FIG. 64. Basal metabolism test 556

FIG. 65. The falling total death rate and the rising diabetic death rate, United States Registration Area, 1880–1930 566

FIG. 66. The mortality rates for diabetes throughout the world 568

FIG. 67. A normal person 569

FIG. 68. Pancreas as seen in a cross-section of the body 570

FIG. 69. How 10 fat and 10 lean men fare as they walk through life 573

FIG. 70. *Left:* A poor, starved diabetic boy, as he looked before insulin was available. *Right:* The same boy as he looked afterward 580

FIG. 71. Administration of insulin to children 584

FIG. 72. Cleaning the skin 585

FIG. 73. Pinching up a fold of skin 585

FIG. 74. Inserting the needle 585

FIG. 75. Injecting the insulin 585

FIG. 76. Portions of different breads and their sugar-forming power 588

FIG. 77. Decline in mortality among diabetics 589

FIG. 78. A diabetic patient untreated 590

PAGE

Fig. 79. A diabetic patient adequately treated   *591*

Fig. 80. Self-subcutaneous administration of insulin by child   *592*

Fig. 81. Insulin map showing regions of body where insulin may best be injected   *593*

Fig. 82. Contrast footbaths   *600*

Fig. 83. From what do diabetics die?   *602*

Fig. 84. Average blood pressure, ages 20 and over   *609*

Fig. 85. Mask for miner   *644*

Fig. 86. Gas mask for protection against poisonous fumes   *644*

Fig. 87. Goggles for safety of eyes   *652*

Fig. 88. Mask for spray painter   *652*

Fig. 89. Skin of the aged   *676*

Fig. 90. Adult head louse (*enlarged*)   *686*

Fig. 91. Body louse   *687*

Fig. 92. Adult Acarus—parasite causing scabies   *688*

Fig. 93. Section of eye from before backwards   *704*

Fig. 94. *Top left:* Rupture of the choroid. *Top right:* Intraocular hemorrhage with greatly increased tension. *Middle left:* Rupture of iris and monocular diplopia. *Middle right:* Traumatic cataract. *Bottom left:* Dislocation of the lens. *Bottom right:* Detachment of the retina   *708*

Fig. 95. Wrong method of removing foreign body from eye   *709*

Fig. 96. A. The outer ear, the middle ear and the eustachian tube.

B. The middle ear, in which are located the drum and the ear bones, the entrance to the mastoid, and the eustachian tube, which leads to the back of the nose.

C. The inner ear.   *716*

Fig. 97. (a) Normal jaw and nasal cavity. (b) Effect long-standing nasal obstruction   *722*

Fig. 98. Palate, uvula, tonsils, pharynx, and tongue   *731*

Fig. 99. Lateral diagram of head showing relation of adenoids, tonsils, nose, ear, and larynx   *734*

Fig. 100. *Upper:* Widely advertised toothbrushes with composition handles badly distorted and made useless by hot water. *Lower:* Every child should have its teeth cleaned regularly   *752*

Fig. 101. Effects of abscessed teeth   *755*

Fig. 102. Food values—calories   *766*

PAGE

FIG. 103. Height and weight at various ages   *769*

FIG. 104. Facts about foods   *771*

FIG. 105. Food values—iron and copper   *772*

FIG. 106. Food values—vitamins   *775*

FIG. 107. Food values—protein   *779*

FIG. 108. Food values—calcium   *781*

FIG. 109. Food values—phosphorus   *785*

FIG. 110. Diagram showing the relation of the head, thorax, and pelvis in the incorrect standing position   *800*

FIG. 111. Diagram showing the relation of the head, thorax, and pelvis in the correct standing position   *800*

FIGS. 112, 113, 114. Exercise 2: To correct faulty posture   *800*

FIGS. 115, 116. Exercise 3: To correct faulty posture   *801*

FIGS. 117, 118. Exercise 4: To correct faulty posture   *801*

FIG. 119. Exercise 5: To correct faulty posture   *804*

FIG. 120. A deep breathing exercise, to relieve the severity of exercise 5   *804*

FIGS. 121, 122, 123. Exercise 6: To correct faulty posture   *805*

FIG. 124. Showing what happens in case of a fallen arch   *808*

FIG. 125. Natural position of bones in normal foot   *808*

FIG. 126. Effect of too narrow, too short, and pointed-toed shoes, showing cramped position of bones in feet   *808*

FIG. 127. X-ray normal foot   *808*

FIG. 128. X-ray normal foot wearing high heel   *808*

FIG. 129. *Left:* Normal feet. *Right:* Defects apparently caused by wearing a shoe too short and too narrow   *809*

FIG. 130. *Left:* Defects apparently caused by wearing tight shoes. *Right:* Deformities apparently caused by wearing short and poorly constructed shoes   *809*

FIG. 131. Footprints indicating quality of the arch   *811*

FIG. 132. Right and wrong foot postures.   *812*

FIG. 133. A good corrective exercise for flat-foot   *812*

FIG. 134. Exercise to strengthen the foot   *814*

FIG. 135. Example of rigid flat-feet   *816*

FIG. 136. Life expectancy   *849*

MODERN HOME
MEDICAL ADVISER

CHAPTER I

The Choice of a Physician
MORRIS FISHBEIN, M.D.

THE FAMILY DOCTOR

Of ALL THE PROBLEMS that may concern the average family, there is probably not one in which the decision is of more ultimate importance for the health and happiness of the family than the choice of the family physician. The family doctor of an earlier day was mostly learned in the school of experience. In many instances he had studied with a preceptor and perhaps had a course of lectures in some medical school lasting six months and devoted but slightly to the practical side of medicine. Such knowledge he obtained by studying cases with his preceptor. He did, however, develop an intimate personal relationship with those whom he served, which is recognized today as the basic feature of the best type of medical practice.

In the old days the family loved, indeed almost worshiped, the family doctor. He was their guide in health as well as in sickness. He alone, of all the community, knew the family secrets, and he could be depended on to keep the faith. True, his remedies were occasionally harsh and his diagnosis largely guesswork, but his record of cures is surprising. He was especially known for his ability to practise the art of scientific observation, using to the utmost his five senses. The physician of today has available innumerable scientific devices for aiding, prolonging, and extending these senses, but unless brains are carefully mixed with the application of the devices the end result may be confusion rather than scientific diagnosis, and the cost far beyond the necessary cost for first-class medical practice.

GRADUATION FROM A MEDICAL COLLEGE

In choosing a physician it is well to have the answers to certain questions which might be called "an aptitude test" for the family doctor. First, is he a graduate of a recognized medical school that requires at least four years of thorough training? There was a time when there were more medical schools in the United States than in all the rest of the world. We had almost 200 medical schools in this country around 1900. Today there are less than 80 medical colleges in the United States, and the vast majority of these are rated as Class A by the Council on Medical Education and Hospitals of the American Medical Association. A Class A college is one with a certain definite number of full-time teachers and with a well-established graded curriculum. It requires at least two years of college education previous to studying medicine, four years of medical education of approximately nine months each, and around one year or two years of internship after graduation before the prospective physician can get his diploma.

LICENSE BY THE STATE

In choosing a physician another point to consider is: Is the doctor licensed to practise medicine in the state in which he has his office? The majority of the states conduct regular examinations for a license to practise, these examinations being given by a group of physicians known as the State Medical Board of Registration and Licensure. In some states the doctor is required to renew his license every year. Before he can get a license he must usually show evidence of his graduation and also undergo a written and practical examination in the basic medical subjects. He must also present certificates of good moral character from at least two physicians who know him.

THE DOCTOR'S INTERNSHIP

A third question to be asked is this: Has the doctor had actual training as an intern in a hospital? Or has he been associated with a practising physician long enough to obtain practical education in medicine? Has he at the time of consultation a direct connection with a good hospital? There are in the United States almost 7,000 hospitals acceptable to the rating boards of the American Hospital Association, the American Medical Association and the American College of Surgeons. Of the 155,000 physicians in the United States more than 100,000 are directly affiliated with these hospitals as members of the staff. The appointment of a physician to the staff of a good hospital indicates that he has been passed upon according to his qualifications by the medical staff of the hospital and frequently also by the board of directors of the institution.

MEMBERSHIP IN THE COUNTY MEDICAL SOCIETY

Fourth: Is the doctor a member of his county medical society, of his state medical society, of the American Medical Association, or of any other recognized, organized body of physicians? The American Medical Association is organized like the United States government. It has county societies which pass carefully on physicians who wish to join. Before a man can belong to his state medical society he must belong to his county medical society. Before he can belong to the American Medical Association he must belong to both county and state medical societies. Before he can belong to any of the recognized special societies, such as those in surgery, diseases of the eye, ear, nose and throat, skin, and other specialties, he must belong to the American Medical Association or to his state and county medical societies.

While membership in a medical society is not an absolute guarantee of honesty or of good faith, the physician who belongs to such a society is subject to the criticism of his colleagues and subject also to being called before special committees to explain actions that are not considered ethical or satisfactory. A patient is much better off with a doctor who belongs to a recognized medical society than in the hands of one who is utterly independent of such organizational control. There are, of course, numerous medical organizations which are not recognized or established or scientific. There is even an organization composed of innumerable quacks who practise all sorts of strange medical cults and promote many unestablished notions.

CHARACTERISTICS OF AN ETHICAL DOCTOR

An ethical physician may be differentiated from a quack by certain well-established characteristics. An ethical physician does not advertise his methods or cures in a newspaper. He does not give out circulars concerning his work or his fees. He does not indiscriminately distribute his picture. He does not put large signboards on his windows or outside his office, advertising his extraordinary merits, or otherwise promoting his wares. A competent ethical physician seldom finds it necessary to travel from town to town to secure patients. He usually has an established place of residence and of work to which patients come when they require his services or to which they send, requesting his attendance when they themselves are unable to travel. The traveling doctor who moves from town to town is not to be consulted or to be considered a safe family physician.

There has been for years a tradition in medicine that new discoveries are freely published to the profession in the various medical periodicals and are not held as secrets by certain men which only they can apply. The public may therefore well beware of any doctor or group of doctors who advertise or publish broadcast the fact that they have discovered a new cure or method of treatment that other doctors do not know about, or who claim they can cure such serious conditions as cancer, tuberculosis, the venereal diseases, or rheumatic disease in a short time by some secret manipulation or by some unestablished method.

THE SCIENTIFIC ADVANCEMENT OF MEDICINE

The advancement of medicine has been associated with the introduction of innumerable complicated devices used not only in the diagnosis of disease but also in treatment. The sense of vision is aided by the microscope which enlarges invisible objects so that they may be seen. There are other instruments such as the cystoscope, the otoscope, the laryngoscope, and the ophthalmoscope which enable the physician competent in their use to look directly into various body cavities. By means of the X-ray, opaque tissues are brought into the field of vision, and by the use of various dye substances combined with the X-ray most of the organs and tissues of the body can now be seen during life.

The development of physics, of chemistry, of bacteriology, and of many sciences on which medicine rests has made it possible for physicians to determine to the thousandth of a gram the content of the blood and of various secretions and excretions of the body, determining thus the presence of sugar, of protein, of various salts, and of other substances related to the functions of the body in health and in disease. In surgery new devices have been developed for cutting tissues without hemorrhage, for keeping the patient quiet or anesthetized during operation, and for keeping conditions so clean that there is no danger of infection.

New methods have been discovered which aid the specialist in diseases of the nose and throat in looking into the sinuses, in determining their contours, in examining the ear externally and internally, and

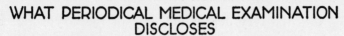
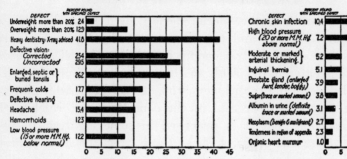

FIG. 1

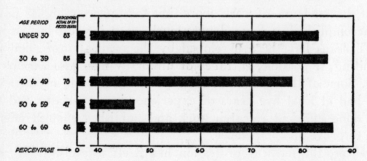

FIG. 2

in peering into the very depths not only of the larynx but even of the lungs.

Development of Specialists

The employment of the special devices used in medical practice requires hours of study and practice for the development of proper technic. As a result of the tremendous expansion of medical knowledge specialization entered the field, so that today not only is medicine practised by general practitioners who, it has been determined, can easily take care of 85 per cent of the conditions for which patients consult physicians, but it is practised in some eighteen to twenty specialties of various types, such as those which concern themselves wholly with internal medicine and diagnosis; surgery, which is divided into orthopedic surgery, genito-urinary surgery, brain surgery, abdominal surgery, and similar branches. There are also specialists in diseases of the skin, in diseases of women, in diseases of children, in obstetrics, in nervous and mental diseases, in diseases of the stomach and intestines, in industrial medicine, in preventive medicine, in anesthesia, and in several other more confined branches.

There is not as yet any legal method for determining who shall be considered competent to practise a specialty in medicine and who shall not. It therefore becomes possible for any physician who wishes to do so to set himself up as a specialist in any medical field. The rewards of specialization are usually beyond those of general practice in the form of shorter hours of work, more time for research, higher pay for work accomplished and, no doubt, much more interest in the work. Various means have been developed by the medical profession itself for limiting, if possible, entrance of unworthy men into various specialties. Some of the specialistic societies will not admit any man until he has had at least five years of experience in a specialty and until he has done sufficient research work and published enough scientific papers to prove his competence.

Moreover, the medical profession has itself established in recent years examining and certifying boards which now undertake, after a young man has been at least five years in practice, to give him both a written and a practical examination and, provided he is qualified, to issue to him a certificate of competence. This movement in medicine is so recent that it is not fair to say that men who do not have the certificate are not competent. It is safe to say that if they have the certificate they have submitted themselves to an examination and have passed it successfully.

CONSULT THE FAMILY DOCTOR FIRST

In the vast majority of cases people who wish to consult a specialist will do well to go first to their family doctor or general practitioner so that he may, after a study of the case, select for the patient such specialists as may be necessary for consultation as to diagnosis or for specialistic treatment. In this way the patient may save himself a great deal of time and money. Numerous instances are recorded in which a patient with a pain in some portion of the body went directly to a specialist, only to find out that the pain which concerned him was not due to an organ within the field of that specialist but perhaps to some entirely different cause.

For instance, such a condition as ordinary dizziness may be due to causes arising in the digestive tract, in the heart and circulation, in the internal ear, or in the brain. Only a careful study of the history of the case, the nature of the symptoms, and similar factors, will enable a physician to see which one of these organs or systems may be concerned. Similarly, bleeding from the throat may be due to conditions in the throat, in which case a general practitioner or a specialist in diseases of the throat might be consulted. On the other hand, it might be due to tuberculosis of the lungs, to a tumor of the esophagus or to hemorrhage taking place in the stomach, in which case a specialist concerned with those organs might be needed. Hence, for the vast majority of complaints the patient should first of all consult a family physician, preferably one to whom he has gone for some time. He may confidently be guided by his advice.

PICKING A FAMILY DOCTOR

When coming into a community the patient may select his physician in various ways. If he will call the secretary of the county medical society the secretary will probably be willing to give him a list of general practitioners in his vicinity. He may then determine by meeting these men and by inquiry into their qualifications whether or not he cares to commit the illnesses of himself and of his family to their care. If the person concerned happens to be a member of any well-established fraternal organization or church, association of commerce, business organizations, or similar group, he may on inquiry among his associates in these groups find out who are the competent physicians in the community, and then, by making his own inquiries as to competence along the lines of the questions that have been suggested earlier in this chapter, determine which of those that have been recommended is suitable to his needs.

Once a physician has been selected and has been found competent to give not only the type of scientific advice needed for ordinary cases, but also to give the personal intimate attention that is the distinguishing characteristic of the best type of family doctor, the patient will do well to cling to that family physician and to recognize in him a friend and a counselor. Remember also that the servant is worthy of his hire. Far too often physicians' bills are the last to be paid because the very nature of the profession has in the past made the physician willing to wait until the bills for food, for clothing, for shelter, for fuel, and the other necessities of life have been taken care of. The physician must himself provide these things for his family. A physician who receives from his patient conscientious and responsible treatment is likely to return to that patient even more conscientious and responsible attention than he himself has received.

CHAPTER II

The Family Medicine Chest
MORRIS FISHBEIN, M.D.

Mᴏsᴛ ᴀᴍᴇʀɪᴄᴀɴs, being independent and individualistic, feel themselves competent to fix defects in the plumbing and almost equally
competent to take care of their own disturbances of health, as well as
to prescribe for more complicated disturbances which really ought
to have prompt medical attention.

A household remedy should be one with a certain definite action;
usually it should contain but one active ingredient. If the thing is
worth keeping in the medicine chest it should be something which is
used fairly frequently. Dangerous poisons have no place in the family
medicine chest. A dangerous poison is one which is likely to produce
serious symptoms or death if taken in even moderate amounts. Prescriptions ordered by the family doctor for a certain illness should
never be kept for the future. If any of the material remains in the
bottle it should be poured promptly into a safe place of disposal.
Since useful bottles are rare around most homes, the bottle may be
thoroughly washed with hot water, dried, and stored away. Few people
realize that most drugs deteriorate with age and that a prescription
for a certain illness is not likely to be useful for the future.

The wise person will go over the family medicine chest at least once
every three months and at that time discard all materials not constantly in use. It might also be well to have the family doctor look at
the materials once in a while to offer his advice as to the materials
worth keeping.

Tᴀᴋɪɴɢ Mᴇᴅɪᴄɪɴᴇ

Medicines rightly used can be of immense aid and comfort to the
afflicted; wrongly used, they may cause serious damage to the human

body. When a doctor prescribes medicines for a patient, they are for that particular patient and not for anybody else in the family. Hence, old prescriptions should not be saved but should be disposed of as soon as possible after they are no longer necessary for the patient for whom they were prescribed.

The doctor usually writes on his prescription, and the druggist

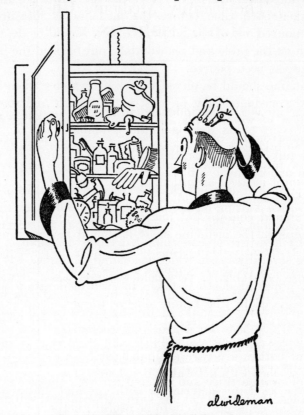

FIG. 3.   Disorderly medicine chest.

recopies on the label, the directions for taking the medicine. It is, therefore, well when giving medicine to a sick person to be sure you know exactly what is on the label of the bottle. If necessary, take the bottle into another room to read the label so as not to be disturbed by conversation with the patient or with anyone else.

Then, when you measure out the medicine, think of what you are doing and pay no attention to anything else. Medicines are usually prescribed in dosages of drops, teaspoons, fractions of teaspoons, and spoons of larger sizes. Because spoons are nowadays in many fanciful shapes and sizes, each family should have a medicine glass with measures of various spoons recorded. When a doctor says any number of drops, the drops should be measured with a medicine dropper and not by guesswork.

If liquid medicine is being prescribed, the bottle should be thoroughly shaken each time before the medicine is measured. When medicine is poured out of the bottle, the cork should be deposited with its top down on the table and immediately put back in the bottle after the medicine has been poured.

Most medicine should be mixed with a little water when taken, but sometimes the medicine may be put in the mouth and washed down with a swallow of water. Pills and capsules should either be handed to the patient from the original package so that he may help himself, putting the pill or capsule on the back of the tongue and washing it down with a drink of water, or else brought to the patient on a spoon so that he may take the pill or capsule from the spoon. In other words, the person who is waiting on the patient should not carry the capsules or pills in the palm of the hand, where they may be softened or disintegrated by moisture or contaminated from the hands.

There are several ways in which medicines of unpleasant taste may be made more palatable. If very cold water is taken, it will serve to cover up the taste. It is not advisable to give medicine to children in foods, particularly in milk, as this may create a distaste for the food or milk which lasts for a long time thereafter.

There are lots of ways to disguise castor oil. One of the simplest is the so-called castor oil sandwich, in which the castor oil is poured on a layer of orange juice and covered up with another layer of the same substance. Water will not mix with castor oil and will not disguise the taste. Nowadays there are available tasteless castor oils and flavored castor oils which serve the purpose without the disagreeable taste.

There are very few remedies which should be kept regularly in the family medicine chest. American people suffer today with overdosage of cathartics and laxatives, and with overdosage of medicine to relieve pain and produce sleep. Physicians are beginning to notice some serious results particularly from overdosing with drugs of the last mentioned type. No one should take such remedies regularly without the physician's directions.

Let us consider now the items that are most commonly found in any first-class family medicine chest. Most families want something to use for moving the bowels in the occasional case of temporary obstruction or slowness of action. Under certain circumstances any laxative or cathartic may be exceedingly dangerous. The most conspicuous example is appendicitis. This is at first just an infected spot on a little organ which comes off the large bowel and which apparently has no

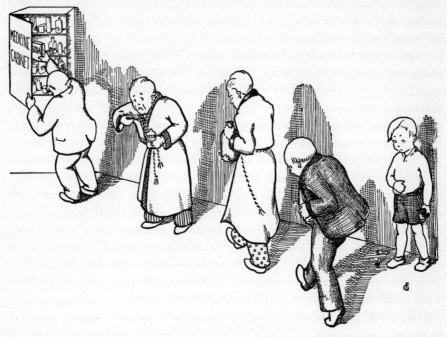

Fig. 4. Never take a cathartic for abdominal pain, unless cause of pain is known. It may be appendicitis.

serious function in the human body. If this infection develops the way a boil develops from a pimple, it is in danger of bursting and spreading throughout the body. When infection is spread in the abdomen the result is peritonitis. Therefore, no laxative or cathartic should ever be taken when the abdomen is exceedingly painful.

The most common laxatives found in a family medicine chest include liquid petrolatum, or mineral oil, which is a mechanical lubricant without possibility of serious harm. Other common preparations much used include, of course, the old-fashioned castor oil, seidlitz powders, milk of magnesia, Epsom salts, sodium phosphate, and aromatic cascara. For the people who use the medicine chest a large sign should be placed indicating that none of these preparations is ever to be used for abdominal pain of unknown cause.

The next most commonly found preparations in a family medicine chest, aside from the cosmetics, are pain relievers. Most of these are used for headaches, although sometimes they are used for what are called neuritis, neuralgia, toothache, and other pains of unknown origin, as well as to produce sleep. Most headache powders bought under patent trade marks contain phenacetin or acetanilid, sometimes in considerable dosage. It is not well to experiment with acetanilid because it may, in large dosage, have serious effects on the body, including particularly the blood and the heart. Too large or too frequently repeated doses will poison anyone who uses them. Moreover, there is a tendency to form the habit of taking such preparations, and such habits are dangerous, since they temporize with what may eventually become a serious condition.

Other drugs much used to produce sleep nowadays are derivatives of barbituric acid of which some of the best examples are veronal, trional, and combinations of barbituric acids with pyramidon such as are included in allonal, and combinations of pyramidon with amytal, dial, nembutal, and ipral. In some countries druggists are not permitted to sell such preparations to anyone without a physician's prescription. This should be sufficient indication of their danger as used by many people without medical knowledge. It is safe to say that the family medicine chest is better off without preparations of this character. The possibilities for harm are sufficiently great to suggest that these preparations be not used except on medical advice.

The most commonly used general pain reliever throughout the country today is acetylsalicylic acid, commonly called aspirin. This preparation has been popularized by extensive advertising campaigns. So far as is known it is relatively harmless except for a few people who are especially sensitive to it. Such people cannot take even small doses. It is important to point out that one aspirin is as good as another, provided it is up to the standard of the United States Pharmacopeia. The original manufacturer claims frequently that the aspirin he manufactures is better than any other. There does not seem to be any good scientific evidence to support this contention.

Among the strongest of medicinal preparations are the narcotics and anesthetics. Narcotics should never be used by anyone without a physician's prescription and, indeed, no drug that has to be administered with a hypodermic syringe should find a place in the average family medicine chest. There are some people with diabetes who have been taught by their doctors to inject themselves with insulin. Even these people should keep their syringe outfit separate from the materials in the family medicine chest.

There are all sorts of antiseptics available for use on the skin, in first aid and also for gargling and for washing various portions of the body. The most widely known skin antiseptics are tincture of iodine and 2 per cent mercurochrome. The Council on Pharmacy and Chemistry of the American Medical Association permits advertising of recognized antiseptics for first aid to the public, and tincture of iodine and mercurochrome are included among the preparations that may be so advertised. This same council, composed of some seventeen authorities in various departments of medicine, has concluded that no antiseptic substance is of value when used as a gargle for the destruction of germs in the mouth and throat. If the antiseptic is applied directly on a swab so that the material is held in direct contact with the localized infection it may have some definite use.

The council has not approved such widely advertised antiseptics as are commonly urged over the radio as being useful in the relief of all sorts of infections of the throat and urged indeed also for the prevention of various types of infectious diseases including colds. There is no scientific evidence that any of the widely advertised antiseptic solutions used as gargles, sprays, or in any other manner will prevent the onset of a common cold. One of the best old-fashioned antiseptic solutions for common use around the home is boric acid solution. Most people prefer to have packages of crystals of boric acid or of the powder, and to make up the solution fresh just before use.

The family medicine chest may also contain aromatic spirits of ammonia which is sometimes given when a prompt stimulant is needed following fainting. Half a teaspoonful in water, in a sudden fainting spell, is a fairly safe thing to give in most cases of emergency. The widely publicized milk of magnesia and sodium bicarbonate, or baking soda, are two preparations which can safely be kept in the family medicine chest and which are frequently advised by physicians for alkaline purposes. Some families keep paregoric as a useful preparation in case of cramps that come on women at periodic intervals.

Really these constitute practically all of the drugs that need to be in any family medicine chest because they are the few materials that can be used safely by most people. In addition, of course, there are the surgical supplies. In these days when everybody takes the chance of needing emergency first-aid treatment because of the common use of the automobile and wide indulgence in sports and gardening, it is well to have a certain minimum quantity of useful supplies around the home.

Among the materials needed for first aid are packages of adhesive tape of various widths, sterile cotton, sterile gauze bandages, sterile gauze pads, scissors which should be kept in the medicine chest and not used for the family sewing or for other emergencies around the home, and the ready-made combinations of a piece of adhesive tape with a tiny piece of sterilized bandage that can be used to cover small wounds or wounds after they have been treated with iodine or mercuro-chrome.

Most people should know that the proper way to stop bleeding of small wounds on the surface of the body is simply to press upon them with a sterile piece of gauze. In case of very serious wounds affecting arteries, and thereby difficult to control, it may be necessary to put a tourniquet around the limb. It is well to realize that the tourniquet should be fastened just tight enough to stop the bleeding and that an ordinary piece of rubber tubing or a narrow towel tied and twisted with a stick will serve most purposes satisfactorily.

In addition to the materials used for first aid, most families will have bed pans for use in cases of illness, glass drinking tubes, syringes for giving enemas, atomizers, and sometimes special devices for creating steam to be medicated with small amounts of tincture of benzoin for relief in various forms of hoarseness or other conditions affecting the larynx and the lungs.

The final materials to be included are the cosmetics. Most modern women prefer to keep their cosmetics in their own boudoirs or sleeping apartments. The man of the house is likely to put his into the family medicine chest. They should include, in most instances, a razor which should be kept in its box and not permitted to lie around loose; also some shaving soap or cream, some face lotion, which may be either witch hazel or some special lotion which he prefers.

It is not advisable to use a styptic in the form of a stick of alum to stop slight bleeding points after shaving. Much better are any of the astringent surgical powders, of which a small amount may be taken from the box at each occasion and applied directly to the bleeding point.

Finally, any good talcum powder may be used with satisfaction after shaving and after bathing, according to the individual preferences of the users.

It is taken for granted that every modern household has a good clinical thermometer, a hot-water bottle, and an ice bag. These are three exceedingly useful devices in any home, and when they are available in an emergency the comfort they give is tremendous. There are certain "don'ts" which may well be repeated in closing this simple account of the contents of the family medicine chest.

They are: Do not save poisonous preparations of any kind, including particularly bichloride of mercury, pills containing strychnine, or solutions containing wood alcohol. Do not keep samples of patent medicines of unknown composition recommended beyond their actual virtues. Never permit any preparation of opium or morphine to be loose in the family medicine chest. Never save any prepared prescription after the specific use for which it was ordered by the physician has disappeared.

EQUIPMENT OF THE FAMILY MEDICINE CHEST

A fountain syringe.

This should be of rubber or of metal. Capacity about two quarts. It will have a long rubber tube and several nozzles of assorted sizes.

A bed pan.

In many illnesses it is not safe for the patient to get up even to attend to the usual body needs.

A rubber sheet.

This is to be placed under the sheet to prevent soiling of the mattress. A piece of oilcloth will serve the purpose satisfactorily for a short time.

Bandages.

These are cheaply purchased. They should be in various sizes from one-inch width to three-inch width.

Adhesive tape.

This can also be purchased in spools of various widths and lengths.

Scissors.

These should always be kept available in the medicine chest.

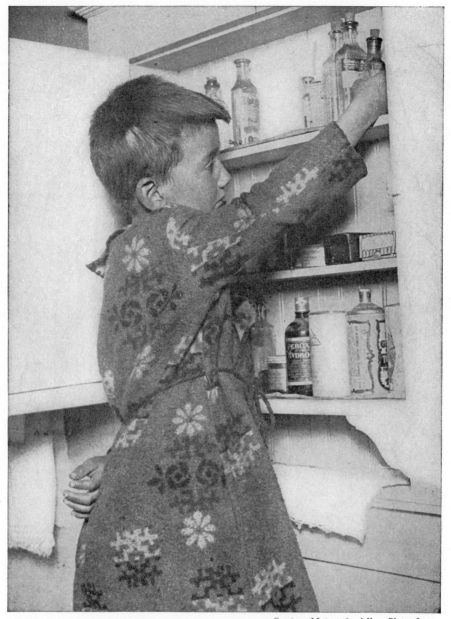

FIG. 5. Danger of medicine chest within child's reach.

Thermometer.

A good clinical thermometer should be available, and preferably two, one for taking temperature by mouth and another for temperature by rectum.

Ice bag.

The ice bag applied to the sore throat is frequently recommended by doctors.

Atomizer.

For spraying nose and throat. A graduated medicine glass for measuring dosages.

The Drugs and Medical Supplies

CATHARTICS AND LAXATIVES:

Epsom salts: An old-fashioned remedy with lots of power. Best taken in the morning on arising. About a tablespoonful in a half-glass of warm water.

Citrate of magnesia: A milder saline laxative. Order a bottle from the druggist. Take a half bottle on arising and the rest later if needed. Anywhere from six to twelve ounces of the solution of magnesium citrate is a dose.

Castor oil: An effective and prompt cathartic but likely to be followed by constipation and therefore not indicated in chronic constipation. A dose is four teaspoonfuls. This can now be had in tasteless and flavored forms.

Mineral oil: A lubricant and the best preparation for most chronic cases of constipation. It is not absorbed by the bowel. Dose: One or two tablespoonfuls. Also used as a spray for the nose.

Mineral oil with agar: This is a modified mineral oil or liquid petrolatum, thickened with agar, a seaweed which adds bulk. Other cathartics and laxatives much used include sodium acid phosphate, phenolphthalein which is the active substance of such advertised laxatives as Feenamint, Ex-lax, and similar products, also the Hinkle pill, the compound cathartic pill, and other mixtures. It is not well to develop a cathartic habit. It is not safe to take cathartics in the presence of undiagnosed pains in the abdomen.

GENERAL DRUGS AND SUPPLIES

Glycerine: Useful for many purposes. A few drops warmed and dropped into the ear are frequently advised for earache.

Vaseline, Cold cream, Zinc oxide ointment: These are useful for abrasions of the skin, chafing, sunburn, etc.

Tincture of iodine: An ideal antiseptic for application to cuts or small wounds of the skin. It is usually painted on, using a toothpick wrapped with cotton.

Boric acid: A concentrated solution is a good home antiseptic solution.

Hydrogen peroxide solution: Diluted about one half with water makes a good cleansing wash for wounds. Diluted one to three with water, can be used as a gargle.

Sodium bicarbonate: Baking soda. Useful as a gargle. Much used for so-called "sour stomach." Good in the bath for itching of the skin.

Aspirin: The great American pain reliever. Much used for headaches. Not safe but much safer than pyramidon, barbituric acid derivatives, acetanilid, phenacetin, and all the other coal-tar derivatives. Dosage: one or two five-grain tablets, repeated in about three hours.

Aromatic spirits of ammonia: Used to bring about recovery after fainting spells.

Surgical powder: A styptic powder, best used on small cuts after shaving.

Petrolatum eucalyptus menthol compound: A nice mixture for use in the nose as a spray.

Paper towels, Paper handkerchiefs: Most useful in sickness. Can be destroyed after use.

The medicine chest should always be kept out of reach of the children. Prescriptions in current use may be kept in the chest, but should be destroyed after the patient is well. Every bottle and package should be clearly labeled. Do not stock up with a lot of cathartics and laxatives, cough and cold remedies. Keep only those regularly used and called for by members of the family.

CHAPTER III

First Aid

MORRIS FISHBEIN, M.D.

WHEN ILLNESS or accidents occur in any home it is well for some-one in the home to be sufficiently aware of what can be done immedi-ately. The certainty of knowledge will avoid the confusion, alarm, and distress that inevitably occur when no one knows just what to do in an emergency.

The emergencies that may occur range alphabetically from acci-dents to the kick of a zebra. No one can be fully prepared for all of these any more than any family is fully prepared for twins or triplets. There are, however, certain supplies that may be kept in every home pending the occurrence of various accidents. The knowledge of the availability of these supplies and what to do with them by the mother, father, or the nurse will be found exceedingly helpful when the emergency arises.

ACCIDENTS

In the United States the number of accidental deaths reaches almost one hundred thousand a year, and it is said that ten million people every year have accidents sufficiently severe to take them from their work. Of the accidents which occur in the home, falls constitute 40 per cent of the total; after falls come accidents from burns, scalds, and explosions; then asphyxiation or strangulation and, finally, cuts and scratches. Most of these accidents are preventable with care, but it is in the nature of the human being not to be as careful as he might.

FALLS

When a person is injured in a fall the first step should be a con-sideration of the extent of the injury. It is necessary to determine whether or not bones have been broken, if there is bruising or hemorrhage and, finally, the extent to which the skin has been damaged. A broken bone usually reveals itself by inability to function. However, the only safe procedure is to call a physician who will take an X-ray picture and ascertain the actual extent of the damage.

Pending the arrival of a doctor it is well to place the injured part completely at rest and, if necessary, to hold it quiet with some suitable splint. A good splint is frequently made by wrapping a large-size magazine, or a newspaper folded many times, with handkerchiefs around the arm or leg to hold the tissues in place. However, unless the person who is applying the first-aid measure knows exactly what he or she is doing, it is better merely to put the injured person at rest and to keep him quiet.

BLEEDING OR HEMORRHAGE

In the case of bleeding there are certain measures which may be undertaken at once. Ordinary wounds can be controlled by pressure with a clean piece of sterile gauze. In case of very severe hemorrhages it is possible to wrap a cloth tightly around the arm or leg above the place of the bleeding. However, tourniquets are so little needed in ordinary accidents about the home that it is hardly worth while to keep a constant supply on hand. A tourniquet is easily improvised by merely tying a loop in a small towel or handkerchief and twisting with a rod of any kind.

If there is hemorrhage from a tooth socket following the extraction of a tooth it can usually be controlled by plugging the socket with sterile cotton or by the application of hot water. Under such circumstances care must be taken to avoid burning or scalding.

NOSEBLEED

Bleeding from the nose is a fairly frequent condition, due either to a purposeful "sock" or to an accident such as running into a door. The simplest measure to stop bleeding from the nose is to place the bleeder in a recumbent position, preferably with the face down. The application of ice water or of hot water to the nose or temporarily packing with sterile clean gauze will help. It will not help particularly, except to distract attention, to pass a key down the back, to inhale smoke, to apply ice to the back of the neck, or to collect cobwebs and stuff them into the nose. If bleeding from the nose is frequent or

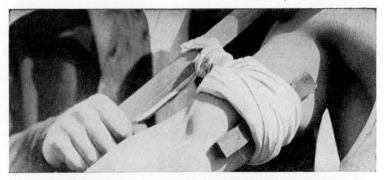

FIG. 6.   Application of tourniquet.

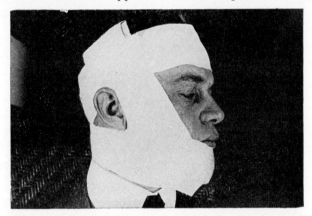

FIG. 7.   Modified Barton bandage. It may be used
with or without plaster.

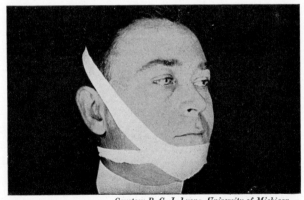

Courtesy R. C. J. Lyons, University of Michigan.

FIG. 8.   Four-tailed bandage in place. This is a good
emergency bandage.

continuous, a physician should make a careful examination of the blood to determine whether or not clotting, or coagulation, of the blood is delayed because of some deficiency. There is no way to strengthen blood vessels to prevent hemorrhage. If there is frequent hemorrhage from the nose a competent specialist in diseases of the nose will be able to look directly into it and to find out whether a dilated blood vessel or an ulcer of any kind is responsible. He can control such a condition by cauterizing the bleeding point or otherwise modifying the conditions responsible.

CONTROL OF BLEEDING

In addition to bleeding from the nose, there may be oozing from wounds elsewhere in the body. If this is continuous it can usually be controlled by pressure with a pad of sterile gauze. Sometimes the application of hydrogen peroxide will stop such oozing. Water as hot as borne may be tried, but merely washing with lukewarm water will frequently increase the bleeding.

Sometimes there is bleeding from a varicose vein of the leg. Under such circumstances the person should lie down, the foot be well elevated, a clean pad of gauze applied and compressed lightly with a bandage. Such a condition, however, is one which demands good medical attention, and a physician should be obtained for handling the condition as soon as possible.

In very severe wounds of any kind packing may be attempted, a sufficient amount of sterile gauze being put into the wound and held in place, but obviously medical attention is demanded immediately when available.

It should be remembered that the loss of blood is weakening. People who have lost large amounts of blood should be kept in bed and all possible movements avoided. They should be given plenty of nutritious food and plenty of fluids. A physician will prescribe suitable drugs and medicinal preparations for building up the blood after a hemorrhage.

One of the most serious accidents that may occur is sudden hemorrhage from the lungs which occurs occasionally in tuberculosis. Under such circumstances the person affected should be put immediately to bed, kept absolutely quiet, and an ice bag applied to the chest. Obviously, such hemorrhages demand most careful study as to the presence of tuberculosis at the earliest available time.

Whenever there is bleeding from the scalp, which is severe, because the scalp is richly supplied with blood vessels, an attempt should be made to stop the blood by applying a pad of gauze. If this does not work satisfactorily a tight band may be applied around the forehead to compress the blood vessels. Tourniquets applied or kept on too long may do much more harm than good. It is well to keep this fact constantly in mind.

Almost anyone can wrap a piece of gauze from a roller bandage around an arm or a leg or the forehead. To put on a bandage that will stay in place, that will be sterile during the process of application and after it is on, and that will serve the purpose satisfactorily is really a job for an expert. The average person should not attempt to learn bandaging. It is as much an artistic performance as playing the piano and probably more artistic than playing the saxophone.

BRUISES

Whenever the tissues of the body are struck with sufficient force there is likely to be bruising. This may come from a blow applied directly or from a fall in which the body moves and strikes against a fixed surface. The first symptom of a bruise is pain; usually this is followed by redness and swelling. Later, due to the blood that has poured out from the blood vessels into the skin, the tissues become black and blue. As the blood is gradually absorbed this changes from brown to yellow and gradually disappears. For most bruises little immediate treatment is necessary. The application of pads wrung out of ice water will lessen pain.

A black eye is a form of bruise especially unsightly and likely to arouse ridicule. The application of iced compresses to the eye will stop the pain and perhaps, to some extent, prevent discoloration. After the blackness appears, the application of heat in the form of hot compresses kept on for half an hour three times a day will hasten the disappearance of the swelling and discoloration. Among things that are not to be done to a black eye are the application of a slice of raw beefsteak, pressure with the handle of a knife, and the application of any kind of strong medicinal lotion or solution.

The danger of injury to the eyeball is far more serious than either the mental of physical pain associated with the ordinary black eye. It is well to have the eye looked at promptly to make certain that the eyeball has not been injured in any way.

FOREIGN BODIES

Among the emergencies demanding first aid is the presence of foreign bodies in the eye, ear, nose, throat, or esophagus. Regardless of how careful mothers may be, children occasionally push foreign substances into various body cavities. When a child chokes there is no time to call a doctor. The mother must act promptly. The mother should remember that the attempt to remove any object in the throat by rough methods may do more harm than good. If the baby is small it should be put face downward, or head downward, and given an opportunity to cough the object out. A very large object can, of course, be pulled out with the finger. A physician removes objects from the throat by the use of special devices developed for this purpose. He has "scopes" of every type with which he may look into the various cavities. He has also special lighted tubes with forceps and hooks for the withdrawal of foreign substances.

When foreign substances get into the nose, more harm is usually done by attempts to dislodge them with improper instruments than by letting them alone until competent advice can be had. If blowing the nose will not remove a foreign substance, sneezing may accomplish it. The physician may wash out foreign substances or by the use of proper forceps seize them and remove them.

Another type of emergency is the foreign substance in the ear, particularly an insect. An insect in the ear may be removed by turning the head to one side and filling the ear with warm sweet oil poured into it by means of a spoon. The insect is unable to live in the oil, and it promptly dies, and then can be floated out with warm water. In syringing the ear with warm water it is best to spray the water against the side at the entrance of the ear rather than directly against the eardrum.

If a child swallows any sharp-pointed object, such as a piece of glass, a bone, or a pin, relief is sometimes had by eating mashed potatoes and bread thoroughly chewed, which aid the passage of the substance down the gullet into the stomach. It is well then to obtain medical advice immediately. By the use of the X-ray the substance may be located and a decision made as to the best method for its removal. Experience shows that in many instances foreign substances that are swallowed will pass from the body by way of the bowel without undue harm.

Foreign substances in the eyes are particularly annoying. With experience, it is possible to locate such foreign substances on the lower or upper lid and to remove cinders or tiny specks with the point of a clean pocket handkerchief. With a little experience it becomes possible for anyone to turn back the upper lid. The simplest method is, first to wash the hands thoroughly; then, with a small match stick or some similar rod laid across the lid, the patient looks down, the attendant grasps the eyelashes, and turns the lid upside down by pulling the eyelashes over the match stick or rod.

No one should attempt to remove a foreign substance from the surface of the eyeball without special training in such first aid measures. It is safer, pending the arrival of expert attention, to merely place a small pad of wet gauze over the eye and to restrain the motion of the eye until attention is available. If any foreign substance has been removed from the eye it may be washed out with a saturated solution of boric acid, made by adding a flat teaspoonful of boric acid powder to a glassful of warm water and stirring until dissolved.

The simplest way to put drops in the eye is with the use of an eye dropper. A small quantity of the drops is drawn into the dropper, the patient sits on a chair facing a good light, the person who is putting the drops in stands in front, pulls down the lower lid, and, while the patient looks away, places one or two drops of the fluid on the outer edge of the lower lid. This will run across the eye and wash the surface. The patient looks away in order to avoid seeing the dropper and jumping when it approaches the eye.

There are all sorts of suggestions for the removal of cinders or other specks from the eye, including rubbing the other eye, blowing the nose, and indulging in similar manipulations. The chief advantage of these manipulations is to avoid harm to the eye from too much inexpert attention.

FIREWORKS AND TOY FIREARMS

Among frequent emergencies demanding prompt attention are explosions of fireworks. Twenty years ago hundreds of people were killed and injured in celebrating the independence of the United States. Following great campaigns of education this type of celebration has been largely displaced by pageants, plays, and exhibits of fireworks under the control of expert showmen.

Air rifles, BB guns, shotguns, and other small-caliber rifles, blank cartridges and cap pistols, sling shots and rubber band flippers, arrows and stones, are responsible for one third of the accidents resulting in loss of eyesight to children. Firecrackers, torpedoes, bombs, and various types of fireworks are responsible for one fourth of the cases of blindness.

Lockjaw or tetanus is discussed elsewhere in this book. The germs of lockjaw develop in soil and in manure and on dirty clothing. Any time an injury occurs in which dirt is forced into a wound and sealed in there is danger of lockjaw. There is the kind of accident that occurs in explosions of cannon crackers, blank cartridges, and toy cannon. The size of the wound is not significant. The tiniest puncture may cause the passing of the germs into the body.

Whenever an injury from fireworks occurs, get a doctor as soon as possible. He will open the wound, clean it, and treat it with suitable antiseptics, and in questionable cases inject the antitoxin against lockjaw to prevent that disease. Never wait until lockjaw develops. After the disease has developed it is one of the most serious affecting a human being. So serious is the possibility of lockjaw that in many cases health departments provide antitoxin without charge to make certain that cases of lockjaw do not develop.

WOUNDS

Whenever the skin is opened, torn, or punctured the injury is called a wound. Wounds may thus vary from the tiniest puncture, such as that of a needle, to severe injuries tearing open several inches of skin and penetrating into body cavities. The greatest danger from wounds, after the immediate danger of hemorrhage, lies in infection. Therefore, the first step of importance in first aid is to prevent infection. Infection may be prevented by disinfection.

In taking care of a wound one must be certain that his own hands are as clean as possible. Surgeons wash the hands thoroughly with soap and water and then wash them in antiseptics, and thereafter wear rubber gloves which have been sterilized by steam under pressure. In taking care of any small wound around the home, it is well to be certain that the hands of the person who is taking care of the wound are as clean as possible. Hence they should be washed thoroughly with soap and water and perhaps also in alcohol. All materials applied to the wound should be sterilized. Such materials are now available in any drug store in packages. If a sterile package of material is not available, it may be made by boiling thoroughly materials available in the home. A freshly laundered handkerchief or towel is likely to be relatively free from germs because laundering, heating, and ironing kill organisms on the surface.

Hundreds of antiseptic substances are now available and are widely advertised. Among the best of the antiseptics is alcohol. Tincture of iodine is widely used as a first aid dressing, as is also mercurochrome, saturated solution of boric acid, hydrogen peroxide, metaphen, and hexylresorcinol solution. When a wound has been contaminated with dirt this should be washed out with a suitable solution. It is not well to apply hydrogen peroxide to a fresh wound because it may cause pain and unnecessary crusting with destruction of tissue.

After the wound has been disinfected by the application of a suitable antiseptic it should be covered with clean sterile gauze and suitably bound. No one should attempt to sew a wound unless he has had medical training. Whenever pus or infection occurs in a wound it should have prompt medical attention. If a person is far removed from medical attention he should realize that it is of the greatest importance to release the pus by opening the wound and then to apply the antiseptic. Wet dressings of concentrated boric acid solution applied for several days are helpful.

Certain types of wounds represent unusual emergencies, among them splinters entering the skin. Small splinters are best removed by using a needle which has been passed through a flame in order to sterilize it; large splinters by the use of a knife blade sterilized in a similar manner, and perhaps also with the aid of a forceps.

When a fishhook gets into the skin it is not well to attempt to pull it out. In order to avoid tearing the tissues it is perhaps better to push the point onward and forward and to let the end of the fishhook follow the point. The barbed end may then be cut off with a wire cutter, and when this is removed the fishhook may be removed by reversing the process.

BURNS

Burns of the skin may be produced by many different methods including the heat from a flame or hot iron, the heat from scalding water or steam, and the heat from electricity. Burns which involve more than one half of the surface of the body are usually fatal. When a person has been suddenly or severely burned he may suffer from

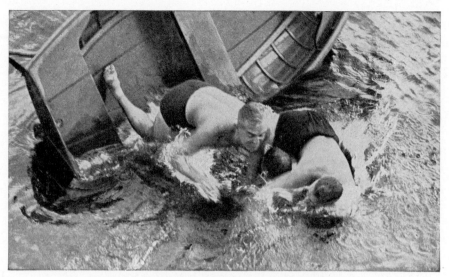

Wrong way of saving a drowning person.

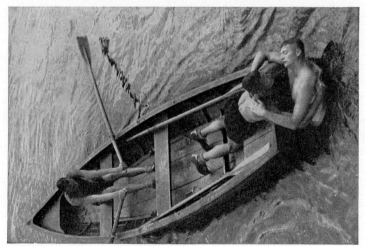

Courtesy of Acme Newspictures, Inc.

Right way of saving a drowning person.

FIG. 9.

shock. This demands immediate attention in order to stimulate him and to save life. He should, of course, be put at rest and the burn suitably covered to prevent continued irritation. Almost everyone now knows that when a person's clothing is actually burning it is well to smother the flames by the use of a blanket, a rug, or any other heavy material that is handy.

In the presence of slight burns or scalds it is preferable to cover the burned portion immediately with cold water, which will check the effect of the heat and stop the pain. If the foot or hand has been burned by spilling hot water, soup, or coffee over it, it is well to put the part burned immediately under water and to keep it submerged until the first effects of the injury have passed. Thereafter it may be covered with sterile vaseline or petrolatum. Loose cotton should not be put on a burn, nor should wide pieces of gauze be applied. It is practically impossible to remove such materials without great injury to the tissues. The gauze may be applied in narrow strips.

Modern methods of treating burns include application of liquid petrolatum, or the application of melted petrolatum, which then hardens and covers the burn. A more recent method involves the use of tannic acid prepared especially for the treatment of burns. This produces a suitable crust or covering under which healing takes place readily.

Burns from acids are among the most serious, particularly nitric and sulphuric acids. The first treatment following a burn by acid is to wash off the acid as quickly as possible with a solution of bicarbonate of soda and to leave the wound in the soda solution for some time. People who work in acids regularly should wear gloves whenever possible. Electric burns are usually deep and severe. They should be treated as are other burns.

RESUSCITATION

Among the most serious of emergencies which may occur, demanding first aid, is resuscitation after asphyxiation, which may result from drowning, from electric shock, and from exhaust-gas poison. Occasionally also there may be asphyxiation from other sources, such as gas escaping from electric refrigerators.

It has been estimated that 25 per cent of men and boys past twelve years of age do not know how to swim, and there are few women who would be capable of swimming long enough or far enough to save themselves in an emergency. When a person has been under water long enough to become unconscious—about four or five minutes—first aid measures are of greatest importance to save life. The practice of resuscitation by the manual method is important because it is the quickest and most readily available. There are numerous devices for artificial resuscitation, but it is usually not well to wait until these come.

Lay the patient on his stomach. Extend one arm directly over his head. Bend the other arm at the elbow and rest patient's cheek on his hand, to keep the nose and mouth off the ground and free for breathing.

Kneel facing forward, straddling the patient's legs above the knees. Place the palms of the hands on each side of his back, just above the belt line and about four inches apart, thumbs and fingers together, the little fingers over and following the line of the ribs and the tips of fingers just out of sight.

With arms straight, lean gradually forward, pressing downward and forward and counting slowly one, two, three. Snap your hands sideways off the patient's back. Swing your body back, counting slowly four, five. Rest. Straighten the arms and repeat the pressure.

To assist in timing the three movements of the straight arm pressure, quickly release and swing back (about twelve per minute), repeat during the period of pressure, "Out goes the bad air"; snap off your hands and repeat during the period of release, "In comes the good." Keep working steadily until breathing begins and continues naturally.

ELECTRIC SHOCK

Following electric shock it is first necessary to remove the electrocuted man from the electric conductor. Employees of electrical corporations do not stop to shut off the current. They take off a coat or wrap and throw it around the patient's body so as to pull him away from the contact. They are told never to put their hands near the pockets of an electrified man nor near his shoes, because the presence of metal materials or nails in the shoes will cause severe shock to the rescuer.

When a person has been shocked by electricity, death may occur instantaneously from paralysis of the centers of circulation of the heart because of overexcitation of the heart muscle, perhaps due to

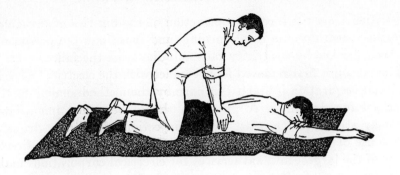

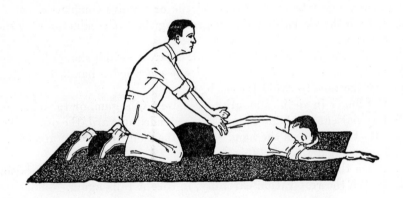

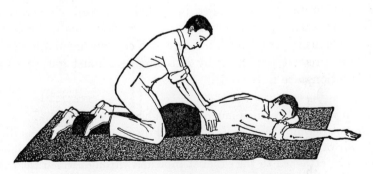

FIG. 10. Technic of artificial respiration.

suffocation from the forcible contraction of the muscles of breathing
Sometimes death occurs from burning, and sometimes the person who
has been shocked by electricity falls and dies from the fall.

The person is first removed from contact with the electrical current.
Artificial respiration is started at once by the method similar to that
described for drowning. A physician should be called immediately
who may stimulate the heart by the injection of suitable drugs or
by the use of methods of massage applied to the heart. The director
of one of the largest first aid services for electrical corporations makes
the following suggestions:

1. Release victim, avoiding sustaining a shock one's self. Any dry
nonconductor may be used to move victim or the live conductor.

2. If both the victim's hands are grasping the live conductor, free them
one at a time.

3. If necessary, shut off the current. Nearest switch should be opened.

4. If it is necessary to cut a live wire, use a wooden-handled axe, turning away the face to avoid the flash.

5. Put finger in victim's mouth to remove teeth, gum, or tobacco.

6. Lay patient on abdomen, one arm extended upward, the other elbow
flexed. Rest the face on the hand so that the mouth and nose are free.

7. Carry out artificial respiration.

8. When the patient revives, keep him lying down. Keep him warm.

9. Watch the respiration carefully, in case it fails again.

Gas Poisoning

Most of the deaths from the inhalation of carbon-monoxide gas
occur from running automobiles in closed garages. However, there
may be suffocation from illuminating gas in the home or from working with various types of machines in which carbon-monoxide develops.
In order to prevent poisoning by automobile-exhaust gas, the following instructions are important.

1. Keep windows open as much as possible.

2. Do not permit the engine to run and discharge exhaust gas directly
into the air of the workroom. Every workroom should have a flexible tube
which can be attached to the exhaust pipe and through which the exhaust
gas may then be carried out of doors.

3. Remember that carbon-monoxide gas has no smell. You cannot,
therefore, know if carbon-monoxide gas is in the air by the smell of the

room or by the cloudiness of the air. These are produced by burning oil and gasoline.

4. If you suffer with headaches report this fact at once so that the conditions of the air may be investigated and proper ventilation established.

5. If you do not feel well, see a doctor at once. You may be particularly sensitive to carbon-monoxide gas, more so than the others. In that case you had better change your occupation. It is not safe for you to be exposed to even very small amounts of the gas.

The Bulletin of the New York State Department of Labor recommends these first aid measures:

If you get a headache, or feel faint, nervous, or irritable, go out into the fresh air at once and stay there until you feel better. When you go out go out slowly and when you get out sit down quietly. Do not go for a walk. You may not have enough oxygen in your blood to permit you to take any additional exercise or exert yourself in any way. Any added exertion at such a time is dangerous and may be sufficient to cause you to become unconscious. Wrap up warmly, therefore, and sit down out of doors until you feel better.

Do not hurry around unnecessarily at your work. The more exercise you take, the more carbon monoxide will get into your blood.

If one of your comrades faints, get him out into the fresh air at once. Put blankets under and over him and surround him with hot-water bottles or hot bricks. Keep him warm at all costs, or he may develop pneumonia. Persons who become asphyxiated with carbon-monoxide gas are peculiarly susceptible to pneumonia. Call up the gas company and an ambulance at once. You must always call both of these, because ambulances are not equipped with resuscitation apparatus. In the meantime the patient should be given artificial respiration, by what is known as the "Manual" or "Schäfer" method. Everyone working in industries where there is a possibility of exposure to carbon-monoxide gas should be familiar with this method of resuscitation. It is very easily carried out. Anyone can learn how to do it. He may thus by his knowledge be able to save someone's life.

Recently the use of injections of methylene blue has been offered as a scientific means for treating patients with carbon-monoxide poisoning. In the presence of such poisoning a physician should be called immediately. He will then determine whether or not any remedies are to be injected. Of the greatest importance is the immediate application of the methods of artificial respiration already described.

FAINTING AND UNCONSCIOUSNESS

Few persons have the slightest idea of what is to be done when another person suddenly becomes unconscious. There are numerous causes for this condition: a blow on the head; pressure on the brain from a large blood clot; a lack of blood supply to the brain; the effects of such drugs as opium, ether, chloroform, or alcohol; or carbon-monoxide gas; but practically all of these are related in some manner to the brain, since the brain is the seat of consciousness.

A physician who is called to see a person who has suddenly become unconscious makes his decision as to the cause of unconsciousness from a number of factors. He feels the pulse to determine whether, by its rate and strength, the difficulty is affecting the circulation of the blood. If the pulse rate is between 76 and 90 and strong, he realizes that there is no immediate danger of death from failure of respiration. He studies the color of the face. If there is great pallor or blueness or a purple color he realizes that there are difficulties with the blood. He observes also if the skin is hot or cold and determines the presence or absence of perspiration. The eyes are noted to observe if the pupils are equal or unequal, if they are dilated or contracted. Unequal size of the pupils is a common symptom of injury to the brain, such as a brain hemorrhage. It may also be desirable to feel the skull to determine whether or not there is a fracture or crushing injury beneath the surface of the scalp.

In the presence of excessive heat, sunstroke may be the cause of unconsciousness. The odor of the breath may indicate the presence of acidosis or the fact that the person has taken a large dose of alcohol or of ether.

Associated with the onset of fainting there may be dizziness or light-headedness. The average human being walks erect and pays no attention to his sense of balance because that is controlled by a number of reflex sensations coming to the brain from various places. The semicircular canals of the internal ear give the human being a sense of his position in space. There is also a feeling associated with the muscles which aids the determination of presence in space. If the body tends to accumulate acid, dizziness is a prominent symptom. Anything that interferes with the coördination between the sense of

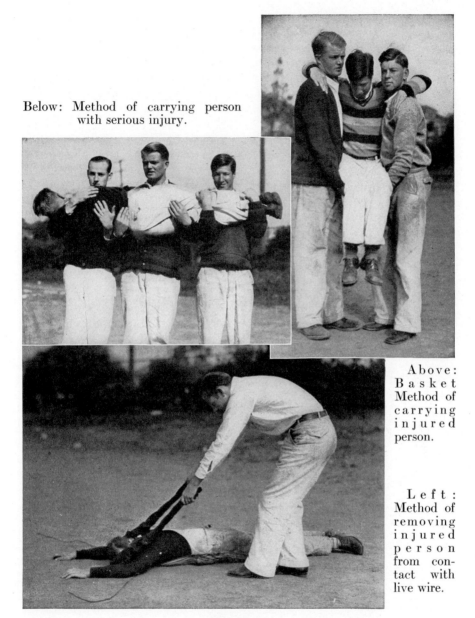

Below: Method of carrying person with serious injury.

Above: Basket Method of carrying injured person.

Left: Method of removing injured person from contact with live wire.

Fig. 11

vision, the muscle sense, and the sensations coming from the semi-circular canals will produce dizziness.

If the sense of dizziness merely comes and goes and yields quickly to proper hygiene such as suitable attention to the diet, the digestion, the action of the kidneys, and correction of disorders of vision, one need not be disturbed. However, if dizziness is repeated again and again it may be due to insufficient blood supply to the brain, insufficient action of the heart, a tumor growing in connection with the semi-circular canals, or some hidden disturbance elsewhere. A feeling of dizziness and fainting, if repeated, demands careful scientific study. Of course, some people faint more easily than do others. Some faint from the slightest emotional shock. Some people faint at the sight of blood, others faint quickly from exhaustion, weakness, lack of air, or similar conditions.

A person who is about to faint realizes it from a feeling of weakness, a blurring of vision, a failure of circulation so that the face becomes pale, and the presence of cold perspiration. The moment a person faints he should be placed flat on the back and his head lowered. The color of the face is an indicator to some extent of the blood supply to the brain. If the face is pale the head should be lowered until the color of the face improves. If, on the other hand, the face is extremely red, it may be desirable to keep the head raised.

A person who has fainted should have plenty of fresh, cool air, cold water applied to the face or chest as a stimulant to recuperative action. Sometimes the inhalation of smelling salts serves to stimulate the breathing of the patient and in that way to aid his recovery. The usual first aid remedy, found in most family medicine chests, for attacks of fainting is half a teaspoonful of aromatic spirits of ammonia given in water. A person who has fainted should be kept quiet and recumbent until fully recovered. If permitted to get up and walk too soon, serious results may follow.

HEAT STROKE

Among the most important problems in first aid is the handling of heat stroke. This occurs not only in tropical countries and in extremely hot weather in the temperate zone, but also at any time in factories, engine rooms, laundries, and kitchens, where people work in extreme heat associated with considerable moisture.

The symptoms of heat stroke may come on suddenly but most

frequently come on gradually. The person who is about to become affected feels weak and tired, gets dizzy and drowsy. The digestion may be disturbed, and there may even be pain in the abdomen. The temperature rises, the fever increases, the pulse becomes rapid, the skin dry, burning, and flushed; the pupils of the eyes are usually contracted, and the breathing fast and noisy. Just before death the pupils may dilate. It is important to be certain of a diagnosis of heat stroke and to make positive that the unconsciousness is not due to drugs, hemorrhage, epilepsy, or diabetes.

The ability to keep cool depends on common sense. One should wear light clothing, loose and porous. Cool baths at frequent intervals aid in making one feel much better. Adequate amounts of sleep keep the body prepared for unusual stress and strain. One should take plenty of water, because evaporation of water from the surface of the body aids the control of temperature. Traveling in hot weather is extremely difficult. It is better, under conditions of extreme heat, to sit in an open coach with a free circulation of air than in the smaller compartments and drawing rooms.

In case of heat exhaustion, the first thing to do is to get the person into a cool place and absolutely at rest, flat on the back. Sponging with cool water helps to control the temperature. It may be necessary to stimulate the circulation with stimulating drugs or coffee to help the patient over the acute condition. Tropical authorities recommend that the person be placed as soon as possible on a bed covered with a large rubber sheet, and then that ice and cold water be rubbed over the body. At the same time that the ice is rubbed, the friction or massage encourages the circulation.

The temperature should be taken regularly and when it falls to 101 degrees, as taken by the bowel instead of by the mouth, one stops the application of cold, covers the patient with blankets, and makes certain that collapse does not follow. If breathing stops it may be necessary to apply artificial respiration. After recovery from heat stroke, small quantities of nutritious food may be given repeatedly in order to aid recovery.

Bite Wounds

The bites of insects, snakes, cats, dogs, and other small animals frequently demand some attention in first aid. The sting of a bee, yellow jacket, or other wasp, should be pulled out, if still in the flesh, and a drop or two of diluted ammonia water applied to the wound. The application of cold compresses will help to stop pain. The sting of a centipede, spider, or scorpion may be more severe than that of a wasp or bee. Bleeding should be encouraged to wash out any material deposited by the bite; then tincture of iodine may be applied and a cold compress used to stop pain.

Most spider bites in the United States are due to the shoe-button spider or the black widow. It is called shoe button because it looks like a black button; and black widow because the female frequently eats the male. The sting of a scorpion is not frequent. A physician usually treats such stings by injecting some anesthetic solution around the bite, including some adrenalin solution to constrict the blood vessels and prevent absorption of the poison.

Flea bites, if painful, may be treated with weak solutions of menthol or camphor.

Dog bites, or the bites of any small animal, must always be investigated to determine the possibility of hydrophobia in the animal that bites. The treatment of the bite itself is ordinarily the same as that for any infected wound. If it seems certain, however, that the animal has rabies, or hydrophobia, the wound should be thoroughly cauterized by a physician.

The scabies, or itch mite, travels rapidly from one person to another. The handling of infestation with the itch mite is really a problem for a physician. It demands thorough cleansing, the application of suitable drugs, and care of the clothing as well.

The bite of the bedbug seldom becomes infected but is an annoyance. The itching is, of course, easily treated by solutions of weak ammonia or very weak menthol.

In the case of every type of insect, prevention is far better than cure. It is necessary to know, first of all, the presence of the insects; second, their breeding habits; and third, special methods for destroying them. If they are once completely destroyed by fumigation or disinfestation methods they are not likely to return soon again, particularly if sufficient watchfulness is exercised to attack them while they are few in number.

HICCUPS

Hiccups to most people is just a temporary disagreeable symptom, but to the scientist who knows of all of the possible relationships of the hiccup as a symptom to various diseases, it constitutes a phenomenon of considerable significance. Between the chest and the abdomen lies a great muscular structure called the diaphragm. Above the diaphragm are the heart and lungs; below it, the stomach, intestines, liver, pancreas, spleen and other organs.

When one breathes, the diaphragm contracts, enlarging the chest cavity and helping the lungs to expand. In order for any muscle tissue to contract, a stimulus comes to it through a nerve. The nerve that controls the contractions of the diaphragm passes from the upper part of the spinal cord in the region of the neck. If this nerve is irritated at any spot it becomes stimulated, and the stimulation causes a sudden spasmodic contraction of the diaphragm that is called a hiccup.

In a recent consideration of the subject, Dr. Charles W. Mayo listed some of the ways in which hiccup can be brought about. In a considerable number of instances it is due to some infection involving the portion of the brain associated with the stimulation of contraction of the diaphragm. In such cases, he has observed the condition affects chiefly men more than forty-five years of age and it tends to follow operation on the colon, the prostate gland, the gall bladder, or the stomach.

Then there are cases which can be classed as chemical hiccup. In these cases hiccup occurs following the eating of highly irritating foods or liquids. Generally such hiccups last only a short time. It is also recognized that tumors of the brain, pressing on the areas associated with stimulation of the diaphragm, may produce hiccup. It is also possible by a sudden dilatation of the stomach to produce an irritation which will result in this symptom. Finally, there are cases of hiccup that have a nervous basis, exactly as hysteria may duplicate almost any disease known to medical science. Then there are cases of hiccup in which the origin cannot be determined.

Everybody has his own cure for ordinary hiccups. In most instances it involves something that will fix the attention on anything except the hiccup. The physician who treats such cases may carry out certain procedures in persistent hiccups which frequently bring relief. One of these is to wash out the stomach; another to prescribe certain narcotics and sedatives that will give temporary relief; a third is to treat the specific infection from which the patient seems

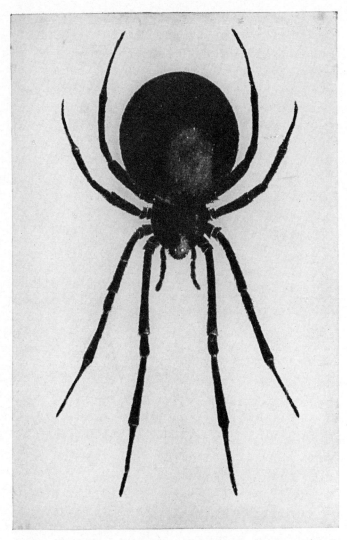

FIG. 12. Black Widow. Coal black, with a red or
yellow spot on the abdomen, identified as *Lathrodectus
mactans;* otherwise familiarly known as the "Black
Widow." She is really our bad spider.

to be suffering. Another method involves the giving of enemas and doses of oil to clean out the entire intestinal tract.

In the case of a baby, it may be held on the shoulder and patted on the back, which will cause it to expel the air which may be distending its stomach or esophagus and thus leading to hiccups. In some cases the stimulation of the nerve results from poisons associated with infections such as infantile paralysis or epidemic encephalitis. The latter condition has been called American sleeping sickness. In these cases the hiccups may be severe and go on for long periods of time; indeed, actually to the point of exhaustion. The treatment of such conditions is a long and serious matter and it is only by the treatment of the fundamental condition that the hiccups are to be controlled.

When every method of treating hiccups has failed and the symptom persists there may, of course, be danger to life. In such cases the surgeon may expose the phrenic nerve and either cut it or place pressure upon it. This will invariably cause the hiccup to stop by interfering with the passing of the stimulus from the irritated center along the nerve to the diaphragm.

Migraine or Sick Headache

Migraine or sick headache is often called recurrent headache. It is called sick headache because it is sometimes accompanied with nausea or vomiting. Sometimes it is found to be dependent on uncorrected errors of vision or sinus disease or on various poisonings of the body. In other words, it seems to be associated with sensitivity to food of one kind or another, or even to serious diseases of the stomach and other organs of the body. On occasion, severe headache is associated with disturbance of the brain, such as tumor or hardening of the arteries. In some instances, the headaches may be wholly on a mental basis.

It is not well therefore to attempt to differentiate one group of headaches as migraine and others as simply headache. Every case of the disease should be carefully studied so that the physician may evaluate all of the different factors that may be concerned. It is perhaps best at this time to consider the headache or the pain as the symptom of a disorder of the human body rather than a disease in itself.

Sometimes the headache is associated with the type of nausea that has been mentioned; sometimes with disturbances of vision in the form of blindness, dullness of vision, blinding flashes of light, or dizziness. In certain cases there are, associated with the pains in the head, emotional disturbances such as a feeling of depression or melancholia. In other cases the headaches are associated with restlessness and irritability, and in still another group with confusion, absent-mindedness, or a sense of unreality. In some cases there are pains in the abdomen which are of the same type as the pain in the head.

Women have their symptoms chiefly at the time of their periodic functions. In many cases the headaches occur frequently, but in the majority about once in two weeks. The type of headache called migraine occurs most often between the ages of eighteen and thirty-five, but may appear at any age. There was a time when it was thought primarily to be a disease affecting women, and some writers have said that it occurs four times as often in women as in men. More recently careful studies seem to show that headaches of this type occur just about as often in men as in women. The reason why it has seemed to be more frequent in women is that they are more likely to consult a physician about the condition than are men, and that the attacks in them may seem to be more severe.

Sometimes the headaches come on without any warning, but in most cases they are preceded by a feeling of depression, by an unwillingness to work or to go about the daily affairs of life. Since there seem to be many possible causes for headaches of this type, the attack on them must be made from various points of view. It is believed that they may on occasion be associated, as has been said, with eye strain or disease of the sinuses. Obviously in such cases careful examination must be made by a competent specialist in diseases of the eyes to make certain that the vision is properly corrected with suitable glasses. It should be made certain that the eyes are not abused by working under conditions of improper illumination. The nose must be examined most carefully and, if necessary, X-ray pictures made of the sinuses to make certain that they do not contain polyps or infection.

The physician will use the ophthalmoscope to look in the back of the eye in order to make certain that there is no pressure within the skull due to any disorder. Sometimes it is necessary to X-ray the skull for possible observation of an abnormality in the brain.

It is believed that migraine is associated with such disorders of hypersensitivity as hay fever, eczema, asthma, and similar conditions.

It is possible in such cases to test the reaction of the patient to various foods and proteins by skin sensitivity tests or perhaps to try elimination diets, in which food substances are eliminated from the diet when their consumption seems to be followed by an attack. Apparently not all cases are due to such sensitivity, but a considerable number may be.

In some instances the attacks seem to come on when the digestion of the person concerned is not working properly. In these instances, it is well to have a thorough study of the gastro-intestinal tract to make certain that there is neither constipation nor a residue of putrefactive matter in the bowel.

In other cases the glands of internal secretion may be involved, and it is necessary to make a thorough study of the body with a view to determining that all of the glands are neither overfunctioning nor underfunctioning. This is merely an indication of the necessity for studying every case of recurrent sick headache with all of the means known to modern medical science.

In a survey of methods of treatment to be applied in headache, Dr. Henry A. Riley points out that almost every method of treatment known to medical science has been applied at one time or another in such cases. He feels, therefore, that some definite change should be made in the life habits of such a patient based on a complete survey of his work, his play, his food, his mental attitude, and his philosophy of life. An inequality of emphasis in the patient's interests and activities should be corrected. He should live a moderate existence, and all excesses should be prevented.

A patient who is constantly indoors and gets insufficient exercise should change his habits in the right direction. Rest and change are particularly valuable for people who are constantly under physical, mental, or emotional pressure. Persons who suffer from recurrent sick headaches should not try to work all the time. They will do well to take at least one afternoon and one day a week for rest or recreation, and perhaps both winter and summer vacations.

In controlling the immediate attack, Dr. Riley suggests that the room be darkened and that everything be kept quiet. Most such patients are so intensely uncomfortable that they do not want to be touched or interfered with. In some instances, an ice bag to the head or a hot-water bottle to the feet may give relief.

The physician who is actively in charge of the treatment of such a patient can do much by controlling the diet, eliminating the substances to which the patient seems to respond with headache. He can also control the actions of the bowels and, on occasion, get results by the injection of various preparations which produce what is known as nonspecific protein reaction. These reactions seem to change the general reactions of the body to all sorts of conditions. The method is, however, wholly experimental, and it is not possible to promise certain results in any instance. The use of various glandular preparations to overcome deficiencies in glands or, in some instances, to oppose overactivity of certain glands is again experimental but is worthy of trial.

In cases which seem to be of this type there arises the question of giving drugs of various types to control the pain. Here it is absolutely necessary to have the constant attention of a physician who is thoroughly familiar with the patient, his habits, his emotional reactions, and particularly his headaches. It is easy to fall into the habit of taking strong drugs constantly, and the physician who understands the patient and his reactions will know how to avoid the danger of such habits.

Metallic and Food Poisoning

The human being is subject to various kinds of possible poisoning from foods and drugs, from mushrooms, and all sorts of similar toxic substances. There are poisons constantly used in industry which may get into the body and thereby produce severe illness.

In any case of poisoning certain procedures are immediately desirable. First, try to ascertain the nature of the poison taken. An empty bottle in the vicinity, the presence of some of the substance in a cup or utensil, or the presence of the poison on the tablecloth or floor or clothing may be a valuable sign. By smelling the breath and examining the mouth of the patient, the physician may determine the presence of stains or burns characteristic of the action of certain poisons. If the patient has taken the poison accidentally he will probably be willing to tell the physician, if he is conscious.

If poisoning is suspected, a physician should be called immediately. Before the doctor comes, it is well to give white of eggs, milk, or strong tea, which are antagonistic to many poisons. In order to get the poison out of the system as rapidly as possible one should provoke vomiting, either by tickling the back of the throat, by giving a cup of warm water mixed with salt, or by washing out the stomach with a stomach tube, if one understands how this is done. If one puts a heaping teaspoonful of salt in a cupful of lukewarm water, stirs until dissolved, and has the patient drink the mixture, repeating the dose every ten minutes until three or four cupfuls have been taken, vomiting takes place promptly, serving to wash out the stomach.

Thereafter the person must be treated as in any case of fainting, dizziness, or shock, the symptoms being treated according to the nature of the case. If the patient is greatly weakened or prostrated he must be kept warm, recumbent, and his general strength sustained.

For many of the common poisons there are special antidotes. However, these are seldom present in the average home, and even when present, few people have time to consult tables of antidotes or know where the antidote is to be found. For poisoning with carbolic acid it is customary to wash out the mouth with whisky or alcohol and water, to have the patient swallow three or four tablespoonfuls of diluted whisky or alcohol and water, and to give a heaping tablespoonful of epsom salts dissolved in water.

Bichloride of mercury is one of the most dangerous of poisons. The physician should be called at the earliest possible moment in order that he may supply antidotes and do everything possible to sustain the patient's circulation and elimination.

In case of poisoning by various narcotic drugs it is customary to provoke vomiting and then to give strong black coffee, at the same time doing everything possible to keep the patient awake. Sometimes it is necessary to walk him about forcefully. As long as he is awake he will continue to breathe, but if he is permitted to sleep, breathing may stop.

There follows a table of poisonings and methods of treatment summarized by the health department of San Francisco:

SYMPTOMS AND TREATMENT OF ACUTE POISONING

SYMPTOMS	ANTIDOTES AND TREATMENT
Acetanilid, Antipyrin, Acetphenetidin (Phenacetin)	
Vomiting (sometimes). Face cyanosed. Skin: cold; profuse sweat; sometimes rash simulating measles, scarlatina, or pemphigus. Collapse; feeble and irregular pulse; slow respiration.	Lavage or emetic. External heat; recumbent position. Caffeine, digitalis. Carbon dioxide-oxygen inhalation, if needed.

Aconite

Tingling and numbness of tongue and mouth and sense of formication of the body. Nausea and vomiting; diarrhea with epigastric pain. Dyspnea. Pulse irregular and weak. Skin cold and clammy; features bloodless. Giddiness, staggering walk; feeling of heaviness. The mind remains clear.

Avoid emetics. Gastric lavage—stomach to be washed with 0.1 per cent (1:1000) potassium permanganate, 250 cc. Reflex stimulants: ether, alcohol (whisky), aromatic spirits of ammonia. Caffeine or atropine. Carbon dioxide-oxygen inhalation, if necessary. External heat; recumbent position with head lower than feet.

Alcohol (Ethyl Alcohol)

Ataxia, cramps, coma, decreased respiration. Abolition of the superficial and deep reflexes.

Gastric lavage. Coffee enema. Carbon dioxide-oxygen inhalation. External heat. Aromatic spirits of ammonia, caffeine or atropine.

Alkalies, Fixed and Caustic (Sodium and Potassium Hydroxide—Lye), Sodium Carbonate (Washing Soda)

Burning pain from mouth to stomach; difficulty in swallowing; sloughed tissues in mouth; vomiting and purging of mucus and blood. Collapse; skin cold and clammy; pulse feeble; anxious countenance; rapid exhaustion; dyspnea. Convulsions. Unconsciousness or coma.

Do not use stomach tube! Give from 100 to 500 cc. of 0.5 per cent hydrochloric acid. Eight ounces of olive oil by mouth. Demulcents such as gelatin, acacia, or flour in water. Caffeine or digitan hypodermically, if necessary. External heat.

Ammonia

Gastro-intestinal symptoms, as in corrosive poisoning. Purging usual, with pain and straining. Body cold, with cold sweat. Countenance anxious. Pulse rapid and weak.

Eight ounces of olive oil by mouth. Large, quantities of water. Neutralization with from 100 to 500 cc. of 0.5 per cent hydrochloric acid. *Do not use stomach tube.*

Anesthetics, Volatile (Chloroform, Ether, Nitrous Oxide)

Rapid heart rate, abolition of reflexes, stoppage of heart or respiration.

Withdrawal of anesthetic. If circulatory collapse persists, ouabain intravenously; epinephrine intravenously or intracardially. If respiration stops, artificial respiration; carbon dioxide-oxygen inhalation; caffeine given intravenously or intramuscularly; atropine hypodermically.

Arsenic

Symptoms usually appear in from a quarter of an hour to one hour. Vomiting profuse, painful diarrhea; thirst; sense of constriction in throat, rendering swallowing difficult; cyanosis; coma.

Abundant gastric lavage with warm water. External heat. Opiate for diarrhea and colic. Infusion of solution of sodium chloride containing sodium bicarbonate (5 per cent), if necessary. Milk diet. Treat patient as potential nephritic patient.

| SYMPTOMS | ANTIDOTES AND TREATMENT |

Atropine, Belladonna

Dryness of mouth. Difficulty in swallowing and articulation; thirst. Skin flushed. Temperature raised. Pulse quick. Pupils widely dilated. Purging. Delirium.

Purified animal charcoal as antidote (2 tablespoonfuls in 250 cc. of water). Evacuation of stomach. Caffeine. Potassium permanganate in 1:1,000 solution, 250 cc.; lavage with the same preparation. Catheterization if necessary. If excitation persists, barbital or paraldehyde. Physostigmine.

Barbituric Acid Derivatives (Phenobarbital, Barbital, etc.)

Coma, circulatory collapse, pulmonary edema, cold skin, cyanosis. Sometimes delirium, twitching and increased reflexes.

Cover patient warmly; apply hot-water bottles. Gastric lavage. Caffeine. Ephedrine. Carbon dioxide-oxygen inhalation.

Bichloride of Mercury

Metallic taste, choking sensation. Pain in stomach, vomiting and purging of stringy mucus and blood. Tongue may be white and shriveled. Skin cold and clammy. Pulse feeble and rapid.

Treatment in Emergency Room: Antidote (by mouth): 10 cc. of 10 per cent sodium hypophosphite in water and then add 5 cc. hydrogen peroxide for each gram (15 grains) of bichloride of mercury. One glass of water. Lavage with antidote (one dose per hundred cubic centimeters of water). Two egg whites, or liberal dry egg albumin in water, and one glass of milk, followed by lavage with water.
Treatment in the Ward: Gastric lavage twice a day with 6 quarts of sodium bicarbonate solution. Sodium acetate by mouth (amount to keep urine alkaline). Use low pressure colonic irrigation twice a day with 6 quarts of solution. (2 drachms sodium acetate to 1 pint of water.) Send urine, vomitus and colonic washings to the laboratory daily for examination for mercury (500 cc. of each). Daily specimens of urine to internes' laboratory. Daily chemical examination of the blood. Administration of stimulants and sedatives as indicated. Treatment continued until symptoms have abated and mercury has disappeared from urine and colonic and gastric washings.

Boron (Boric Acid, Borax Solutions)

Epigastric pain, abdominal cramps, vomiting, diarrhea, weak pulse, cold clammy skin, sometimes cyanosis and collapse. (Boric acid, 3 to 6 gm., has been fatal to infants, and 15 grams has been fatal to adults. Thirty gm. of borax, likewise, has been fatal to adults.)

Keep patient warm, in recumbent position. If taken by mouth, gastric lavage; or, if given by rectum in enema, rectal lavage, warm water. Caffeine may be given, and the kidneys should be protected by the administration of alkali (1.0 to 5.0 gm. sodium bicarbonate and alkaline drinks or fruit juices) and by the administration of sodium thiosulphate.

SYMPTOMS | ANTIDOTES AND TREATMENT

Camphor (Camphor Oil; Spirit of Camphor)

Characteristic odor of breath; burning pain in stomach; colic; giddiness; pulse rapid and weak. Impulsive movements; delirium. Face flushed. Sometimes convulsions. Collapse. Coma.

Apomorphine, hypodermically. Gastric lavage repeatedly with warm water. Inhalation anesthesia to check convulsions; then barbital by mouth or intramuscularly to check excitation. Caffeine or digitan hypodermically, if necessary. External heat. Artificial respiration, if required. Convalescence may be prolonged.

Cantharides

Burning pain in throat and stomach; difficulty in swallowing. Vomiting and diarrhea; mucus and blood may contain shining particles of the powder. Salivation and swelling of the salivary glands. Burning in urethra; frequent micturition. Urine contains albumin, casts, and blood. Pulse weak and slow; collapse.

Gastric lavage; mucilaginous drinks; opiate for pain. No oil by mouth. Treat as for potential nephritis (alkalies and milk diet).

Chloral Hydrate

Vomiting, collapse, delirium, fall of temperature, cyanosis, dyspnea or slow respirations. Coma.

Gastric lavage with potassium permanganate 1:1,000, 250 cc. External heat. Caffeine, then digitalis. Carbon dioxide-oxygen inhalation, or artificial respiration, as needed.

Cinchophen (Atophan)

Poisoning generally subacute or chronic, but toxic symptoms may become rapidly severe during or in absence of administration of drug.
Symptoms of cinchonism; nausea and vomiting; persistent abdominal pain; diarrhea. Jaundice; liver pain or tenderness; stupor. Urine colored red to brown. Collapse. Coma.

Gastric lavage. Magnesium sulphate. Withdrawal of administration of drug. Camphor oil, caffeine or digitan, if necessary. Continue with treatment for hepatitis; injections of dextrose and insulin; carbohydrate diet; bicarbonate by mouth for acidosis.

Cocaine and Procaine Hydrochloride

Anxiety, fainting, pallor dyspnea, brief convulsions and apnea. With smaller doses, confusion, laughter, vertigo, motor excitement, tachycardia, irregular respiration, pallor, dilated pupils and exophthalmos, paresthesia, delirium and dyspnea. If death does not occur in a few minutes, recovery always follows.

Gastric lavage with 1 liter of 0.1 per cent (1:1,000) potassium permanganate (if taken by mouth). One-half per cent potassium permanganate solution if stomach is empty; otherwise, tannic acid (5 gm.). Soluble barbital intravenously.

SYMPTOMS | ANTIDOTES AND TREATMENT

Cyanides (Sodium or Potassium; Hydrocyanic Acid)

Characteristic odor of poison. Dyspnea; rapid pulse; unconsciousness; tremors; violent convulsions; dilated pupils; absence of cyanosis. If patient survives an hour, recovery may occur.

If poison has been swallowed, give sodium thiosulphate, 10 per cent in water, 500 cc., using stomach tube if necessary. Inject intravenously 50 cc. methylene blue (1 per cent in 1.8 per cent sodium sulphate solution), repeat in 15 minutes, if necessary. Or, try sodium nitrite, 10 to 20 mgm. per kg. body weight (12 to 24 cc. 5 per cent sodium nitrite solution) intravenously. Epinephrine into heart.

Digitalis

Vomiting; diarrhea. Slow pulse; cardiac irregularity. Lassitude; muscular and sensory derangements.

Gastric lavage with potassium permanganate 0.1 per cent (1:1,000) or tannic acid, 1 per cent. Horizontal position. External heat. Atropine hypodermically. Quinidine for cardiac irregularity.

Ergot

Pale skin, small and rapid pulse, constricted arteries. Hallucinations. Cyanosis of the fingertips and toes. Sensory disturbances. Ascending gangrene of the extremities.

Gastric lavage in acute poisoning; withdrawal of administration of ergot. Nitrites. Warm room. Periodic inhalation of carbon dioxide and oxygen.

Fluoride (Roach and Insect Powders)

Nausea and vomiting; burning, cramplike abdominal pains; diarrhea. Sometimes tremors or convulsions. Grayish blue cyanosis. Urine and blood show presence of fluoride.

Copious gastric lavage with limewater or weak calcium chloride solution. Calcium gluconate intramuscularly, or calcium chloride, 10 cc. of 10 per cent. in water, intravenously. Digitan hypodermically; artificial respiration, if necessary. External heat.

Formaldehyde

Odor. Sore mouth. Dysphagia. Severe abdominal pain. Unconsciousness and collapse. Later diarrhea and tenesmus.

Swallow a tumblerful of 0.2 per cent ammonia. Lavage with dilute ammonia followed by raw egg, or egg albumin in water.

Gas (Garage Gas, or from Defective Flue Fumes, Carbon Monoxide)

Giddiness and singing in the ears. Lividity of face and body. Loss of muscular power. Unconsciousness and collapse.

Carbon dioxide-oxygen inhalation, or artificial respiration, if needed. Bleeding followed by transfusion if indicated. External heat. Oxygen tent if available. Digitalis.

SYMPTOMS   ANTIDOTES AND TREATMENT

Hydrochloric Acid

Gastro-intestinal symptoms, coffee-ground vomitus. Purging usual, with pain and straining. Body cold, with cold sweat. Countenance anxious. Pulse rapid and weak.

Magnesia magma 100 to 400 cc. White of egg or olive oil as a demulcent; external heat; camphor oil, caffeine or digitan hypodermically, if necessary.

Iodine

Pain and heat in throat and stomach. Vomiting and purging, vomitus being yellow or blue if starchy matter is present in the stomach. Stools may contain blood. Intense thirst. Giddiness, faintness and convulsions.

Sodium thiosulphate by mouth (1 to 10 gm. in water) as an antidote. Then lavage with 1 per cent sodium thiosulphate. Later, thin starch paste or flour soup. External heat; camphor oil, caffeine or digitan hypodermically, if necessary.

Lead

Metallic taste, dry throat, intense thirst. Abdominal colic. Constipation, dark feces. Vomiting may occur. Giddiness, stupor, convulsions, coma.

Magnesium sulphate in solution as antidote. Lavage with 1 per cent sodium sulphate, mucilaginous (acacia) or egg albumin drinks. External heat. Cathartic after lavage.. Calcium gluconate intramuscularly. Opiate for colic.

Morphine, Opium

Coma, gradual in onset. Symmetrical pinpoint pupils that dilate terminally Respirations slow and shallow. Body cold. Cyanosis; convulsions.

Potassium permanganate 0.1 per cent (1:1,000), 250 cc. by mouth. Gastric lavage with some solution of potassium permanganate. Black coffee. Try to keep the patient awake by suggestion. Carbon dioxide-oxygen inhalation. Artificial respiration, if necessary. External heat. Caffeine or atropine hypodermically, if respiration fails to improve.

Mushrooms

Colic, vomiting, purging. Mental excitement followed by coma. Extremities cold. Pulse slow. Respiration stertorous. Pulmonary edema. Pupils dilated.

Gastric lavage. External heat. Atropine.

Nicotine and Tobacco

Severe depression, prostration and muscular weakness; severe nausea and vomiting. Marked dyspnea. Weak rapid pulse. Pupils first contracted then dilated. Muscular tremors, followed rapidly by convulsions. Coma.

If free vomiting has not occurred, wash out stomach repeatedly with potassium permanganate, 0.1 per cent (1:1,000), and warm water. Strong coffee. Caffeine or digitan hypodermically, if necessary. External heat. Artificial respiration, if necessary.

SYMPTOMS	ANTIDOTES AND TREATMENT

Nitric Acid

Pain in throat and stomach. Vomiting of whitish, flaky matter that blackens on exposure to light.

Magnesia magma, from 100 to 400 cc. White of egg, or egg albumin in water, or olive oil (250 cc.) as a demulcent. External heat. Camphor oil, caffeine or digitan hypodermically, if necessary.

Nitrites and Nitroglycerine

Collapse, unconsciousness, cyanosis or pallor, low blood pressure, slow pulse, irregular respiration. Sometimes vomiting and convulsions. Persistent cyanosis. Methemoglobinuria.

Recumbent position. Gastric lavage if poison has been swallowed. Guaiacol 0.5 gm. and Berlin blue 0.5 gm. together, gastrically or orally, 3 to 6 times daily. If necessary, epinephrine intravenously; digitan hypodermically; oxygen inhalation. External heat.

Oils, Volatile and Ecbolic (Tansy, Pennyroyal, Santal, Absinthe, Turpentine)

Characteristic odor of breath; burning, nausea, vomiting; eructations; colic; diarrhea. Skin rash; jaundice. Convulsions; dilated pupils; rapid stertorous respiration; pulse slow and feeble. Unconsciousness. Coma. Sometimes, uterine hemorrhage, abortion, hematuria.

If vomiting has not occurred, repeatedly wash out stomach with warm water. Demulcents: acacia, starch, or flour in water. Magnesium sulphate unless diarrhea is present. Opiate for colic. Camphor oil, caffeine or digitan, if necessary. External heat. Barbital for excitation. Later, treatments for nephritis and hepatitis; abortion.

Oxalic Acid

Gastro-intestinal symptoms as in corrosive poisoning. Purging, in most cases, with pain and straining. Body cold, with cold sweat. Countenance anxious. Pulse rapid and weak.

Calcium lactate (10 to 20 gm. in 250 cc. of water). Potassium permanganate, 0.1 per cent (1:1,000), 250 cc. by mouth. Gastric lavage with same permanganate solution. Demulcents. Heat applied to abdomen. Camphor oil, caffeine or digitan hypodermically, if necessary.

Paris Green

Symptoms usually appear in from a quarter of an hour to one hour. Burning heat and constriction or choking in throat, rendering swallowing difficult. Nausea and incessant vomiting and purging. The vomiting matter may be green from bile, or, in the case of arsenic, black from the admixture of soda, or blue from indigo. Pain in the stomach and abdomen. Cramps in the calves of the legs. Urine may be suppressed. There may be delirium or paralysis. Collapse; skin cold and clammy, sometimes showing eczematous rash. Pulse small, quick and irregular, or imperceptible.

Abundant gastric lavage with warm water. Infusion of solution of sodium chloride if necessary. Tincture of opium for diarrhea and colic. Caffeine, strychnine or atropine, as needed, for circulatory and respiratory stimulation. Milk diet. Treat as for potential nephritis.

SYMPTOMS   ANTIDOTES AND TREATMENT

Phenols (Carbolic Acid, Lysol, Cresols, "Sheep-Dip")

Characteristic odor present. Burning sensation in mouth and throat; burns on lips and in mouth; nausea and vomiting. Abdominal pain. Faintness; collapse; pulse slow and weak; face livid; cold sweat; respiration depressed; unconsciousness. Coma. Urine scanty with smoky color.

Gastric lavage with 10 per cent ethyl alcohol in water, 1 quart; continuous lavage with warm water. Infusion of physiological salt solution; epinephrine intravenously or intracardially. Caffeine or digitan hypodermically. External heat. Artificial respiration if necessary. Later treatment same as for after effects of corrosives.

Phosphorus

Symptoms usually appear in three stages: (1) A few hours after administration, there develops a garlic taste, gastro-intestinal irritation, burning pain, thirst, swelling of the abdomen and vomiting of blood (green or black). The vomit has a garlic odor and in the dark may be phosphorescent. The patient may die, or there may be: (2) An intermission of symptoms for three days or more, with a feeling of malaise followed by: (3) The final stage, characterized by intense jaundice, enlarged liver and distended abdomen; great prostration, cold sweat, an anxious look, feeble pulse, muscular twitching, coma.

Two hundred cubic centimeters of 0.2 per cent solution of copper sulphate by mouth. Lavage with from 5 to 10 liters of the same solution followed by lavage with 1 liter of 0.1 per cent potassium permanganate; followed by the administration of 100 cc. of liquid petrolatum. No fats or oils should be given, as they aid absorption. External heat. Treatment continued for liver injury—high carbohydrate diet; dextrose and insulin.

Quinine and Quinidine

Ringing in ears, disturbed vision, photophobia. (Later deafness and blindness.) Nausea; vomiting. Faintness. Difficulty of speech, somnolence; unconsciousness, alternating with delirium and coma. Pulse slow and feeble. Sometimes convulsions.

Tannic acid by mouth. Gastric lavage with potassium permanganate 0.1 per cent (1:1,000). Epinephrine intravenously or intracardially, if necessary. Caffeine or digitan hypodermically. If excitation persists, barbital by mouth.

Strychnine, Nux Vomica

Feeling of suffocation and lividity of the face. Tetanic convulsions, with short intermission, causing sweating and exhaustion, opisthotonus, risus sardonicus, staring eyes, fixed chest, and hard abdominal muscles. Hearing and sight are acute, and consciousness is retained. The muscles of the jaw are not affected until late.

Early: Give by mouth or with stomach tube purified animal charcoal, from 1 to 2 tablespoonfuls in a glass of water. Gastric lavage with potassium permanganate, 0.1 per cent solution (1:1,000). *Later (with muscular hypertonicity):* Arrest hyperexcitability or convulsions with inhalation anesthesia (ether or chloroform) and then inject intramuscularly soluble barbital, 1 gm. (20 cc. of 5 per cent), later by mouth; or pentobarbital, 1/10 gr. (6 mgms.) per pound body weight as the first dose and one half this amount for succeeding doses. Do not use any methods

SYMPTOMS   ANTIDOTES AND TREATMENT

Strychnine, Nux Vomica (continued)

that excite spasm, such as attempting in-travenous injection. The patient should be isolated and kept absolutely quiet. Ether inhalation should be given if convulsions continue. Artificial respiration, if respiration fails.

Thallium (Depilatories; Rodent Poisons—"Thalgrain")

Abdominal colic, nausea, vomiting, and diarrhea; constipation; stomatitis; alopecia; peripheral neuritis; central nervous involvement (ptosis, strabismus, convulsions, choreiform movements, optic atrophy). Evidences of liver damage, nephritis; sometimes pulmonary edema. Thallium in urine.

Early: If emesis has not occurred, copious gastric lavage with 1 per cent sodium or potassium iodide (in water); catharsis (avoid sulphates). If shock is present, 25 gm. (50 cc. of 50 per cent) dextrose intravenously; external heat; reflex stimulants, epinephrine, caffeine, or digitan hypodermically; artificial respiration if necessary. *Later:* Rest in bed; control mobilization of thallium in body by daily intravenous injections of sodium iodide, about 15 to 40 cc. of 2.3 per cent, in water (freshly prepared) (about 0.3 to 1 gm. NaI) until urine test shows absence of thallium; dose of iodide may gradually be doubled. Daily chemical examination of urine: collect and evaporate to dryness 24-hour urines for thallium test—absence of, or only slight, green color on flaming residue. When symptoms of thallitoxicosis subside, proceed cautiously to increase elimination of thallium by intravenous injection of sodium thiosulphate, 0.3 to 1 gm. (6 to 20 cc. of 5 per cent in water; freshly prepared) for adult, alternating with sodium iodide solution intravenously, if necessary. Pilocarpine (promotes secretion), calcium lactate, if necessary; dilute hydrochloric acid for achlorhydria; bland ointments for dermatitis; barbital or codeine for restlessness and pain; treatments for liver injury and nephritis, if necessary.

CHAPTER IV

Hygiene of Women
MORRIS FISHBEIN, M.D.

As DR. THURMAN B. RICE points out in another section of this book, the boy and girl, until the age of twelve, may be reared in much the same manner. Their health problems are approximately the same. Thereafter, however, the problems of the girl are distinctive. It is at this period in her life that her organs begin to differentiate in such a manner as to prepare her for her functions as a mother. It is taken for granted that the mother will have prepared the daughter suitably for recognition of the changes that are to come. In the majority of girls these changes take place so gradually that they are not noticed.

The startling change which appears is the development of the menstrual flow. In far too many instances, notwithstanding the advance in health education that has been made in the last quarter century, girls still come to this phenomenon without any knowledge, and some of them sustain mental shocks which mark their lives thereafter. Until menstruation appears, the girl is not likely to bear children; with the coming of menstruation, the organs develop and the possibility exists.

Before that time, the body configuration of most girls has been much like that of the boy. After puberty, which is the time when the menstrual flow appears, the breasts, the pelvis and neck enlarge, hair develops in the armpits and over the sexual area, and the voice changes.

The onset of the menstrual flow is not always an abrupt and complete development. The first flow may be very brief; it may disappear and not appear again for weeks or months; it may, at first, be irregular and then later regular. Just as soon as the flow appears regularly at a definite interval for several months, the menstruation may be said to be established.

Associated with this physical change, there are also mental changes

Many of these changes are associated with new interests in the male sex, in more mature occupations, in a different type of reading, and in many similar matters. For this reason, parents should have surveillance over their daughters and use proper understanding of the nature of the change that is occurring.

However, our views have greatly changed in the last quarter century. Girls used to be sick in every sense of the word during the menstrual period. Nowadays they are likely to go through without the slightest alteration in their habits. There are, of course, instances in which the function is accompanied with severe pain or with physical disturbance. When these occur, they should have the attention of a physician. The hygiene associated with minor disturbances will be discussed in later paragraphs.

The adolescent girl is undergoing rapid development. For this reason her posture must be carefully watched. If she grows too rapidly and is somewhat tall, there may be an inclination to slump the shoulders forward, the abdomen out and the chest in. Such posture is bound to lead to a poor figure later in life. Exercises, described in the article on posture in this book, will help to develop a proper position when standing and when sitting. The chin and abdomen should be kept in and the chest forward. Many young girls worry about the development of the breasts and, not understanding the changes that occur, attempt to hide them. Poor posture may result from holding the shoulders in such a manner as to draw in the chest.

The girl, at this period of life, needs plenty of sleep; ten or eleven hours in twenty-four is not too much. Extra relaxation in the form of a nap in the middle of the day, such as is given to smaller children, may be exceedingly useful in maintaining her body tone. There need be no special attention to the diet other than the certainty that it contains the necessary proteins, carbohydrates and fats, mineral salts and vitamins that are necessary in any well-balanced diet.

Many girls passing from adolescence into adult age feel that it is necessary for them to adopt sophisticated habits. Whereas they have formerly avoided tea and coffee in favor of milk, they want to partake of these beverages as giving them somewhat more of a status in the family. It should be remembered that tea and coffee are mild stimulants and may be undesirable, particularly at this period. Smoking cigarettes is not necessary, and again may be considered as a habit to be controlled until it can be indulged in with intelligence.

Some girls at this age put on so much weight that they are seriously disturbed. The weight may increase so rapidly that the skin of the abdomen stretches and red marks appear along the curves of the hips. These should not cause worry because they will fade when the weight of the body is more definitely adjusted. For the control of the tendency to overweight, a suitable diet with a lowered amount of carbohydrates is desirable. Nowadays most people have learned enough about calories and carbohydrates in relationship to overweight to exercise a certain amount of control over this danger.

Special attention should also be given at this period to the condition of the thyroid gland. In some children there is a tendency to over-activity of the gland, which is marked also by rapid heart, nervousness, perspiration, and similar symptoms. If any sign appears of overactivity of the thyroid gland, the basal metabolism should be determined by a competent doctor and the condition of the thyroid gland controlled in relationship to the results. If there is overweight or underweight, the basal metabolism test should also be made to determine whether or not the activity of the thyroid gland is related in any way to this unusual development.

In the Great Lakes area and in the Northwest, the water and the soil lack iodine, hence there is a tendency among young children to develop simple enlargement of the thyroid gland that is known as simple goiter. There is a special chapter on this condition elsewhere in this book. Any tendency of the thyroid gland toward enlargement should, of course, be studied by the family doctor. In most cases, however, intelligent parents nowadays give small doses of iodine regularly each week to supply the iodine deficiency and thus effectively prevent the appearance of simple goiter.

DISORDERS OF MENSTRUATION

As I have already said, menstruation may be occasionally irregular during the first year without causing any anxiety. Certainly, by the end of the first year it should be regular, in the majority of women, occurring every twenty-eight days. Menstruation occurring regularly anywhere from twenty-one days to five-week intervals may be considered within normal limits.

Sometimes, in connection with the first appearance of menstruation, the usual signs of adolescence appear, including pimples and black-heads on the face, back, and chest, soreness and swelling of the breasts.

and headache. These may appear as the result of the changes in the glands that occur at this time.

Ordinarily menstruation should cause no more pain than any of the other functions of the body. When the pain occurs, it is usually associated with a disturbance of the circulation or of the glands. Sometimes failure of the bowels to act properly is a complication, which may be easily corrected by establishment of regular habits, sufficient rest, drinking of plenty of water, and the other measures suggested in the section on digestion.

EXERCISES

Various exercises have been described for use by growing girls at this time. Some of these simple exercises involve not only the usual bending and standing, which are good for posture, but also standing in the knee-chest position, walking on the hands and feet as the monkey or cat walks, and other postures which help to develop the ligaments which hold the organs of the pelvis in position. Dr. Josephine H. Kenyon points out there are many simple factors which influence menstruation and which will easily control it.

Emotional shocks and nerve shocks may tend to be associated with pain at this time. A change in the altitude, extraordinary changes in the diet, over- and under-exercise, and many similar factors may yield difficult symptoms. For this reason, the routine of the girl's life during the menstrual period should be disturbed as little as possible.

She may take her baths daily as always, preferably a warm bath; but if she is in the habit of taking cold baths, she may take these also. There is no good reason why most women should not take a bath during the menstrual period. If the flow of blood is profuse, strenuous swimming may make it excessive; also a very hot tub bath may increase the amount of blood lost. A very cold bath taken just before or at the beginning of menstruation may occasionally stop the bleeding. The danger of infection from the water is very slight.

Indulgence in competitive games during the menstrual period should, of course, be carefully controlled. Such games involve emotional stress and high tension. They place a considerable burden upon the heart. They bring about shocks and jolts to the internal organs for which these organs are not competent. It is particularly important that every girl indulging in athletic sports have a physical examination in relationship to her feminine constitution.

Painful Menstruation

There are a tremendous number of remedies which have been suggested for painful menstruation. This indicates also that no one of them is specific. Sufficient rest and sleep, proper hygiene and treatment for anemia, if that is present, are especially important. Some patients get immediate help from rest in bed and the use of an enema for emptying the bowels. Others are relieved by placing a hot-water bag over the painful area. Aspirin and similar drugs which relieve pain are used by many girls and are not harmful, if taken in small doses and preferably under the direction of a physician.

Sometimes it is necessary for the doctor to make certain modifications of the glandular mechanism of the patient. The administration of suitable glandular substances which are known to have control over the menstrual functions sometimes yields successful results in eliminating pain.

In the process of menstruation at least three organs are involved: the pituitary gland, the ovaries, and the uterus. Regular bleeding from the uterus, called menstruation, is nearly always dependent on proper functioning of the ovaries. These, in turn, are controlled by a portion of the pituitary gland in the brain. The pituitary gland has been called the motor of the ovaries. When there are unusual symptoms during the menstrual period, such as flushing, numbness of the finger tips, fainting spells, and crying, it is the glands and their secretions which are ordinarily responsible.

Because of the tendency to bleed at this period, some women bruise more easily during the menstrual time; others suffer with nosebleeds. These symptoms usually disappear when the menstruation ends.

When menstruation is exceedingly scanty, the state of the blood should be studied as to whether or not there is anemia. There should also be an investigation of the basal metabolism and the general nutrition.

During menstruation the vast majority of women wear a simple cotton pad, such as is now commercially available in many different forms in this country. There is seldom any necessity for any type of medication in connection with these pads. Where there are unusual odors of any kind, a careful investigation should be made by a competent doctor to determine the presence or absence of infection. In most cases, annoying odors are a sign of infection, and they cannot be corrected by application of deodorants or powders of any kind.

More recently, cotton packs or tampons have been developed. It is doubtful whether these are desirable for women who have a profuse flow. This applies also to various types of rubber cups that have been devised for controlling the menstrual flow. For persons in the theatrical profession, for acrobats, and women who indulge in sports of various kinds, such devices may be desirable.

The medical profession has not settled definitely the question of the advisability of using douches before and after the menstrual period or at any other time. About an equal number of specialists in diseases of women are arrayed on each side of this question. Women who are not infected in any manner and who do not have excessive discharges of mucus and other material from the genital tract need not employ douches regularly. Ordinary bathing will suffice for the purpose. However, in cases in which there are excessive discharges, or in which, as has been mentioned, there is an odor present, a physician should be consulted in order to determine the presence and nature of the infection. The infection should be treated by the means that the physician will recommend. This recommendation will in most instances involve the use of suitable cleansing and antiseptic agents used in the form of douches and in similar ways.

ABSENCE OF MENSTRUATION

Most people know that menstruation disappears when a woman becomes pregnant and is to have a child. It disappears also at a period known as the climacteric, which is also an important epoch in the life of women. This period is also called the menopause, as an indication of the fact that the menstruation disappears at this time.

There are, of course, other factors which occasionally produce a change in menstruation and in some instances even a temporary absence. A change of geographical location, which involves chiefly a change of climate and perhaps of altitude, not infrequently produces alterations in menstruation. Usually the flow may stop, but in some cases the amount of blood lost is excessive. Because the process of menstruation is controlled by glandular action, disorders of menstruation, including stopping for no apparent reason, are generally assumed to be due to some glandular difficulty.

Women who do not menstruate are not in any way inferior to those who do. They rarely show any abnormal symptoms, and their sex life is about the same. The whole difficulty lies in the minds of such women. They feel they are subnormal; they may become exceedingly disturbed mentally worrying over the condition. Frequently a physician can bring about menstruation in such patients by the experimental use of various glandular preparations.

The discontinuance of menstruation at the menopause is, of course, a different matter. The average duration of menstruation in women is from 30 to 32 years. The average age for the beginning of the climacteric or menopause in the temperate zone is about 47 years. However, there is an enormous variation in the ages at which the symptoms of climacteric may arise. Cases are known in which the change of life occurred as early as 27 years of age and as late as 59 years. Usually in the United States the discontinuance of menstruation occurs between 45 and 50 years of age in 50 per cent of women; between 40 and 45 in 25 per cent; between 35 and 40 in 12½ per cent, and between 50 and 55 years in 12½ per cent.

In most instances there is a definite association between the onset of puberty, or the beginning of menstruation, and the time of the appearance of the menopause. In general, the earlier the menstrual function begins, the longer it will continue. Girls who have an early puberty will have a long, potential, reproductive career and a late menopause. A physician named Gallant published a chart of approximate ages as to when the menopause would appear, based on the age of the onset of puberty. The table, which is for healthy women, follows:

Year in Which Menstruation Appears	Menopause Should Occur
10	Between 50 and 52 years
11	Between 48 and 50 years
12	Between 46 and 48 years
13	Between 44 and 46 years
14	Between 42 and 44 years
15	Between 40 and 42 years
16	Between 38 and 40 years
17	Between 36 and 38 years
18	Between 34 and 36 years
19	Between 32 and 34 years
20	Between 30 and 32 years

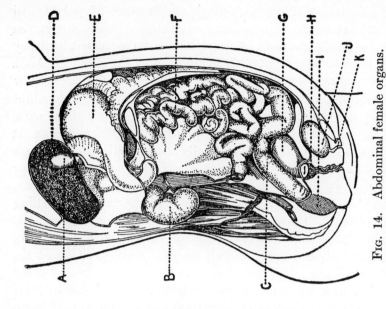

Fig. 14. Abdominal female organs.

A. Gall bladder. B. Kidney. C. Large intestine. D. Liver. E. Stomach. F. Small intestine. G. Uterus or womb. H. Vagina. I. Rectum. J. Bladder. K. Urethra.

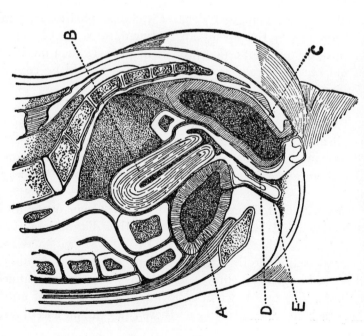

Fig. 13. Lateral view of female pelvic organs.

A. Bladder. B. Uterus or womb. C. Rectum. D. Vagina. E. Urethra.

Exactly as parts of the body change at the onset of puberty, so also do similar changes occur at the menopause. Usually the spleen and lymphatic glands decrease in size. There is an increased tendency to constipation, because of changes in the wall of the intestine. Most women have some physical discomfort and some mild mental or nervous changes, but some women cease menstruating with slight inconvenience. As a rule, the woman may miss one or two or more periods, then will have menstrual periods that seem almost normal; then she will miss other periods, and finally the periodic flow will cease altogether. This variability is due to the fact that the glandular changes which are occurring take place gradually.

There may be, during this period, slight inflammation and swelling of the sexual parts. These are, however, of little significance. The most difficult symptom which may develop at this time is excessive bleeding. Whenever excessive bleeding occurs, however, either at the menopause or at any other time, a physician should be consulted immediately so that he may make a study of the condition and determine its cause. It is well established that the appearance of blood is sometimes associated with the appearance of cancer. The only way to make certain is to have a direct examination of the tissue to guard against such a possibility.

Occasionally there is a good deal of itching, particularly after bathing. In such cases the use of an ointment, such as 12 per cent boric acid in an ointment of rose water, is helpful. If such mild treatment does not secure a good result, a physician should be consulted for the prescribing of something more powerful.

While it is true that states of mental depression and other abnormal mental states occur somewhat frequently at or about the age of menopause, it must be remembered that these are not really important abnormalities, and that they occur also in men around the age of fifty. Unless they are extreme, there is nothing to do in the way of treatment.

Since many different forms of mental disorder may occur at this period, it is always advisable to have a scientific diagnosis as to the character of the disturbance that occurs. In some women there seems to be increased sexual desire at this period. In such cases also the treatment is good hygiene, including also the avoidance of any unnecessary stimulants. The avoidance of coffee, and a good deal of outdoor exercise may be helpful. In other cases there is a gradual loss of sexual desire. This also may be quite temporary. Many women continue to be sexually active for considerable periods after the menopause. Not infrequently there is a mild degree of overactivity of the thyroid gland, and, associated with this, increased excitability. There may also be a slight elevation of the blood pressure.

All of these symptoms, however, are associated with the gradual change in the glandular mechanism and, unless severe, need not be considered seriously. [New substitutes for missing glandular substances may be prescribed by the doctor to overcome symptoms.—Ed.]

The changes associated with this period demand slight modification of the general hygiene of the body. Usually older people will want less food. Because of the difficulties of digestion, foods rich in carbohydrates, including sugars, cake, candy, preserves, and jelly, should be taken with moderation, as also foods that are known to cause indigestion in many cases; for example, foods fried in a good deal of grease, hot breads, pastry, cheese, and similar substances.

Since there is a considerable amount of congestion in the abdomen, the care of the bowels should be a special problem. A daily, free evacuation of the bowels is essential to health. The use of mild laxatives may bring a good deal of relief. The kidneys must be especially watched for the onset of any degenerative changes.

It is necessary to keep the skin in good condition by bathing—sometimes alternate hot and cold baths. Massage is helpful in toning up the nervous system and the circulation. Exercise daily in the open air is helpful in steadying the nerves and stimulating the body generally.

From the point of view of the mind, it is particularly necessary at this time of life that some pleasant occupation be followed. Usually by this time children will have passed the age when they need constant supervision, and the mother must take relaxation from her home cares. Many women at this time of life become expert bridge players or golfers, although previously they may have taken but little interest in such diversions. Any mental occupation that will take the woman into a new interest is the best possible safeguard against the slight mental difficulty which develops in some women at this period.

[The estrogenic hormones will aid in overcoming such symptoms as headache, hot flashes, and melancholia, which are so distressing at this time. These substances, however, should never be taken except when prescribed, and in the dosage prescribed, by the doctor.—Ed.]

The Rhythm of Menstruation and the Safe
Period for Prevention of Conception

In connection with the study of menstruation, it has been found that there is a definite relationship between the time a woman menstruates and the time when an egg cell or ovum passes from the ovary into the uterus. If a woman menstruates regularly every twenty-eight days, it is usually impossible for her to conceive between the first and tenth day of her menstrual cycle, the first day being the one on which the menstrual flow begins. She can conceive on the eleventh day and up to and including the seventeenth day, but she will not be able to conceive from the seventeenth day on. Therefore, the days on which conception is most likely are the days from the fourteenth to the sixteenth day after the first day of menstruation. This is the period in which the mother cell or egg cell is produced by the ovary. In a woman who menstruates every twenty-eight days, the egg cell comes from the ovary on the fourteenth day.

The period of nine days, referred to as the period when conception is most likely, includes three days for the production and discharge of the egg cell, one day allowed for variability, and two to three days for the survival of the fertilizing power of the male cell. It has been definitely shown that the male cell will not survive much over three days, unless it meets the egg cell of the female and brings about conception. The extra three days added to these seven are in the interests of safety against any irregularities.

Records have now been kept of many thousands of cases in which women have observed this safe period, and failures, when absolute observance prevailed, are exceedingly few. Of course, the matter is complicated when the menstrual cycle in the woman is more or less than twenty-eight days. For the majority of women, therefore, it will be necessary to determine the exact dates and variations of the menstrual cycle. This is done by keeping an accurate record for several months of the exact dates on which menstruation begins, how many days it continues, and the number of days from the first day of menstruation to the first day of the next menstruation. All sorts of calendars and devices have now been developed for keeping records of this kind.

It is known that a good many women have occasional variations in their menstrual cycle. Thus one authority said, "The only regular thing about menstruation is its own irregularity." Just as soon as the cycle is definitely established, it becomes possible for the woman to calculate the periods when she is likely to conceive, or the fertile period, and the period when she is not likely to conceive, or the sterile period.

The simplest method of counting is that which begins with the first day of the last menstrual period, rather than counting backward from the last menstrual period. The first period of sterility includes nine days, including the first day of menstruation. The period of probable fertility includes the next ten days, and the next period of sterility is the time until the next menstruation. In the ten-day period of probable fertility, there are the first two days and the last two days which are less probable than the six days intervening. The fourteenth day before the next menstruation is the day of most likely fertility.

Women should learn that it is not well to depend on the memory for such data, but that an actual record of the dates on a calendar is more certain. According to the Knaus method, the safe periods have been calculated for women with menstrual cycles of from twenty-three to thirty-four days, as follows:

For women with a twenty-three day menstrual cycle:
Ovulation may occur from the sixth through the tenth day after the first day of the preceding menstruation;
Probable conception may occur from the fifth through the twelfth day after the first day of the preceding menstruation;
For irregular women conception is possible on the first to the fourth day.

For women with a twenty-four days menstrual cycle:
Ovulation may occur from the seventh through the eleventh day after the first day of the preceding menstruation;
Probable conception may occur from the sixth through the thirteenth day after the first day of the preceding menstruation;
For irregular women who conceive easily conception is possible from the second through the fifth day.

For women with a twenty-five day menstrual cycle:
Ovulation may occur from the eighth through the twelfth day after the first day of the preceding menstruation;

Probable conception may occur from the seventh through the fourteenth day after the first day of the preceding menstruation;

For irregular women conception is possible on the third through the sixth day.

For women with a twenty-six day menstrual cycle:

Ovulation may occur from the ninth through the thirteenth day after the first day of the preceding menstruation;

Probable conception may occur from the eighth through the fifteenth day after the first day of the preceding menstruation;

For irregular women conception is possible on the fourth through the seventh day.

For women with a twenty-seven day menstrual cycle:

Ovulation may occur from the tenth through the fourteenth day after the first day of the preceding menstruation;

Probable conception may occur from the ninth through the sixteenth day after the first day of the preceding menstruation;

For irregular women conception is possible on the fifth through the eighth day.

For women with a twenty-eight day menstrual cycle:

Ovulation may occur from the eleventh through the fifteenth day after the first day of the preceding menstruation;

Probable conception may occur from the tenth through the seventeenth day after the first day of the preceding menstruation;

For irregular or fruitful women conception is possible on the sixth through the ninth day.

For women with a twenty-nine day menstrual cycle:

Ovulation may occur from the twelfth through the sixteenth day after the first day of the preceding menstruation;

Probable conception may occur from the eleventh through the eighteenth day after the first day of the preceding menstruation;

For irregular women conception is possible on the seventh through the tenth day.

For women with a thirty-day menstrual cycle:

Ovulation may occur from the thirteenth through the seventeenth day after the first day of the preceding menstruation;

Probable conception may occur from the twelfth through the nineteenth day after the first day of the preceding menstruation;

For irregular women conception is possible on the eighth through the eleventh day.

For women with a thirty-four day menstrual cycle:

Ovulation may occur from the seventeenth through the twenty-first day of the preceding menstruation;

Probable conception may occur from the sixteenth through the twenty-third day after the first day of the preceding menstruation;

For irregular women conception is possible on the twelfth through the fifteenth day.

For women whose menstrual cycle REGULARLY *falls from twenty-six to thirty days:*

Ovulation may occur from the ninth through the seventeenth day after the first day of the preceding menstruation;

Probable conception may occur from the eighth through the nineteenth day after the first day of the preceding menstruation;

For irregular or fruitful women conception is possible on the fourth through the seventh day.

For women whose menstrual cycle REGULARLY *falls from twenty-eight to thirty days:*

Ovulation may occur from the eleventh through the seventeenth day after the first day of the preceding menstruation;

Probable conception may occur from the tenth through the nineteenth day after the first day of the preceding menstruation;

For irregular women conception is possible on the sixth through the ninth day.

CHAPTER V

Sex Hygiene
THURMAN B. RICE, M.D.

INTRODUCTION

THE INVESTIGATIONS *of recent years indicate how profoundly various aspects of sex hygiene affect our lives not only from the physical but also from the mental point of view. The chief contribution of the Freudian psychology has been the emphasis which it has placed on the extent to which the inhibitions of previous generations have operated to establish many neuroses and sexual disorders. Certainly, there is good evidence that some conditions which were formerly thought to be wholly physical in character have a mental basis, and that this mental basis is established by failure to develop proper relationship between the sexes.*

Much of the background of these disorders is established in childhood and in adolescence. It is therefore important to recognize the significance of proper education in the facts of sex early in life. In the section which follows, Prof. Thurman B. Rice, of the Department of Preventive Medicine and Hygiene in the Indiana University School of Medicine, considers the whole problem of sex education beginning with the instruction of the child in these important matters and carrying his subject through to relationship during courtship, marriage, and wedded life.

Professor Rice is also an author of a series of pamphlets for children of various ages which is published by the American Medical Association, and which parents may turn over to their children in order to inform them properly on these subjects. Some of the material included in this chapter has also been published in Hygeia, *the health magazine published by the American Medical Association. The response to it, particularly from educators in the various school grades throughout the United States, has been excellent. A proper appreciation of the relationship of sex to health and to daily life is essential for satisfactory living.*

M. F.

THE CONTINUATION OF LIFE itself is directly dependent on the functioning of the fundamental instincts which bring men and women together in an infinitely important relation known as the family or the home and into which are born other human beings like unto themselves. Sex is everywhere about us. We see it in the clothes we wear, in the occupations we serve, and in the sports and games by which we seek relaxation. Short stories, novels, poetry, art, sculpture, music, and the drama constantly remind us of the fact that men and women are different and that they behave as they do largely because of this difference. If we would know what it is that motivates men and women and boys and girls; if we would understand the psychology, the hopes, the desires, the lusts, the passions of our neighbors; if we would know what it is that makes one man a hero and another a beast, we will do well to look into this matter of sex. Sex is omnipresent; it is everywhere about us; it touches us from a dozen angles; it is actually the *sine qua non* of our existence.

Is it not strange, then, that there should be so much misunderstanding of this vital subject? Is it not amazing that intelligent men and women should be in so many instances utterly ignorant of the true significance of this, the basic fact of life?

THE IDEALS AND PURPOSES OF SEX EDUCATION

There are many reasons why every child and every adult should understand, as well as he may, the various complicated functions by which the race reproduces itself and by which the family comes into existence and is held together as a unit. How this information may be transmitted correctly and decently to the younger generation is a problem of the utmost consequence.

The layman needs comparatively little detailed information concerning the minutiæ of the process of reproduction. He needs rather a broad understanding of the general principles involved. He should regard the understanding of sex as being of the nature of an art rather than a science, the science being needed only that he may practise the better the fine art of living broadly, deeply, and well. Sex and life are inseparable; each is the origin and the end of the other. Happy is the man or woman, the boy or girl, in whom sex is a well-rounded part—*and nothing more*—of the whole purpose and philosophy of life.

Sexuality has been confused with sensuality. A mere incident in the program—an incident that corresponds to the carrying of the pollen by the bee—has been regarded as the whole program. It has been supposed that sex is selfish and seeks only its own self-gratification when actually nothing is so unselfish as the love of a mate for a mate or a parent for a child. It has been said that sex has ruined many a man or woman, but it has been forgotten that it has brought out the best that was in countless millions of others. It has made men and women of foolish boys and giddy girls. Sex can inspire an ordinary swain to poetry; it can make heroes of us all when our children or loved ones are in danger.

Our young people are demanding a positive education. They will not take "don't" as a rule for conduct. If "mother knows best," they think that mother should be able to give a reason for thinking that she knows best. Negative education tends to produce a pedagogic vacuum which will speedily be filled with something, be it good, bad or indifferent. When the minds of children—and adults—are loaded high with positive facts and principles based on the assumption that sex is natural, good, beautiful, and entirely proper, there will be nothing to be feared from the untruths and half truths which may be so disastrous. Once the mind is filled with pertinent facts it is satisfied and goes about its legitimate business untempted by morbid or lascivious curiosity. We much prefer to have our children turning toward the beauties of virtue rather than fleeing from, or likely toward, the ugly—sometimes not so very ugly—mien of sin.

Particularly is it important that the child should never be frightened when this subject is discussed. The method of imparting sex education whereby the mother calls the child to her side and tells him or her that she went down to death's door in order that the child might be born is most vicious. Children cannot understand the fact that suffering and sacrifice may make a thing precious. The normal child may be told that the benefits of a dental operation are immeasurable, but, just the same, the fact that "it will hurt" outweighs.

to him, every conceivable gain. The mother who associates sex with pain is often laying the foundation for an unsatisfactory or even destructive attitude toward life. Likewise, the parent who makes the subject ugly or disgusting or vulgar is injuring the child instead of helping him. Some suppose that it is necessary to do this in order to guard the virtue of the unmarried young person. Virtue is far better guarded by those who have a thorough understanding and appreciation of its worth.

Sex is a red-blooded thing; it throbs with high passion; it lives, and loves, and fights; it is a giant who constructs or destroys, makes or breaks, according as it is understood or not. Pink pamphlets for pale people will hardly serve the needs of the robust men and women who make the world go around. As well say "naughty, naughty" to a hurricane as to prescribe certain anemic books as a means of helping young people to control the powerful forces which surge within them. Most publications of this sort have been written by persons who have never known *la grande passion* or who, having seared themselves in its flame, are now devoutly wishing "to save the young people from what I have gone through." The services of such are not needed in the present purpose. This is a task for men and women who have felt the divine urge to create, have gladly accepted the challenge, and have not betrayed the trust.

We shall make no attempt to anticipate the questions which some bright-eyed child may ask, but are merely hoping that we may be of aid in preparing the parent so thoroughly in the basic principles of the subject that he or she may be able to feed and to satisfy the perfectly natural childish curiosity which brings a child to his parent with vital questions. Possibly the vocabulary which we use may be of value, inasmuch as the lack of the proper word to use is often a serious difficulty. The method of approach may be of value to some who know well enough the subject matter but not the pedagogic methods for putting it across. The parent need not expect to learn or build up a philosophy of sex and life in a moment. He will need to study long and seriously before he will be skillful in the handling of so delicate a matter. Unless the parent has had a reasonably satisfactory understanding of, and attitude toward, the subject, he need hardly expect to become expert in teaching his children concerning it. This is particularly a subject to be taught by example as well as precept. The man who treats his wife as if she were an inferior creature will have difficulty in instructing his boys, and the nagging wife will fail utterly in leading her offspring to a beautiful conception of sex life.

REPRODUCTION IN THE PLANT AND ANIMAL KINGDOMS

Those who would understand the marvelous process by which plants and animals may produce other plants and animals of the same sort, and, in particular, would like to understand the matter of sex as it is manifested in the reproduction of the human race, can do no better than to study the phenomenon as it is manifested in simpler forms of life. The process as it is observed in man is so complicated as a result of various social, moral, and ethical relations that it is necessary first to study the subject in some easier form. As a matter of fact, every phase of the process may be scrutinized in this way without arousing the various prejudices and suspicions which have so clouded the issue. Many parents are anxious to initiate their children into the mysteries of the subject, but are deterred by the lack of suitable means of expression.

A fairly complete understanding of the phenomenon in lower forms of life will give the parent or teacher poise and resourcefulness which will be greatly needed in teaching the subject and in developing a satisfactory philosophy of life. Not infrequently the parent or teacher needs more than anything else concrete illustrations for the explanation of the various difficult points, and usually a vocabulary is sadly lacking. We insist that he or she who teaches must himself or herself have reached some degree of mental poise and decision on these matters. There is no better way to do this than to become acquainted with the elementary biology of sex as it is manifest everywhere about us.

Obviously each species must have some adequate way of reproducing itself, otherwise it would long since have perished from the earth. The continuation of the species is the most fundamental instinct of every plant and every animal species. Most plants begin to die as soon as the seeds are well along toward maturity, and all animals except man are ready to die as soon as the end of the reproductive cycle has been reached. It is sometimes supposed that the self-preservative instinct is strongest in man and beast, but everyone must have seen men and women risking life, reputation, health, social standing, wealth—everything—in order that they might express themselves sexually or take care of their offspring, and so we must conclude that the instinct for reproduction is really basic.

Two general methods by which the species may be reproduced are observed in nature: the sexual and the asexual. Animals, except in the very lowest forms, use the sexual method. The same is true of most plants, but there are a considerable number of them which have dispensed with sex as a means of procreation. The bacteria, for example, merely divide in the middle, making two new individuals which are exactly alike and like the parent cell. In a sense the different individuals in a bacterial culture are really different fragments of the same original germ. Even high in the plant kingdom we see essentially the same thing. A twig from a willow tree becomes itself a willow tree. It is like the parent tree for the good reason that it is a part of the parent tree. A number of cultivated species of plants are propagated by tubers, roots, bulbs, cuttings, and grafts, which are all asexual means, though these plants have sexual organs as well. Seed potatoes represent a use of the asexual method, while potato seeds (occasionally found in small pods where the flowers have been) are of sexual origin. Several of the very low forms of animal life can reproduce themselves merely by dividing or being divided. We need not discuss this phase of the subject, however, for the good reason that we are wishing as quickly as possible to make the application to the human race.

Even though some forms of life may use the asexual method of reproduction, it is now believed that all of them have some sort of sex, rudimentary though it may be. Bacteria, until recently, have been considered as being exceptions to this general rule, but now a great many authorities believe that even they manifest an extremely primitive activity which is to be regarded as being truly sexual. Inasmuch as Nature has used this particular plan in the life of every one of her products, the conclusion is inevitably forced upon us that there must be some most excellent reason for the phenomenon. Let us suppose that every individual of a given species were free to reproduce himself by asexual means for an unlimited number of generations. It is easy to see that a given strain might come rather soon to be quite different from the original species. In this way there would arise an enormous number of varieties, and a condition approaching chaos would result. This is, indeed, exemplified by the fact that those plants which are reproduced by bulbs, cuttings, and tubers commonly have a great number of varieties: roses, dahlias, gladioli, etc. Nature seems, however, to hold the majority of species more constant, and so each time the act of reproduction is repeated it is necessary that a given individual fuse his heredity with that of another individual of the same species. In this way each separate drop of living matter is merged with the great ocean of related living matter, and wide deviations from the type species are rendered much less likely to occur.

However that may be from a theoretical standpoint, it certainly is a practical fact that sex is fundamental to the continuation of all higher forms of life. It is the warp of life into which an infinite variety of patterns may be woven by manipulation of other factors which may be called the woof. Sexual reproduction is the masterpiece of Nature. Into this process she has poured her sweetest perfumes: the flower, for example, is the sex organ of the plant. About it she has drawn her most beautiful patterns. Into it she has dumped her paint pots, as witness the colors of the mating bird, the butterfly, and the flower. Music and poetry are called upon to adorn it. Sex is motivated by the most precious of all passions, conjugal and parental love. Young girls are as enticing as possible; young men are handsome and valiant. The young of most species are charming—or, if not that, are at least interesting. Everyone loves the puppy, the colt, the kitten, or, most of all, the baby. Who can be so blind as to fail to see in this thing the very essence of life itself?

If we look into even the simpler and most familiar forms of sex, we may discern opportunities for the teaching of human problems to children. There is the flowering plant; for example, the bean. Every child is familiar with the seed of the bean, and if not accustomed to seeing the growing plant, it is quite a simple matter to plant a few beans and see them grow. (Beans bought for food purposes have often been heated so that the germ of life has been killed; therefore beans intended for planting should be used for this purpose.) A flower pot in the window will serve if there is no room for a garden. The child will be much interested in planting the seed and in seeing it grow. Finally the buds and then the flowers will appear. They are the most beautiful part of the plant. Insects will visit the flowers and will go from one to another sipping the nectar and transferring the pollen as it sticks to their legs. Even a crude dissection of the flower will reveal two sets of organs in the heart of the blossom. The one set, the stamens, carry at their tips a yellow powder (pollen) which is the male element; while the other, the pistil, is the female portion of the plant and has a sticky spot on the end to which the pollen will adhere if it should touch.

The insect, in visiting one flower after another, carries the pollen of one plant to the pistil of another. The pollen grains sprout and grow down the entire length of the pistil and carry the tiny cells which unite with the egg cells to form the seeds which are essentially new individuals. The growth of the seeds in the pod—the body of the mother plant—may be easily followed. Essentially the process is the same as is observed in the higher animals, except that the two points that are hardest to get across to children are much more simply explained. Most important is the fact that the part of the process which corresponds to the mating of the sexes is the apparently trivial visit of the bee who carries the male element to the female organ of the next flower. In teaching children it is usually this point that puzzles most parents. Possibly the use of the bean plant as an example may make it easier to explain this part of the process. Emphasis must, of course, be put upon the significance of the whole program and not upon this particular episode. The purpose of the process is the reproduction of the species and not to make an opportunity for bees.

Other plants may be used in somewhat the same way. For example, the flowers of the members of the melon family—muskmelons, pumpkins, cucumbers—are not all alike. Some of them have only the female organs, while others have only the male. In this respect they are more like the higher animals with which we are particularly concerned. In the case of strawberries and certain fruit trees there are some barren plants which are male. These plants never have fruit, but if they are all pulled out the other plants will be worthless as well.

The nesting habits of fish furnish an excellent example for teaching purposes. The females lay their unfertilized eggs over a clean spot on the bottom of the lake or stream. The male then comes to the nest and pours over the eggs a secretion known as "milt," which consists of millions of the sperm cells. When one of these sperm cells unites with an egg cell a new individual life begins. Obviously the method is exceedingly wasteful, but it is the best that fish can do. The young are compelled to get along as best they can after they are hatched, and, as a matter of fact, great numbers of them perish. In consequence, it is necessary that thousands or even millions of eggs be laid. By paddling slowly in a boat about the edge of a lake during the spawning season, the nests of sunfish may easily be found as clean round spots on the gravelly or sandy bottom, over which the parent usually hovers. The parent fish keeps the area clean and will chase away enemies who may come to destroy.

The mother frog does somewhat better. Her eggs are put out in a gelatinous material that protects them considerably. Then, too, they are black above and light below, making them harder to see. The dark color absorbs the heat of the sun and hastens the hatching process. The male fertilizes the eggs at about the time they leave the female's body. When the young tadpoles are finally hatched they are usually compelled to get along as best they may in a cruel world and many of them serve as juicy tidbits for birds, fish, and other animals.

The turtle illustrates a marked step in advance. The eggs are fertilized before they are laid and are held in the body of the female until a considerable quantity of food has been stored up in them and a firm shell is built about the food and the living portion of the egg. The eggs are then laid in and covered with the sand near the water's edge. There the heat of the sun stimulates growth. They will not be hatched until they are in a rather advanced state of development as compared with the young of the fish and the frog. Far fewer eggs are laid, for the good reason that the few that are laid are better equipped. Even so, there is no care on the part of the parents, and the young have strenuous times finding food and escaping the myriad dangers which beset their paths.

Birds do still better by their young. The parent birds mate and build a home—a most interesting home, indeed, as may be found by the simple expedient of sitting quietly and watching. The egg is retained in the mother's body until it is large and loaded with food for the young bird. It is then laid in the carefully prepared and concealed nest, where it is faithfully guarded for days by the mother, who hatches it with the heat of her own body. In the meantime, the father bird has protected the nest by driving away enemies, or has attracted attention and danger away from the nest and to himself by flashing his bright colors and brilliant song from a tree safely remote from the nest. When the young are hatched, the parents bring food, the mother keeps the nest clean and picks lice and other vermin off the young. She hovers over them when they are cold or when it is storming; she powders them with dust from the road, thereby discouraging insect pests; she never rests in her untiring efforts to feed and protect them; she teaches them to fly and to find food for themselves.

A most interesting subject for children to study is the nesting habits of the birds. City children need not often be at a disadvantage in this respect, for robins nest everywhere, and canaries can be had for a small sum. The larger cities may have fewer natural facilities, but such cities have zoölogical gardens and museums where there are unusual opportunities for such study. Parents who are awake to the possibilities can always find opportunity for such instruction in nature —and sex.

Higher in the scale the mammal takes even better and longer care of the young. The egg is developed as in the case of the other animals mentioned, but is never entrusted to the dangers of the outside environment—being far too precious—and so the young develop in the body of the mother. When the time comes that they must be delivered, Nature has provided for them a food which is taken from the mother's body and is the perfect food for the growing baby animal. The protective instincts of the mother are easily observed. Here is an example of parental love which is easily recognized even by a young child. Unfortunately, the function of the father is often much less inspiring, inasmuch as the male of the most easily studied mammals is generally apparently little interested in his offspring. There are, to be sure, instances in which the mammals have something somewhat like a human family, but most of these are in animals not easily observed by the child.

It is for this reason, in our opinion, a mistake to say too much about the male parent when referring to mammals. The example of the birds is better and more easily observed. By this we do not mean that the act of fertilization is any the less proper, but as we are teaching human children it is better to use examples which are more nearly like human customs. It is not that we would attempt to conceal the facts, but only that we would not call attention to them. There are authorities on sex education who advise that children be deliberately shown every phase of reproduction, as may be easily shown in dogs, for example. Personally, we are inclined to think that it must be rather hard to make the demonstration edifying. We believe that this is a phase of mammalian life that had best be left to accidental observation. If the child, after having been properly instructed in such matters as indicated above, asks questions about the more obvious facts of mammalian life, the whole matter should be discussed with him, and the social need for discretion in the mentioning of such matters should be explained.

Even a child must have observed that the human being is an animal, and as such has many of the ways of an animal. Even a child must learn early that the human being is much more than a mere animal, however, and should conduct himself or herself accordingly. Human children are precious. They must be given tender care over a long period of time. In this way the child can be made to see the reason for the family as we have it. In this way he comes to appreciate the rôle of the father and the mother, who have built about him a home that is stable, safe, and the very core of his existence. The functions of the father and the mother in that home seem widely different, but each is equally important and each has for its purpose the preservation of the child himself. The child sees his father working, bringing home food, paying for coal, furnishing a house in which to live, protecting him from injury, giving elemental care, playing and romping with him, planning with him, helping him, and advising him in ways that help tremendously. Every boy and girl should believe that his or her father is of the nature of a god, and so in this way the human father lifts himself above the level of the father of a puppy. The child sees—or should see—the father and mother exchanging embraces and words of affection. He realizes that sacrifices are being made, and so he comes to the way of thinking that anything that his father does must be quite all right—and as a matter of fact the father's position in the family will be much easier taught when everything that the father does *is* quite all right.

We are here giving much attention to the father for the reason that his rôle is commonly considered to be the hard part to explain. It is hard to explain, probably, for the reason that the male of most of the lower species have so little to do that is exemplary in terms of human conduct. Unfortunately, for one reason or another, a considerable number of human fathers also do little that is exemplary by the same standards, and so their purpose is rather hard to explain to the innocent child.

The function of the mother is much more obvious and needs no particular elaboration here. One point is important: The actual deliverance of the child from the body of the mother is usually a considerable ordeal and may easily become a family catastrophe. It is hard to make the child understand why such a process is necessary if he knows all of the sordid details. For that matter, it is hard to make adults understand why the bearing of children should be so difficult.

Why must childbirth in the human be so much more difficult and dangerous than in the lower animals? The reason is to be found in several relations which are not very obscure. In the first place, there is the matter of the erect posture, which has done so much to change the configuration of the pelvis in many women, and particularly in those who may have suffered as children from the disease known as rickets. This disease allows the abnormally soft bones to be excessively distorted by the weight of the body, and, in consequence, the birth canal is too narrow. Erect posture is, however, a fundamental advantage to the human race and is not to be lamented. Secondly, the nervous development of the human mother makes her much more susceptible to pain than are the lower animals. Human beings are not clods, and so they feel more keenly. Frankly, we would not have it otherwise. In the third place, the human child is so precious that Nature strives to hold it as long as possible in the place where it is safest. The newly born human infant is exceedingly helpless even then, and would be dangerously so if it were born any sooner. For this reason the mother must carry the child a relatively longer time. Finally, the development of the head which is made necessary by the large size of the brain enormously complicates the act of delivery. But that marvelous brain is the one really great characteristic of man, and we must not find fault with that which makes us great among the creatures of Nature. Thousands of those brains are now actively engaged in devising means of making childbirth easier and safer, and are succeeding, too.

We are presenting these facts for the enlightenment and instruction of adults, but *for the sake of the child*. In our opinion it would be a great mistake for a mother to call a child to her side and initiate instruction in these matters by telling him how "mother went down to death's door and suffered horribly in order that her baby might be born." The child knows nothing, and can understand very little, of sacrifice and suffering. He does not know that things that are precious are also expensive. He is often shocked and frightened. Pain is always bad to the child and to be avoided. Entirely too much has been said about the sacrifices of motherhood, and far too little about the privileges. No parent worthy of the name begrudges a reasonable personal sacrifice which he or she has been compelled to make for the sake of a bright and healthy child. Then why talk about it? Particularly is it bad to throw the matter in the face of the child itself.

We are in great need of an understanding of sex as a normal physiological function of the greatest consequence to the perpetuation of life on the earth. When assigned to its proper place in the scheme of things, and when interpreted properly, the understanding of this subject adds enormously to the meaning of life. Unfortunate, indeed, is the child—or adult—who is led to believe that sex is a *risqué* or low experience that lies out on the edge of things—a subject to be hushed and covered at every turn. Fortunate is the child whose parent so understands the subject that he may lead the child by gradual steps to a realization of the importance of sex and who arouses in him a determination to protect and conserve this vital force which unites in him the glorious past and the still more glorious future. There is no better way to attain such a position of wisdom and understanding than by studying the manifestations in those species which represent the steps by which we have attained our present position of eminence in the world of living things.

The Anatomy and Physiology of the Reproductive System

Before one may expect to teach the subject of reproduction to his or her children, he or she should be thoroughly grounded in the elemental principles of anatomy and physiology by virtue of which the miracle of life begins. It is not at all necessary that the layman should know all of the great Latin names for every little part or that he should hope to understand the chemistry and physics of the whole process, but he does need to know something of the amazing things that take place in the months preceding the birth of a child, and he needs to understand the system well enough to be able to give it the care that hygiene demands. Very badly indeed he needs a vocabulary by means of which he may discuss these matters without the faintest taint of vulgarity or obscenity.

The generative system in either of the two sexes consists of two portions: 1. The sex glands themselves (ovaries in the female, testicles in the male). 2. A system of tubes which carry the sex cells, and later, in the female, protect and nourish the developing child. Strange as it will seem to the layman, the organs of the two sexes are really much alike, each organ having its exact but poorly developed homologue in the opposite sex.

The sex glands of the male, the testicles, consist of a great number of microscopic tubules which are lined with cells which are constantly undergoing cell division after the individual has attained sexual maturity. These cells become the spermatozoa or sperm cells, which are tiny little living bodies with long slender tails which whip about and in this way propel the sperm in its search for the egg cell. These sperm cells carry the entire inheritance which a given child will or can get from his father. The spermatozoa may live for several days in the tubes of the male, or may even live for some time after they have gained access to the female organs. They begin to be produced when the boy reaches puberty (about fourteen years of age), and continue to be formed until senility has been reached. During the period of sexual maturity they are commonly produced at the rate of millions per day.

In addition to the above function of the testicles, there is another that is nearly or quite as important as the production of the sex cells. Between the tubules which produce the spermatozoa there lie certain cells which are called the interstitial cells. They secrete a substance which is absorbed by the blood and is responsible for the development of the secondary sex characteristics of the male. Everyone is familiar with the fact that the body of the man differs from that of the woman in other respects than the appearance of the sex organs themselves. The beard of the male, the deeper voice, the heavier bones, the narrowness of the pelvis, the texture of the skin, the scantiness of the subcutaneous fat, the lack of development of the breasts are all the results of this secretion. Unfortunate, indeed, is the man who does not have enough of this secretion to cause such a differentiation of his body that he may be immediately recognized as being definitely masculine in appearance. It is because of the loss of this substance that the castrated male (known as a eunuch) loses the characteristics of a manly man. Such individuals are commonly held in contempt by normal members of both sexes.

The ovaries of the female serve a purpose in the female exactly comparable to that of the testicles in the male, though there are, of course, differences in the details. The egg cells are already pretty well formed in the ovary at the time of birth, or shortly afterwards. They need to be matured, and stocked with a small supply of food, and then are ready to be extruded from the ovary. At the age of puberty (age twelve to thirteen years) the girl begins to produce mature egg cells at the rate of one (occasionally more) per menstrual month (twenty-eight days). This is continued until the menopause (change of life) is reached. This means that, on the average, less than five hundred egg cells are actually released in a lifetime.

As in the testicle, the ovary contains interstitial cells which produce a secretion that is responsible for the secondary sex characteristics of the female. The soft skin, the abundant subcutaneous fat, the development of the breasts, the higher pitched voice, the wider pelvis, and a great many other typically feminine attributes are too familiar to need enumeration. Women, because of loss or atrophy of the ovaries, or because of some other glandular disturbance, occasionally lose much of their femininity and may develop a beard or coarse, man-like features. Such a misfortune is distressing, indeed, to the individual herself, and greatly disfigures her in the eyes of others.

The testicles and the ovaries are the essential organs of reproduction. Indeed, as we have seen, many of the simpler animals and plants have hardly any other organs of reproduction than just these. Even in somewhat higher animals, as the fish and the frogs, the eggs are simply turned out into the water, and the spermatic fluid is spread over them there. The accessory organs of reproduction in such case are exceedingly simple, and sex, as we commonly think of it, can hardly be recognized. The episode which is considered by the thoughtless person to be the whole of the process becomes a trivial part of the program—merely the spreading of the milt of the male over the eggs laid in the water by the female.

As the higher forms of life are studied, it is noted that more and more care is given the fertilized egg. The reptiles and the birds lay large eggs containing abundance of food so that the young may attain considerable size and development before they need to begin to fend for themselves. The mammals give their young even better care, and for weeks and months the female carries the young in her own body, and then, after releasing them, suckles them for another rather long period. Obviously such an arrangement has necessitated an enormous increase in the complexity of the system. The entire body of the female is modified to take care of the fertilized egg and to nourish the young. The body of the male is likewise modified so that it may be able to impregnate the female and protect her and the young during the critical months before and after the birth of the young. Sex as we commonly think of it is highly developed in these animals.

The human species is characterized by the fact that the infant has an unusually long period of gestation, infancy, and dependency. It is this long period of comparative helplessness that allows the child to develop countless possibilities which would have been quite out of the question had he been compelled to look after himself from the first. Likewise it is this which has made necessary the tremendous changes in body structure of the two sexes, and the even more complicated development of the human family life, upon which the happy and efficient functioning of so much in the life of the child depends. There is here a most vital point which is often overlooked by superficial students of sex and its problems. They seem to think that the work of the reproductive organs is finished as soon as the child is born or weaned. Actually this is by no means the case. The child needs a highly stable and secure home until he or she is at least grown.

Anything that tends to hold the father and mother together in a tight and rugged union until after the child is born and reared is of tremendous advantage to the individual and the race. This is, then, also a function of the reproductive organs. Fortunate indeed is the child whose parents have learned such functions of the reproductive system that they may derive exquisite pleasure and enjoyment therefrom. That child is safe because he will have behind him a father and mother who love each other and are devoted to him. Such a child will usually go much farther than the one from a broken or loveless home.

The accessory sex organs of the male consist of a long tortuous tube from each of the testicles to the corresponding seminal vesicles or reservoirs, where the spermatic fluid and the sperm cells are stored until such time as there may be opportunity for extrusion (ejaculation); the prostate gland, which secretes a mucus-like fluid which carries the seminal secretion and makes a medium which will permit the spermatozoa to live and reach their objective; and the penis, which is an erectile tube capable of depositing the mixture of spermatic and prostatic secretion into the vault of the vagina near the mouth of the womb.

The accessory organs of the female are necessarily much more complicated for the reason that they must not only protect the egg cells but must provide a home for the developing child for nine long and eventful months. Essentially they consist of two tubes (Fallopian tubes or oviducts) which are open at the upper end and receive the egg cells when they are extruded from the ovaries. These tubes open into the womb, which is a muscular, hollow organ capable of enormous expansion. The womb in turn empties into the vagina, which is for the purpose of receiving the seminal secretion, and later of serving as a passageway for the child at the time of birth. The external female organs are called collectively the vulva. The breasts nourish the newly born child until it is old enough to eat other food.

The egg cell, after being released by the ovary, passes into the Fallopian tube, where it may or may not be fertilized by coming into contact with sperm cells. In case it does not make such a contact it lies there for a few days and then passes down into the womb and finally to the exterior. If it is fertilized it begins at once to divide rapidly and grows apace, utilizing the food that is stored in the egg cell and probably also some food absorbed from the surrounding tissues. It now migrates down into the womb and attaches itself to the inner wall of the womb (uterus) as would a parasite. After a time a placenta is formed. This organ is the point of contact between the mother and the child. The bloods of the two individuals remain separate, both the mother and the child having a set of closed vessels in the placenta, but fluids and gases can freely pass from the one to the other through the vessel walls by the process of osmosis. The mother furnishes food, water, oxygen, and other requirements; the child gives off waste materials of various sorts to the mother. No nerves pass from the one to the other. Various membranes for the protection of the child are also produced. These membranes and the placenta are delivered after the child is born and are collectively known as the "afterbirth." At the time of birth the walls of the womb contract strongly and expel the child and the "afterbirth."

The life of a new individual begins when the living egg cell of the mother is fertilized by the living sperm cell of the father. Really, then, the human child is approximately nine months old when it is born, and more has happened in the development of the individual during that nine months than will take place in the next nine years. There are many who suppose that life begins in the child at about the time that the mother may feel the movements of the child in the womb. Indeed, it is customary to refer to these movements as the "beginning of life." This phenomenon is usually observed at about the middle of the pregnancy. Actually, however, the child is alive from the time of the union of the egg and the sperm.

As soon as it is known that a baby is expected, parents are usually greatly interested in the speculation as to whether it is a boy or a girl. There is good reason to believe that the sex of the child is unalterably determined at the time of fertilization. To date there is no reliable means of controlling the sex of the offspring, and there is no accurate way of knowing until the child is born whether it is male or female. According to the most widely accepted theory of sex determination, each cell in the body of the female contains two determiners for sex (chromosomes), while each cell in the body of the male has but one such determiner. When the egg cells are produced, each cell contains one of these determiners; when the sperm cells are made, half of them have one sex determiner and the other half have none. If, then, the sperm with one sex chromosome meets an egg cell which always contains one, the fertilized egg cell will have two and is therefore female. If the sperm cell has no sex chromosome, then the fertilized egg cell will have but one—the one from the egg cell— and the sex is then male. If this theory is correct, and there is little doubt about its being correct, it would seem that the control of the sex of the unborn child by any practical means is probably quite outside the range of possibility. Many attempts to control sex have been tried, but none have as yet succeeded.

Even though the sex of the child is determined from the very first, it will be weeks before the differentiation of the organs is such that the sex might be recognized, even if the child could be examined closely. By such careful examination it is possible during the third month of fetal life to determine whether or not the child would have been male or female if it had lived. Previous to this time, the sex organs appear exactly alike, and, even in adult life, it is possible to find in each sex the exact homologue of the organs of the opposite sex. In the early months of fetal life the one or the other set of characteristics begins to be accentuated, and the opposing organs begin to atrophy.

In case a developmental error is made on the part of Nature it may be rather difficult to say without careful examination—and examination which sometimes requires an abdominal operation—whether the full-grown individual is male or female. These unfortunate persons are called hermaphrodites and are looked upon with considerable disdain and pity by their normal neighbors. Usually they are decidedly more like the one sex or the other, though, as mentioned above, there are some who present considerable difficulty in diagnosis. These individuals are practically always sterile, either as males or females, and never are they actually able to function as both father and mother at the same or different times.

Obviously the matter of reproduction is of the utmost consequence both to society and to the individuals concerned, and for that reason it is extremely important that every person of mature age should understand something of the complex phenomena which take place during the months of pregnancy, the hours of actual confinement, the days of the lying-in period, and the months of lactation. It is, furthermore, most essential that this information shall be highly authoritative. If these relations were well understood, a vast amount of suffering, distress, and danger to the mother and child might be avoided. The matter has been well covered in another part of this book. The race must go on, and there is positively no other way by which it may do so.

There are three proper functions of the reproductive system in the human species: 1. The production of and the bringing together of the sex cells. 2. The production and the protection of the child, whether it be before, during, or after birth. 3. A means whereby a man and wife may express affection for each other, and on that solid foundation build a home which is, in turn, the foundation of society. All of these functions are absolutely legitimate, proper, and respectable when exercised according to the laws, customs, and ethics of the time and domain.

THE TEACHING OF SEX TO THE YOUNG CHILD

We need hardly point out that the process which brings an innocent child into the world and reproduces the species is inherently clean. The parent who attempts to instruct a child in the marvels of sex must thoroughly convert himself to a firm belief in this fact, self-evident though it may seem. The process is right, and the child is pure. If, then, there is anything wrong about it, the difficulty must lie in the parent or his understanding of the situation.

It is most unfortunate, for the sake of the child, that we cannot assume that persons about to become parents have become familiar with the fundamental facts concerning the process which has brought the child into existence. Even before marriage they should have talked over these matters and should have sought to learn through legitimate channels the facts about so important a matter. Surely there is no further excuse for hesitancy after marriage. During the months between conception and the birth there are many reasons why intelligent persons will wish to know something of what is going on. Between the time of birth and the asking of the first question there is a period of two to four years, during which time one might be expected to prepare himself or herself for the time when the child will want to know something of vital matters, and yet a large percentage of parents find themselves utterly unprepared for the inevitable time when the intelligent child begins to ask questions. Mothers are shocked when the first question is asked. They seem to think that the child is still a babe in arms. Fathers tell the distressed mothers to explain matters to the children, but usually have no suggestions as to what to tell or how to tell it.

Long before it is time to begin to teach the child by word of mouth about these matters, there are other responsibilities which must be met. Within the first few days of life the genital organs of the baby should be carefully examined for evidence of defects or abnormalities. In case such defects are found they should be corrected when possible, inasmuch as such peculiarities are often responsible for irritations or abnormal stimulations which may greatly complicate the sexual life of the child when he or she is older. The tissues of the infant are still highly plastic, and it frequently happens that corrections made early are unusually successful for this reason.

The boy baby should be carefully examined to see if he needs circumcision. If the foreskin can be completely and easily retracted most authorities think that circumcision should not be done, but when there is the least doubt about the matter decision should be made in favor of the operation, which is a trivial one when done within the first week or two of life. When the foreskin is tight or adherent there will accumulate under it secretions which will produce bad odors and cause pain and itching. Such a child is likely to get into the ugly habit of pulling at and handling the genitals and may develop habits which are harmful and unsightly. In case circumcision is not done, the mother or nurse should carefully retract the foreskin each day and see that the organ is thoroughly clean. Many "nervous," restless, and "fidgety" boys can be helped by circumcision, provided there is real reason to think that they need such care.

At an early age boys should also be examined to determine whether or not the testicles have descended into the scrotum. These essential organs of sex are developed in the abdominal cavity, but at the time of birth or rather soon thereafter they should have descended. If they can be felt in the scrotum or can be gently pressed down into the scrotum there is no need for apprehension. If, on the other hand, they cannot be found, attention should be given to the matter—without causing too much curiosity on the part of the child—and the advice of a physician obtained. If descent does not take place, an operation to transplant the testicle into the scrotum should be performed before the boy reaches puberty. Undescended testicles commonly atrophy, and if both are in this condition sterility may result.

The girl baby also should be carefully examined for abnormalities. In not a few instances she may be in need of an operation which is essentially the same as that of circumcision in the male. Other defects may be present. In the washing of the female infant, care must be taken. Sometimes the hymen may be ruptured by rough handling. While it is true that the presence of an intact hymen is by no means proof of virginity, or the absence of it proof of sexual experience, there is still a large percentage of people who believe that such is the case, and so care must be taken to prevent an accident which might later put the babe, grown to womanhood, in an embarrassing position. Washing of the parts should be done in such a way that the friction will not cause erotic stimulation and in this way lead the child to the habit of playing with herself.

It is well known that crying babies, male and female, will nearly invariably hush when the genital organs are manipulated. This is an old, old trick of careless nurses and ignorant mothers. Under no circumstances must it be practised, as it may lead promptly to the practise of masturbation. Masturbation is probably far less harmful than has been supposed. Still, it is certainly an ugly habit, and every reasonable means of preventing it from establishing itself should be taken. It is doubtful if mothers have often practised such means of quieting their babies, but others to whom the child may have been entrusted have been less conscientious. The routine care of a child should never be delegated to someone else when it is physically possible for the mother to see to it herself.

During the period when the child is too young to be given definite instruction, much can be done to lay the foundation for sound health and useful habits. The child who learns cleanliness and regularity of body function will be much more likely to respect the purposes of the reproductive system when grown than will a person who as a child was permitted to abuse or neglect the various bodily functions. The strictly normal individual is less likely to develop improper habits or perversions than the one who suffers from various biases or abnormalities. Childhood is the time for health training, and health is the sound base upon which rest normal reactions with regard to sex.

Much of the difficulty in teaching and training children in these matters concerning sex is due to the mistaken idea that children do not manifest interest in such subjects until they are several years old. Sex is far too fundamental a thing to lie dormant for so long a time. The excretory organs are inseparably related to it, and indeed, it has its effect upon the entire body. Regularity in sleep, in eating, and in going to the toilet; pleasant manners and polite speech; love of beauty, truth, and decency; play in the open air; development of a natural attitude toward other children; modesty and respect for one's self are every one of them developed in large measure—if they are developed at all—before the child is four years old. Every one of these traits is of the greatest value in the development of an admirable sex life. It is hard to see how the child that hears and sees vulgarity and lives as a waif can get a fair start in the understanding of so pure and chaste a subject.

Great care will be needed in teaching the child that the social conventions are necessary without instilling in him or her the idea that the sexual organs are ugly, unclean, or sinful. The nude baby is proudly exhibited to admiring relatives and friends, the nude child of four is to be seen by the family only, and the boy or girl of eight is expected to be careful about such matters even in the bosom of the family. A fine sense of modesty is of the utmost consequence in the social training of the child. On the other hand, there are times, as when medical examinations must be made, when what has been called modesty is really prudery. The development of poise in these fine qualities is of the utmost consequence. It can be taught only when the child has been led to regard the sexual apparatus with respect rather than shame. Dignity and modesty are closely allied here as elsewhere. The child is made to understand that there are some things that are sacred and for that reason not to be cast before swine; there are some things so fine that they must not be permitted to become common. The child is shown that grown-ups, men and women, cover themselves, and that if he or she would be like them he or she must do so as well. Reserve rather than shame, pride in something that is too important to be left lying around, is the motive to be emphasized.

Many of the difficulties attendant to the teaching of sex are immediately solved when the child is taught the proper, the dignified names for the parts of the body. It would be hard to understand how a child could use the vulgar names which are commonly heard without deterioration of dignity and respect. Hardly better are the baby names and the meaningless terms which are often given them in the vain attempt on the part of the mother to save the child from what she supposes to be vulgarity. The child must acquire a dignified vocabulary if he is to keep the subject clean. It is hard to see why it should be more embarrassing to the mother to have the child come to her saying that he wishes to go to the toilet than to have him use some of the other expressions which are equally evident in their meaning under the circumstances. A frank acknowledgment of these things and their meanings is the very basis of future understanding of them. Hypocrisy and prudery have had their day and have made a mess of it.

During this impressionable period of life the attitude of the father and mother toward each other will have a profound effect on the character and sexual behavior of the child in later life. The child who sees his father treat his mother with chivalry and respect is much more likely to treat girls and women in the same way. The little girl who sees in her own mother a beautiful character is unconsciously receiving an education in these matters which is infinitely more effective than all the carefully planned precepts which might be memorized from books or articles on sex education.

But while it is really the generalities which count in the training of the child it is the details which are more perplexing to the parent in charge. This is because the details have a way of demanding immediate attention. What shall the mother or the father tell the child when he asks the highly pertinent and searching questions which have perplexed parents for so long? There is but one thing to tell them. It is the *truth*. By this I do not mean that it is necessary to tell a child of four the entire truth, or that it is necessary to give him the detailed truth. As a matter of fact, that would be impossible for the good reason that not even the wisest man knows the entire or the detailed truth about these matters. When the child asks a question he does not expect the scientifically complete answer, but in later life he will greatly appreciate the fact that he was told the truth in so far as he was able to understand it at the time.

When the child notices the difference between his or her body and that of the opposite sex it is an easy matter to explain that there are two sorts of people, and two sorts of everything else that is alive. That is so that each little child and each little baby animal may have a father and a mother to care for him and make a home for him. It is pointed out that birds of certain kinds are different in color and appearance, and that there are differences in function which correspond to this difference in appearance. By all means arrange for him to see a bird's nest, if possible, and understand something of what goes on there. He will have observed that fathers and mothers have different purposes in life, and there are marked differences in dress, in habit, and occupation. The whole process is perfectly natural, and when naturally told to a normal child will give rise to no morbid curiosity whatsoever. It is merely an interesting fact about the most interesting thing in the world—life.

A momentous question is that concerning where the baby came from. It is a question that every child should have asked by the time he is four or five years old or even sooner. The most ridiculous substitutes for the beautiful truth have been given him—most of them extremely unconvincing. What a pity that mothers have seen fit to tell children that babies—they themselves, indeed—are found in garbage pails, in the straw pile back of the barn, under the leaves in the woods, in a hollow log, in the doctor's satchel, and in other monstrous places. Hardly better is the "made in Germany" story of the stork, except that it is somewhat more dignified. The children of Germany love and respect the stork, but the small children of this country know nothing of such a creature.

Children are invariably tremendously interested in babies and commonly are asking their parents if they may have a baby brother or sister. They see no evil in the possibility, as, indeed, there is none.

The question that is most dreaded is, "How did the baby get in the mother's body?" Here is something that is supposed to be hopelessly vulgar. Well, for those who think it is so we can understand that the problem is difficult. When, however, the father and the mother have loved each other as they should, the act that is the expression of that love and the act that enables them to bear beautiful children is not vulgar in any sense. The child—bear in mind that this is a young child—can be told that as a result of the love which the parents bear for each other and for the child the baby began to grow in the body of the mother. An older child will need more information, to be sure, but this is as essentially the truth as the most tediously accurate and scientific account of the union of egg cells and sperms.

The difficulty of explaining the rôle of the father will fade into nothing at all if the child believes that his father is a great hero who can do no wrong. When the child has seen his father caressing his mother nothing could be more natural—as indeed nothing is more natural—than that they should desire and have children. It is most unfortunate that so many fathers live and treat their families in such a way that the children may learn to know that their acts are selfish. In such case the teaching of sex will be difficult. In the main, however, small children believe that their fathers are great persons, indeed, and that whatever they do is just right, and in such case nothing could be easier than proper instruction in these matters. The rôle of the mother is easily taught. As it is perfectly natural for the child to develop in the mother's body, it is perfectly natural that the child should accept the method as the ancient and honored way of life, and that is all there is to it.

After the child is old enough to understand the simple anatomy of the two sexes, it may be explained that the sperm cells of the male are introduced into the body of the mother and there combine with the egg cells somewhat as the pollen of the male plant fertilizes the female. It should then be explained that such transfer of the male to the female must take place only between married persons, else a child may be born when the parents cannot make a home for it. It may easily be explained that the process is one that is perfectly proper when the man and woman are married and much in love with each other, and that it is an act of the utmost intimacy and delicacy.

When the child asks the *details* of birth—as he or she rarely will—care must be taken that he or she is not frightened by morbid details. No small child can understand the forces which come into play in such an event. It is a serious mistake to worry him with the harrowing details in such case, then. It is enough to know when the time comes that the mother worked hard and is very tired. She will need to rest in bed for several days and must be shown every possible deference and affection.

The most important principle in the training of a child in these matters is that the native curiosity of the child should be satisfied, and satisfied with something that can serve as a basis for subsequent teaching. The child must learn that it can depend *absolutely* upon the father and mother as a source of honest and authentic information on this subject, just as he can go to the same source for food, for shelter, and for help of any sort. The child should never be repressed when asking honestly concerning such matters. Once the demand for the truth is filled, the child can then go about his or her normal activities without being bothered with things he or she is too young thoroughly to understand. At this age interest may be keen for a moment, but when satisfied will soon turn to other things more closely related to the development of the child. There is not the least reason for the artificial stimulation of an interest in the subject, but there is good reason for quieting the natural interest by satisfying it. Questions put by the child should be answered when possible, but they need not be provoked. Generalities are sufficient for small children. Mention of pain, danger, or sacrifice should never be made, for the good reason that they cannot be understood.

In case questions which cannot be answered are asked, the parent must make it clear that the question is perfectly proper if it is honestly asked. If the subject is one that cannot be answered but can be looked up, it is the duty of the parent to tell the child that he will investigate the facts and inform him later. If it is one that cannot be answered, the point should be explained as well as may be and the incident used as an example of the greatness and intricacy of the whole marvelous process. Frequently the ingenuity of the parents will enable them to restate the question so that the child can be satisfied though the direct question was not really answered. Always the teaching and the example set should be on the highest possible plane that the child can understand and appreciate. Parents who understand the process and live the part will have no difficulty.

The imagination and resourcefulness of the parent will do better than any "canned" information. It is not necessary that every bit of the information be absolutely scientifically up-to-the-minute provided it is earnestly and truthfully set out as the best that the parent knows on the subject. The development of a philosophy of life and living is much more needed than are the latest scientific details.

Whatever is done or taught, the idealism of the child must be preserved. The rôle of the father as hero, provider, and protector; the part of the mother as one who will love and protect whatever may happen, cannot be too strongly emphasized. The child easily understands such teaching and responds eagerly to idealism of this sort. The love of the father and mother for each other and for the child is the means by which the child came into existence and is as essentially the truth as if every detail were explained in full.

The School Child

The school child is no longer under the eye of his parents. He will hear and learn of sex. The pertinent question is not "Will he learn?" but, rather, "Where and of whom will he learn?" It is a foolish parent who thinks that a boy or girl in school will remain ignorant of these matters, and it is, indeed, a trusting parent who is willing to turn the instruction of his son or daughter in these matters over to ignorant companions. The child of this age is getting started to school and is beginning to feel that he knows something of life. Quite naturally he wants to understand things as they are. Fortunately he has not yet reached the age of puberty with its many perplexing problems and disturbing urges which will furnish an additional motive for sex interest.

Except that it will be necessary to give these children more information than was given the pre-school child, the problems are not greatly different from those that have just been discussed, for the good reason that the sexual system is still relatively undeveloped, and the child has only a passing interest in such matters. The teaching is still indirect and should consist of principles rather than details. It is a matter of ideals and of idealism. Questions should be answered fully and frankly—in so far as the child is able to understand or is interested—but questions are not to be raised in the mind of the child.

This is the time when children are so tremendously interested in nature, and it is easy, indeed, for them to have observed most of the essential phenomena of sex before they have become involved in the complex social phenomena which so muddle the issue in the human race. The parent who understands the fundamentals of sex and life as they are manifested in plants and animals will have an enormous advantage in the teaching of his children.

An important matter during this period is the teaching of a sense of modesty without at the same time teaching shame. Parents all too often shame their children into a state of mind that is mistaken for modesty. Shame, except for some improper act, is an emotion that should never be utilized in teaching. There is nothing about the reproductive organs for which a child need be ashamed. He learns to cover himself because it is the custom to do so, and because the older persons whom he wishes to emulate do so. There is nothing wrong about the genitals, but rather they are so important that they must be protected. They are so intimately one's real self that one must not go about exposing in a cheap and common way that which is so essentially private. Nice manners prescribe that care must be taken in these matters, and the child soon learns to take this view.

Nearly all normal children have their little love affairs during the first years in school. Since it is so obviously true that one of the most important tasks in later life is the selection of a worthy mate, it is well that even children should be gaining a little proficiency in so vital a matter. Just as the kitten playing with a ball is really learning to catch mice, so these children are practising the greatest of all arts. It is a grave mistake for parents or others to tease children about their love affairs. Such teasing puts the idea into the head of the child that there is something inherently wrong about the whole matter and that he or she has done something that is improper. When, subsequently, a real affair is developing, it will be carefully concealed from the parents, and in this way the parent loses his opportunity to be of service in teaching the child how he or she may select the best companions. Furthermore, the curiosity of the child teaches him to seek the evil which he has been led to believe is in the apparently harmless relation which he or she has with another of the opposite sex. With such stimulation he will all too soon find the evil.

Parents who tease their young children about their beaux and seek to deter them from making dangerous alliances should look about them and learn that the best way to insure against these play love affairs going too far is merely to let them run without resistance. Children are far too fickle as a rule to do more than toy with a passion which they are much too young really to understand. Soon it will be forgotten. On the other hand, the parent who attempts to break up such an affair is assuming a grave responsibility. He will be almost sure to intensify it. There is no more certain way to drive a young— or older—couple into each other's arms than for some dumb parent to personify the well-known bull in a china shop and "set his foot down on the whole business." The reason for this is easily seen. We naturally tend to protect out friends when they are attacked, and we invariably learn to love those whom we protect. Not only are the children being set into mischief when they are teased, but the parents are accomplishing exactly the opposite result from that which they desire when they indulge in so low a form of correction—or amusement.

The parent who allows his or her children to assume natural relations with other children of the same or opposite sex need rarely fear that mischief will be done. The child, being still undeveloped sexually, gives no thought to the grosser manifestations of the subject unless they are suggested to him by his elders. When the relation is perfectly natural and the parent has abstained from teasing, the child will be free to talk about the matter, and so the parent may keep himself informed concerning the course of events. In case, then, the child gets on dangerous ground, a frank discussion of the matter is possible and will not be resented if skillfully handled. The parent may be able to point out in a kindly manner the good and bad traits in the favored friends, and in this way may be of real service in the important matter of picking the permanent mate a few years later. God knows the young people need all of the aid they can get in so difficult a project. It is rather evident, too, that many of them have no knowledge whatever about how to go about it—if one may judge by the results.

Boys and girls will frequently play "father and mother" games. Though it may seem far-fetched to some, they are actually gaining much experience which may be of great benefit to them in later life. It is not at all unusual to hear children of this age express themselves as to what they will do when they are men or women, as the case may be. For the most part they will do well if they later come up to these expressed ideals. It is also common to hear children say what they will do when they have children of their own, or what their children will or will not do. The wise parent at such a time may well listen and note. It is possible that he or she may learn something. Under no condition may the children be ridiculed or teased at such a time. Here is manhood and womanhood in the making, and it is mighty serious business.

So long as such games are strictly spontaneous they are splendid. They may become most sordid, however, when the elders attempt to help.

Much worry has been needlessly suffered by devoted parents who have failed to understand children of this age. Boys and girls are curious. They will naturally examine their bodies, or, if the opportunity presents itself, the body of another of the same or opposite sex. The misguided parent thinks that this is exactly the same as if an adult should do so and gets all excited about it. Frankly, we would be inclined to question the mentality of a child who has not done so. The best way to draw the teeth of such a possible menace is to allow the child to satisfy that fine sense of curiosity which impels him to try to find out how things are made, and, having found out, lets him go on to something else. Two little girls in a closet were caught discussing these matters, and the mother was needlessly alarmed. It was explained to them that such conduct is not considered to be good social form, and no more was said about it. They had satisfied their curiosity, and the episode was ended. It is likely that they rather soon forgot about it. If they had been severely punished, however, they would have had good reason to remember and to wish to continue the experience when the opportunity to do so without being caught presented itself.

Frequently children will get into the habit of playing with or pulling at the genitals. Such children—both boys and girls—may be in need of a thorough examination by a competent physician. It is not unlikely that circumcision is needed. If there is no pathologic basis for the habit, the child should be taught that it is bad manners to do so and that an ugly habit may be formed. With help, rather than scolding, he may soon break himself. Parents should remember that no one can break a habit except the person who has it, and that the task is one that sometimes requires patience and perseverance beyond that which a child may be expected to have. Little boys and girls are occasionally found to have developed the practice of masturbation. Normal children of this age will rarely go to excess unless they are being stimulated by some older person. If a child of this age masturbates frequently a careful watch should be made, not so much of the child as of its older associates. The reason for this is evident, as the child is not sufficiently developed for the habit to have arisen from within.

Children of this age should be interested in many things, and when they are so one need not worry about their being too much concerned about an instinct which is far from being mature. All sorts of healthy activities are to be encouraged. Exercise in the open air is far more conducive to good results than excessive poring over books. Regular habits in matters pertaining to health will lay the best possible foundation for a normal sex life in later years. The child should grow in "wisdom and stature" during this time. He or she should develop the body as it was intended to be developed. School interests, play, club work of all sorts, scout exercises, athletic teams, and kindred activities permit little time for those forms of sex activity that might really be dangerous.

Of vast importance during this period and before is the development of self-control. We cannot understand how a subsequent marriage is going to be successful if either partner is unable to control his or her temper or selfish inclinations. Parents are doing the consorts of their children a grave injustice when they permit children to grow up in such a way as to cause them always to consider their own welfare first. This may seem to some as if it were a subject that had nothing whatever to do with the subject of sex, but actually it has everything to do with it. The child that must have his own way, that must have everything that he wants, that has never been taught to give up, that doesn't know how to work, is going to make a mess of marriage.

The question as to how much direct sex instruction should be given during this period is a rather knotty one. Sex during this period is probably less to the fore than at any time since babyhood, provided the curiosity of the pre-school child has been properly satisfied as discussed in the preceding chapter. If the child knows in a general way about these matters, he will let it go at that until the problems of adolescence begin to assert themselves. Matters pertaining to sex in its simpler forms should be frankly discussed by the family in the presence of the child. Questions are answered, and basic principles underlying proper conduct are deeply implanted, and that is about all that is necessary.

The boy of this age is intensely idealistic. He has his heroes—men of action and high accomplishment. He dreams of hazardous stunts and impossible accomplishments. All too often he is attracted as a moth to the flame by the supposedly brave exploits of the gangster and the gunman. In many cases this is because his own good parents and relatives are so unromantic as to bore him to death. Fathers need more to appreciate the intense desire that their sons have to be able to brag about their dads. The father should attend to his most important business—that of being a "real guy" in the eyes of his children.

Girls are being encouraged to be teachers, stenographers, concert pianists, prima donnas, lawyers, doctors, nurses. As a matter of fact, most of them—fortunately—will become housewives and mothers. Why cannot these objectives be held up as ideals? Then, when they have a home of their own, they will find in the monotonous routine a purpose toward their ideal. In case, however, they have been taught that they are to have some glamorous career and then find themselves washing dishes for a family, they are nearly sure to despise their task. There are those who suppose that a career as a mother is a narrow experience as compared with that of typing letters for a concern that sells lumber or vacuum cleaners. Some suppose that a mother needs less education than a teacher who does nothing but teach a single subject in a high school. The mother must be a nurse, a physician, a teacher, a legal adviser, a cook, a dietitian, a financial genius, a diplomat, an authority on child psychology, and a hundred other things—at least, she should be. Why cannot this be made a career toward which girls can be pointed with pride?

Psychologists tell us that the child is half educated long before he even starts to school. His mother has taught him—or so often she hasn't—the mother tongue, his habits, his manners, his attitude toward life, his self-control, his reliability, his respect for truth and right, his religion, his patriotism—and yet the task of a mother is considered too lowly to serve as an ideal! A wife, who has the responsibility of five children, once lamented that she envied a woman of her age who had attained a degree of success in bacteriology. She should be reminded that the other woman grew bacteria in culture tubes, while she was growing men and women in a home. All of this is very important in sex education. Indeed, it is the very heart of the whole thing. The girl who has been brought up to regard her womanhood as a career, the boy who is thoroughly instilled in the principles and practice of manliness, will probably not make great mistakes in their sex lives.

The pre-adolescent age is a period which is immensely important in the orientation of the boy or girl. Orientation is possible at this time for the reason that the strong sex impulses have as yet not taken definite direction because of their relatively immature state of development. A little later they will be so strong that they may take the bit in the mouth and run away. Happy is the adolescent who has been set in such a direction that he or she can permit his or her sex to run away for the good reason that it is running in the direction of the greatest advantage. Those driving men and glorious women who make the world go round are the ones, in large measure, who got their correct bearings in the pre-adolescent period and were able to drive full speed ahead into the business of being someone and of doing important things.

The Period of Adolescence

While a great many sex problems have their origin before the age of puberty and adolescence, the problems which arise at these times are much more urgent and difficult than those of the earlier years. This is the period of anxiety for parents.

This is the time when young people really need help and understanding. It is a time when powerful and utterly new forces are arising in them. New impulses are driving them they know not where. Elated with the new sensation of being comparatively grown up, and intoxicated with the previously unknown freedom which is usually granted them, they go plunging from one extreme to another. While there is some doubt about the matter of their maturity they must do everything possible to prove that they are grown up, and so the boys learn to smoke and to swear great and supposedly manly oaths. They affect deep knowledge of women and girls and tell of their conquests with this and that and the other one. They rarely, if ever, drive a car under seventy miles an hour, if one is to believe everything that he hears. It is, of course, obvious to those who understand something of the psychology of the period that they are overcompensating for their all too evident inexperience—whistling to prove that they are unafraid.

The girl usually passes through a "boy-struck" period. She giggles and makes herself conspicuous. Unless carefully controlled or endowed with unusual reserve, she is likely to go in for excessively high heels, extremes in dress, and large use of cosmetics. During this period 'of unrest she is sadly in need of intelligent and sympathetic guidance. Such guidance, however, is likely to be extremely distasteful to her. It will be impossible for parents who have neglected the matter of sex education until this time to pick up the reins of control and go serenely forward. Only those children who have been gradually led up to a realization of the forces at work within themselves will be in a position to appreciate the advice that wise parents can give. How may a mother who has told her daughter that babies slid down rainbows now hope to get control of the situation? Long before the time of adolescence the children have learned that their parents *are* sources of accurate information on the subject, or that they *are not* sources of accurate information. They may be expected to behave accordingly.

In continuation of sex education into the period of adolescence the parent or teacher must know that generalities are no longer sufficient. It is not enough to tell them to behave themselves and be good children. A concrete and detailed instruction in vital matters in which they may be concerned now becomes a necessity. By this we do not mean that every episode in sex life must be carefully diagrammed, but rather that the problems which the boys and girls are likely to meet should be discussed with them in a perfectly natural manner. It will, indeed, be well if the instruction is so natural and so unassumed that the boy or girl is hardly conscious that he has been instructed. Young people of this age should be included in the family conversation about many matters related to the subject of sex.

Let us assume here that adolescent boys and girls have had their minds thoroughly satisfied concerning the positive and beautiful phases of the subject. They are then ready to have some of the negative phases mentioned. This part of the education must not be made so graphic that it shocks or alarms, but these young people should know about the possibilities of conception out of wedlock, and that under such circumstances the mother and child are sure to suffer severely from the social stigma which such a birth imposes. They should know something of venereal disease, which is perfectly capable of ruining them, their loved ones, and their careers. They should know of the depreciation of character which invariably follows the cheap promiscuity which seems so enticing under certain circumstances. These are not pleasant matters to explain, but children of this age should be treated somewhat as men and women, though they are still boys and girls. Life is coming to be real at this period; it is getting to be rather earnest. Young people will appreciate the confidence that is shown when such matters are frankly discussed, and they will really be grateful, though they may seem not to be so.

In case the young people have had no proper instruction in matters pertaining to sex during their earlier years; if they have no dignified vocabulary in terms of which these matters may be discussed; when they see in sex only the possibility of sensuous gratification, it will be difficult indeed—or well nigh impossible—to correct the omission. Still, one can do no less than try. In such case one must of necessity begin with many of the negative phases of the subject.

It is perfectly possible for boys and girls of the age under discussion to be parents of children. When such is the case, the careful parent can do no less than explain to his children something of the details of the sexual act. Only those who are willfully blind will pretend that it is possible or desirable to keep young people of this age ignorant of so vital a function. If there were any assurance that they might get such information in a relatively truthful form, there would be less need to insist upon parental instruction, but there is absolutely no such assurance. It is doubtful if there is so much misinformation on any other known subject. It is not so much that parents are ignorant, but rather that they "know so much that ain't so." They should be made to understand that sexual relations are of the utmost consequence to the welfare of the individual, the family, and the race, but that they are only for those who are sufficiently mature to bear and rear children, and are married so that they can do so. Unless this can be done in a way that convinces the young people themselves, it had as well not be done at all. Merely to admonish them in abstract terms is of little or no value.

Provided the biology teacher of the high school has an appreciation of the possibilities of his subject, we strongly suggest that at least one course in this subject be taken in high school. Young people are usually safe when they are on familiar ground. It is possible in a biology class to discuss fundamental matters of sex in the most casual manner and in this way to lay an impersonal foundation for a sound understanding of the subject. When home influences and parental instruction then supplement scientific instruction, little concern need be entertained concerning the welfare of youths and maids who have normal poise and self-control.

Of much importance to the youth of this age is an appreciation of the fundamental reasons for the existence of a stable family life. Without the carefully integrated family the human infant or child is placed at a serious disadvantage and may not be able to overcome the handicap. While it is perfectly possible for persons to live in a satisfactory manner without wedlock, it is evident that marriage is fundamentally necessary, and in spite of the fact that many marriages go on the rocks, it is rather certain that men and women are normally better satisfied and happier in that relation than out of it. Marriage should then be held before young people as a probable goal, and careful thought and planning may well be given to the matter. All too frequently boys and girls break out into a scarlet rash as soon as marriage is mentioned. Giggling and protesting, they disclaim any such intentions. As a matter of fact, this behavior is a discredit not so much to these boys and girls as to their parents, for it shows clearly they have not frankly discussed such subjects with their offspring.

The sanctity of marriage may well be taught and illustrated at any age of development, but it is important that it be increasingly emphasized as the child approaches the age when he or she may be expected to enter into such a contract. Unfortunately there are a great many people who cannot understand the reasons why marriage should be more than a mere civil contract. The reason why marriage is more than a civil contract is to be found in the fact that children will probably result from such a union. Conventional marriage is the foundation on which is built the home, and the home is the basis of every one of the other social institutions—the school, the church, the government, industry, and social relations. Without the home it is hard to see how we could get along in any sort of acceptable manner. A community of good homes invariably has good schools, influential churches, thrifty, industrious, intelligent, educated people, and an acceptable government. A community of bad homes is hopelessly in the mire. These are facts that can be made plain to young people, who will consciously or unconsciously adjust themselves accordingly. Happy marriages and healthy homes are not the products of accident, the writers of melodrama to the contrary. They are worked out by persons informed in matters pertaining to real human values.

We shall do well, before we criticize the young people of today, to consider the difficult position in which we place them. They develop sexually earlier than they should and would were it not for the omnipresent sex stimulation which they are constantly receiving. They see moving pictures of the most sophisticated sort; they pick up *risque* books or hear such books discussed; they see all sorts of irregularities. At an early age they have been more or less intimately introduced to the urges and passions, but are not permitted to marry until they are well into their twenties, as a rule.

In contrast to this situation is that of our parents, who were not let out into society until they were sixteen or seventeen, and were solidly married, frequently, at the age of eighteen or nineteen. In the early months of the period of courtship they were so awkward and green that they could hardly get into serious mischief, and by the time they were well out of that period marriage was usually consummated. If we are going to bring children up in such a way as to avoid the awkward and green stage, we are under obligation to help them take care of the passions which are aroused but may not be gratified. The awkwardness of the adolescent boy or girl is a protective device of no mean consequence. It is likely that those children who come through this adolescent period slowly and naturally will be better adjusted than those who are hurried through by socially ambitious parents.

It is for this reason that athletics are so important for boys and girls of this age. Many suppose that athletics are for the purpose of developing the physique. They are of much more consequence when they develop character. As a matter of fact, strenuous athletics at this time in life may, and frequently does, actually injure the body when not properly controlled. Play and recreation, rather than high-powered competitive sports, are needed. The boy who plays tennis, basketball, baseball, or engages in any of the many other wholesome sports, is not in much danger of giving too much thought to the girls. Very often, indeed, he has a fine scorn for the members of the so-called weaker sex because they cannot equal him in the manly sports. He plays until he is tired enough, when he goes to bed, to go promptly to sleep. He has something to think about; he has training rules to keep; he learns to give and take.

Girls will usually be somewhat less interested in athletics, though there are many exceptions. The reaction of girls toward athletics is essentially like that of boys, but there are certain differences which should not be entirely forgotten. There are, for example, the limitations imposed by the regular recurrence of the menstrual period. We do not wish to make invalids of girls, but insist that some consideration be given this matter. This point will be discussed later. The pelvis of the girl is broader and more loosely jointed than that of the boy. This is a relation which is necessary, as the pelvis must be built in such a way as to sacrifice strength for the contingencies of future childbirth. Heavy or excessive muscular exercise can for this reason more seriously injure the girl than the boy. Furthermore, there is an adjustment of the blood supply that is of much consequence. Nature insists that the demands of the reproductive system shall come first. For this reason the blood supply of the pregnant or nursing woman is commandeered for the reproductive organs and the breasts. If a girl is allowed to develop herself too highly in athletic lines she is able, in not a few instances, to train her muscles so that they will make such a drain upon the blood supply as will cheat somewhat the reproductive organs. It is well known that rather poorly developed women often have beautiful babies, while it is also well known that women of the muscular type are often sterile or have puny, poorly nourished (from the breast) babies. An analogy is seen in the fact that beef (muscular) cattle give poor milk and little of it, while the bony Jersey and Guernsey cows give large amounts of rich milk. We strongly believe in athletics for girls, but insist that they should be somewhat less strenuous and competitive. Girls do much better with the types of games that are mostly individual endeavor; boys need the highly coöperative games. This is in line with their probable needs in later life, when men, as a rule, work with others, while a housewife for the most part does her work alone.

Every child of adolescent age should have a hobby. Parents should make the way easy for the development of any special interest that the child may have. Collections of all sorts are made by interested young people: butterflies, beetles, plants, stamps, match-box covers, marbles, buttons, and a thousand and one other things. What a vast amount of mischief can be avoided by such means! The exercises prescribed by the Scout Manual have been of incalculable value in keeping boys and girls in pursuits which permit them to come along without too much attention to the developing forces within them. Of two boys of our acquaintance, one spent his spare time loafing on street corners, while the other was constantly looking for new plants for his herbarium, which already numbered several hundred specimens. It is not hard to guess which was developing best.

The parent who calls the child in from play in order to give him his weekly instruction in sex is entirely out of step. Sex is life. It is just plain wholesome living and doing. Therefore the teaching of this subject must be casual and matter of fact, except under certain conditions, when it must be highly idealistic and romantic. The wise parent will know when to look the other way and likewise when to set up the sanctuary. The best that the adolescent can do is to grow and develop. When the new-found powers begin to assert themselves, they must be met with frankness and understanding—a sacred trust—a hostage to the future.

The habit of masturbation is likely to be developed during this period. The practice is certainly in bad taste and something of which no one can possibly be proud. Otherwise it is of little consequence unless the boy or girl worries about it or is degraded by it. The best that can be done is to arouse interest in other things, so that it and the memory of it will be forgotten. If masturbation caused only a small part of the ailments of which it has been accused, the human race would be in a bad way, indeed. Forget it.

Boys are frequently alarmed by the occurrence of seminal emissions or discharges of prostatic and seminal secretions while asleep. Mothers finding the stained sheets are sometimes greatly alarmed. It means nothing except that the boy is developing properly and is not indulging in masturbation or sexual relations. It is sometimes said that sexual relations are necessary after a certain age is reached, else the organs of the male will atrophy from disuse. Nonsense! Nature is not so dumb as to permit such a misfortune to that system which she so highly cherishes. She has provided the reproductive organs with a safety valve in the form of these seminal emissions. They are perfectly normal, and are indeed an accurate indication of proper and safe development. In the same category are the voluptuous dreams which boys and occasionally girls may experience. Think nothing of them.

Before she is twelve years old the girl should have the phenomenon of menstruation explained to her. Otherwise she is likely to be frightened by it and may be ashamed to say anything about it if she is not accustomed to confide in her mother. Formerly it was the custom of careful mothers to put their daughters to bed for a day or two at each menstrual period and to interdict all activity and bathing during this time. The girl was taught that she was "sick" and that she might expect for the next thirty years to be an invalid once a month and then to pass through a "change of life" that would probably kill her. In all too many instances the girl and woman lived up to the program expected of her. She was taught to be an invalid. Recently we have seen the absurdity of such a method, and now it is customary to go nearly as badly to the opposite extreme. The girl is told to pay no attention to it except to protect her clothing from soilage and to go ahead and do *anything* that she might otherwise do. Some girls can get by with this program just as some got by with the other.

A much more sensible approach is that which takes into consideration the altered condition of the parts but does not emphasize the condition as being morbid. Menstruation is a normal process, but in many respects approaches the pathological. Bleeding, for example, is otherwise always associated with pathology of some grade, as also is pain. The uterus of the menstruating woman is congested, and there are marked changes in the distribution of the blood; the nervous system is often considerably more unstable at such a time, and there are other evidences of altered physiology. Moderate exercise is rarely harmful; exposure to fresh air at such a time will be of no consequence unless there is chilling; bathing in warm water will rarely have a bad effect. It must be borne in mind that chilling of the skin usually tends to increase internal congestion of some sort, and so judgment must be exercised. Certainly the girl should be taught that the menstrual function is essentially physiological and that it should be treated as being such except when there is reason to believe that it is definitely pathological.

Children frequently experience rather intense love affairs. The adolescent is, of course, considerably more inclined to such attacks of "puppy love." On the other hand, some young people become so self-conscious in matters pertaining to sex that they go to the opposite extreme. Either reaction is easily understood and may be regarded as normal. Boys who are so delighted with their developing manhood are likely to become rather contemptuous of girls who have not their virile qualities, and so they sometimes think girls are quite impossible. It is not unlikely, however, that at times they may admire mightily from a distance. Girls who are becoming more careful of many little fine points of life are sometimes inclined to regard boys as being hopelessly uncouth. These reactions are also quite natural and do not presage a continuance of such feelings. As a matter of fact, rather the opposite is true as a rule, inasmuch as overreactions are common. Concerning all of these manifestations we can only say that they are normal, and strictly the affair of the individual concerned. For the rest of us, "Hands Off." The boy or girl should be allowed to develop his or her own individuality provided he or she is not taking a route that leads to deviations from what is considered to be a normal reaction.

Adolescence is a period of much dreaming and idealization. Children at this period are frequently dubbed lazy because of their propensity for dreaming and also because nature is protecting their rapidly growing and developing bodies from injury that might be inflicted by too energetic parents wishing to capitalize on the apparent—but more apparent than real—strength. The spirit of the youngster must not be injured by telling him that he is shiftless and will come to nothing. High ideals and religious motives are characteristic also of this period and may be utilized in helping to hold the young people to trends of action that may be considered safe.

The Mating Period

There comes a time in the life of every normal youth and maid when he or she is vastly interested in members of the opposite sex. The urge to mate, first in a process of courting and later in a solid marriage, becomes the dominant factor in the determination of conduct. Older and younger persons may marvel why otherwise sensible persons should appear so foolish, but the young people themselves are intent on having their fling and their fun while they may.

In this country, particularly, is the way of the lover made easy. Young people may choose their own mates almost without any help from their elders. Free choice is the inalienable right of every young person. No one is so unpopular as the stern parent who frowns on the dashing young dare-devil who for the moment sends his daughter into a state of ecstasy. In many other countries the young people have little or nothing to say about the matter and must mate according to the wishes or convenience of the parents.

Young people should be taught before the mating period is too urgently upon them that it is important indeed to look their companions over pretty carefully before allowing themselves to get in too deep. This is what is meant by "falling in love intelligently." We commonly speak of "falling in love" as if it were a sheer accident against which there was no protecting one's self. It is said that "love is blind," but surely this is a time for having the eyes wide open

How may we hope to teach young people to use more discretion in the vital matter of marriage selection? Who is a suitable mate, anyway? How may one know whether the particular person is going to wear well or not? Obviously these questions are capable of being answered only in the most general of terms. Certainly the following points are extremely important:

1. The prospective mate should come from a family that is free of serious hereditary defects. Inasmuch as this is not a textbook of eugenics we shall not attempt to describe them. Furthermore, the family should be one of intelligence, industry, thrift, and such social standing as will be compatible with the status of the person making the choice.

2. The matter of the health of the individual is very important. The marrying of an invalid is a mistake that is rarely corrected. Physical attractiveness is of some importance, but exceptional beauty need not be required or particularly desired.

3. Similarity of interests and cultural background should by all means be considered. A vivacious wife and a phlegmatic husband are hardly likely to be happy. Likewise a boob, a boor, a clown, or a gigolo will be badly miscast among "in-laws" of the opposite type. Character, industry, thrift, honor, sobriety, and kindred qualities are by no means to be disregarded.

4. Education should be considered. By education we mean the ability to know what should be done in a given set of circumstances and when and how to do it. We have little respect for mere "book-learning" or diplomas in the present connection. Acceptable manners are a part of education, as are cooking, sewing, and the ability to earn funds and use them wisely.

5. It is well to know how the given individual treats the members of his or her family, and how he or she is regarded by the other members of his or her own and the opposite sex.

6. Each party should understand the attitude of the other toward children, toward sex, and toward sexual morality.

7. Misgiving is sometimes expressed when the prospective husband is much larger than his mate. It is feared that she may have difficulty in giving birth to his children. This is much less serious than was formerly the case, for the good reason that obstetrical science is now far more proficient. Cæsarean section offers a solution in case trouble should arise. In general, it is better for the couple to be near the same size, but a match need not be called off because of difference of this nature. The small wife of a large man should in all cases see her physician as soon as she finds herself pregnant.

8. An accurate inventory of cash on hand, assets, liabilities, the ability to maintain or take care of a home, and a frank understanding of the financial status is essential. By this we do not mean that we would condemn marriage to a person who is financially poor, but we are merely insisting that the situation be understood and soberly considered.

9. It will be much better if the individual has long been known and if the courtship has been long enough and under diverse conditions enough that the wearing qualities have been tested reasonably well before the marriage is actually consummated.

10. In general it will be much better if both of the mates are of the same race and social level. In some instances differences in religion, and even in politics, may cause trouble.

11. Concerning the matter of love for the individual there must be no doubt. One must be willing to make any sacrifice for the loved one, and to prefer him or her above all others. Anything short of a mutual unselfish devotion will almost surely break down in the stress and strain of married life.

It is not expected that many young people will have the discretion soberly to count the debits and credits of the suitor after the love affair has developed, but children who have had such ideals held up to them from an early age will be somewhat less likely to err in so vital a matter when they are older. Young people who understand and appreciate something of the nature of the problems of married life will be much more likely to use judgment. It is too much to expect that children who have had no instruction in sex and character will listen to their elders when they are in the heat of a fervid love affair.

Strangely enough, most parents, when they try to exert an influence upon the choice of mates which their children are making, produce an effect which is just the opposite of that which was desired. An undesirable young man brings daughter home from a function of some sort. The next morning she is questioned, and there is a scene. She is frequently told that he is worthless, good-for-nothing, and altogether impossible. She defends him, of course, and the thing is done because we come quickly to love those whom we defend. There is nothing which will so certainly drive a couple into matrimony as will the idea that the poor dear one is being mistreated and persecuted. It is human nature that we should desire that which we are told we cannot have. An uncouth young man, or a silly girl, can much more easily and certainly be eliminated by inviting him or her into the home and allowing the daughter or son to see him or her in comparison with persons of known value and merit. Many an unhappy marriage has been contracted because the young people have revolted against what they considered an infringement of their sacred right to choose.

Naturally the parent feels that he has some rights in the matter— as indeed he should have, if he has sense to be worthy of the opportunity—and as indeed he does have, if he has made the most of his opportunities in the training of the child. Does not a parent have the right to have some say as to who shall be the other parent of his grandchildren, in whom he will be tremendously interested? Does he not have some rights in saying who shall share the property which he will leave to his child? Does he not have the right to protect his child from what he believes is a disastrous marriage? The answer is that he does have some rights, but that he will have to use all the diplomacy and tact in his possession to get those rights. This is no place for the bungling despot of the home to "lay down the law" or "set his foot down." This is the prerogative of him who has spent two decades or more in preparing a son or daughter for the most important decision that he or she will ever make.

The superior experience of parents *should* make them capable of real aid to the young people, but in a great many cases the judgment of the young is much better. The mother who insists that her son or daughter shall consider social standing above everything else, and the father who demands a fat bank roll, think that they are looking after the welfare of son or daughter, but are really setting up obstacles which will be cleared with difficulty if at all. Loveless, sordid marriages made with an eye on the bank book will rarely be made by the young people themselves, and may be regarded as a legal form of prostitution. On the other hand, young people are rather prone to the "love-at-first-sight" sort of infatuation which may lead them into hasty, ill-considered marriages which rarely turn out well.

A difficult matter in modern courtship is that concerning the payment of expenses. Formerly it was possible for a couple to spend evening after evening in the most delightful companionship without the expenditure of a cent. There were no shows to attend, no gasoline to buy, no sodas, no expensive presents, no boxes of candy, no flowers. Now the matter of expense is one of considerable consequence. As likely as not the girl is earning as much or nearly as much as the man, but the old relic of chivalry demands that the man shall pay the bill and that he shall be ever so generous. Many girls are slipping a coin to the boy-friend sometimes, or are asking him not to spend more than is absolutely necessary, but there are others of the "give-me" type who are bleeding their consorts to the limit and are looking for boys with fat allowances and beautiful cars.

It is most unfortunate that there are expenses to be considered. Sometimes girls have been led to believe that they are under obligation to repay in ways that are destructive to morals and character. So long as the girl was entertaining in her own home, and furnishing lemonade or home-made fudge, she might bid her suitor begone when he made improper proposals; when, however, she has accepted a theater ticket, a soda, and an automobile ride and finds herself miles away from home in her friend's car, the situation is considerably more complicated, and it is not a matter of astonishment that an inexperienced girl who wishes to continue the theater parties, sodas, and rides will sometimes solve the problem in the wrong way. There is also a strong temptation for a sexually aggressive young man to take advantage of the situation. He reasons that he should have something in compensation for the outlay he has made. Being uninstructed in sex ideals, as are most boys, the form of the compensation desired is easily guessed.

Certain organizations in the large cities are giving parties and entertainments which will have the effect of throwing young people together with the express purpose of making it possible for courtship to progress as naturally as possible. Coeducational colleges serve a most useful purpose in this connection. Various church organizations and societies serve the same end. Rooming houses and girls' dormitories usually have some sort of parlor where a degree of privacy may be had. Private homes should give some thought to the matter of providing a place where the daughter may be the hostess and therefore in control of the situation. A midnight lunch from the family ice box will be deeply appreciated by the young chap who has none too much money to spend. It will also put him under a wholesome obligation to be a gentleman, whereas under a different set of circumstances the girl might feel obliged to repay him for favors received.

The matter of privacy is one of some consequence. In this country a young couple expects as their right a degree of privacy which is nearly equal to that which they will enjoy after they are actually married. Whether this is right or wrong, there is apparently little or nothing that can be done about it. To deny it would be to drive them to places where they could get privacy under much less favorable circumstances, or to appear to persecute them, which would have the effect of making them tend to wish to abuse whatever opportunities for privacy they might have. The use of a living room from which other members of the family are not entirely and rigidly excluded would seem to be a proper medium.

Interesting is the fact that the city mother used to worry when she had reason to believe that her daughter was alone with her friend on country roads. All sorts of terrible possibilities arose to worry her, though she felt no such qualms when the couple were alone in the city. The country mother, on the other hand, thought nothing of her daughter driving alone with a young man in the country, but was afraid for them to go to the city unless someone went with them. Each mother rather intuitively understood that the young people were most in danger when they were in unfamiliar surroundings. Now that the distinction between city and country has mostly been wiped out, this reaction of mothers is less familiar, but it is still a fact that the young people are most likely to get into trouble when they are treading unfamiliar territory. This is the reason why they should be instructed thoroughly—but not morbidly—in matters pertaining to sex. Just as a democracy must educate the citizens who are the electorate, so must we educate our young people in these matters if we are safely to allow them the privacy that is customary in this country.

Some have supposed that they can control the relations of the two sexes by the use of chaperons. It is true that they can control the more obvious forms of indecency, but that is all. A chaperon thinks that she is saving the virtue of a girl when she compels a couple to use some restraint in their dancing positions. If the results were not so serious the idea would be humorous. The couple that wishes to dance in an indecent manner will not be restrained by a chaperon who all too often has been a prissy old maid, or a prim dowager who hasn't the slightest idea what the whole thing is about. We need chaperons, and lots of them, but the chaperons should be built into the character of the young people themselves; otherwise they are simply figureheads who believe that there is no mischief simply because they have seen none. The conventional chaperon, of course, serves a useful purpose when she prevents couples who are improper from suggesting such activity to those who otherwise would have had no thought of it.

We must remember that our young people are tremendously stimulated. We give them dancing lessons early so that they will quickly pass through the awkward age; we show them stimulating and *risqué* motion pictures; we have on our tables books that are written to sell and consequently made as "sexy" as possible; we scoff at conventions and laws which do not happen to suit our tastes; we wink at vice, graft, and illicit liaisons. Furthermore, after stimulating our young people in such manner, we will not as a rule permit them to marry until they are much older than was the evident biological intention of Nature. According to Nature's standards a couple is ready to marry when fifteen or sixteen years old, but the requirements of conventional society sets the time much higher. Under such circumstances we marvel that there is no more immorality than there is.

Love between the two sexes is a pure and fine emotion, and those who cast their pearls before swine will soon lose them. For an individual to simulate the expressions of deep affection when such feelings are really not held is to invite an inevitable deterioration of character which will eventually rob that individual of the power of fine and noble emotions of this sort. A girl will soon find herself marked as one who has been pawed over; a boy will soon lose his respect for clean and sweet womanhood. He who cheapens so precious an emotion as love will rue it if he has any of the finer sensibilities. He who sincerely and deeply loves another and who has earned the right to legitimate favors is entitled to them, but this presupposes that he would wish to bestow his affection only upon the favored one.

Marriage is of such consequence that it should be carefully considered. The couple expecting to make such a contract should thoroughly discuss every phase of the subject before doing so. All reliable sources of information should be sought, and notes should be compared. Each should frankly tell the other what he or she expects. The desirability or undesirability of having children must be thoroughly threshed out before going ahead. Whether or not sexual relations for other than reproductive purposes will be desired or permitted is an important matter. Agreement upon a date that will fit into the menstrual cycle may well be made. Arrangement for the use of contraceptives in the early days of the marriage, and an understanding of such use, is rather important unless the couple is willing to risk the possibility of pregnancy which might be terminated prematurely. If the bride-to-be is anxious that sexual relations not be consummated at once, that point should be understood—and respected.

There is nothing finer and more beautiful, nothing more useful, nothing more pure than those prenuptial agreements and arrangements which insure that the couple are really ready to marry and to assume the sacred obligations which marriage entails.

The Honeymoon

The honeymoon is the period between the marriage ceremony and the time when the young people shall have become more or less settled into the routine of a married couple. It is frequently used to designate a trip that is taken for the purpose of getting away from prying eyes. It is a period of adjustment to the new regimen and may be wisely or unwisely spent. Not a few marriages are utterly wrecked during this time, and a great many others are so strained as to weaken or damage the prospect of future happiness and usefulness. It is a time of high emotional tension and needs to be rather soberly considered. The obvious purpose of the honeymoon is to grant to the newly married lovers an unusual degree of privacy while they are experimenting with the new status in which they find themselves.

It is unfortunate that there have grown up so many ugly customs about so beautiful a thing as a wedding. Pranks without number are played upon the couple; many of these pranks are in exceedingly bad taste, and not a few are positively indecent.

Wealthy families are inclined to make much of a wedding. There are parties, showers, receptions, and elaborate ceremonies, and finally a long and tiresome honeymoon is planned. A trip to Europe or a tour around the world seems like an ideal wedding present, but is entirely too long and tiresome. On such a trip the lovers are thrown entirely too much into each other's company and may utterly exhaust themselves and their interest in each other. The fatigue of travel and of sightseeing, added to the strain of adjustment and the enervating effects of excessive sexual exercise, is entirely too much. It would be better if the trip were short and the demands made upon physical and emotional resources were light. A cabin in the woods, or a room at a summer or a winter resort, according to season, is likely to be much better. It is easy also for the pair to lose themselves in a large city, where hotels afford any degree of seclusion that may be desired, and the myriad diversions of the city furnish opportunity for any degree of activity that may be needed.

Families in moderate circumstances often exceed their means in attempting to give their young people a big and elaborate wedding and trip. The worry as to whether the funds will hold out, and the consciousness that the rocket-like celebration is going to end with a thud, make a bad start. Better no honeymoon at all than one that cannot be afforded.

The most important relations of the period, however, are not those which are commonly called the honeymoon. They are those which take place in the very first days and nights of married life. The happiness and even the health of the couple may be seriously crippled by the bungling caresses of one who is not ready for real marriage or is utterly lacking in understanding of the processes involved.

Biologic marriage and conventional marriage have entirely different purposes, but the two are supplementary to each other and are best consummated at approximately the same time. In case the biologic marriage has lagged and one or another of the pair is not ready for the actual union, the process of courtship should continue until the mate—usually the bride—is really ready for sexual relations. Theoretically, legal marriage gives each the right to the body of the other, and many men have been crass enough to insist on those rights as soon as the privacy of the bedroom has been reached. Embarrassed, shocked, frightened, and even subjected to physical pain, the bride is essentially forced by one who has but a short time before promised to love and cherish her. Under such circumstances she is set against the whole process and, indeed, may never learn to take a normal attitude toward a relation which should be exquisitely pleasurable to both partners. In a short time the husband, being disappointed in the fact that his wife is no longer a lover, may become disgusted and seek mistresses who can take an interest in such things. Modesty is fine and splendid, but a ruined marriage is too big a price to pay for *mock* modesty.

Every prospective bridegroom should understand that, unless he has positive and first-hand assurance to the contrary, the bride will probably wish to delay the climax of the ceremony which has just been performed. Brides without previous sexual experience may be reluctant indeed, in spite of the fact that they are intensely in love with their new husbands. In such case there is nothing for the *gentleman* to do but bide his time and divert himself in the gallant and romantic manner which has so far won her approval that she has been willing to take his name and hand and share her life with him. The rights which the law gives him are as worthless as dust until they have been ratified by her approval. "Women first" is the code of the gentleman. If this fact could be impressed on the consciousness of bridegrooms most of them would be only too glad to wait until the loved one is ready to invite them. Young people, when newly married, are in a highly idealistic and romantic state and are more liberal and unselfish probably than at any other time in their lives. But the young man, being intensely stimulated himself and never having been told that the feeling of the bride may be different, supposes that she as well as he is eager to bring about the consummation of their marriage. If she is so, very well! There is not the least reason for formality in cases where courting has progressed to such a stage. When, however, the bride is reluctant, courtship must be continued, and courtship only.

All or most of these difficulties can be avoided by a frank prenuptial understanding. The couple who are so excessively modest that they cannot discuss this subject had better grow up a little, learn something about themselves, and really get in love before going ahead with a wedding. If the girl seems reluctant, her fiancé can make her happy and reassured if he will promise her that he will consider her wishes in these matters as well after marriage as before. She, in turn, should assure him that she understands the purpose and nature of marriage, and that she will do her best to become interested in that which is so vital to happiness and unity.

In times past there is reason to believe that such an understanding has often not been attained, and that a green, inexperienced, awkward youth and a shy, embarrassed, undeveloped girl were commonly thrown together in utter ignorance of all the arts of conjugal life. Such, indeed, was considered to be the ideal condition, and mothers were prone to boast that their daughters knew absolutely nothing about such matters. It is no wonder that so many marriages went on the rocks. Probably the only reason that so many escaped is that the daughters were rarely so dumb as fond mamma supposed. Young people are much better prepared in this respect for marriage nowadays. There are opportunities to learn; there is a vocabulary in which they may speak to their prospective mates; there are books, pamphlets, and lectures from which they may learn much; and in most instances there is the practice of those intimacies which are the proper prelude to marriage.

Sheer clothing, athletic uniforms, and brief bathing suits have accustomed both sexes to the general appearance of the body of the other sex. It is to be hoped that this has helped greatly to prevent excessive embarrassment in the act of disrobing, and that it also will tend to temper somewhat the excitement of one or both. To one who stands in great reverence of the significance of the marriage relation it seems that a couple intensely in love and entering into a relation of such significance and beauty might find an exquisite delight in coming frankly and gladly together devoid of every covering and artifice. This is no time for silly giggling and undressing in the closet. It is a time for truth, dignity, and that fine sense of self-respect that is proud to proclaim to all the world that this man and this woman are taking their places in the long line of those who have lived and loved, and have nourished and cherished the spark of life that has come down without a break since the day of Creation.

The accomplishment of the first act of sexual congress is by no means without its hazards. In case the male organ is of unusual size care will need to be taken, particularly if the wife is small. After some time adjustment will be made and normal relations may be assumed, but until that time the husband may have to practise restraint. The first union will be facilitated considerably if some lubricant is used. Vaseline will serve in this capacity, but a surgical jelly is better. The hymen of the young wife will occasionally present real difficulty: it is so resistant in some instances that considerable effort may be required to break it. In rare cases it may even require the aid of a physician to remove this obstruction. Occasionally there will be some pain, and there may be slight bleeding as a result of the first union. When such is the case the greatest care must be taken, and the wife should by all means be granted the privilege of being the active party. An aggressive husband essentially attacking a sensitive, frightened, and unprepared wife and hurting her may completely wreck all hope of a full and happy married life. He must let her be the aggressor while he with infinite patience and tenderness is still the gentle lover subject to her slightest whim.

Concerning the hymen there is need of exact information, else innocent wives may be accused of having had previous sexual experience. At one time it was supposed that the hymen was considered an infallible proof of virginity. It is now known that many virgins have lost the hymen as a result of athletic activities, accident, horseback riding, or manipulations incident to bathing. On the other hand, there are women who are no longer virgins, but have an intact hymen. Ignorance of these facts has many times caused the most cruel injustices to be committed.

Many people who should know better suppose that all of these delicate relations can be trusted entirely to the instincts and that for this reason there is no need to discuss them. Nothing could be further from the truth. Nature has furnished us with certain instincts, it is true, but they are the "law of the jungle." It is these instincts which have caused so much trouble in times past for the reason that instinct is utterly disregardful of anything except the desire of the male to consummate sexual relations at every possible opportunity, and to bring about fertilization as quickly as possible. As well go back to the practice of clubbing our wives into unconsciousness and chaining them to the tent pole to keep them from running away. Modern marriage is—or should be—on a different basis. In no other species than man is the pleasure or welfare of the female given more consideration than is necessary to gain her physical acquiescence, but man is more than a beast and should behave accordingly.

Because sexual relations as they are practised by men and women serve another function than merely that of reproduction they cannot be successfully practised from instinct alone. They are of the nature of an art; they express fine and noble emotions just as do the other arts. Because they constitute an art they must be learned and practised before a high degree of proficiency may be attained, even after many years a well-matched couple may still be improving in technic and in appreciation of the legitimate pleasures of conjugal love. There are books to be had which give the most detailed description of every phase of the copulative function, but one can hardly expect to learn to play the piano by reading about it. If definite difficulties arise, such information may be of service, but otherwise the couple should be somewhat less sophisticated in the early stages of the honeymoon period. It is only necessary that both remember that *the act is perfectly proper* and that the spirit of love demands that *each shall show the utmost solicitude for the comfort, happiness, and pleasure of the other*. With this as a guide it is hard to suppose that many marriages could go wrong.

The Young Married Couple

Much has been said about the advisability of the wife working after marriage. Until the couple can get a start there can certainly be no objection to the wife's holding her former job or getting another one. It will mean extra hours of work and less leisure now that she has the care of a home or an apartment, but it is all for the good of the cause. It would be a poor wife, indeed, who would not put her shoulder to the family wheel and help to make it turn.

Unfortunately, however, there is more to the matter than just that. It will be hard later for her to give up the outside job and devote herself exclusively to home-making with its comparatively intangible rewards. We need not be surprised that she is loath to give up the independence that comes with a check at the end of the week. There are so many things that are needed and can be had only if the wife as well as the husband earns.

So it is customary to put off, and put off, and put off the real purpose and culmination of marriage—children. If two have trouble making ends meet with two salaries—as two commonly do—how shall three or four or five live on one salary? And so by sex repression, which often eats into the hearts of both, by the use of more or less distasteful contraceptive methods, or sometimes by resort to criminal abortion, the couple more or less successfully cheats Mother Nature of her due. From month to month, with fear and hope combined, the coming of the menses is awaited as if its failure would be a world-wide catastrophe. Years pass, and the couple are still in need of both pay checks. Educated tastes have been developed and seemingly must be pampered; children are forgotten, or are pushed farther and farther into the future. Usually they say that "some day" they want children but hardly see how they can manage it just yet. "Some day" they are going to have beautiful blue-eyed boys and golden-haired girls, but when "some day" comes Nature has all too often become tired of being turned away, and the Gate of Life is closed.

It is hard to criticize a couple who gradually work their way into this predicament. Nothing could seem more logical than that they should have made the decisions that they did. Society as it exists in a civilized community puts a premium on the childless marriage. Just the same, such a ménage is not really a home. A generation of such homes and there would be nothing. The error that young people are so likely to make is to believe that parties, shows, elegant furniture, and sport roadsters can bring more happiness than children. Once they have had the children they would know that nothing can bring the soul-satisfying rapture that a baby brings, but, of course, they haven't had such experience, and quite naturally cannot appreciate it. Such marriages are easily broken. With no children, with little property investment as a rule, with both having an income, the slightest friction is likely to cause a serious split. Interesting is the fact that families in which the wife continues to work for years after marriage rarely become well-to-do. If the husband had had to shoulder the responsibility of a growing family he might have waded in and made more of his opportunities. Breezing along, though, with the help of the wife, he has taken it easy and got nowhere.

If the wife works there should be a definite understanding concerning the time when she shall be promoted to the much more important work of real home-making. Marriages when both parties are poor but in good health and willing to work are frequently the very best of marriages. Stories told of the hard times that grandfather and grandmother had in the old days are familiar family lore, and will be a century hence. We frequently see the young wife working to help her husband complete his education, and it makes a most inspiring picture. Likewise, the wife may continue her education after marriage. These are the young people who know what an education is. They will get along.

Health is of the utmost importance to the welfare of the home builders. In the first place, only those who have health are fit to marry. It is foolish indeed for a young person to marry an invalid or semi-invalid—immensely romantic in some instances, and highly idealistic, but nevertheless foolish. It is much like marrying a drunkard to reform him. Better reform him first! Besides, it is most selfish for a sick person to fasten himself or herself upon another person and call it love. Marriage is a big job at the best. It is entirely too much for sick people. When sickness comes after marriage, as of course it is probable that it will eventually come, there is nothing that honor can condone except to see it through, but even so it may and often does utterly wreck the family.

There are several particular health hazards which must be considered by people of this age group. Tuberculosis finds in them its most susceptible victims. The bearing, nursing, and caring for children undermines occasionally the health of the mother, particularly if the children come too close together. Hard work on the part of both in the years when they are so anxious to get a start, accepting extra jobs, taking few vacations, worrying, and falling for the temptation to avoid the expense of doctors' bills when there is real need for professional attention, all take their toll. Nervous breakdown from overwork, pneumonia, organic heart disease, occupational diseases, and other related conditions are prone to attack this group. Health is a matter of much more than personal concern to these people. It involves the welfare of the entire family and for that reason deserves to be considered seriously in this place. What one of us has not heard our fathers and mothers wondering, "What will become of us if one of us should get sick?"

Life, accident, and health insurance have proved themselves of the greatest possible consequence in solving the problems which inevitably arise when health is impaired. It is said that the total amount of life insurance in force in the United States is well over *one hundred billion dollars*. The effect of such a fund is beyond comprehension. During the recent depression life insurance has been the only form of investment aside from government bonds of the better sorts which has not suffered depreciation. As soon as the family can possibly afford to do so, investment should be made in some form of time-tried insurance. When there are children there is particular need of such protection.

In this place we need no more than mention the importance of a firm economic basis for so important an institution as the family. Unless there is a dependable income, unless the housewife and her husband know how to manage so as to keep within that income and have a little to spare for savings, there is trouble ahead. A savings account, a house to live in, a few life insurance policies and other conservative investments, are absolutely essential to the welfare of a home. It may seem a little strange that these should be mentioned in a discussion of sex education, but in the sense that we are using the term they are as much a part of the program of raising a family as is the incident which is commonly regarded as sex. Everything which helps young people to understand the problems of a family is in a very true sense sex education.

One of the biggest questions which the young couple must decide is that concerning children. Will there be children? And, if so, how many? There are, to be sure, many excellent reasons why a particular couple should not desire children at a given time, and there are even reasons why they should not have them at all. There is, for example, the couple which dares not have children because of some hereditary taint. They act wisely in taking precautions which will prevent them. On the other hand, it is most unfortunate that they did not find out about such matters before marriage and act accordingly. A given couple may feel that the health of one or the other is such that the burden of parenthood should not be added. This is, of course, a legitimate reason, though many of these persons were ill before marriage, and really because of that unfit for marriage. The economic position of the family is often such that children might be endangered by being brought into the home at such a time.

We have no desire to say what should be the size of family which a given couple should seek. Circumstances will need to be consulted. It requires an average of more than three children to the couple for a given stratum of society to maintain itself numerically. Any family of less than four is, then, on the average, falling behind. This is a serious matter or not, according as the group is a useful one or not. Unfortunately, those families which should have no children usually have many, and those that might be expected to bear and rear superior children as a rule have few or none. The loss to society is great, and the loss to the individuals themselves is even greater.

For those couples who cannot for some reason bear children there are infinite possibilities in the adoption of orphans. With care the adopted child that has come from a good family has an even chance with the blood descendant of the same age and physical opportunity. It cannot be shown that adopted children turn out worse than others. They may on the average do better, when they have been carefully selected. A careful physical and mental examination should be made of all children who are being considered for adoption. Couples without children may also satisfy their parental instincts and do a great service by taking up some phase of work which has to do with the welfare of children and young people. It is the only way to stay young and keep sweet. "Suffer little children to come unto Me and forbid them not, for of such is the Kingdom of Heaven" is no idle dogma. It is the essence of life.

The care of the children after they are born is enormously important. It is discussed in succeeding chapters.

There are many problems which are sexual in the sense that the term is usually used. A husband and wife, a man and woman, in vigorous health and living in the intimacy which is properly granted to a married couple, have many opportunities for expressions of love and affection. Shall we deny them the privileges of sexuality except for purposes of reproduction? Certainly not! They will need to learn well the art of love so that they may know the exquisite pleasures of conjugal love. The stability of the marriage will depend largely on this ability, though, of course, there are other factors serving toward this end.

In most cases where there is dissatisfaction with the conjugal relation at this stage in life the cause is to be found in the fact that women are more slowly aroused and require a longer time for gratification than is the case of the man. Husbands are prone to forget that courtship is as necessary after marriage as before. Quickly aroused and quickly satisfied, they are inclined to forget that the partner in everything else should also have her share in the emotions of sex, else she will become disgusted and intolerant of the whole process. Part of the trouble is also due to the fact that a large percentage of women suppose that sex gratification is not for them and that there is something akin to vulgarity in any manifestation of pleasure or interest in it. With the husband as considerate as he should be and the wife convinced of the propriety of legitimate conjugal relations there should be little difficulty in building a sex life that will bind the family together with hoops of steel.

Considerable effort has been made to determine in an accurate way the limits of safe and proper sexual indulgence. The frequency with which the act may be safely performed without injury to health or vigor is not something that can be reduced to formula. It will vary widely in different couples, and it is impossible for an outsider to set out rules. So long as the act is mutually pleasurable, and both the partners are able to go about the usual day's work without unusual fatigue or lassitude, it is evident that no harm is being done. In case either partner feels the strain, moderation must be practised. The average among Americans is two to three times a week. As in the case of everything else, it is better to err on the side of too little than too much. No one would wish to give up the pleasure of eating food, but everyone is disgusted with gluttony. Hardly anything can be so revolting as sexual gluttony. The love embrace is too sacred a thing to be made common.

In practically every family at some time it is considered best that conception should not take place in the immediate future. Improper methods may on one hand fail to control the size of the family, or on the other may cheat the couple of such sexual experience as is essential to health and happiness. The pair that lives in constant fear of pregnancy can hardly be happy and can hardly do the task that so much needs to be done. There are individuals who by virtue of strong wills, or who by lack of the normal desires, may solve this problem by refraining entirely from intercourse, but the vast majority of couples cannot go along happily on such a regimen. In such case, one or the other of the pair is likely to seek gratification outside of the family, and a whole train of dangerous possibilities are born forthwith.

Common opinion takes it for granted that sexual appetite is something that cannot be controlled. It is astonishing how many people suppose that a "red-blooded" individual is utterly at the mercy of any sexual passion that may chance to blow. The attitude of irresponsibility for sexual misconduct is a convenient alibi for those who have not the strength of character to stand by their guns. Such is not a strong and manly attitude, but is a sign of weakness in those who cannot or will not be strong. It isn't smart, or strong, or clever, or evidence of broadmindedness; it is a blow at the very heart of society and the home. A yellow cur can follow any vagrant female who may pass. Indeed a yellow cur *will* do just that.

Marriage is not a lark. There is no more serious business in all the world than that of building a home and rearing children. Prospective husbands and wives had better grow up before undertaking the honorable responsibilities that come to those who assume the social and biological status known as marriage.

Sex in Middle and Advanced Life

Most men and women experience a considerable shock as they approach and pass the age of forty. They have learned to look upon "fat and forty" as being the zero hour of romance. As young people they have supposed that one so old has lost every good reason for living. To be a solid burgher or thrifty housewife of forty has been supposed to be the end of everything, and now to find one's self at the halfway place or a little beyond seems incredible. Actually, however, a large percentage of people are happier after this age than before. Particularly is this true of those who have lived and loved wisely and not "too well." The individual who can adjust his life and thinking to the fact that he is no longer a gay and irresponsible young thing will find many compensations for the fact that he can no longer swim across the lake or beat the young fellows at tennis. The woman who can relax a bit at this time and smile indulgently at the mad struggle for beauty and youth has before her many happy days of comparative quiet and serenity.

Of great importance in this process of adjustment is that which has to do with sex. Ordinarily people of forty and above do not bear children. A few children are born of mothers above this age, but it is a rather risky adventure, as some of the children are hardly up to the standard of their brothers and sisters born at a more vigorous period of life. A small percentage of these children are definitely defective and are called "exhaustion products." It is also said that an unusual number of these children are of exceptional ability, but the likelihood is rather in the direction first mentioned. Men may continue to be fertile for a long time past the forty mark, but there is some objection to men being fathers after they are much above forty. The possibility that the children will be left orphans in such case is quite obvious.

Are we to suppose, then, that all of the functions of the reproductive apparatus have been filled? Not at all. Usually there are children to be raised. The family still has a purpose. Couples who have enjoyed the embraces of earlier life will still continue to enjoy them and will not need to consider the possibility of pregnancy and additional children with their many responsibilities. With the children from underfoot it is not unusual to see a couple much more attached to each other than when they were so busy. It is, indeed, not unusual to see them almost like two young lovers, or perhaps more often as Darby and Joan contentedly living a life of placid, uneventful domesticity.

It is difficult for younger people to see in this period anything but a tiresome and monotonous existence, and there are many who find themselves at forty or above in an openly rebellious attitude. They want one more fling at "life" and may do foolish things in the effort to get it. The man who has been circumspect and careful about all such matters may get sympathetic for himself and think he has missed a great deal. Somewhat bored with the faithful but unromantic wife, ne is prone to yearn for a younger and more vivacious companion. If some degree of affluence has rewarded his labors, he is in a position to indulge himself—and be an easy mark for gold-diggers who really hold him in contempt. Occasionally a woman of forty retains her youth better than her husband and may be tempted to "step out" a bit with a snappy "gigolo" or a neighbor whose "wife doesn't understand him." She yearns for a lover instead of a tired workhorse who prefers his house slippers and shirt sleeves to a "tux" and a ballroom. It is not unlikely that this period offers more urgent temptations than does any other. Certain it is that the opportunities for making a fool of one's self during this time are unexcelled.

Likewise the unmarried person of this age is in danger. The unmarried woman who is approaching the end of what would and should have been the reproductive period of her life sees her youth slipping. Until this time she has usually hoped that the opportunity for family life would come, but she now rapidly resigns herself to the prospect of a lonesome and not unlikely bitter old age. She feels cheated. Life is going without ever having really bloomed or borne fruit. Something of the same feeling is experienced by married couples who have had no children. Fortunate indeed are such childless persons who have attained a vicarious parenthood either by adopting children or by interesting themselves in the children of their friends or in young people. It is easy for unattached persons to get self-centered and in this way to become the typical "old maid." Mothers do not become "old maids" for the good reason that they are more interested in their children than they are in themselves. Because they are interested in other people, other people are interested in them, and everyone has a good time. In case the opportunity for marriage first comes in middle or advanced age, the problem of adjustment will be difficult, to say the least.

It is not uncommon to hear men say that when they are no longer interested in a pretty face or figure they will be ready to die—life will no longer be worth living. The loss of virility in men is looked on as a calamity of the highest degree. Such an attitude reveals an utter lack of understanding of the real meaning of life.

Loss of virility is Nature's way of insuring against "exhaustion products"; it is her way of making sure that fathers will probably live until the work of raising the child in accomplished; it is her protection for the weakened and wasted organs of the body which in the wear and tear of life have likely become injured to such an extent that ardent wooing and frequent sexual embraces are dangerous. What a fool is the man who seeks rejuvenation by some sort of gland operation or transplantation! Even if gland transplantations were successful, which they are not, little good could come from such meddling. It is like putting a powerful new motor into a rickety old chassis in the expectation of roaring along at eighty m.p.h. Of course something breaks—usually an artery in the brain—and there is real trouble. "New wine in old bottles" has been a dangerous combination for so long that it looks as if the fact might be better appreciated.

The elderly widower gets himself a young wife. How can a young woman be really in love with a man thirty or forty years her senior? For that matter, how can a man of that age who understands things be truly in love with a young woman? Ten years more will find him an old man while she will be just starting. Clashes between the wife and his children—as old as she—are inevitable. The suspicion that she loves his money rather than him; the fear that she may be stepping out with younger men; the painful effort to entertain her as a young wife deserves to be entertained; the fear that children may be borne at a period in life when children would be a burden; and a dozen other fears real and imaginary, take away every iota of the tranquillity that should be the heritage of him who has lived long. Much wiser indeed is he who chooses a companion who is near his own age.

Respect for gray hairs is a duty of the young. It is even more the duty of those who have the gray hairs. The young people are right when they tell grandma to "be her age." By this we do not mean that men and women of middle age should don the funereal black that used to be the custom, and that they should fold their hands and get ready to die. Quite the contrary! Dyeing the hair, having face-lifting operations, refusing to wear the glasses that they need, nervously driving themselves to act as if they were mere girls, these wretched women fool no one and wear themselves out trying to make the stream of life start over at the source. If it could be done there would be some excuse for the effort, but of course they always lose. Almost any young girl can be pretty or even beautiful, but it takes a "heap o' livin' " to make a beautiful old face. The lines of age are simply the character lines that have been developed through years of habitual smiling; or frowning; and constitute real beauty—or ugliness. The beauty of youth is skin deep, but the beauty of age really goes to the bone.

There is nothing which is so capable of building real character as a full understanding and appreciation of sex and its obligations. In times past women have been taught to avoid sex as if it were vulgar and ugly. In consequence, many of them, as soon as they were married, have been careless of their personal appearance and have grown into the slatternly, careless type which is still seen everywhere about us. Some of them have seemed rather to be proud of the fact that they were unattractive. Ugliness has been supposed to be a sign of virtue or of something or other; it has removed them from temptation—most effectively.

The opposite extreme, and one that is just as disgusting, is the woman who never forgets her "sex appeal" and goes to every sort of artificial means to hold her youthful appearance. Life to many of these women seems to be nothing except a struggle against the onslaughts of age. Hours are spent with hairdressers, beauty experts, and beauty doctors of all sorts. Sex to these women has not meant the bearing of children, as a rule. They have emphasized that phase of the program which is merely a preliminary to the real purpose, and in consequence is shallow and superficial. On the other hand, the woman who has loved her mate frankly and honorably, who has borne and reared his and her children, who has sacrificed everything for her loved ones, who has borne pain for them, who has known the pangs of unutterable dread and fear when they were in danger, who has felt her heart bursting with pride of them, who has smiled when she wanted to cry, who has loved and lived, develops in middle and advanced life a beauty which is the beauty of the Madonna.

For those who are at middle age and are capable of reading it, nothing is so valuable as a little book by Aldred Scott Warthin, for forty years professor of pathology at the University of Michigan. The book is entitled *Old Age* and is the life philosophy of Dr. Warthin written when he was old and wise. It is for the intelligent layman and is written in nontechnical language. Warthin points out that at every age some part of the body is old and worn out and is making way for something else. Even before birth some parts have atrophied and have made way for growing structures. At the time of birth the senile afterbirth is dropped as worn out and no longer needed. It has served its purpose and is cast aside as useless baggage. The thymus of the child is old, or should be, when the child is adolescent; the womb and the ovaries are old at forty-five; the prostate and the testicles are commonly old in the sixties; the body as a whole is old at seventy or shortly thereafter. Those who are religiously inclined—and religion is a great asset at this or any other age—will see in old age and death a further sublimation in which the earthly body is dropped, as was the afterbirth, as being a useless encumbrance to the spirit, which is immortal.

Senility and death are seen by Dr. Warthin as being perfectly natural processes provided they do not come too soon. Death is, indeed, quite as necessary as birth. If there were no deaths there soon could be no births, because the earth would be full and running over with old people living in the past. The aged must make room for those who are younger and more vigorous. Even this is a part of the reproductive act. We must do our best to get our children ready to do the work of the world, and then we must get out of the way so that they can do it. Unjust? Not at all! As young people we took the places of those who were older and as old people ourselves we can expect the same inevitable fate. In the relay race that is life each runner is expected to do his best and then pass the torch to his successor. Having done so, he can perform a last and valuable service by getting out of the way and taking care of himself in such a way as will not divert the attention of the one who is at the time carrying the responsibilities of the race. Everyone who understands the purpose of life knows that "the game is the thing." It's a poor sport that wants to carry the ball every time and unwillingly submits to a substitution when the coach calls him to the bench.

A philosophy of this sort is more than may reasonably be expected of those who are constantly thinking of themselves and are ever looking for their own pleasure and advantage. To some it will seem harsh. Those who have children should understand, however, and should be glad to make way for their children—just as they have always made way for their children in other matters. Even this, then, is a part of the reproductive instinct, using the term in its broadest sense. Inasmuch as the end of life must come, it is much better to be philosophical about it and not be like a small boy who has eaten his cake and is crying because he cannot still have it.

The purpose of life is not primarily that we as individuals shall be royally entertained. It is too much to suppose that God, or Nature, or Call-it-what-you-will has created the universe in order that we as individuals may have full stomachs and sexual gratification. Obviously one of the purposes of life is that the species may be propagated. Another, apparently, is that we may use our wits to control the forces of Nature about us and possibly make something of ourselves. A misunderstanding of the real purpose of preventive and curative medicine and of life itself is responsible for a great deal of trouble and worry. Under our present system, for example, a physician is obliged—and rarely questions the essential wisdom of it—to save and prolong human life as long as possible. He is honor bound to keep the idiot alive, though the life may be worse than useless. The physician can do no less, and we would not wish him to do otherwise, but the real emphasis should be upon the preservation and creation of those individuals who will be an asset to the community and the race. It is not that we object to the saving of the lives of human derelicts, but rather that we wish to emphasize the main objective, the improvement of the general average.

It is commonly said that health is more important than anything else. This is exactly the same sort of false philosophy that is responsible for the despondency which comes to those who are attaining advanced age. Health is not, or should not be, an end in itself but merely a means to an end. The earnest parent is anxious to remain well, not so much because he or she is afraid to suffer as that he or she wants to be able to take care of the children until they are able to take care of themselves. When a parent dies the neighbors lament not so much the loss of a friend and neighbor as they look with apprehension upon the fact that he or she left little children. The parent who would not jeopardize his own health or safety for the sake of his child is not a real parent but a miserable imitation. And so the aged person who appreciates and understands his rôle is much happier and more reconciled to the part which he must play whether he likes it or not.

The individual with this outlook will be buffered against the shock that comes at the age of forty, and the despondency which comes at a later age when it seems that everything is going to pot when actually it is merely the changing of the guard. He will see in his waning sexual powers a reason and a purpose, and will therefore more easily be content that it should be so. He is willing to allow someone else to carry the ball, and is happy if the cause for which he has lived and fought is being advanced by the younger and stronger hands of those who come after.

The Purpose of Marriage

From the standpoint of society, the real purpose of marriage is the creation of a home into which children may be born legitimately and reared in decency and self-respect. We do not mean by this statement that young people should have in mind only such a purpose in the selection of a mate, but we do mean that they should carefully consider the responsibilities of parenthood before they enter into a relation of such consequence. The fitness of a given individual to be a father or a mother is really more important than the fitness of the same individual to be merely a husband or a wife.

The prospective bride or bridegroom should consider the family tree of himself or herself and of the preferred mate. It will be well to consider whether or not a given man is likely to be able to provide for a family, or whether a given girl is of the domestic or maternal type who will enjoy caring for babies. The couple contemplating marriage should frankly discuss the probability of children being born and should come to some agreement in such matters before the ceremony of marriage has been performed. It will be well also if by some means they may attempt to determine whether or not they are probably sexually compatible. In other words, young people should "fall in love intelligently," a phrase which has been much ridiculed by those who believe that love and marriage should never be considered in any other light than that of the moon. Many will protest that we are seeking to take the romance out of marriage. On the contrary, we are really trying to preserve the romance so that it may last and last and last. In our observation the marriages which have been carefully worked out are more likely to be permanently and solidly "romantic" than those which have been consummated in a fever of something or other which passes in the moonlight as true love.

It is the nature of the young of the species to desire the company of the members of the opposite sex. In our eagerness to disclaim everything related to sex we have tried to make ourselves believe that the purposes of such an attraction are entirely or largely idealistic and platonic. Scientific candor forces us to admit, however, that the real purpose of such an attraction is that the species may be reproduced. Nature has no other purpose. If Nature alone were consulted, there would be no such thing as conventional marriage, and as a result there would be no such thing as the civilized home, and, indeed, no such thing as civilization itself. Marriage, by which we mean conventional marriage, has been evolved by man as a means of rising above the chance mating of the animals and as a device for placing about human offspring the care and protection of parents who continue to love each other after the heat of sexual passion has waned.

However much we may disdain the methods of Nature, we cannot divorce ourselves entirely from them. The wise couple will not even attempt to defeat the purposes which Nature has in bringing them together, but will try to sublimate and use those purposes and in this way attain the purposes both of Nature (that there be children) and of convention (that they and their children be properly established in a real home).

Strangely enough, there are persons who, though they are perfectly capable of normal relations as a parent, are exceedingly anxious to avoid such responsibilities and privileges. We believe this to be an unnatural attitude for the reason that if it were universalized it would mean the end of the biological species to which we belong. All animals and plants have the urge to reproduce themselves, and we must agree in such case that the instinct is natural and fundamental. Many species of animals do not, however, breed well when domesticated, and man, the most domesticated of all, responds somewhat in this way. As men and women become more divorced from natural settings and pursuits, as they become more artificialized, more "educated," more "civilized," they tend to have smaller and smaller families, and for that reason the race has been and still is dying out at the top. Personally, we doubt if such "education" is really education, and if such "civilization" is really civilization in the highest sense, but such is the custom of the times. It is doubtless the reason why many people consider the bearing of children to be common and plebeian.

Since the day of creation our ancestors have every one of them been hardly enough to live to the age of sexual maturity. Every one of them has escaped a thousand accidents which, had they had less wit or strength, would have been fatal not only to themselves but to their progeny as well. Every one of them has had the normal instinct to reproduce himself or herself and has been sufficiently comely to be sought and accepted by a member of the opposite sex. If one should believe that man was created some six thousand years ago, the fact that our ancestry goes back to the day of Creation without a break is quite remarkable, but if one believes that man and animal life has existed for millions of years and that during that entire time there has been no break in the continuity which leads to you and me the fact becomes amazing. In the gigantic relay race that is life, a billion ancestors have passed the torch from one to the next in never-ending sequence until the present generation is reached. It is almost unbelievable that men and women should fail to see the significance of, and that they should seek to avoid taking a place in, so extraordinary a procession.

The real, the primary purpose of marriage, then, is children. That two persons should enjoy the constant society of each other is most fortunate but is really of little concern to anyone but themselves, unless there are children. When there are children we have the setting for an ideal home. That two persons should quarrel and fight is again of little importance to anyone except themselves, unless there are children. When there are children in such a distraught home there is tragedy. The couple without children is very likely to separate for some trivial reason, and such marriages are commonly highly unstable. Judges are much more free in granting divorces to childless couples than to those who have dependent children to consider. For a long time the courts have been considering a childless marriage somewhat in the light of a "companionate marriage." If a particular marriage is fruitless from the standpoint of the propagation of the better elements in society it is worthless except as a medium of convenience for two individuals.

When one considers the importance of the relationship which the person to be married is about to assume it makes him wonder why society has been so careless in permitting any Tom, Dick, or Mary who can find a willing mate to enter into such a contract. The parent, in addition to his or her duties as a provider or housewife, must furnish the biological inheritance, must serve as nurse, physician, dentist, teacher, preacher, legal adviser, companion, administrator, and adviser to the child. The parent should be an authority on mental hygiene, infant care, dietetics; he or she should speak the mother tongue with accuracy, beauty, and force; he or she should train the child in proper habits, in obedience, thrift, industry, appreciation of truth, beauty, and virtue. The parent who has usually had not a word of scientific or even practical training in child care and guidance is responsible for the education of the child before he goes to school and all of the time during school except for about six hours a day, five days in the week, and six to nine months in the year.

In spite of all these facts, society requires of the applicant for a marriage license less than of the applicant for an automobile driver's license, and much less than it asks of a man who is applying for a job sweeping the streets or hauling the garbage. Obviously we must not demand too much of the applicants for a marriage license, but surely it is not unreasonable to demand *something* of them. In most states of the Union, or more likely in all of them, anyone can get a marriage license if he is persistent and can find a partner. It is said that in times of old, parents had the power of life and death over their children and could make away with them or sell them into slavery. Atrocious! Nevertheless, parents *still* have the power of life and death over their children. Parents can neglect their young, and frequently do neglect them, so that they die of the results. We have in mind parents who are probably ruining a child by refusing to have him circumcised; another parent who will not permit a child's tonsils to be removed, though they need removal badly; another parent denied a child antitoxin and the child died. Other parents are condemning their children to slavery to vicious habits, or to physical defects that could be corrected, or to modes of living that will make their lives miserable. The parent *still has the power of life and death over his children,* and for this reason should be a person who can and will administer such power wisely.

In consideration of the great importance to society and to the individual it seems as if the schools would have worked out a method long before this time of imparting instruction that would really "help solve the problems of life." Children are taught nearly everything except what might be expected to help them support or care for a home and a family. In recent years girls are being taught domestic science—which is the most important of all sciences—but many such courses are quite impractical. Biology courses can, and occasionally do, give a valuable insight into the problems of life. As a rule, however, they are as barren of living relations as is the Sahara.

The family is the real unit of society; the home is the place where the unit lives, and marriage is the bond which holds the family together until the task is really finished. A community of good homes is one with good schools and churches, flourishing business enterprises, and loyal community interest. The teachers have little trouble at school; and policemen patrol the district only to protect it; there are no riots, no antisocial manifestations, no need of the strong arm of the law. A community of vicious or wretched homes, on the contrary, is a constant menace to every good thing. All the policemen, all the teachers, all the jails, all the hospitals, all the correctional institutions in the world will not be able to undo the ills that are bred in those ugly homes. It is impossible to purify a stream by planting flowers along its banks and leaving the source foul. Likewise, society can never rise higher than its source—the family in the home.

Society is compelled in various ways to try to assume the relations which should have been assumed by the parents. But so often the parents will not, or cannot, or do not accept their responsibilities, and in such cases organized society can do no less than to attempt to palliate the evil. We go to great expense to stand *in loco parentis* for these children who are obviously unfit for the problems to be met in modern life. There is nothing else to do about it. We have permitted these people to be born and to be abused; now we must take care of them. It seems that at present they are rather rapidly increasing, and society is assuming more and more responsibility for them. All of which costs money and much money.

The ultimate purpose of marriage is superior children. Legal marriage gives these children a name; it gives them property rights; it gives them citizenship; it establishes their legal status; it places the protection of the state about their home where they may be born and reared in security. In addition to these legal bonds there should be other bonds which hold father, mother, and child in a tight and compact unit. Any relation which will strengthen that bond is of the greatest possible consequence, while any relation which endangers the bond is pregnant with dire results for the individual and for society at large.

An ideal family is like nothing so much as a beautiful flower. There is present in each a male or father element and a female or mother element. Beautiful in design, arrangement, color, and fragrance, the parts of the flower act together as a unit for the production and preservation of seeds—children—until they have attained such a degree of maturity that they may be safely entrusted to the dangers of the outside environment. By such means the perpetuity of the species is insured so long as the flower shall continue to exercise its primary function—the production of seeds—the rearing of children.

ABNORMALITIES OF SEXUAL FUNCTION

In spite of the teaching which we have received to the contrary, the individual with normal emotions and sensibilities regards his (or her) sex as the core of his (or her) personality; he looks upon this thing as being the most intimately personal of all his attributes. For this reason any deviation of sex from normal as seen in others or as experienced in self is sure to make a profound impression and to arouse most unpleasant emotions.

MASTURBATION

Masturbation is admittedly an ugly habit. Millions of people claim to believe that it causes insanity, feeble-mindedness, epilepsy, loss of virility, pimples, specks before the eyes, and a dozen other symptoms which are more or less terrible. As a matter of fact, it does nothing of the sort. A great many wild animals practice some form or another of self-sexual stimulation (auto-eroticism). At some time in life nearly all men and boys have practised this form of self-gratification, and likewise a great many women and girls. If it were really a cause of insanity there would be mighty few sane persons. It is likely that the reason so many people so vehemently deny ever having practised masturbation is because they really have done so and are so thoroughly ashamed of it.

The bad effects of masturbation are the indirect results of the act and of the attempt on the part of the elders to stamp out the practice. Children are shamed, they are whipped, they are spied upon, they are threatened with insanity and all sorts of dire consequences, they are led to believe that they are lower than the dirt, and, as a result of these clumsy attempts at correction, they really are injured. The constant reminder of these awful consequences keeps the child thinking about what it is much better to forget.

When children are taught early that the reproductive organs are clean and wholesome; that sex is something that has a great and beautiful usefulness; that it is something to be kept unspoiled for the future, and that it serves a purpose that is all but sacred; when children are kept busy with wholesome play and work and planning, and when they are loved and understood in matters such as these, there will possibly be a little masturbation, but inasmuch as that little will be speedily forgotten there will be no harm done. Be sure the children are healthily tired when they go to bed. Be sure that there is no need of circumcision, or if there is that it is corrected. Be sure the organs are clean so that they will not be irritated by foul secretions. Be sure that tight underwear does not demand constant pulling at the clothing.

Excessive masturbation is, of course, injurious in itself, but is rarely seen except in the mentally defective or in those who are driven too much into themselves. It is usually the *product of* rather than the cause of mental deficiency.

Persons who are extremely restless because of urgent sexual desire may possibly be more injured by the racking and the loss of sleep than by the act that will permit them to obtain relief. Husbands or wives who make excessive demands on their mates might well practise masturbation rather than wreck their home life by insisting upon their rights. As the potent male rather regularly has seminal emissions if he has no other sexual outlet, it is evident that masturbation becomes merely a waking instead of a dreaming activity. Physiologically, its effect, when not in excess, is no greater than emissions, which are obviously merely an overflow. Psychologically, the effect is nil, bad, or extremely bad, according as no, some, or much attention is paid to it.

EXCESSIVE SEXUALITY

A dangerous form of sexual abnormality is that which puts excessive emphasis on the subject. The male of this type is sometimes referred to as being a satyr. The damage which such a person can do is incalculable. He spreads venereal disease, he seduces wives and maids, he becomes the father of illegitimate children, he may commit rape or other crimes of sexual violence. No woman or girl is safe while he is about.

When the female displays excessive sexuality she is known as a nymphomaniac. The nymphomaniac is not to be confused with the normal individual who quite properly desires a relation that is legitimate. The term would, of course, have different meanings in different communities and in different times, inasmuch as in some places and times any woman desiring sexual relations would be considered such. In case the individual seems utterly unable to control the urge and exposes herself in a wanton manner she should be subjected to thorough medical examination. It is possible that there is local irritation of the genital organs or some internal glandular disturbance that may be corrected. Proper sex education of little girls will probably be of aid in preventing cases which are not on a pathologic basis. Dissatisfaction with existing marriage relations may be a cause that can occasionally be corrected. Incarceration may become necessary when other means fail.

SEXUAL FRIGIDITY

At the opposite extreme are those women, many of them married, who either have no desire for sexual experience, or are even definitely adverse to it. In times past this has frequently been accounted as a virtue, but with a fuller understanding of the subject it is recognized both as a personal tragedy and a cause of serious difficulties in the family.

There are many causes of this condition, which is commonly called *frigidity*. In the first place, the instruction which many girls receive from their mothers is such as would produce in them an intense distrust of the male of the species, and would repulse any normal instinct with regard to sex. The mother often deliberately teaches the daughter to take this attitude, doubtless thinking that she is protecting the girl from temptation. She does not realize that she may be preparing the daughter for an unhappy marriage. The girl whose father has been crude and repellent is quite likely to develop in an unnatural way as a result of the harsh treatment he has shown his wife and children.

Probably the commonest cause of frigidity is lack of preparation for marriage on the part of inexperienced girls. Awkward bridegrooms thinking that inasmuch as marriage has taken place there were no further reasons for gentlemanly restraint, have frightened, shocked, shamed, and even injured their brides at a time when the destiny of the marriage was in the balance. With such a start, and with the same act repeated as often as the new husband is able or may wish, the wife is set strongly against the whole program and is likely to develop into a woman who has the most intense disgust for anything of a sexual nature. It is extremely important that wooing should continue until the conventionally married couple are really ready for biological marriage. When this is done and patience is practised—when the bride is shown the same deference as the fiancée—

there will be very few women who will fail to develop a strong desire for the conjugal embrace.

Another common cause of frigidity is fear of conception. Wives may have ever so many excellent reasons why they do not desire children at a given time. Frequently most or all of the responsibility for the prevention of conception is placed upon them. They dread the long months of pregnancy with their pain, nausea, dragging discomfort, and danger. Frequently there have already been more children than is best for the welfare of the family or the mother. Under such circumstances the wife is under the constant dread of another conception and as a result wishes to avoid every possibility of such a happening. In a similar relation is the woman who has reason to believe that her husband is unfaithful to her. She resents the fact and fears the possibility of venereal disease which he may have contracted.

Sometimes religion, sometimes training, or lack of it, sometimes abnormality of the organs, sometimes a disproportion between the organs of the two mates, sometimes psychological incompatibility between the two may be responsible. Whatever the cause, it is pretty certain that a couple will be unhappy if the wife is frigid. If there are children the couple may hang together but furnish the children a decidedly bad environment; if there are no children divorce or separation is nearly inevitable. Not only does a satisfactory relation pay large dividends in personal enjoyment, but it enables couples to form a strong and stable marriage which will insure that their children have a good home until they are old enough to take care of themselves.

SEXUAL COMPLEXES

An interesting relation is that which is known as the Œdipus complex. It is seen when there is an unusual attachment between father and daughter or mother and son. This does not mean an improper relation. As a matter of fact, these children are often cited as being particularly praiseworthy. These excessive attachments may do serious harm to the exemplary young men and women who are so unfortunate as to get caught in their mesh. Parents—particularly parents of a single child—should watch for this trap into which an adoring child may be lured. Particularly if the father lives alone with the daughter or the mother with a son there is danger. Likewise there is danger if the child resembles in appearance and character the dead parent.

Much has been said concerning repressions of various sorts, and of sexual repressions in particular. Some have seen fit to follow blindly the teachings of Freud and to see in every sort of dream, in every sort of twist in character, and in nearly every sort of mental deviation a tangle of repressions which are basically sexual. There is no doubt that there is much truth in the theory which has been developed, but it is quite certain that the whole thing has been grossly overdrawn. Some have even advised that one should not attempt to control or repress the impulses that arise for the reason that terrible complexes may develop if such is done. This position is, of course, quite impossible since society could not exist if everyone simply followed any urge that he might feel. On the other hand, it is a fact that spinsters, bachelors, and persons who have been disappointed in love or have strongly loved someone under conditions which made it necessary to conceal the feeling are very subject to all sorts of disturbances which may seriously undermine the body and mind.

Extremely important is the matter of suggestion or of direct teaching of irregular practices. A child who has wrong ideas about such matters can ruin a school or a neighborhood. Children who have never had filled the vacuum in their minds regarding sex are easily led into almost any sort of abuse of the sexual apparatus, and irreparable damage may be done in a short space of time. Children who have had adequate sex instruction will be far less attracted to perverted persons and also much less likely to follow improper suggestions. As in every other instance, we can best overcome evil with good. *Disgusting practices are in most instances more directly to be charged to the parents who failed to instruct the child than they are to be held against the unfortunate victim of distorted perspective in these matters.*

The Hygiene of the Reproductive System

A fine watch does best when it is meddled with least. The same is true of any complicated mechanism and in particular of the generative apparatus. A policy of "hands off" is hard to beat in this connection. There are, to be sure, elemental points in the care of the organs which should be understood by everyone, but further than this the layman should not go. There has been so much ignorance and misinformation concerning the sexual apparatus that the layman may hardly trust anything that he has learned from the usual sources. When there is reason to believe that something is really wrong, the family physician or a specialist whom he may designate should be consulted at once. It surely is needless to say that the physician should be furnished with a full and frank history of the ailment and its possible causes. Furthermore, he must be permitted to make such examinations as he thinks necessary.

CLEANLINESS

The first principle to be considered in the hygiene of the reproductive system is cleanliness. By this we do not mean to imply that lack of cleanliness will often jeopardize the physical health of the individual. Actually there is more danger that meddlesome methods of attaining cleanliness will cause disease than that lack of cleanliness will cause it. This is particularly true in the case of the female. But there is more to this matter of hygiene than mere maintenance of health. The reproductive organs must be clean; they must be free of odor; they must be wholesome; they must not offend. They are so exceedingly important to the welfare of the race, the self-respect of the individual, and the happiness of family, and yet they are so likely to be regarded as being vulgar by those who do not understand that there must not be any question whatever about them.

Odor is undoubtedly of first consideration. The fact that we wear clothing complicates the matter for the good reason that the clothing does not permit the free ventilation that would carry away odors before they become concentrated and would permit the rapid evaporation of perspiration. Clothing should be as light and as well ventilated as comfort will permit. Great improvement in underwear has been made in recent years. Undergarments should be changed as often as one's finances will permit and should of course never be worn after they are definitely soiled. Night clothing should entirely replace the underwear that has been worn through the day. This will give opportunity for airing and drying of the various garments which would be most likely to offend.

Frequent washing of the external genitalia is of course extremely important. It is the *external* organs that need washing and not the internal. Much harm has undoubtedly been done by the use of antiseptic or even cleansing douches as many women use them. In the first place they are not necessary from the standpoint of preventing odors for the good reason that the odors of the vagina proper are practically never concentrated enough to cause trouble if the external organs are clean. The normal vagina nearly always contains great numbers of germs which are known as Döderlein's bacilli. These germs are not only harmless, but actually beneficial, because they prevent the growth of other germs which can really cause trouble. Incidentally these germs are closely related to, or by some are considered to be identified with, the germs that are deliberately put into acidophilus milk which is much used for restoring healthy conditions in the bowels. There is not a bit of doubt that Döderlein's bacillus is of positive value in the vagina. If it is frequently washed away with cleansing douches or inhibited with antiseptics, abnormal conditions develop in the vagina, and real trouble may ensue. Furthermore, strong antiseptics frequently irritate the mucous membrane and make it more susceptible to invasion by other bacteria. Not a few of the commonly used douches are definitely irritating or even poisonous when used in too concentrated form or when used frequently. This is particularly true of bichloride of mercury and lysol.

Sometimes, particularly in the male, it is impossible to hold down odors merely by washing the external genitalia. In some individuals the foreskin is so tight about the end of the penis that it cannot be retracted and the groove beneath it cleaned of the white secretion—known as smegma—which accumulates there. This secretion is of an oily nature and easily becomes rancid, producing exceedingly bad odors and also irritation of the mucous membrane. At the time of birth every male child should be carefully examined to determine whether or not he is in need of circumcision which consists in removing the foreskin. When done in the early days of life the operation is a trivial one. Later it is somewhat more serious, but never dangerous when performed by a competent surgeon. Even those individuals who are not in need of circumcision should retract the foreskin and clean the groove beneath it carefully at least once a day. A child in need of circumcision is often made nervous by the irritation of the rancid secretions and will be constantly twisting, squirming, and pulling at himself. He may also develop the habit of masturbation as a result of the irritation which induces him to handle his penis. We do not advocate that all boys and men should be circumcised, but are emphatic in recommending such treatment when there is difficulty in keeping the parts clean otherwise. Girls are also occasionally in need of circumcision, or what is essentially the same thing.

Occasionally discharges of various sorts from the genital organs will greatly complicate the habit of cleanliness. In *every* case in either sex the cause of any discharge should be ascertained if possible. The family physician or a reliable specialist should be consulted, *always*. *Never* should patent medicines or home remedies be used as a substitute for careful examination and treatment by a physician. *Never* must the patient go to an advertising physician or to one who is known or suspected to be a quack. In case the discharge can be cured and the cause removed the problem is solved. When the condition cannot be corrected, the greatest of care will be needed to prevent offensive odors and a disgusting local condition.

MENSTRUATION

The peculiar demands of menstruation call for attention in a discussion of hygiene. There is first to be considered the necessity of caring for the actual physical needs. During this period the pelvic organs of the female are considerably congested, and for this reason are more subject to infection and circulatory disturbances. It is for this reason that excessively long hours of standing on the feet, dancing, strenuous athletics, and similar activities are not advisable for many women. Likewise sexual excitement will intensify the effect, and may cause trouble. Bathing was formerly interdicted, but is now permitted in most cases if the water is warm. There is, of course, additional need of cleanliness at such a time, and local bathing is always perfectly safe. There are many women and girls who can even swim in cold water while menstruating, but such chilling of the skin is nearly sure to drive the blood inward and increase the internal congestion or cause severe cramping.

In case the menstrual periods should cease in a girl or woman who is probably not pregnant, careful physical examination should be made to determine the cause. In earlier times this cessation was supposed to cause tuberculosis. Now we understand that in most such cases tuberculosis is already present and the checking of this drain is a means by which Nature seeks to conserve the patient's strength. Patients with anemia of any sort or those with nervous disturbances are also likely to cease menstruating until they are restored to their normal condition. Of great importance is the mental attitude of the woman toward her menstrual periods, and toward the "change of life," at which time the periods gradually cease from natural causes. In times past girls were literally taught to make invalids of themselves, and women were led to believe that "the change" was something greatly to be dreaded and a time of danger. We understand now that menstruation is a perfectly normal process, and that the menopause need cause little apprehension if it is approached with understanding and poise. The fact that women are now so much less embarrassed in visiting a physician about such matters has opened a way of escape from many of the dangers and discomforts. The frank consideration of all subjects relative to sex and the far more natural attitude toward them has in large measure taken them out of the limbo to which they were formerly assigned.

With so much advertising of absorbent pads and other aids to feminine hygiene it is hardly necessary to describe in detail the means by which women may avoid the soiling of their clothing with the menstrual discharges. As stated elsewhere, young girls should have these matters explained before they are twelve years of age, or by the time they are ten or eleven if they are somewhat precocious in their development. It is important that the girl be taught so that she will not be frightened by the first appearance but will come to her mother for aid and advice. This is, of course, an excellent opportunity for the mother to explain something of the nature and purpose of the genital organs and to impress the girl with the value of the process of which the menstrual cycle is a part.

DISEASES OF THE GENITAL ORGANS

There are various serious diseases of the genital organs which need to be understood so that they may be detected at the earliest possible moment. We shall not describe the venereal diseases in this place, as they will be discussed in a later chapter. Various other chronic inflammations and injuries resulting from childbirth or injury usually manifest themselves by symptoms or pain of some sort. Of greatest importance are the various forms of cancer which may be found. Unfortunately cancers are not painful in their earlier stages. To be sure, they are terribly painful later, and this fact may mislead persons who are really in danger and will not believe that they are so because they are not in pain.

At the present time about one woman in seven above the age of forty years is dying of cancer of one kind or another. About one third of these cancers are of the womb, usually the mouth of the womb. We shall not attempt to give such a description as will enable the layman to make an unerring diagnosis of cancer of the womb, but merely call attention to the fact that any sort of unnatural bleeding from the privates should be investigated thoroughly. Excessive bleeding, bleeding after the change of life, continuous bleeding, or the passing of clotted blood, constitute "unnatural" bleeding. These signs do not mean that a given person surely has cancer, but they do mean that there is something wrong, and that a thorough examination is needed. The physician should be required to prove that it is not cancer before the investigation is ended. Once the diagnosis of cancer is made, treatment in the hands of a reliable surgeon is the only hope. It is believed that unrepaired tears of the mouth of the womb may be the cause of cancer in many instances, since they cause long continued irritation. The wearing of a pessary for long periods of time may also serve in this way.

Another third of all deaths from cancer among women is from cancer of the breast. These growths are always small before they are large, always localized before they are generalized, and always painless before they are painful. The growth usually manifests itself as a lump or nodule in the breast, or sometimes as a thick place in the skin reminding one of a piece of bacon rind. It is usually irregular in shape, attached to the skin and deeper tissues, and solitary in number in the earlier stages at least. As the breast is moved the nodules cause dimpling. If near the nipple, they commonly cause the nipple to be drawn in. The chances for recovery are good if the diagnosis is made early and the appropriate treatment begun at once. If surgical treatment is delayed, the operation is much more severe, and there is less chance of cure. Rarely cancer of the breast is seen in the male.

Cancer of the prostate and bladder are fairly common in the male. The earliest symptom is usually blood in the urine or difficulty in emptying the bladder. These symptoms should call for an immediate examination to determine the cause.

The reproductive system of the female is much more complicated than that of the male and is for this reason more subject to disease and injury. It furthermore is under far greater stress in the performance of its function of childbearing. For this reason care must be taken to avoid as many as possible of the dangers which beset the sexual life. In the first place, women—and men, too, for that matter— should not marry unless they are reasonably sure that they are free from disease and deformity. Women who have suffered from rickets as children should make sure that the pelvic opening is large enough to permit the passage of a child at the time of birth. In recent years it has been possible for such women to bear children by submitting to Cæsarean section, but even in such case it is better if the obstetrician knows beforehand that the child cannot pass through the birth canal. Women who have reason to believe that they are suffering from active or recently arrested tuberculosis should refrain from childbearing both for their own sake and for the sake of the child.

We believe there is no legitimate excuse for an intelligent woman to go into maternity without informing herself thoroughly concerning the risks and the means of reducing those risks to the minimum. Certainly there is no excuse for delay after she finds herself actually pregnant. She should consult her family physician or the specialist of her choice as soon as she becomes aware of her condition. If the pregnancy is the first, there is additional reason for such professional care. Likewise the women beyond the age usual for childbearing and those who have reason to believe that they may have weak hearts and kidneys should take extra precaution.

SEXUAL INTERCOURSE IN PREGNANCY

Many couples wonder if sexual intercourse may be indulged during the period of pregnancy. This will depend upon several factors. Certainly it should not if there is a feeling that the act is degrading during this time. Likewise it may only be practised when both mates desire it. There is good reason from the standpoint of the possibility of infection for refraining during the last few weeks of the pregnancy. In case the wife seems to have been injured by marital relations on previous occasions, or if she is one who is easily aborted, continence is the only safe rule. In those instances—and they are many—in which the wife desires the relation at this time and does not seem to be injured by it there is no real objection. The fear that the child may be injured is quite without foundation except in those women who are easily aborted. Unfortunately we must take into consideration the fact that many husbands might seek other mistresses if they were required to refrain from sexual relations at home. The danger of venereal disease in such case is probably greater than the danger of injury to the wife as a result of intercourse, provided the wife is not definitely pathological.

CONTRACEPTIVES

Strange as it may seem at first thought, there is often more danger in attempting to prevent conception than in going through with the pregnancy. Several of the contraceptive measures are definitely hazardous. Contraceptive devices and their dangers may be roughly classified as follows:

1. *Antiseptic douches used after the sexual act.*

If these douches are irritating or poisonous, or if they disturb the normal bacterial growth of the vagina, we are sure that they may do harm. Bichloride of mercury and lysol are particularly to be feared. All such means are frequently ineffective.

2. *Vaginal suppositories or injections containing organic acids or substances which kill the spermatozoa.*

These are probably not often dangerous. They are frequently put up in a cocoa-butter base, and there is some objection to oily applications to mucous membranes. These methods are by no means surely effective.

3. *Pessaries of some sort are much used.*

Pessaries that are left in position for long periods of time are always irritating and may cause serious trouble. They may cause infection, or the chronic irritation resulting from their use may possibly lead to cancer. Those that are inserted at the time are a nuisance and likely to be regarded with considerable distaste.

4. *Rubber devices to hold the semen from contact with the womb.*

These devices considerably diminish normal sensation and are unpleasant to use. They are likely to cause dissatisfaction and incompleteness of the act, which may in turn have a bad effect upon the nervous system.

5. *Incomplete act of coitus.*

This method of preventing conception is nearly sure to cause dissatisfaction with the marital state if it is used habitually The method is not very effectual in many instances.

6. *Sterilization by surgical means.*

In the instance of those who have very good reasons for not having children, or of those who are adjudged by society as being unfit for propagation, this method is excellent. Sterilization does not unsex the individual. He or she can still indulge in sexual relations with pleasure.

ᅠ

7. *Continence*.

The prevention of conception by refraining from the sexual act is recommended for all *unmarried* lovers. It is, however, a somewhat dangerous means in the instance of married couples unless there is mutual agreement concerning it. Most couples practise continence or some of the less drastic forms of contraception during the period in the menstrual cycle when conception is most likely to occur. These methods have much to commend them.

ABORTION

In many instances when contraceptive measures have failed, criminal abortion is practised. This is always a more or less dangerous procedure. When done even under the most careful conditions it is still dangerous, because Nature revolts strongly against such practices. In addition to the physical danger there is also the mental side to be considered. Maternal nature receives a severe shock when scheming villains undertake the deliberate death of the child which by all rules should be the joy of the mother's heart. When abortion is done by ignorant persons under urgent necessity of concealing the act and not quite free to call the physician as needed it is exceedingly dangerous and often ends fatally for the mother as well as the child.

SEXUAL STIMULATION

The health of the reproductive system can be injured also by various attempts to stimulate the sexual function. The elderly or weakly man attempts to boost his waning powers by some sort or other of gland therapy. The eating of the testicles of castrated animals, the taking of tablets purported to contain dried testicle of slaughtered animals, the transplantation of monkey, or even human, glands is familiar pseudoscience in recent years. The effects are transient if they exist at all, and it is quite likely that they are entirely psychological. Even if there were a definite increase in sexual power, it is likely that the operation would be dangerous to the degree that it was effective. Old men's bodies are not able to stand the strain of highly active glands. The use of drugs which are supposed to stimulate sexual desire is another dangerous mirage. Cantharides (Spanish fly) is particularly dangerous and must *never* be used for this purpose, as it is an intense kidney irritant. Furthermore, it is not able to do the things which popular tradition claims for it.

Of the utmost importance in sexual hygiene is temperance in the exercise of the various functions. It is doubtful if there is a more disgusting creature than the sexual glutton. On the other hand, the individual who does not permit, or cannot enjoy, the reasonable use of the reproductive system, misses the really biggest thing in life. The man or woman who has short-circuited the reproductive act and so has escaped the responsibilities of parenthood has cheated himself of the high points of existence.

CHAPTER VI

Care of Mothers before and after Childbirth
J. P. GREENHILL, M.D.

INTRODUCTION

IN PREVIOUS GENERATIONS *the woman who was about to bear a child kept the matter a secret, even from her husband, until well along in the course of the event. As the time approached when the child was to be born, she would notify the physician. In many instances, however, even this did not occur, but the doctor was called posthaste at the moment of childbirth. Then, in the home, with the aid of a neighbor or a relative, the child would be brought into the community.*

The advances of scientific medicine have greatly changed our points of view in relationship to what is proper in childbirth. Nowadays the intelligent woman may consult her physician even before proceeding with the idea of having a child. She finds out whether or not her health is such as to permit her to have a child without seriously injuring herself and without danger to the prospective child. When the physician's examination has revealed that her condition is satisfactory she may proceed.

Nowadays the intelligent woman consults her physician also as soon as she realizes that she is pregnant. He then examines her again to make certain of the diagnosis. This he confirms by various tests in the laboratory as well as by physical examination of the patient herself. During this period her life must be regulated according to her condition. It is important to control her diet, her exercise, her rest, her work, and every other factor of her existence. Examinations are regularly made of her excretions in order to determine whether or not the organs are functioning satisfactorily.

Such prenatal care in childbirth is of the utmost importance for lowering the death rates associated with this condition, and also for bringing into the world healthy and normal children.

M. F.

147

More than twenty thousand women lose their lives in the United States each year as the direct or indirect result of childbirth. Most of these deaths are preventable, and a good deal of the blame may be attributed to the unfortunate women themselves. Because of ignorance, negligence, territorial inaccessibility, financial distress, or other reasons, thousands of women in this country fail to be examined by a physician while they are pregnant. These women do not call in expert aid until the child is actually ready to be born. Since more than half of the total deaths from childbirth may be prevented by proper care before the baby arrives, every woman who is to have a baby should visit a doctor long before the expected date of confinement. Not only will the lives of thousands of mothers be saved, but countless other women will be spared temporary or permanent invalidism. Furthermore many thousand babies will be born alive who would certainly perish in the absence of prenatal observation. The care which a woman receives before the baby arrives is known as prenatal or antenatal care. In contradistinction to this is the care after the child is born, and this is spoken of as postpartum or postnatal care.

Really a confinement case begins at the time of conception. Hence the woman should consult a physician as soon as she believes she is going to have a baby. The ideal arrangement would be for a woman to have a thorough examination before she decides to have a child, because not infrequently abnormalities are found which, unless corrected, may make childbearing a hazardous undertaking. Occasionally a disturbance is found such as serious heart, kidney, or lung trouble, which absolutely precludes pregnancy. A woman should know this before she conceives. Then she should seek a physician who has a sympathetic nature and one in whom she can have utmost confidence. Faith in the doctor is important to allay the fears which young prospective mothers frequently have. Advice should be sought from the physician and not from well-meaning but misinformed friends and relatives, many of whom instill fear rather than dispel it.

If a woman cannot afford the services of a specialist in obstetrics or an experienced general practitioner, she should visit one of the numerous prenatal clinics to be found in every large city and in many small ones.

SIGNS OF PREGNANCY

A woman may suspect she is to become a mother in a number of ways. The most important sign is absence of the monthly flow, especially in a young woman who has usually had regular monthly periods. A second significant sign is morning sickness or nausea and vomiting. Frequently the breasts feel full, they are tender to the touch, and they have peculiar sensations such as tingling or throbbing. The skin around the nipples becomes darker in color, especially in brunettes. Another sign is a desire to pass urine at frequent intervals. Not one of these symptoms by itself indicates pregnancy, but a combination of two or more is presumptive evidence that a baby may be expected. A woman does not usually feel the baby move around until the sixteenth or eighteenth week of the baby's development. At this time the abdomen is usually enlarged sufficiently to verify the suspicion of a pregnancy, and a physician can feel the baby and hear its heart beat. After the fifth month a baby or at least parts of it may be shown on X-ray pictures.

VISIT TO PHYSICIAN

When an expectant mother visits the doctor the first time, he will take a complete family history and make a thorough examination. The latter includes not only external and internal investigation of the organs directly associated with childbearing and the measurements of the bones, but also an examination of the teeth, thyroid, breasts, nipples, legs, arms, and other organs. The blood pressure and temperature should be taken, the urine examined for kidney and bladder complications, the weight recorded, and the blood studied for anemia, and in many cases also for syphilis. The latter social disease is found with sufficient frequency to warrant an almost routine Wassermann examination of the blood of pregnant women. This disease is not a stigma of immorality, for in about half the cases women acquire it innocently.

A woman should visit her doctor at least once every three weeks during the first seven months of pregnancy and at least once every two weeks thereafter. If abnormalities exist, the patient may have to see her physician more often. At each visit she should bring to the physician a three- or four-ounce bottle of urine obtained from the first urination of the day of the visit. The bottle should be carefully washed before it is used, because its former contents may be the cause of false tests. Once a week it is advisable to measure the amount of urine passed in twenty-four hours. If there is a considerable reduction in the amount usually passed and the patient has been drinking the customary amount of fluids, this fact should be reported to the physician. It may indicate a disturbance of the kidneys. A label should be attached to the bottle giving the patient's name, the date the specimen is collected, and in certain instances the amount of urine passed in twenty-four hours. If a specimen of urine is to be mailed to a doctor, a teaspoonful of chloroform should be added to the specimen before it is sent.

Serious Symptoms during Pregnancy

During each visit the doctor will ask the patient certain questions concerning her health and the baby and listen to any questions or complaints. He will usually inquire about the following symptoms: nausea, vomiting, swelling of the hands, feet, or face, headaches, constipation, dizziness, pain in the abdomen or legs, spots before the eyes or other visual disturbances, bleeding from the vagina, movements of the baby, shortness of breath, nervousness, and other symptoms. He will observe the patient's blood pressure, the pulse rate, abnormal swellings, excessive gain or loss in weight, and the results of the examination of the urine. It is not necessary to be examined internally at each visit, but at least one examination should be made in addition to the first one, and this preferably about four weeks before the expected date of confinement.

Estimating the Day of Birth

It is impossible to predict accurately the day when a baby is to arrive. However, the approximate date can be estimated in a number of ways.

1. Add seven days to the first day of the last monthly flow and subtract three months. Thus if the last menstrual period began July 10th, add seven days, giving July 17th, and subtract three months, which gives April 17th as the approximate day labor may be expected. In most cases the confinement will take place within a few days before or after this calculated date.

2. A woman having her first baby may add twenty-two weeks to the

day she first feels the baby move. A woman who has already borne children should add twenty-four weeks.

3. If the exact day of conception is known, 273 days added to this will give the approximate date of confinement.

4. By repeated examinations, a physician can usually tell within a few days when a baby will be born.

THE DIET

The child in the womb depends on its mother for its supply of food. The nourishment is not given to the child directly, because there is no direct connection between the mother and her child. The latter lies in a sac filled with fluid which permits the child to move about freely. In one part of this sac is an organ known as the placenta or afterbirth. This is made up of myriads of small projections known as villi, in each of which is a small blood vessel. These villi dip into a collection of the mother's blood, and it is the coverings of these villi which extract from the mother's blood the food which the child requires. The nourishment which the villi take up is transported from the small blood vessels in the villi to large blood vessels which pass through a tube connecting the afterbirth with the child. This tube is known as the umbilical cord, and it usually contains one vein and two arteries. The vein carries fresh blood containing nourishment to the child, whereas the arteries carry blood containing waste products from the baby to the afterbirth. This impure blood is transmitted from the afterbirth to the mother's blood, and the mother purifies this blood in the same way she cleanses her own blood, namely, by eliminating the waste products through her bowels, kidneys, lungs, and skin.

Since the connection between the mother and the child is as intimate as just mentioned, it is obvious that the child's development depends to a large extent upon the mother's diet. The child's growth is not entirely dependent on the mother's food intake, because if the diet is lacking in certain substances which the child requires, these substances in many instances will be extracted from the mother's tissues, usually to her detriment. A common example of this is the loosening and decay of the mother's teeth during pregnancy, due to the fact that the mother does not eat enough calcium and phosphorus to supply the growing child. Hence it is important that the mother's diet contain both the proper quantity and quality of food each day to supply all the demands of the fetus.

Not only is the mother's diet important for the baby, but it is important also for her own benefit. In order to avoid trouble there should be certain additions and restrictions to the diet the expectant mother has usually followed. As a general rule it may be said that the expectant mother should eat a well-rounded diet, just as she eats in the non-pregnant state, except that she should drink plenty of milk, eat more fresh fruits and vegetables, and less meat, fish, eggs, and condiments. A woman should not make the serious mistake of overeating because she believes she must eat for two individuals. The excess food is not transferred to the baby but is stored in the mother. This may lead to serious consequences, not the least of which is difficulty in giving birth to the baby. However, women should not starve themselves in an attempt to keep down the weight of the baby, because the weight of a newborn baby is not dependent entirely or even in great part on the amount of food its mother eats. The food should, of course, be chewed thoroughly and slowly.

A proper diet during pregnancy contains the following:

1. *Water*, which serves many functions. At least eight or ten glasses of liquids a day in one form or another should be taken.

2. *Proteins*, which build and repair the tissues of the body. These are found chiefly in meat, eggs, milk and milk products, and such vegetables as peas and beans.

3. *Fats*, which furnish fuel for heat and energy. These are found in cream, butter, cheese, oils, and fat meats.

4. *Carbohydrates* or *starches*, which also supply fuel. They are found chiefly in sweets, sugar, bread, potatoes, cereals, milk, and rice.

5. *Minerals*, which are the most important substances for the growth of the bones and teeth. They also increase resistance to disease, and they keep the blood in good condition. They are found especially in milk, certain fruits, and most vegetables. If vegetables are cooked, the water should not be thrown away but should be used for soup. The chief minerals necessary during pregnancy are calcium, phosphorus, and iron.

6. *Vitamins*, which regulate the growth of the body and in some instances prevent miscarriages. They are found in milk, eggs, meat, whole wheat, fruits, vegetables, cod-liver oil, viosterol, and halibut-liver oil. In the winter months cod-liver oil takes the place of sunshine.

7. *Iodine* in certain regions of the country is necessary to prevent the formation of a goiter in the mother and the child. It is found chiefly

in such sea food as oysters and salmon. Iodized salt or iodine tablets may be used, but only under the direction of a physician.

It will be observed that milk is the ideal food because it contains water, proteins, fat (in the cream), sugar, minerals, and vitamins. It is easily digested in all its forms (sweet, sour, or buttermilk). At least a pint of milk should therefore be taken every day not only throughout pregnancy but also after the baby comes as long as the baby is nursed at the breast.

In some cases pregnant women have a strong desire for unusual foods out of season or odd things. Chief among these are pickles, highly seasoned foods, and chalk (calcium). This perversion of appetite is known as "pica," and unless these foods disagree with the mother, they may be indulged in.

It is best for the expectant mother to avoid alcohol altogether or to restrict its use to a small amount. It is likewise advisable to limit the number of cigarettes smoked to a maximum of four a day.

SPECIAL DIETS

During the first three months of pregnancy at least 50 per cent of all women suffer from nausea or vomiting or both. These women should not attempt to eat the usual three meals a day but should take small amounts of solid food, especially starches and sweets, every two or two and a half hours. If part or all of the food is vomited, more solid food should be eaten immediately. Water should not be taken with these meals but between them. The following diet may prove useful:

Before getting out of bed:
  Crackers or dry toast.
One half-hour later breakfast consisting of the following:
  Orange, grapefruit, stewed prunes or apricots.
  Cereal with cream and sugar.
  One soft-boiled egg.
  Thin buttered toast (with unsalted butter).
  Milk, cocoa, weak tea or coffee with sugar.
10:00 a.m.:
  Glass of milk with crackers (graham, nabisco, oatmeal, etc.).
Lunch:
  Cup of cream of celery, asparagus, spinach or potato soup.
  Soup crackers.

Salad of lettuce, tomato, endive, etc., with sugar and few drops of lemon.

Whole-wheat bread, or toast, buttered.

Ice cream, water ice, or custard.

4:00 p.m.:

Milk, cocoa, chocolate or weak tea.

Small piece of cake, crackers, or wafers.

Dinner:

Cup of bouillon or vegetable soup, especially tomato.

Soup crackers.

Small lamb chop, broiled steak, or veal chop, well done.

Baked potato, mashed potatoes, or carrots.

Thin bread, or toast, buttered.

Lettuce or tomato salad.

Ice cream or water ice.

At bedtime:

Glass of hot milk, chocolate or malted milk.

Graham or oatmeal crackers.

The nausea and vomiting usually cease spontaneously after the fourth month, and from this time on the following diet is recommended:

Breakfast:

Fruit, such as orange, grapefruit, stewed prunes, or baked apple.

Cereal with cream and sugar.

One boiled or poached egg.

Two slices of crisp bacon.

Buttered toast, roll, or corn muffin.

Cup of cocoa, chocolate, weak tea, or coffee, with sugar and cream.

10:00 a.m.:

Glass of milk.

Fresh fruit or fruit juice.

Lunch:

Cream of celery, tomato, or asparagus soup.

Crackers or wafers.

Baked potato with butter.

Lettuce or tomato salad with sugar and small amount of lemon juice.

Ice cream or blanc mange.

4:00 p.m.:

American or cream cheese sandwich.

Glass of milk or malted milk.

Dinner:
  Celery, pea, spinach, or corn soup.
  Salt wafers.
  Small lamb chop, steak, or equivalent in fish.
  Mashed or baked potato, carrots, peas, beet tops, or spinach.
  Lettuce, tomato, endive salad with sugar and lemon.
  Cheese and crackers or toast; nuts.
  Ice cream, jelly roll, plain cake or fruit.
  Cup of weak tea or coffee with cream and sugar.
At bedtime:
  Glass of hot milk or malted milk.
  Crackers.

If a woman finds that certain foods disagree with her, she should eliminate them from her diet for a while. If the distressing symptoms reappear when she resumes eating them, these foods should not be eaten for the remainder of the pregnancy. In general it is advisable to avoid highly seasoned, spiced, greasy, fried, or fatty foods, rich pies, pastries, and other desserts, too many sweets, strong condiments, alcohol, and strong coffee and tea. A woman who is underweight when she becomes pregnant may eat more than one who is overweight.

Most of the water should be taken on arising in the morning, between meals, and before retiring at night. On the day the twenty-four-hour specimen of urine is measured, the amount of water taken should also be recorded, and both of these figures should be given to the doctor.

CARE OF THE BOWELS

A pregnant woman should have at least one bowel movement every day, in order to eliminate not only her own waste products but also those of the baby in the womb. If the bowels are not emptied daily, poisons accumulate in the system, and an extra load is placed on the kidneys, which already have a great deal of important work to do during pregnancy. As a general rule, women have a strong tendency to be constipated while carrying a baby. Constipation is still more likely to occur in women who do not drink enough fluids and do not eat the proper kinds of food, and in those whose bowels did not move regularly before pregnancy supervened.

In order to prevent constipation as much as possible and also to overcome it when present, the following rules should be observed:

1. An abundance of water should be taken upon arising, during the day, and before going to bed.

2. Every day an attempt should be made to have a bowel movement at exactly the same hour. The best time for this is after breakfast, and one should have patience. However, there should not be too much straining. A glycerine suppository inserted into the rectum may stimulate the bowels to move.

3. The diet should contain a large amount of fresh fruits and vegetables. The fruits should include apples, apricots, cherries, figs, grapes, ripe olives, oranges, peaches, pears, pineapple, plums and prunes, raspberries and strawberries. The vegetables should include asparagus, beans, cabbage, carrots, celery, corn, lettuce, onions, peas, spinach, tomatoes, and watercress. Other foods which may help are bran, cereals, and bread. Tea should be avoided if there is marked constipation.

4. In some cases it may be necessary to inject four to six ounces of warm olive oil into the rectum before retiring. This is to remain overnight, and its purpose is to soften the stool, protect the lining of the rectum, and prevent or remove a spasm of the bowel.

5. If the above measures do not prevent or relieve constipation, drugs must be used. In nearly every case such simple substances as mineral oil (one tablespoonful night and morning), or milk of magnesia (one tablespoonful every night), usually suffice. In more stubborn cases it may be necessary to take a teaspoonful of fluid extract of cascara sagrada each night. An enema should be the last resort, and the fewer that are taken throughout pregnancy the better. The simplest enemas consist of weak salt solution or a very weak soapsuds solution.

CARE OF THE KIDNEYS IN PREGNANCY

The kidneys have an extra amount of work to do during pregnancy, and they frequently give rise to serious disturbances. If a woman knows she has or has had kidney trouble she should visit a physician before she plans to have a baby and let him tell her whether it is safe for her to bear a child. Women who have serious kidney disturbances, such as chronic nephritis, should not attempt to have children, because the kidney trouble will nearly always be aggravated, and the baby in many instances will not be born alive. However, if a woman has only a mild degree of nephritis she may go through a pregnancy without complications provided she is carefully watched by a competent physician.

Women with normal kidneys should have a specimen of urine examined at least once every three weeks, and towards the end of pregnancy more frequent examinations are advisable. However, women with kidney disturbances should have their urine examined at least once a week, and they should measure their urinary output every day. At least three pints of urine should be passed daily, and if the amount decreases the doctor should be informed.

If swelling of the feet, ankles, hands, or face is noticed, the doctor should be notified. Frequently these swellings indicate some abnormality in the function of the kidneys.

Chronic nephritis is not the only kind of kidney trouble which occurs during pregnancy. There may be a condition known as pyelitis, in which part of the kidney is inflamed and the urine contains pus and bacteria. Examination of the urine will also reveal whether diabetes or a tendency to diabetes is present.

TREATMENT OF KIDNEY COMPLICATIONS

If chronic nephritis is present it is necessary to curtail in the diet the amount of meat, fish, eggs, peas, beans, spices, and alcohol, but table salt should be eliminated almost entirely. In the majority of cases the blood pressure is high, hence this as well as the urine must be carefully controlled by the physician.

If pyelitis is present, it is necessary to drink as much water and fruit juices as possible and to follow the same diet as for nephritis. Other medication will be prescribed by the physician.

Women who have diabetes or a tendency to it must abstain from sweets and starchy foods. Naturally a woman with any kind of disturbance should be under the care of a physician.

CLOTHING IN PREGNANCY

The manner in which an expectant mother dresses herself is important. Comfort should not be sacrificed for the sake of appearances. In cold weather sufficient clothing should be worn to keep warm, whereas during the hot months the clothing should be light. In some regions it is important to be prepared for sudden changes in the weather in order to avoid chilling. Most of the clothing should be simple and should be washed frequently. None of it should hinder free movements of breathing or of the arms and legs. There must be no circular constrictions anywhere; hence it is important to give up using round garters, belts, tight corsets, or tight skirt bands. Round garters are the worst offenders, because they may result in varicose veins or swelling of the legs. Side elastics attached to a maternity corset are the proper type of garter.

Underclothing should always be worn, the kind and amount depending upon the weather. It may consist of one or two pieces, but it is best that the drawers be closed. The under-garments should be changed every day or as often as possible, because they absorb the waste matter eliminated by the skin. All clothing should be well aired at night.

Up to the end of the third and sometimes the fourth month the usual type of corset may generally be worn. After this time the customary type of corset compresses the abdomen and may lead to harm. Hence after the fourth month it is best to wear some type of maternity corset, the chief purpose of which is to support the growing womb. It is more important for a woman who has already had one or more children to use a maternity corset than for a woman who is going to have her first baby. The reason for this is that most women who have given birth have some weakness of the abdominal wall, and this requires support. Women who have a flabby abdominal wall must wear a proper maternity corset constantly, or they will have a good deal of discomfort, especially backache. On the other hand, some women carrying their first baby may be comfortable throughout pregnancy without a corset.

Most women must wear a support for the breasts, or the latter will be painful. This support should not be tightly applied, but should elevate the breasts.

Proper shoes are essential. The usual narrow, high-heeled shoes not only cause pain but are actually harmful. During the latter months of pregnancy the feet spread and enlarge somewhat, hence slightly larger shoes must be worn. Furthermore, as the abdomen continues to grow, there is a tendency to pull the body forward. To overcome this, the woman instinctively throws her shoulders back. If the woman wears high heels, the body is pushed still farther forward, and to save herself from falling she must throw her head and shoulders much farther backward. This causes a good deal of backache, discomfort in the lower part of the abdomen, and fatigue. The proper shoe for a pregnant woman is one which is sufficiently wide and has low broad heels somewhat on the style of the Cuban heel, or one still lower and wider. Rubber heels lessen the amount of jarring while walking.

It is natural for women to want to prevent the ungainly shape and "high stomach" which some of them have after giving birth to a child. Most of this is due to relaxation of the skin and the rest of the abdominal wall and to markings on the skin known as striæ gravidarum. Much can be done to prevent these by wearing a proper maternity corset, avoiding constricting bands, wearing proper shoes, and massaging the abdominal wall with mineral oil or olive oil every day during pregnancy. Beginning a few weeks after the baby comes, this should be continued, and likewise systematic body exercises. Regular bowel movements are essential to prevent this also. However, it must be borne in mind that in some women with an inherited predisposition to flabbiness, little can be done to prevent a "high stomach" or striæ gravidarum. Furthermore, women who never indulged in athletics in their youth may not be able to prevent these disturbances.

EXERCISE IN PREGNANCY

A woman who expects a baby should take a certain amount of exercise daily, unless there are special reasons for not doing so. The benefits derived from exercise are improvement in the circulation of the blood, better appetite and digestion of food, better elimination of waste products of the body, more restful sleep, and an opportunity to divert the mind from household responsibilities.

The amount and kind of exercise for an expectant mother depend to a certain extent on the individual woman. One thing is certain, however: the expectant mother should never exercise to the point of fatigue. She should stop as soon as she begins to feel tired. The nearer the day of confinement, the more readily does fatigue set in. Women who are accustomed to participate in strenuous sports can tolerate more than women who lead an indoor and sedentary life. Women who have many household duties to perform do not need as much exercise as women who do not have such duties.

WALKING

Practically the only active exercise available for expectant mothers is walking, and this should be outdoors, except during inclement weather. For this purpose, broad, low-heeled shoes with wide toes should be used, because high-heeled shoes may cause backache and missteps. It is best to walk during the hours of sunlight, because the sun's rays are beneficial. They help the body utilize the minerals in the food. However, during the summer months the expectant mother should be cautious about taking a walk in the hot sun. While walking, it is advisable to proceed leisurely and to avoid crowds. Long tramps are too strenuous for most women. About two or three miles is a fair average daily walk.

If even a short walk produces a tired feeling, the expectant mother should not walk much but should rest in the open air. While resting, the mind may be occupied with reading, knitting, or chatting. At least two hours each day should be spent outdoors. This time is best divided into two periods, one in the morning and the other in the afternoon. When the weather is unusually bad, a walk should be taken at home, either on an open porch or in a room with all the windows wide open. In winter, warm clothes should be worn for this, just as if one were on the street. It is needless to emphasize that the home should be well aired at all times, night as well as day. It is advisable to take five or six deep breaths night and morning before an open window. Likewise, while walking outdoors, deep breathing should be practised for short periods each day.

VIOLENT EXERCISE

Violent exercise in any form should be avoided. This includes running, tennis, golf, swimming, cycling, skating, and horseback riding. Dancing should be indulged in only occasionally and for short periods of time; but the prospective mother should never dance in a crowded room.

TRAVEL

Driving an automobile should be given up, and motoring should be restricted as much as possible. If automobile rides are taken, rough roads should be avoided.

It is inadvisable to take long train rides or steamer voyages. Certainly women who have lost babies before full term on previous occasions should avoid traveling whenever possible and should undertake a journey only after consultation with a physician. The dangerous period of travel is that time in each month when menstruation would ordinarily occur. At this time more than any other, overexertion of any kind may produce premature birth of the baby. When railroad travel is imperative, the smoothest road and the most comfortable accommodations should be chosen. One should recline as much as is convenient.

HOUSEWORK

A certain amount of housework is not only permissible but is desirable. Here also the expectant mother should never proceed to the point of fatigue. Only light work should be done. Going up and down stairs quickly or often may be harmful, as may be lifting or moving heavy articles. Sewing on a machine that requires the use of the feet should not be done. If there is a young child at home, the expectant mother should not lift and carry him around any more than is absolutely necessary. By observing these precautions many backaches and much fatigue will be avoided.

When an expectant mother has much housework to do and finds that the additional walking outdoors makes her tire quickly, she should take only a short walk and spend most of the outdoor allotment of time sitting and resting, especially when the sun is shining. This will insure not only physical but also mental relaxation.

The prospective mother should learn to rest frequently, especially if she does housework. Most women, and more particularly those who tire easily, will find an afternoon nap of an hour or more of great help. Even if one does not actually sleep, complete relaxation in a reclining position will prove refreshing. To obtain the full benefit of such relaxation, it is essential to undress and go to bed. Where there are young children in the home, the mother may take her siesta when the children take theirs. If exercise is taken during the day, there need be no fear that an afternoon nap will prevent sleeping at night.

It may not be amiss to add a word about modesty. Not infrequently women refuse to leave their home, even for a short walk, during the last few weeks or months of pregnancy because they are sensitive about their appearance. This attitude is entirely unwarranted. Women should be proud that they are to become mothers, for there are women, and unfortunately they are numerous, who would give a part of their lives for the ability to give birth to babies but who cannot have children.

Places of amusement may be visited, but those that are poorly ventilated or overheated should be avoided. Jostling in crowds is, of course, bad.

Massage during pregnancy is rarely necessary and is permissible only on the advice of a physician. Women who must remain in bed for a few weeks during pregnancy usually need massage.

BATHING

Many people firmly believe that bathing during pregnancy is harmful. This is a pernicious belief. The skin should be kept clean at all times, but more especially during pregnancy, because the activity of the skin is greater than usual at this time. This is due to the increased elimination and excretion of the body during pregnancy, and the skin constitutes an important organ for these purposes. The expectant mother must eliminate not only her own waste products but also those of the child within the womb.

The skin contains myriads of openings called pores, which lead to sweat glands. By means of these pores certain excretory products of the body are eliminated. If these pores become clogged, proper elimination is prevented, and the expectant mother suffers in consequence.

The water and waste products that cannot be thrown off by the sweat glands remain in the blood until the kidneys, the bowels, and the lungs do the work. An unpleasant odor usually develops. To keep the pores open, to remove the accumulation of degenerated skin, dirt, grease, and dried perspiration, and to keep the skin functioning, it is necessary to wash the entire body with soap and water, and this must be done daily.

KIND OF BATH TO TAKE

The kind of bath is important. One may take a shower, sponge, or tub bath, but the water should be neither too hot nor too cold. Very hot baths cause fatigue. The water should preferably be at a temperature between 85 and 90 degrees F. Even the woman who is accustomed to a cold bath each morning should increase the temperature of the water during pregnancy; for while a cold bath is stimulating, it is not as efficacious as a warm bath for actually cleansing the skin. However, women who are accustomed to a cold shower or tub bath may take such a cold bath in the morning and leave the cleansing bath for the evening.

Since the object of a bath is not only to cleanse the skin but also to stimulate the circulation, it is advisable to rub the whole body with a rough towel fairly vigorously. A "salt towel" may be more effective for this purpose, especially if there is profuse perspiration. A "salt towel" is made by immersing a coarse bath towel in strong salt solution and wringing it as dry as possible.

WARM BATH DAILY

It does not matter much whether the daily warm bath is taken in the morning or in the evening before retiring. However, for women who do not sleep well, it is best to take the warm bath at night, because it is soothing and will promote sleep. If the warm bath is taken in the morning or during the day, at least an hour should elapse before one goes outdoors. If the bath is taken in the afternoon, at least two hours should have passed after the midday meal.

Sponge baths and shower baths may be taken up to the time of actual confinement, but not tub baths. The latter should be avoided during the last four weeks of pregnancy, and sponge and shower baths substituted. Tub baths are shunned during the last month of pregnancy because there is danger of the bath water gaining access to the organs and causing infection. This danger is much greater in women who have already borne children and is more manifest the nearer the time of confinement. When taking tub baths, women should be especially cautious to avoid slipping or falling while getting in and out of the tub.

The following types of bathing should be avoided by most women: cold tub baths, cold plunges, cold showers (except for those who are accustomed to such baths), ocean bathing, and Turkish and Russian baths. Hot sitz baths should be taken only on the recommendation of a physician. Sweat baths should also be shunned except on the physician's recommendation, because they usually prove to be too exhausting. They rarely do any good in normal women.

CARE OF THE BREASTS

Special attention should be paid to cleansing the breasts and nipples. Care must be exercised to avoid compression of and injury to the breasts; this holds true not only during pregnancy but also during the entire life of the woman, from early infancy. Certainly beginning with puberty, the breasts should be protected from excessive pressure and from injury.

During pregnancy a breast supporter should be used, especially if the breasts are large. The skin of the breasts should be washed with soap and water daily just as the rest of the body. Special precautions should be taken to remove the scales that frequently cover the nipples. These scales are due to drying of the discharge which normally exudes from the nipples during pregnancy. The nipples may be anointed daily with cocoa butter, cold cream, or lanolin. Astringents, such as alcohol, should not be used because they harden the nipples, thereby favoring the formation of cracks, which may become avenues of infection.

If the nipples are flat, they may be drawn out for a few minutes each day during the last few weeks of pregnancy; but this must be done with the utmost gentleness and after demonstration by a physician or nurse.

CARE OF THE GENITAL ORGANS

The genital organs likewise require some special attention. During pregnancy there is increased secretion, but this does not require removal. On the contrary, this increased secretion is a helpful measure and should not be disturbed. If, however, the discharge is profuse or has a disagreeable odor, the doctor should be told about it. Douches should never be taken without consulting the doctor. Sexual intercourse should be restricted as much as possible during pregnancy and entirely eliminated during the last six weeks.

CARE OF THE HAIR

The hair should be washed once a week, using a mild soap for this purpose. The lather should be worked into the scalp before rinsing. The scalp should be massaged and the hair brushed daily. If the hair is dry or there is dandruff, olive oil should be rubbed into the hair and scalp.

CARE OF THE TEETH

It is important for every expectant mother to have her teeth examined and cleaned at least twice during her pregnancy. If the dentist finds defects which he can remedy, it is perfectly safe for him to correct the abnormalities. But he should not do more than is absolutely necessary. He may fill (using temporary fillings), clean, and pull teeth, but not make gold fillings, inlays, or bridge work which require a long time and cause a good deal of discomfort.

In many pregnant women the teeth decay and loosen, and in practically all of these women this abnormal process may be corrected by eating an abundance of calcium (chiefly in the form of milk), phosphorus (chiefly in the form of eggs), cod-liver oil, viosterol, fresh fruits, vegetables, butter, and whole-grain cereals. These foods will help not only the mother's teeth but also the teeth of the unborn child. Likewise an abundance of sunshine is essential in order to enable the body to utilize the calcium and phosphorus which are eaten. The teeth should, of course, be carefully brushed at least twice a day and dental floss used to remove particles of food lodged between the teeth. If the gums have a tendency to bleed they should be vigorously massaged with the fingers two or three times a day.

The Mind

The expectant mother should try to lead a quiet, cheerful life and avoid mental as well as physical upheavals. There is usually nothing to fear about pregnancy and labor, and the best proof of this is that millions of women constantly go through these physiologic processes without harm, all over the world. It is best to avoid contact with friends or relatives who relate tales about difficult obstetric cases they know. If a woman has any fears she should speak to her doctor about them. He will usually be able to prove there is no basis for them, and if there is good cause for the fears the physician will be able to correct or overcome the cause. Reading cheerful books helps a great deal.

Signs of Trouble

There are certain signs and symptoms which arise during pregnancy and which may be forerunners of trouble unless attention is paid to them. The following is a list of them, and when any of them are present they should be called to the attention of the physician without delay:

1. Persistent vomiting of most of the food eaten.
2. Stubborn constipation.
3. Frequent or persistent headaches, especially if associated with dizziness and marked constipation.
4. Swelling of the feet, ankles, hands, eyelids, or face.
5. Rapid gain in weight.
6. Diminished output of urine.
7. Blurred or double vision, or spots before the eyes.
8. Shortness of breath or inability to sleep unless the head is elevated on a few pillows.
9. Vomiting after the fifth month.
10. Frequent fainting spells.

11. Any infection or fever.

12. Failure to feel the baby after it has been definitely felt for a while.

13. Escape of bloody or watery discharge from the vagina with or without cramps in the lower part of the abdomen. During the early months of pregnancy these are symptoms of a threatened or beginning miscarriage or abortion. Should they occur, someone should notify the doctor and the patient should get into bed. Her feet or the foot of the bed should be elevated and an ice bag placed on the lower part of the body. The patient should not become excited, because nothing serious can happen during the first few hours, and a doctor can surely reach her during this time. It may happen that the fetus and afterbirth are expelled spontaneously. All tissue, including blood clots, which is passed, should be saved in a towel or in a jar so the doctor may see whether all the parts came away. This is important, because if part or all of the afterbirth is left in the womb, it may have to be removed with instruments.

MINOR AILMENTS DURING PREGNANCY

HEARTBURN AND BELCHING

Many women are greatly disturbed by frequent attacks of heartburn or belching or both. In spite of its name, heartburn has nothing to do with the heart. It is a peculiar burning sensation in the chest and throat, accompanied by the presence of a bitter fluid which escapes from the stomach into the throat. Sometimes heartburn may be prevented by drinking a glass of a milk and cream mixture a few minutes before meal time. The fat in the cream and milk prevents the secretion of acid in the stomach. However, when heartburn is actually present, fats will not help. In fact, they may even aggravate the condition. The best remedies for heartburn are a half-teaspoonful of baking soda (sodium bicarbonate) in a half-glass of water, a teaspoonful of milk of magnesia, or two or three soda-mint tablets. These substances neutralize the acid which causes the heartburn.

FAINTING AND DIZZINESS

It is not uncommon for pregnant women, especially those who are anemic, to have attacks of fainting or dizziness. The condition is not serious; hence, there is no cause for alarm or worry. If a woman feels faint she should immediately lie down on a couch or bed. If she is in a place where there is no bed or couch, she should gently slip down to the floor and lie flat. The faintness will pass away in a few minutes. If the attacks are frequent, it is a good thing to keep spirits of ammonia or smelling salts in the house within easy reach or in the purse. If a woman becomes dizzy she should sit down and lower her head to her knees in order to permit more blood to reach the brain.

VARICOSE VEINS

Women who have varicose veins on the legs and thighs should keep the legs up on a chair or a stool while they are sitting down. They can read, sew, or fulfill most sedentary occupations with their legs elevated. This relieves the distended veins of the extra load of blood they must carry when the patient is standing or sitting with her feet lowered in the usual position. Care must be exercised not to injure varicose veins, because they may bleed or become infected. In cases where the veins are unusually large, a rubber stocking or elastic bandage must be worn. This should be long enough to extend above the highest visible varicose vein and should be put on the leg in the morning before the woman gets out of bed.

HEMORRHOIDS OR PILES

Many pregnant women are troubled by piles. The usual symptoms are pain in and bleeding from the rectum while having a bowel movement. Piles are a special form of varicose veins, and they are always made worse by chronic constipation and straining at stool. They are much more common in women who have had children than in those who are pregnant for the first time. It is important to eat the proper kinds of food and to go to the toilet at the same time every day. In addition, a tablespoonful of mineral oil should be taken by mouth morning and evening. If the piles are much swollen, ice compresses will help. If the hemorrhoids do not readily go back into the rectum, they should be pushed back with a lubricated finger, because there is danger of obstruction and infection of these veins. If they cannot be pushed back or if they bleed frequently the doctor should be notified.

CRAMPS IN THE LEGS

Cramps occur rather frequently, especially in the second half of pregnancy, and they may come on during the night as well as during the day. They may be relieved by changing position, by rubbing the cramped part, by applying heat or cold, by bending the foot at the ankle, and by standing on a cold slab such as the floor of the bathroom. In some cases the cramps are due to disturbances in the mineral balance of the blood, and in these cases viosterol helps considerably.

PREVENTION OF GOITER

In all pregnant women the function of the thyroid gland is increased, and, because of this, slightly more iodine is needed during pregnancy than otherwise. If insufficient iodine is eaten, the thyroid gland of both mother and baby may enlarge. In most parts of the country there is ample iodine in the drinking water and in the vegetables and grain grown in these regions. However, in certain localities like the Great Lakes region there is a lack of iodine, and the expectant mothers in these places must take iodine in some form such as iodine tablets, iodized salt, or Lugol's solution. However, none of these should ever be taken without orders and strict supervision by a physician, because harm may result.

PREPARATIONS FOR CONFINEMENT

The large proportion of women in cities have their babies in a hospital because of the numerous advantages gained thereby. The doctor or the patient may make the necessary arrangements. Since premature delivery is not uncommon, it is a good plan to have certain articles packed in a suitcase a few weeks before the expected date of confinement. These articles should consist of two nightgowns, a bathrobe, two pairs of stockings, a pair of slippers, a few handkerchiefs, a toothbrush and toothpaste or powder, and a comb and brush. In most hospitals the baby's clothes are supplied by the hospital until the child is ready to leave. Hence the day before the patient expects to depart from the hospital, the husband or someone else should take to the hospital for the baby a shirt, a band, a petticoat or bathrobe, a pair of stockings, safety pins, a few diapers, a sweater, a cap, and two blankets. Of course these are only a few of the things which the expectant mother should have bought a few weeks before the baby arrives. The following is a list of clothes necessary for a baby. Since newborn babies quickly outgrow their clothes, not much is needed at the time of birth. In warm weather the material should be cotton or cotton and silk, whereas in cold weather wool or wool and silk is preferable.

Fall and winter:
>3 binders (if not at hospital).
>3 silk and wool shirts with sleeves.
>3 pair silk and wool stockings.
>3 long nightgowns.
>2–4 dozen diapers.

If mother wishes to dress baby:
>3 muslin slips.
>3 muslin dresses.

For outdoor wear:
>2 caps.
>2 sweaters.
>1 bunting.

Spring and summer:
>3 binders (if not at hospital).
>3 cotton shirts with sleeves.
>3 shirts without sleeves.
>3 pair cotton stockings.
>3 long knit gowns, light-weight.
>2–3 dozen diapers.

If mother wishes to dress baby:
>3 muslin slips.
>3 muslin dresses.

For outdoor wear:
>Bonnet.
>Sweater.
>Light bunting or coat.

For the crib:
>1 good hair or felt mattress.
>3 mattress protectors.
>1 rubberized sheet.
>2–6 quilted squares.
>2 woollen crib blankets.
>6 cotton sheets.
>1–2 washable spreads.
>3 cotton flannel wrapping squares.

Toilet necessities:
>1 bathtub.
>1 dressing table.
>1 hairbrush and comb.
>1 tray and bottle set for toilet articles.
>4 knit wash cloths.

4 knit face towels.
3 large bath towels.
Other needed accessories:
1 beam scale (may be rented).
1 diaper pail (to soak soiled diapers).
1 room thermometer—to keep temperature right—68 degrees by day,
    55 degrees at night, 72–75 degrees in the bathroom.
1 clothes horse.
Small-necked nursing bottles for water or formula.
Anti-colic nipples and bottle caps.

WHEN TO CALL THE DOCTOR FOR CONFINEMENT

Labor is the term applied to the process of giving birth, and there are usually three signs by which the beginning of labor may be known:

1. Rhythmic contractions of the womb which the woman experiences as abdominal cramps. These may be felt by placing the hand on the abdomen, because the latter becomes hard during a contraction and relaxes when the cramp subsides. At first these cramps or labor pains are irregular in frequency and intensity, and they begin in the back and radiate to the front. Later they become more frequent, more regular, stronger, and located in the abdomen. "False pains" are weak contractions which occur a few days or a few weeks before actual confinement. They may be distinguished from true labor pains by the fact that they do not increase in frequency, intensity, or duration, and they subside after a while.

2. The escape from the vagina of water which is not urine. This is due to rupture of the bag of waters in which the baby lies. Labor pains usually do not begin for a few hours after this starts, but it is advisable for the patient to remain in bed while waiting for the pains to begin. Better still, she should go to the hospital after notifying the doctor.

3. A thick, mucous, bloody discharge from the vagina, known as the "show."

Only one of these signs is usually present at first, and it is sufficient to warrant notifying the doctor. Then the hospital should be informed that the patient is on the way. Abnormal symptoms may sometimes arise just about the time of confinement, and the doctor must be told about them without delay. These symptoms include bleeding from the vagina, a sudden fainting attack, severe persistent cramps in the abdomen, vomiting, disturbances in vision, and muscular twitchings.

It is a good thing to keep the telephone numbers of the doctor, his assistant if he has one, and the hospital, in a place where they can be obtained without delay.

What to Do if the Baby Is Born at Home before the Patient Can Go to the Hospital

The average duration of the first labor is between sixteen and eighteen hours, and the length of labors after the first one is from eight to ten hours. Hence there is no need to be panic-stricken when labor begins. With few exceptions there is always ample time to get to the hospital. Occasionally, however, for one reason or another, especially in the case of a woman who has had a few quick labors, the entire duration of labor may be so short that the baby is born at home. When it is obvious that the child will be born in the home, the patient's physician should be informed of what is happening. If he cannot be reached, his assistant or another physician should be called to act in the emergency. A kettle of water should be placed over a full gas jet to boil, and a small pair of scissors and two pieces of tape or string dropped into the water.

The cleanest room should be chosen for the patient, and there should be sufficient warmth, especially for the sake of the baby. The expectant mother should, of course, remain in bed. If a baby can come in such a short time, the process is nearly always normal and easy. As soon as the baby is born, if it cries spontaneously, nothing need be done except to wrap a warm, clean towel around its body to keep it warm. There is usually no harm in leaving the child in bed just as it is, provided it is breathing normally and its color is pink. If the doctor is informed of what happened at home he will usually be able to arrive in time to clean his hands properly to tie the cord and see that the afterbirth is delivered.

If the baby does not breathe or cry immediately after birth, someone should thoroughly wash his or her hands and fore-arms with soap and water and then with alcohol and should rub the baby's back up and down with two or three fingers. If this does not produce crying, the baby should be held up by its feet, and its buttocks gently spanked a number of times. This usually causes the baby to cry. Then it should be kept covered with a clean warm towel.

If the afterbirth should be expelled before the doctor arrives, someone should thoroughly scrub his or her hands with soap and water, and with the two pieces of boiled tape or string, tie the umbilical cord in two places. The first should be about one inch from the baby's body and the other about one inch farther away. Before tying the two tapes, iodine should be applied on the part of the cord where the strings are to be tied, and the strings should be saturated with iodine. Great care should be exercised that none of the iodine touches the baby's body, because it may produce a burn. The cord should then be cut between the two pieces of string with the pair of scissors which is in the kettle of boiling water. More iodine should be applied to the cut edge of the cord which is attached to the baby. It is important to be sure there is no bleeding from this end of the cord. If there is bleeding, another piece of string should be applied tightly.

The afterbirth and the sac should not be thrown away but should be saved for the doctor to see. It is important to know whether all of the afterbirth and the sac came away intact. If a piece is left behind, it usually causes hemorrhage and frequently infection unless it is removed immediately.

POSTNATAL CARE

By the term puerperium is meant the interval of time which extends from the birth of the baby until the organs of reproduction return to their normal condition. This interval usually lasts from six to eight weeks, but may take much longer.

During the first two weeks of the puerperal period the mother and the newborn babe are usually under the direct supervision of a physician, either in a hospital or at home. Physicians differ in their attitude towards the activity of their patients during the first two weeks following childbirth; but it may safely be said that most obstetricians have rightfully given up the custom of keeping a patient flat on her back during the first ten to fourteen days. Patients are now allowed a great deal of freedom, and beginning with the fourth day a series of mild bed exercises which involve the arms, the legs, and the abdominal muscles may be tried. The woman may sit up in bed on a back rest after the fourth day, and in a chair on the tenth or eleventh day, if everything is normal. Patients are usually permitted to leave the hospital three or four days after getting out of bed.

When a patient leaves the hospital she is advised not to walk the steps leading to her apartment if one or two strong-armed males can carry her. If the patient must walk, it is advisable for her to walk slowly and to rest frequently. If there are a number of landings on the way up, it may help to have a chair transported from landing to landing so the patient may sit while she is resting. Since there is considerable excitement incident on dressing the baby, packing suitcases, saying good-bye to nurses, riding home, meeting neighbors, and so on, it is best for the patient to go to bed as soon as she reaches home and to remain there until the following morning. It is probably best for the patient to leave the hospital in the afternoon because of the advantage of traveling during the day and because by the time home is reached there are not many waking hours left. Once in the home the patient should not attempt to walk steps until the end of the third week. She should not go out into the street until the end of the fourth week.

Probably the most important factor necessary to safeguard a happy household in which there is a newborn child is a calm and unperturbed mind for the mother. On that depends to the largest extent the health of the baby. As has been said, the day of departure from the hospital is one of excitement, and in consequence of this the baby not infrequently loses weight on that day. After the first day at home the mother must learn to be more or less callous to disturbing influences. Certainly, petty inconveniences should not be permitted to interfere with the peace of mind. If a nurse is at home, she, of course, assumes a great deal of responsibility in the care of the baby. The strict routine of caring for a newborn baby, especially in a small apartment, may tend to upset some young mothers, but there is no reason to be alarmed. Tranquillity of mind and absolute regularity in feeding the baby will usually guarantee a thriving infant. Normal-sized babies are fed every four hours, beginning at 6 or 7 A.M. and ending at 10 or 11 P.M., and are not given a night feeding. When a mother has not enough breast milk for the baby, usually made manifest by a crying spell immediately after nursing or by a failure to gain weight, complementary feedings of cow's milk should be given; but only after consultation with a physician. The baby should be given about an ounce of water between feedings three or four times a day. If a baby gains six or more ounces a week it is doing satisfactorily. One should not make the mistake of dressing the baby too warmly, and whenever possible it should be kept outdoors on a porch.

The matter of sterilization of articles used for the breasts and the baby need not be detailed here; but it cannot be emphasized too strongly that surgical cleanliness is important. Special precautions should be taken to keep the nipples clean. Sterile dressings should be applied to the nipples until the baby is at least ten weeks old.

During the puerperium the mother should have an abundance of sleep and in addition should rest in a reclining position for definite intervals of time both morning and afternoon. While resting, it is advisable to lie on the abdomen for periods of fifteen to twenty minutes, just as we ask our patients to do when they are in the hospital.

During the first few days at home, tact is necessary to avoid visitors or to cut short their stay. The same holds true for telephone calls, especially if there be at the other end of the wire a garrulous individual or one who wants to impart information concerning some dreadful occurrence. Visitors who have colds or infections should not be interviewed and should by all means be kept out of the baby's room. If the mother herself has a cold, she should cover her mouth and nose with a handkerchief or a mouthpiece when nursing or bathing the baby. No medicine should be taken by the mother or given to the baby without the sanction of a physician. Where there are other children in the home it is prudent to keep a sharp lookout, since three- or four-year-old children are prone to be jealous of a newcomer. This is because nearly all the attention of the mother is showered on the new arrival and the older child is no longer the cynosure. It is, of course, obvious that showing the baby off before relatives and friends is harmful.

A nursing mother should for the first few weeks after childbirth consider herself in the light of a convalescent invalid. This does not mean, however, that she should fear to do any kind of housework or lack confidence in her ability to take care of her baby. More consideration must be given to general rules of health than is customary, and the diet should be abundant and varied. The mother should avoid highly seasoned foods and foods which are found to produce disturbances in the baby. Plenty of liquids should be imbibed, especially milk. The bowels should be looked after. Water, fruits, vegetables, and coarse cereals help to maintain regular bowel movements, and if a laxative is necessary, mineral oil or milk of magnesia may be used. Alcohol and smoking may best be avoided. Fresh air is important, and where a porch is available, the mother should be on it while resting and especially at that time of day when there is an abundance of sunshine.

When nursing the baby it is better to sit up than to recline. A very important thing to avoid is constant observation of the baby while it is at the breast; for this not only strains the eyes of the mother and produces headache, but also strains the muscles of the neck and back, which likewise become the seat of pain.

For the woman with a lax abdominal wall an abdominal support of some kind is helpful. Tub baths are best not taken until after the fourth week, but showers and sponges should be used instead.

Unless the weather is unusually pleasant it is best not to go out for a ride or a walk until the baby is four weeks old. After this time it is advantageous for the young mother to leave her home for at least one or two hours each day and spend this time sitting, walking, or riding in the open air, especially when the sun is shining. Strenuous exercise, such as playing golf or tennis, swimming, skating, or driving a car, should be avoided during the puerperal period. Social functions during these weeks should likewise be reduced.

The return of menstruation varies in different individuals. In those who do not nurse their babies, the flow usually returns at the end of six weeks, while in those who do nurse their babies the first menstrual period appears any time after the third month. In some, however, the menses do not return until the baby is weaned. The first period is usually profuse, sometimes enough to cause alarm. At the time of the first period, the woman had better keep off her feet as much as possible; but if the flow is too profuse, the advice of a physician should be sought. In fact, if the mother has any doubt concerning herself or the baby she should consult her physician rather than take the advice of well-meaning but often misinformed friends and relatives. Cracked or bleeding nipples or painful breasts call for immediate notification of the physician.

It is customary for a patient to return to her physician at the end of the puerperal period, namely, six to eight weeks after the birth of the baby, for an examination. At this time the physician will examine the breasts and nipples, the abdominal wall and the condition of the reproductive organs, and see if hemorrhoids are present. If the patient had a high blood pressure or kidney trouble during pregnancy, the doctor will take the blood pressure, examine the urine, examine for swelling of the legs and hands, and perhaps make other tests. If any abnormality is detected the physician will tell the patient what to do, and he will make an effort to correct it. Generally this examination is designated as the final examination. This is unfortunate, because both the physician and the patient regard it as the final contact until a new pregnancy begins. Since many women have abnormalities or develop them after childbirth, it is advisable for women to see their physicians again six months after the baby is born, and again when the baby is a year old. Women who have abnormal conditions should, of course, visit their doctors as often as they feel it is necessary.

WEANING THE BABY

The time when a baby is to be weaned varies considerably. Women who have an abundant supply of breast milk should nurse their baby for eight or nine months. However, not all women have a supply of milk which will last as long as this. Women with ample breast milk should not wean the baby during the first few months without an urgent reason. Breast feeding is important for the mother as well as for her child, because it helps to restore her organs more quickly and more completely than otherwise. A doctor's advice should be sought before a woman with a good supply of milk decides to discontinue breast feedings.

Nursing at the breast should be eliminated gradually. First a bottle of cow's milk, or better still a cereal feeding, should be substituted for one breast feeding. This is best started at about the sixth month. During the seventh month a vegetable meal and some cow's-milk mixture may be substituted for another breast feeding. In the eighth or ninth month the child may be weaned completely. However, if the baby has been ill, if the source of cow's milk is not very good, or if the weather is unusually hot, it may be better to postpone complete weaning for another month. Cow's-milk mixtures should be substituted for all the breast feedings if the baby gains on the former. When this takes place the breasts should be bound gently but firmly with a sheet or smooth towel and fluids should be restricted to a minimum. These measures are taken to prevent the breasts from filling up too much and causing a great deal of pain. Ice bags will relieve the pain, and if the bowels are not freely movable Epsom salts, or citrate of magnesia may be taken. These will remove more fluids from the body.

Superstitions and Misconceptions about Childbirth

From the dawn of history there have been innumerable superstitions associated with childbirth. The ancients held such peculiar notions about reproduction that laymen of today who are familiar with these ideas consider them ludicrous. However, the vast majority of the laity who today scoff at the credulity of the uncivilized and the semicivilized hold fast to enough erroneous beliefs about childbirth to make phy-, sicians laugh at them in turn.

There is an almost universal belief among the laity in so-called maternal impressions. This expression signifies that a child in the womb may be marked in some obscure way by what the mother thinks, feels, or sees during pregnancy, especially if the experience is disagreeable or shocking. This belief is one of the oldest in history. Not only was it prevalent among the uncivilized peoples, but many of our most prominent literary celebrities used it as a theme for their writings. Among the latter may be mentioned Goethe, Scott, Dickens, and O. W. Holmes. When a child is born with a birthmark, those who believe in maternal impressions make an effort to detect a special form in the birthmark and link it up with some frightful occurrence which the mother experienced during the last few months of pregnancy. However, there is absolutely no support for the belief in maternal impressions. In the first place birthmarks and other defects are usually accidental aberrations in the growth of the child. These abnormalities begin to manifest themselves when the fetus has been in the uterus only a few weeks, because the child is almost completely formed by the time it reaches its eighth week of development. Hence nothing which happens to the mother in the latter part of gestation can possibly affect the child in the womb. Secondly, there is no direct contact between the mother and the baby in the womb, by way of either the nerves or the blood. The nerves connect the mother with the womb but not with the baby; hence the worst thing which can occur is stimulation of the uterus, with subsequent interruption of pregnancy. Even this occurrence is uncommon. The baby receives nourishment from the mother, but only because the afterbirth extracts the necessary ingredients from the mother's blood. Thirdly, in most instances where the child presents defects, the mother was never frightened or upset in any way. In spite of the horrors to which women abroad were subjected during the World War, there were no more "marked" babies than are usually born.

Another common belief is that a baby born during the seventh month of its intrauterine existence can live, whereas one delivered during the eighth month cannot. This is incorrect. The truth is that the longer a baby remains in the womb before it is born, the more advanced is its development, and hence the greater its chances for survival. The few exceptions do not disprove this rule.

There are many misconceptions concerning the determination of the sex of a child before birth. It is commonly held that if a baby's heart tones are more than 140 per minute the baby is a girl, whereas if the heart rate is less than 140 the child is a boy. This belief is based on the fact that large babies usually have slower heart rates than smaller ones, and since boys are generally larger than girls it is assumed that slow heartbeats indicate boys. The truthful physician will tell his patients that he guesses the sex of babies incorrectly almost as often as he guesses it correctly. Normally about 105 boys are born to every 100 girls, and this ratio holds true regardless of seasonal variations and geographical divisions. Hence, if a physician guesses boys more often than girls, over a long period of time, his correct guesses will be slightly greater than his incorrect ones. Among premature babies the proportion of males is higher than 105 to 100, and among fetuses which are expelled during the early months of pregnancy the males are still more predominant. There is as yet no satisfactory explanation for this phenomenon.

Some people believe that the sex of a baby depends on the time in the menstrual cycle when conception takes place. This is wrong. In human beings the sex is determined at the time the female egg is fertilized by the male spermatozoön or sex cell. It is the latter which determines whether a child is to be a male or a female. There are two types of spermatozoa, one of which produces males and one of which is responsible for females.

Some individuals believe that a woman who has only one ovary is capable of having only male or only female children. This belief is not true, because women with only one ovary may give birth to babies of both sexes. Likewise these women have a menstrual flow every month, and not every second month. In other words, women with one ovary are just as capable from a reproductive point of view as women with two ovaries.

There is an almost unanimous belief that a woman who has a Cæsarean section must have all her subsequent babies delivered in the same way. This is erroneous, because many women have babies through the natural passages after having had a Cæsarean section. Of course, if the first operation was performed because a woman has small pelvic bones, the operation will have to be repeated for each baby unless the babies are unusually small. On the other hand, if abdominal delivery was resorted to because of such complications as hemorrhage, convulsions, etc., and this complication is absent during subsequent pregnancies, delivery may readily be accomplished in the natural way. However, if natural delivery is awaited after the old type of Cæsarean section, there is a distinct risk of rupture of the uterus. This hazard is extremely slight after the new type of abdominal delivery.

Another misbelief is that a Cæsarean section cannot be performed until a woman is in actual labor. However, this operation may be done at any time during pregnancy, even weeks and months before the time of the calculated confinement. Likewise it may be performed at any time during labor, but the longer a woman is permitted to have labor pains before the operation is resorted to, especially if the bag of waters has ruptured, the greater the risk of infection.

Some individuals are of the opinion that a woman can have only two Cæsarean sections. The truth is that there is no limit to the number of these operations a woman may have. In fact, there is a case on record of a woman who had ten babies by Cæsarean operation. Fortunately this is a unique case. Because every abdominal operation carries with it some risk, usually most physicians sterilize a woman after her third Cæsarean operation, and even after the second one if this is desired by the patient and her husband. Sterilization as performed today does not prolong a Cæsarean operation greatly and does not increase the risk of the operation. Even if the womb is removed after delivery of the child, there is no increased hazard. The womb is practically never removed unless it is diseased.

Contrary to a common notion, sterilization as now performed has absolutely no deleterious effect on a woman in after life. If she were not told that she can no longer have babies she would not know she was sterilized. All her normal functions, including menstruation, continue except the ability to conceive. It is only when the ovaries or the uterus are removed by operation or their function is destroyed by radium or the X-rays that the menstrual flow ceases and the symptoms of the change of life set in.

A fairly common misconception is that which maintains a woman is incapable of becoming pregnant as long as she nurses a baby. Many women have had an opportunity to learn otherwise. Conception is possible at this time regardless of whether a woman menstruates or not. Most women begin to menstruate within a few months after their babies are born. Those who do not nurse their babies usually have the first flow at the end of about six weeks, whereas those who nurse do not begin to menstruate until a few months later. Strange as it may seem, pregnancy is possible not only during the period of nursing but also before a young girl of twelve or thirteen years begins to menstruate, and also at the end of the reproductive career for a year or more after a woman ceases to menstruate because of the change of life. In other words, even though there is no monthly flow, the ovaries may produce and expel ova or eggs which are capable of being fertilized.

A common belief not only among the laity but also among some physicians is that the size of the baby at birth is dependent for the most part upon the amount of food the mother eats during gestation. While this appears to be logical, it has not been proved. There is no constant ratio between the gain in weight in the mother and the size of the baby. The size of babies depends chiefly on heredity but also in some cases upon abnormal conditions in the mother. For example, women with kidney trouble usually have puny babies, and mothers with diabetes frequently have abnormally large offspring. Physicians carefully control the weight of obstetric patients because an excessive gain is primarily deleterious for the mother and only secondarily for the baby.

Since the baby is in reality a parasite, it takes all the nourishment it needs from its mother's blood. If the mother's food does not contain all the ingredients a baby requires, the child will obtain these substances at the expense of the mother's tissues. Hence it is important for a pregnant woman to take not only the proper amount of food but also the right kinds of food, minerals, vitamins, etc. While this is true, there is no reason for women to believe in the false notion that a pregnant woman should eat for two individuals, herself and her baby. It is unnecessary for an expectant mother to eat more than usual, because her body metabolizes the food she eats in a much more economical way than in the nonpregnant state.

Of lesser extent is the belief that one can tell the sex of a baby from the shape of the mother's abdomen. Thus a high prominence is said to indicate a boy, whereas a more even distribution to the sides and to the back is said to be indicative of a girl. These notions have absolutely no truth in them. Likewise there is no basis for the belief that if a woman extends her arms upward to reach for objects the baby will be born with a loop or cord around its neck. In the first place, stretching cannot result in lassoing the child around the neck because the baby moves about freely in a spacious sac of fluid. Secondly the finding of one or more loops of cord around a baby's neck at birth is fairly frequent and usually has no significance at all. Only rarely does a loop of cord wound around a child's neck produce trouble.

It is frequently said that a child will be lucky if it is born with a caul or veil, that is, with the sac in which it lies throughout pregnancy. Maybe so—but it has never been proved.

Many women and physicians believe that a tight binder applied to the woman's abdomen after childbirth will result in the restoration of a normal figure. Unfortunately this is not true. No matter how snug a binder or bandage is applied, it cannot restore tonicity of weak abdominal muscles. On the other hand a tightly applied abdominal binder may result in harm. A loosely applied binder helps to steady the enlarged uterus when the patient moves around in bed, it relieves the feeling of emptiness in the abdomen, and it allays the minds of those women who believe that the binder will restore their anteconceptional figure.

CHAPTER VII

Care and Feeding of the Child
PHILIP C. JEANS, M.D.

INTRODUCTION

INVESTIGATIONS INDICATE *that the boys and girls entering college these days are on an average two inches taller and from seven to ten pounds heavier than their parents and grandparents who entered these same institutions at the same ages in the previous two generations. The fact is significant because it shows what preventive medicine and hygiene have done to build better bodies. In an earlier day children just "growed" like Topsy in* Uncle Tom's Cabin. *Nowadays the diets are regulated, as well as the hours of sleep, the hours of exposure to sunshine and fresh air, the clothing, and all of the other factors of the child's hygiene.*

The reason for such regulation lies, of course, in the change in the habits of civilized man. In a previous generation, children were raised largely in rural populations where they had plenty of sunshine and fresh air, plenty of fresh vegetables and milk, and all of the circumstances combined to promote the growth of a healthy little animal. As human beings moved into great collections of humanity in cities, the sunlight and fresh air began to be shut out. Because of the difficulties of transportation, it became necessary to depend largely on food from cans and on materials transported over many hundreds of miles before they were used by the consumer. The more food and milk are handled, the more likelihood is there of contamination from the hands of those who bring them to their final market.

Hence, there has developed the necessity for a regularly ordered hygiene of childhood, which is presented in the two articles which follow, by P. C. Jeans, professor of diseases of children in the University of Iowa, and by Dr. F. F. Tisdall of the University of Toronto in Canada. There will be found in these two articles some duplication

182

of information, but it seemed to be desirable to present it from two points of view for several reasons. The article by Dr. Jeans is extensive and covers all of the different aspects of the subject. The article by Dr. Tisdall is concentrated and represents the barest outlines of what every mother must know in this field.

M. F.

Development of the Infant

IN ORDER TO KNOW whether a baby is normal and developing as he should, it is necessary to have certain standards for judgment. In setting up any such standards, it must be remembered that individual babies will vary somewhat from the average. To say that a baby should weigh seven pounds at birth is stating an approximately average value which everyone knows is strictly true for only a few babies. Babies at birth may weigh six, eight, or nine pounds and be perfectly normal. Extreme variations from the average are of significance. A baby weighing five pounds or less at birth must be classed as a delicate or premature baby requiring special care. Similarly moderate variations from the average in all of the other criteria of growth and development are not to be taken seriously in themselves. The weight or development at any particular period is not of as great significance as the progress which the baby makes from time to time. The infant should show constant and steady progress as indicated by the various standards.

A baby of average weight at birth should double the birth weight by five to six months and treble it by one year. These are average values. A baby who is well fed with ample food will grow faster than this. If the diet has been a balanced one, it is probable that the larger baby is physically superior. The baby may be expected to gain six to eight ounces a week in the first six months and four to six ounces a week during the second six months. After this time the weight gain is much less.

The body length of the baby is also a criterion of growth, but it is not always used in routine evaluation of progress, because of the greater extremes of food quality and quantity required to affect growth in length.

The head grows rapidly in size during the first year, increasing two and one-half inches in circumference in this period. The bones of the skull are relatively soft and may be moulded readily by permitting the baby to lie in the same position. Many infants' heads have become permanently misshapen because the mother did not take care to see that the baby's position was changed frequently. A good practice is to turn the baby on the left side after one feeding and on the right side after the next one. The soft spots or fontanels of the skull represent areas which have not yet calcified. The small one at the back of the head is usually hard by three months. The large one in front should close by eighteen months, but in many vigorous, well-nourished babies, the anterior fontanel has disappeared by one year of age.

The first or deciduous teeth are twenty in number. These begin to erupt at about six months of age and should be completely erupted by two and one-half years. They tend to erupt by pairs, the lower central incisors coming first, then the two upper centrals, followed by the upper lateral incisors. These six incisor teeth should be erupted by one year of age. Moderate variations in the time of eruption of teeth may indicate nothing abnormal. Marked variations may be indicative of rickets.

The muscular movements soon after birth are few, but activity increases rapidly, though in the beginning the movements seem purposeless. By three months the neck muscles are strong enough to support the head. At three months the infant will attempt to grasp objects though with poor muscular control. The grasp becomes accurate at five to seven months. Vigorous well-nourished babies sit alone at six months with occasional falls: they usually sit securely at eight months. Though babies may stand awkwardly earlier, they usually are able to stand well when supported at nine months. The usual time of first walking is sometime between twelve and fifteen months. Between the ages of sitting and walking, most babies accomplish progression over the floor by creeping or otherwise, though a few normal babies do not.

Babies are able to laugh and coo sometimes at two months, sometimes not until several months later. They do not say understandable words until the latter part of the first year. By the end of one year usually several simple words are in the vocabulary. By two years simple short sentences are used. Many entirely normal children are late in talking. In a few instances this delay is of several years, often it seems because a child has felt no necessity for speech, in that

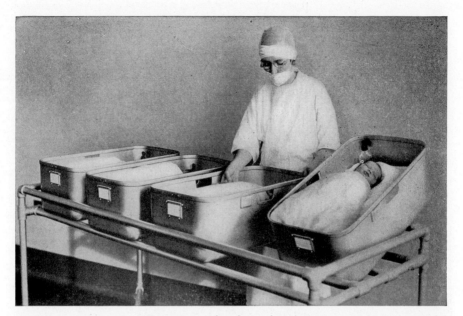

FIG. 15. Aluminum bassinet.

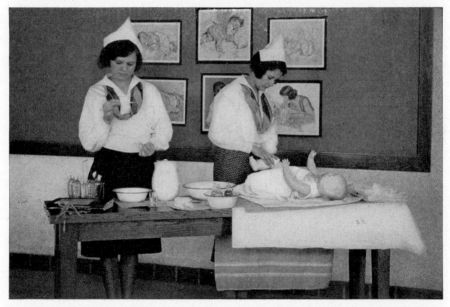

FIG. 16. Taking the baby's temperature, and bathing (sponge bath).

Fig. 17. Washing the baby's eyes.

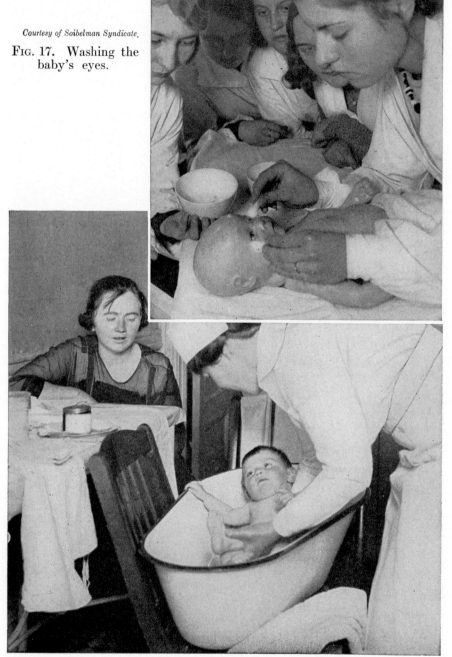

Fig. 18. Bathing the baby (tub bath.)

all desires are anticipated. Parents should not use baby talk to children, as they learn only that kind of speech which they hear.

The infant's vision seems quite imperfect in the beginning. It is not until five or six weeks of age that he pays attention to objects held in front of him. He does not follow with his eyes until he is three to four months old, at which time, or soon thereafter, he makes combined purposeful movements of head and eyes and recognizes people and objects familiar to him. At about this time, or a little earlier, he will turn his head toward a sound and be able to recognize voices.

The mental development of the infant in the first year or two is judged largely by the criteria of physical development which have been discussed. A baby may be slow in sitting, standing, and walking, for the reason that he has been ill or has been poorly fed; or it may be because he is mentally backward. With good food and in the absence of illness, mental backwardness should be suspected when purposeful motor behavior of all types is abnormally delayed or when the infant is inattentive to familiar sights and sounds.

Physical Care and Hygiene

The baby should always have his own bed. Whenever possible he should have a room exclusively for his own use. The room which he occupies should be well ventilated or the air changed frequently During his waking or play hours the temperature should be in the neighborhood of 70 degrees F. During sleep time the temperature can be 10 to 30 degrees lower than this, depending upon the age, size and vigor of the baby. When the room is kept cold for sleep it is advisable to have available a warm room to which he can be taken when necessary. When properly supervised and protected, a baby can spend much of his time out of doors after two weeks in summer or after three months in winter.

In the first weeks after birth the infant will sleep practically all of the time except when he is bathed and fed. At two to three months he sleeps fourteen to sixteen hours daily, and lies quietly for possibly two hours more. At six months the average baby sleeps about fourteen hours and at one year very little less than this. After eighteen months one expects a twelve-hour sleep at night with an additional daytime nap. The baby not only needs no pillow, but usually is better off without one. During a long nap it is advisable to see that the young baby is turned several times; the older baby will turn himself.

The daily bath should be given before one of the morning feedings. After the cord comes off, this should be a tub bath. The room should be warm, not hot, and without drafts. The temperature of the bath water is best at about 100 degrees F. for the young baby, gradually decreased to 90 degrees F. at one year. Unnecessary exposure is to be avoided, especially for the young or delicate infant. This may be accomplished by lifting the baby directly from the tub onto a large bath towel. Whether the baby is dried on the mother's lap or on a table matters little, though usually the procedure is more quickly performed on a table. The use of talcum powder is not a corrective for poor drying. Babies would be fully as well off without this accessory. In very hot weather it is often advantageous to give the baby one or more sponge baths in addition to the morning tub bath. Routine care concerning the eyes, ears, nose, mouth, and other details of body cleanliness, is given at the time of the morning bath. The only care needed for the eyes is possibly the cleaning of the inner corners. This can be done with a piece of cotton wet with boric acid solution. In cleaning the ears there is no need and some danger in entering farther than the tip of the canal. If it is necessary to clean the nose, this may be done by using a small piece of cotton wrapped firmly on a toothpick and dipped in mineral oil. The mouth ordinarily needs no attention until the teeth appear. Then all that is required is to keep the teeth clean. While the teeth are few, this can be done readily with cotton on a toothpick, perhaps with the aid of a tooth-paste (not powder). While the baby is young the hair and scalp are washed daily at the time of the bath. This is done with soap and water, as for the remainder of the body. In case there is a milk crust on the scalp, some simple oily preparation, such as mineral oil or vaseline, may be placed on the scalp at night and the scalp washed as usual in the morning. At the time of the bath also the genitalia should receive attention. Boys are prone to have adhesions of the foreskin to the glans, and a material known as smegma accumulates back of the glans. If the foreskin is retracted each day and a small amount of oil applied, the part is kept desirably clean and adhesions are prevented. If the foreskin retracts with difficulty, a physician should be consulted in order that the difficulty may be corrected. Smegma accumulates also in the vulva of girls, and this part should be cleansed daily. Cleaning is desirable only of the visible parts.

Very young babies often have a small amount of milk in their breasts. The only importance in this fact is that it be recognized as normal, and all that is required is to let the breasts alone.

It is desirable that the baby's buttocks be washed with soap and water after each stool. Occasionally the buttocks become reddened or even excoriated. This is due to one of two causes. One of these is the strong acid present in diarrheal stools; the other the formation of ammonia from the urine as it remains for a period in the diaper. In either case it is useful to keep the baby's skin protected with some simple ointment. When due to diarrhea the trouble will cease as soon as the diarrhea is controlled. Since the ammonia is formed by the growth of certain bacteria in the urine as it is kept warm next the body, and since it is not possible always to change a diaper immediately it is wet, the management of choice is to place some antiseptic in the diaper which will prevent bacterial growth. A most effective antiseptic is bichloride of mercury (corrosive sublimate) which is used in solution as the final rinse water for the diapers. The solution is prepared by dissolving one 7½ grain tablet in 2 quarts of water. This material is highly poisonous when taken internally and must be kept out of reach of irresponsible persons.

In the care of the diaper much has been said against the use of laundry soaps and washing powders, because it was felt that these were instrumental in causing ammonia formation and excoriations. Since these are not the cause of such difficulties, diapers may be washed in the same manner as all other clothes, and then should be well rinsed.

CRYING

A certain amount of crying daily serves a useful purpose. It is a form of exercise and constitutes a large part of the exercise a young baby gets. Also, in the very young, crying helps to expand the lungs and keep them expanded, overcoming the state of collapse which is normal before birth. However, crying is sometimes excessive. Such crying is usually due to discomfort, which may be from hunger, extremes of temperature, colic or other pain. Though babies cry from fright and anger, these are not causes of habitual crying. It must be admitted also that babies cry sometimes in order to get the attention which they find that crying brings them.

EXERCISE

Exercise is essential for good development. In the early weeks, when the infant is relatively helpless, sufficient exercise is obtained by the usual carrying around of the baby by the mother, though some mothers have been taught to leave their babies too much alone for fear of spoiling them. As muscular development progresses the baby gets his exercise by kicking and other movements while lying unrestricted on his bed. Later he sits, plays, creeps, and walks. After the first few weeks, if permitted, the baby usually will obtain sufficient exercise for himself, but care must be taken that he is at liberty to do so. Among the baby's toys and playthings objects of such a size as may be swallowed have no place.

TRAINING

The training of children begins in early infancy. Babies are born without habits, and those which they get are either accidentally acquired or are taught to them. In infancy small things lead to habit formation. Regularity in feeding and in everything done for the baby is conducive to good habits. The baby should become accustomed to going to sleep without the presence of the mother, and certainly he should not be rocked to sleep. He should become accustomed to sleeping without a light at night and if he should awaken at an unusual time and cries, he should be allowed to "cry it out," if it is reasonably certain nothing serious is wrong. The age at which babies can be trained to the toilet is early in proportion to the amount of teaching energy spent in this direction. At three to four months of age, sometimes sooner, the bowel movements tend to occur at rather regular times each day, viz., immediately after the morning bottle. It is a good plan to place the baby over a small vessel regularly at this time. He is thus encouraged to develop a regular habit which will save the mother much inconvenience later.

The harm of thumb sucking is chiefly the resulting jaw and tooth deformity. This habit in moderation probably does not harm, but since it is impossible to state any dividing line between that which is and that which is not harmful, the safest plan is not to permit it in any degree as a habit. Numerous appliances for the correction of thumb sucking are available. The simplest measure, often effective,

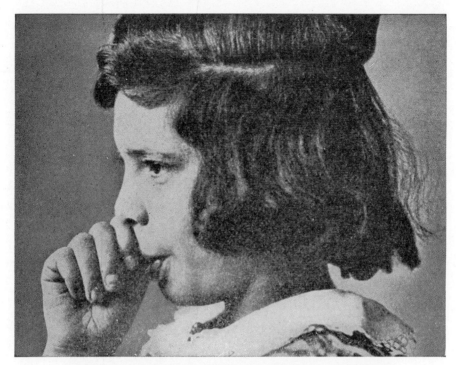

FIG. 19. Thumb sucking.

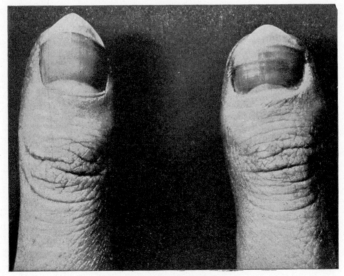

FIG. 20. Thumbs deformed by sucking.

is the application of a few turns of adhesive tape lightly about the thumb. Little excuse exists for permitting a baby to have a pacifier.

Nutrition of the Infant

INTRODUCTORY DISCUSSION

Nutrition deals with the food we eat and the structures which the body makes of it. A diet which is adequate to maintain the body in good nutritional health must include the essential food materials. These essentials are known as protein, carbohydrate, fat, mineral salts, water, and certain substances known as vitamins.

The body needs all of these various food materials at all ages of life, though the amount and the form in which they may be offered vary according to the age. The infant, the child, and the adult need exactly the same essential food elements. The foods chosen to supply them must be adapted to the digestive capacity and the relative need of the individual. For example, meat contains an excellent quality of protein, but it is not adapted to the digestion of the young infant, whereas milk also contains an excellent quality of protein and is a food which is digested by the infant with relative ease. Milk is not a perfect food, but it is more nearly so than any other natural food, and is the basis upon which the infant's diet is constructed.

In the life processes of the body, certain materials are constantly being broken down to simpler ones; the process is comparable in some respects to the burning of fuel in a furnace. This combustion takes place even when the body is in complete repose, and it is increased by activity in proportion to the degree of muscular exertion. In the process of combustion, heat is liberated. This is what keeps the body warm. Heat produced in this manner can be measured. The measurements are made in heat units or calories. A known amount of food will give rise to a definite amount of heat, which can be calculated. Thus it is that food is often measured in terms of calories. If insufficient food were furnished, the body would consume itself to the point where life would be impossible. It is necessary therefore to supply energy (food capable of producing energy) to the body for the purpose of maintaining life. In order that the infant may grow and develop properly, it is necessary to supply energy in addition to that which will only maintain life. Growth takes place only when food is supplied in excess of the amount needed to replace that which is burned to maintain the body. The infant's need for energy is relatively (per unit of body weight) far greater than that of the older child or adult and the effects of an inadequate supply show themselves more quickly. Between 85 and 90 per cent of the infant's energy needs are supplied by fats and carbohydrates, this being the chief function of these two food materials. The remainder of the energy is derived from protein.

Protein is an essential part of all cells; without it, life would be impossible. Plants can form protein from substances which they are able to obtain from the soil and the air. Man and the animals cannot do this but must have the constituents of protein supplied to them either from plants or from other animals. For existence a certain amount of protein must be supplied in the diet, and for body increase (growth) an increased amount is necessary. Since no other food element can replace it, protein is an essential part of the diet. A sufficient amount may readily be supplied by the milk of the infant's diet providing the amount of milk offered is adequate. A moderate deficiency of protein causes slow growth and feeble musculature. Gross deficiencies will eventually lead to death. Proteins from different sources differ in their chemical structure. When a protein has all the components necessary to build the kind of protein needed by the body it is called a "complete" protein. Milk protein may be considered as complete. It is characteristic of the vegetable proteins that they are not complete and as a consequence are not as adequate for producing good growth as are the proteins from animal sources.

The food materials which have been discussed (fat, carbohydrate, and protein) are present in food in gross amounts, and their presence may be determined by relatively simple chemical tests. Certain other essential food materials are necessary to the body and present in foods only in minute amounts, and their presence cannot be determined by chemical tests. These materials have been grouped under the general term of vitamins, though they differ widely from each other in their nature. They are identified chiefly by the effect which their absence from the diet produces, and for lack of better names they are designated by letters of the alphabet.

Vitamin A is necessary for growth. A marked deficiency of A causes characteristic changes in the mucous membranes of the eye, nose, and throat and elsewhere. These changes predispose to bacterial invasion and secondary infection. Thus it is that a gross deficiency of

A may be a factor in frequent colds and in nasal sinus disease. It is to be remembered, however, that infection in this region is often due to other causes, and further additions of A to the diet may be of no benefit if the amount already present is adequate. Vitamin A is present in milk fat, egg yolk, and in the glandular organs (such as liver) of animals. A yellow pigment, carotene, which the body is able to transform into A, occurs in small amounts in certain vegetables and in citrous fruits. Vitamin A is not widely distributed in foods nor present in any food in large amount. Since it is present in milk fat, there are many who consider that the infant receives an ample supply from this source. However, this has not been demonstrated, and it would seem the part of wisdom to supplement the infant's diet with a concentrated source of this material. Such a supplement is usually in the form of cod-liver oil, which contains both vitamins A and D.

What has been known as vitamin B is now known to consist of several vitamins. It is becoming customary to designate the old vitamin B as B complex, one of the factors B or B_1 and the other G or B_2. Both of these dietary factors are necessary for proper growth. A gross deficiency of B_1 produces the disease beriberi, and changes in the intestinal tract which result in poor function and in loss of appetite. A deficiency of G produces the disease pellagra. Vitamin B complex is present in fruits and vegetables and to a lesser extent in milk, meats, and eggs. The amount of this vitamin in human milk depends in a large measure upon the amount in the diet of the mother. The diet of many mothers is so incomplete that the B in the milk is often dangerously low. For this as well as other reasons the diet of the infant is advantageously supplemented at an early age with B-containing foods. Although a deficiency of B leads to a loss of appetite, not all babies have their appetites improved by addition to the diet of vitamin B preparations, for the reason that other causes for poor appetite are also common. If fruits and vegetables are included in the infant's diet at an early age it is rarely necessary to give special vitamin B preparations.

Vitamin C also is present in fruits and vegetables. For the young infant either orange juice or tomato juice is relied upon as an adequate source, and the diet should be supplemented early with one of these food materials. Deficiency of vitamin C in the diet leads to the disease scurvy, a condition which is not rare among infants even in this enlightened day. As with vitamin B, the amount of vitamin C in the milk depends upon the amount in the diet of the mother. The amount of C in fresh cow's milk may be sufficient to protect the artificially fed infant, but this never should be relied upon, as vitamin C disappears rather rapidly from milk with the lapse of time and especially when milk is pasteurized or kept hot for longer than a few minutes. It is not advisable to feed to an infant fresh cow's milk unless it has undergone some heat treatment. It is a good general rule, therefore, to supplement the diet of every infant with vitamin-C-containing foods, such as orange or tomato juice.

Vitamin D is essential to the body for the proper use of calcium and phosphorus with which to build bone and teeth. A deficiency of this vitamin in infancy leads to rickets, a condition in which the bones become soft and often crooked. Rickets, at least in a mild form, is relatively common, especially among artificially fed babies. Vitamin D is present to some extent in milk fat, egg yolk, and the glandular organs of animals. This vitamin is not widely distributed in foods and is not present in any common food in very large amounts. A well-known and moderately concentrated commercial source is cod-liver oil. Fat-like substances (sterols) which are normally present in the body may be converted into vitamin D by the action of ultraviolet energy. The common source of ultraviolet energy is sunshine, which explains the infrequency of rickets in the summer and its prevalence in the winter and spring. The very short energy waves which are classed as ultraviolet are easily filtered out of sunshine by clouds and dust, and they do not pass through ordinary window glass. Special lamps have been devised for the production of ultraviolet energy, some of which give off this energy in an amount considerably greater than that obtained from sunshine. Ultraviolet energy converts certain sterols into vitamin D wherever it may come into contact with them, whether it be in the body, in food material, or in some concentrated state. Thus certain foods which have been exposed to ultraviolet rays take on the properties of vitamin D. The substance ergosterol, when irradiated, becomes the most concentrated form of vitamin D which has been prepared. This preparation is known as viosterol. Whenever growth is rapid, as it is in infancy, it becomes desirable to supplement the diet with some preparation containing vitamin D in larger amounts than are ordinarily found in the food. Cod-liver oil is the usual form in which this substance is given. Recently there has been a general tendency to fortify cod-liver oil with viosterol or to make a complete substitution of viosterol for cod-liver oil. In this connection it is necessary to remember that viosterol contains only one vitamin, whereas cod-liver oil contains two, both of which are essential to the body. Though vitamin A may be present in the diet in sufficient amount in some instances, viosterol is not to be considered a substitute for cod-liver oil, nor are the virtues of ultra-violet lamps to be evaluated on the basis of much of their advertising and exploitation. The usefulness of these lamps is limited, and with the exception of special cases, the expense is not justified.

Vitamin E is unimportant for the infant because of its wide distribution and the improbability of any infant's receiving an inadequate supply. It may be related to some cases of habitual abortion.

Under usual circumstances it may be considered that all of the mineral salts necessary to the body, with the exception of iron, are supplied by the milk of the diet. Normally the infant is born with a store of iron which will serve his iron needs for several months. Certainly not later than six months after birth, and preferably sooner, iron or iron-containing foods should be added to the diet. The addition may be by means of egg yolk, beef juice, ground boiled liver, vegetables and fruits, or if desired by iron salts used as a medicine. Babies born prematurely do not have the usual iron stores at birth, and babies who are ill during the early months may have their iron stores exhausted sooner than the normal expectation. Calcium and phosphorus are essential minerals which are supplied by milk in relative abundance, but are markedly deficient, as compared to milk, in all other foodstuffs. This fact becomes significant and important in those instances in which in later infancy the baby is permitted to refuse milk and to substitute other articles of food.

Water is essential for the storage and combustion of food, for the excretion of waste products, and for many other life processes. The baby's needs for water are relatively much greater than those of the adult, and he shows the harmful effects of deprivation or loss much more quickly and more seriously. This fact becomes important in certain illnesses, such as diarrhea with marked water loss in the stools, and vomiting with failure of water retention. Sometimes a baby becomes so dehydrated (dry) that its life is threatened for this reason alone. In health and on a good diet the amount of water ingested usually need be no cause for special concern since the infant's diet normally contains such a high proportion of water. Water, in addition to the regular diet, may be indicated in hot weather or in case of sweating from any cause. Because of the difficulty of determining when a baby is thirsty, water can be offered regularly at suitable intervals as a routine measure, but frequently it will be found that the baby will refuse it.

DIGESTION

It is common knowledge that the digestive capacity of the infant is limited. Many foods served to adults would cause digestive disturbances if fed to an infant. The basic food of an infant's diet is milk. The stomach of the newborn baby seems to have acid and digestive juices adequate to digest human milk without difficulty. Unmodified cow's milk tends to cause more or less digestive difficulty in the early months of infancy. The common modification of cow's milk, such as boiling, acidification, or dilution, makes it better adapted to the digestive capacity of the infant.

The young infant has relatively little capacity to digest starchy foods. Babies who are fed cereals or other starches in the early weeks usually have no difficulty from them, as the undigested part of the starch merely passes through as a harmless foreign body. Only occasionally are fermentative processes set up with their consequent distress.

Other foods commonly offered to infants (fruit juices, fruits, sieved vegetables, cod-liver oil) usually cause no digestive difficulties, though sometimes the coarser parts of some of these foods are not digested and are passed in the stools.

The emptying time of the infant's stomach is of some importance. The stomach usually is empty in from two to three hours after a feeding of human milk; and two and one half to three and one half hours are required for cow's milk in the usual modifications. It is inadvisable to feed babies at such short intervals that the stomach at feeding time still contains some food from the last feeding. Too frequent feeding leads to digestive disturbances. Illness from any cause tends to delay the emptying of the stomach and to affect the digestive capacity sufficiently to cause digestive symptoms. Sometimes when the digestive symptoms (vomiting or diarrhea) are prominent and the responsible illness somewhat obscure, the illness is attributed erroneously to the digestive tract.

STOOLS

The first passages from the bowel after birth are dark green. As soon as food is given, the character of the stool begins to change and usually by the fifth day it has assumed the type characteristic of infancy. When the baby is breast fed the stools are usually passed two to five times daily; they are soft, bright yellow, acid in reaction, and have a slightly sour cheesy odor. The stools from cow's milk are less frequent (one to three daily), somewhat firmer, a less brilliant yellow, and with a more disagreeable odor than those from human milk.

When milk is the principal food, the color of the stool depends in a large measure upon the speed of passage through the bowel. If the passage is rapid, as in cases of diarrhea, the bowel movements do not have time to turn from their normal green to a yellow color, and the stools then are green. If the rate of movement of the intestinal contents is very slow, the stools may become gray or white in color. These various colors are of no significance except as indicators of the speed of movement of intestinal contents. If for any reason the baby is deprived of food, the stool color becomes brownish and increasingly dark and finally dark green, depending upon the degree of starvation.

Probably much more attention is paid to curds in the stools than their importance deserves. The curds most frequently observed are composed of soaps which have been derived from the fat of the food. A moderate amount of these curds may be considered normal for the baby receiving human milk. Usually with cow's-milk feeding, the intestinal contents are moved along more slowly, and the soaps are drier from absorption of water and are pressed more firmly together so that they do not appear as curds. Anything which causes diarrhea or increases the frequency of stools allows the passage of soaps in the form of small masses or curds, so that usually their presence has no greater significance than an indication of more rapid movement of intestinal contents.

The significance of mucus in the stools is also commonly misconstrued. Mucus appears in the stools when the intestinal tract is irritated for any reason. Diarrhea is commonly associated with irritation and consequently with increased mucus. Most cathartics are irritative and are productive of increased mucus, and the common idea of continued catharsis for the purpose of getting rid of mucus is absurd, for the reason that the greater the amount of catharsis, the greater the amount of mucus.

BREAST FEEDING

It seems unnecessary to present arguments that every mother who can should nurse her infant, and most mothers can, at least for the first few months. It is in these early months that natural feeding is of greatest importance. Despite the fact that human milk is such an excellent food, it must be recognized that the milk varies in quality with the diet and habits of the mother. For example, the various vitamins cannot be present in the milk unless they have been taken in adequate quantities by the mother. In order that her milk be at its best and serve well its intended purpose, the mother must observe the common rules of good hygiene and diet. These rules are fully as necessary for her own health as for that of the baby. Mothers frequently develop cavities in their teeth during lactation, because they secrete more calcium in the milk than they ingest. It is desirable also that the mother have sufficient sleep and moderate exercise but never to the point of fatigue. Worry and other nervous states often have a harmful effect which may be reflected in the quality of the milk.

The diet of the mother may be quite varied, and any food is permissible unless it causes digestive disturbance. The avoidance of acid foods is a fallacy. Examples of a well-balanced diet for the pregnant and nursing mother are given.

Sometimes it is found that the mother is unable to secrete adequate quantities of milk. If the mother's diet already is good, the milk supply cannot be increased by increasing the diet, though the milk may be increased by improving the diet when this has not been satisfactory. The best stimulus to maintaining or increasing the milk is regular and thorough emptying of the breast. When milk accumulates in the breast because of incomplete emptying, parts of the breast tend to become hard and painful from the pressure of the retained milk. This condition is often called caked breasts. The surest way to decrease the milk is to permit the breasts to become and remain caked.

There are very few good reasons for the mother not to nurse her baby. She should not nurse it if she has tuberculosis or a serious chronic illness. Nursing should be suspended temporarily during a severe acute illness. Menstruation is not a good reason for weaning, even though the baby may be uncomfortable for a day or two. Should the mother become pregnant the baby should be weaned gradually to avoid overtaxing the mother. Medication taken by the mother need not constitute a reason for weaning, for no drugs given in customary doses are secreted in the milk in harmful amounts.

TECHNIC OF NURSING

It is customary to place the baby to the breast six to twelve hours after birth and every six hours during the next twenty-four hours and every four hours thereafter. During these first few days little is obtained by the baby, but the nursing helps to stimulate the flow of milk. Water or 5 per cent sugar solution is offered every four hours. The milk usually is secreted after the third or fourth day. The nursing interval then should be either three or four hours, depending upon the quantity of milk available. More milk is obtained with the shorter interval, and this is usually the better choice in the beginning. Whatever interval is chosen, the schedule should be followed with regularity. The baby should be nursed at one breast at one nursing and the other breast at the next. The average time at the breast is about fifteen minutes. More than half of the milk is obtained in the first five minutes, and the greater portion of the remainder in the next five minutes. Usually something is wrong when the baby nurses longer than twenty minutes.

All babies swallow some air with the milk. This may be a cause of vomiting or of discomfort. It is desirable therefore to hold the baby upright after each nursing and to pat him gently on the back until eructation of the air occurs.

The care of the mother's nipples is important. They should be bathed before and after each feeding. A fissuring of the nipples may occur. This is always painful and sometimes leads to breast abscess. Fissuring of the nipples has the same cause as chapped hands, and can be prevented in the same manner, viz., keep them as dry as possible as far as milk is concerned, and if necessary keep them greased with some simple ointment such as vaseline or cold cream.

DIFFICULTIES

The difficulties encountered in breast feeding are few. Some babies are overfed. This may be evidenced by a large weight gain and intestinal discomfort often of a colicky nature. There may be unusual regurgitation of food and increased frequency of stools. Since most of these symptoms may be produced by other causes as well, it is desirable to make certain of the diagnosis by weighing the baby before and after nursing. The remedy for overfeeding is simple. The baby should be placed on a four-hour schedule. Usually this is sufficient. If it is not, the time at the breast should be shortened. Another measure is to give the baby water immediately before nursing so as to satisfy his hunger sooner.

Relatively large numbers of babies are underfed. This often happens in milder degrees without the mother being aware of it. The chief symptom is a slow or negative weight gain. There may be evidence of hunger, or intestinal discomfort, colic and regurgitation from swallowed air. Air swallowing tends to be greater in underfed babies. Weighing before and after nursing to determine the amount of milk taken will disclose the difficulty. The remedy in underfeeding is to give food in addition to the breast milk, and not to wean the baby. A suitable formula prepared from cow's milk should be given after each breast feeding. In some instances enough human milk may be obtained by feeding the baby at both breasts each nursing.

Whenever the baby becomes ill from any cause, he is likely to have gastro-intestinal symptoms, even though no primary disease exists in the intestinal tract. Thus, one should not be too ready to blame these intestinal symptoms upon the milk and to overlook the real causative factor. So often when the milk "disagrees," the difficulty is entirely unrelated to the milk.

WEANING

In general it is the choice of wisdom to wean the baby from the breast at the age of eight to ten months. This may be done gradually by substituting an increasing number of bottle feedings. If the baby has reached the weaning age without being accustomed to a bottle, it often happens that he will refuse it as long as he can get the breast. Thus abrupt weaning is necessary at times. In the case of abrupt weaning, when the baby is unaccustomed to cow's milk, it is usually preferable to have the formula slightly weaker for a few days than it would be normally for the baby's age. Weaning in the summer is still feared by many mothers. There need be no such fear if the milk formula and other foods are appropriate for the baby and are properly prepared.

ARTIFICIAL FEEDING

Human and cow's milk are similar in many respects. They have the same constituents, but the proportions are different. It is chiefly because of these differences in proportion that digestive difficulties occur when unmodified cow's milk is fed to young infants. The milk of all cows is the same except for the quantity of fat. For infant feeding it is generally advisable to use milk of medium or low fat content. Holstein milk or milk from a mixed herd is preferable. Milk from Jersey or Guernsey cows should be partially skimmed.

Milk is readily contaminated in the milking and handling and is an excellent food for the growth of bacteria. All harmful bacteria and most of the others are killed by pasteurization. Boiling milk for several minutes also kills the bacteria and in addition alters the milk in such a way that the casein forms a finer curd and is thereby more easily digested by the infant. For this reason it is generally preferable to use boiled milk, and when this is done pasteurization is unnecessary.

Evaporated milk is ordinary fresh cow's milk which has been concentrated to slightly less than half of its volume by the evaporation of the water. It is then sealed in cans and sterilized. It has been shown to be an excellent, safe, and convenient food for the artificial feeding of infants. For use it may be diluted back to its original volume with water and used in the same manner as fresh milk. The sweetened varieties of evaporated milk (condensed milk) are not suitable for the routine feeding of infants, as the protein content of such milk when diluted for use is so low that it does not permit proper growth of muscle tissue.

Dried milk is milk which has had practically all of its water removed. It is useful in infant feeding, though usually more expensive than fresh or evaporated milk. Some dried milks are prepared from skimmed milk instead of from whole milk. Dried milk is used frequently in a community which cannot obtain fresh milk or when a milk of low fat content is desired. To obtain a product similar to whole milk it is necessary to add one part by weight of the dried whole milk to seven parts of water.

SUGARS AND CARBOHYDRATES

Milk alone is not a suitably balanced food in early infancy without the addition of sugar, and when the milk has been modified by dilution sugar is necessary to satisfy the energy requirements of the infant. Thus some variety of sugar is always used in the milk formula. The sugars commonly used are lactose (milk sugar), cane sugar (table sugar), and derivatives of starch (dextrin, maltose, dextrose, and mixtures of these). All of these serve the baby equally well after they have been absorbed from the intestinal tract. The choice of sugar is based upon its cost and upon its behavior in the intestinal tract of the infant. Certain sugars are more laxative than others. For example, lactose is absorbed relatively slowly and usually passes far down the intestinal tract before complete absorption. This long presence in the tract has a laxative effect. At the other extreme is dextrose, which is absorbed quickly and consequently is a good sugar to use in cases of diarrhea. Corn syrup is a mixture of dextrin and maltose and has found favor because it is inexpensive as well as useful, though it is less convenient to handle than the dry sugars. Dry dextrin-maltose mixtures are extensively employed.

DILUENTS

One of the chief objects in the modification of cow's milk to make it more suitable for young infants is to alter the casein in such a manner that it forms a fine curd in the stomach. This object is very commonly achieved by dilution with water. Sometimes cereal water, usually barley water, is used for this purpose. Such diluents do no harm but provide little food value. Limewater, so commonly used in the past, is now seldom employed as a diluent.

SYNTHETIC FOOD MIXTURES

Several manufacturers have prepared mixtures of milk and sugar in proportions thought to be suitable for infant feeding, and these may be obtained in a dry or liquid form. All that is required for use is the addition of water in specified proportions. All of these mixtures are relatively expensive. In most instances an attempt has been made to make these synthetic foods similar to human milk. Because of their low protein content, many such milks are not well suited to the rapidly growing infant. Malted milk and sweetened condensed milk are examples of milk and sugar mixtures which are quite ill suited for infant feeding, because of their high sugar content.

FORMULAS FOR WELL BABIES

In the usual methods of infant feeding, the need for protein must be satisfied by milk. At least two ounces of milk for each pound of body weight is given each twenty-four hours. By the time the baby is taking a quart of milk a day, other foods may be added to supplement the diet in such a way that more milk is unnecessary.

The amount of sugar added to meet the total food requirement is usually one ounce daily during the first two months and one and a half ounce during the succeeding four months. More or less than this may be indicated under special circumstances.

The amount of diluent (water) used should be sufficient to bring the total volume to that which the baby will take conveniently in twenty-four hours. In general it may be stated that a baby should take at a single feeding two to three ounces more than his age in months. Seldom is it desirable to give more than seven ounces at a feeding at any age, for by the time the baby is receiving seven ounces he is taking also other foods than milk.

As an example, a baby four months of age weighing twelve pounds, might do well on a formula containing twenty-four ounces of milk, one and one half ounces of sugar, and water sufficient to make five feedings of six and one half ounces each, or six feedings of six ounces' each, as seems best suited to the individual baby.

During the first two weeks of life the milk dilution usually should be a little greater than that which has been specified until the baby becomes accustomed to the cow's-milk feeding. The original mixture should never be less than half milk, and this should be used only for a few days. It is frequently customary to start with two thirds milk and one third water.

A feeding schedule which will be found suitable for the majority of well babies is as follows:

Age	Wt. lbs.	Milk oz.	Sugar oz.	Water oz.	Feedings oz.	Interval Day hr.	Interval Night hr.
1 wk.	7	10	1	4	7 x 2	3	4
2 wks.	7	14	1	7	7 x 3	3	4
1 mo.	8	16	1	8	6 x 4	3	8
2 mo.	10	20	1½	10	6 x 5	3	8
4 mo.	12	24	1½	9	5 x 6½	4	8
6 mo.	14	28	2	7	5 x 7	4	

If corn syrup is used as the sugar, an equal volume of water is omitted.

Sugar Equivalents

1 ounce by weight of cane sugar = 2 level tablespoons.
1 ounce by weight of lactose = 4 level tablespoons.
1 ounce by weight dried malt sugar = 4 level tablespoons.
1 ounce by volume of corn syrup = 2 level tablespoons and contains 1 ounce of sugar.

It must be remembered that the formulas and schedules given are calculated for the average baby and that adjustments frequently will be necessary for any individual baby. A baby who is hungry, not gaining as he should, and who is having no digestive difficulties should have more food than is indicated in the schedule. Often minor adjustments in the quantity or type of sugar will make the difference between constipation and loose stools. For these and many other reasons it is highly advisable to have the infant's feeding under the supervision of one who is expert in such matters.

FORMULAS WITH UNDILUTED MILK

Cow's milk may be altered in other ways than by dilution so that it is readily utilized by the infant. One of the methods of accomplishing this is by the addition of an acid in carefully regulated quantities to milk which has been previously boiled. Lactic acid (the acid of naturally soured milk) and citric acid (the acid of citrous fruits) have been used extensively for this purpose. Milk which has been soured by bacterial growth under laboratory control is excellent when it is available. The feeding of undiluted acid milk permits a greater food intake and thus a more rapid growth is brought about. These babies exceed the averages in height and weight. In the light of some of our more recent knowledge this would seem to be an advantage. The following table gives an approximate feeding schedule for the average well infant using undiluted acidified milk:

Age	Milk oz.	Sugar oz. (vol.)	Feedings: oz.
1 wk.	12	½	6 x 2
2 wks.	15	1	6 x 2½
1 mo.	21	1½	6 x 3½
2 mo.	25	2	5 x 5
4 mo.	30	2	5 x 6
6 to 10 mo.	35	2	5 x 7

If corn syrup is used as the sugar, an equal volume of milk is omitted.

THE PREPARATION OF FORMULAS

Sweet Milk Dilutions

The milk, sugar, and water should be mixed and then boiled from one to three minutes with constant stirring. It should be poured immediately into boiled nursing bottles, stoppered and cooled rapidly, and placed on ice until ready for use.

Lactic Acid or Citric Acid Milk

The milk and sugar should be mixed and boiled for two minutes while stirring. It should be cooled rapidly; when quite cold the acid is added slowly while constantly stirring. It should then be poured into nursing bottles, stoppered, and placed on ice.

The amount of citric acid required is usually four grams to the quart of milk. Citric acid may be purchased as weighed tablets ready for use. These are dissolved in a small quantity of water and the solution stirred into the milk.

Lactic acid is purchased as an 85 per cent solution. One teaspoonful or one hundred and twenty drops is required for each quart of milk.

Sometimes orange juice is added to the milk. The amount required to bring a quart of milk to the proper acidity is about three ounces.

Acidified Evaporated Milk

One pint of water and the amount of sugar specified are boiled for three minutes. When this is thoroughly cold, two thirds of a teaspoonful of lactic acid is added to it. This mixture is then added to one pint of evaporated milk. The product is then approximately equivalent to one quart of acidified fresh milk.

CHOICE AND CARE OF BOTTLES AND NIPPLES

It is preferable to have as many nursing bottles and nipples as there are feedings in the day. Both the bottles and the nipples should be of such a type that they can be readily and thoroughly cleaned. The bottles and nipples should be washed with soap and water and boiled for five minutes. The bottles are then ready for filling and the nipples for clean storage.

Any funnels, spoons, pans, etc., used in the preparation of the formula should be boiled each time before use. If possible it is advisable to have one set of utensils for use in the preparation of the baby's formula only.

TECHNIC OF FEEDING

For feeding, the milk should be warmed to body temperature by placing the bottle in a vessel of hot water. Care should be taken not to heat acidified mixtures much above body temperature for the reason that the curd is likely to clot and settle out. The size of the hole in the nipple should be such that when the bottle is inverted the milk drops out rapidly but does not flow in a steady stream. The baby should be fed in arms and in a position in which the shoulders are higher than the buttocks. Any milk refused should be discarded. After feeding and before being put to bed the baby should be held in a position which will permit regurgitation of any swallowed air. Gentle patting on the back will assist in eructation of the air.

ADDITIONS TO THE MILK DIET

Neither human nor cow's milk is a perfect food. Babies fed exclusively on either for a long period will develop certain nutritional diseases. Iron and vitamins C and D and possibly B and A particularly are likely to be deficient. Food materials which supplement the milk diet in these respects should be given early.

Orange juice should be started during the first month. Two tablespoons of orange juice should be diluted with an equal quantity of water and given once or twice daily. This amount is gradually increased to the juice of half an orange at three months of age and then to that of an entire orange daily. In some instances it is advisable to substitute tomato juice for orange juice. When this is done a somewhat greater quantity of tomato juice should be used.

Cod-liver oil should be started early in infancy. In the beginning the amount can be one half teaspoonful twice daily and gradually increased until one teaspoonful is given each time. However, one teaspoonful daily of a high-grade cod-liver oil will be found sufficient for most babies. It is probable that the baby needs cod-liver oil in the summer as well as in the winter, for during the hot summer months it is not always possible to give him sufficient sunshine. Iron in some form should be given the baby before he is six months of age. Although it may be given in the form of medicinal iron, it is usually preferable to administer it in some iron-containing food. Egg yolk and

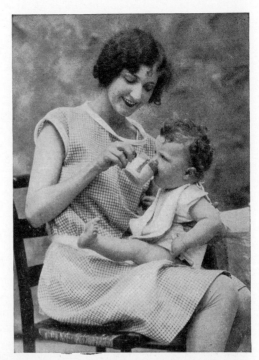

FIG. 21. As soon as possible, the child should be taught to drink from a cup. This is an aid to weaning.

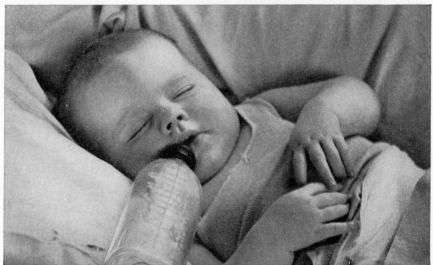

Courtesy of Ruth Alexander Nichols.

FIG. 22. Permitting child to sleep with nursing bottle in mouth may deform face.

green vegetables are the common foods chosen for infants. Certain fruits also are of value. This is especially true of apricots and peaches. Therefore egg yolk, vegetables, and fruits are offered to infants at increasingly earlier ages.

It is customary to give various cereals to infants beginning at six to seven months. Cereal is entirely satisfactory as an infant food, though it is probably not as important as are the fruits and vegetables and egg yolk. Consequently it seems more advisable to have the infant well established on these other foods before cereal is started.

Care of the Sick Infant

The illnesses of an infant are usually of an acute rather than of a chronic nature, and the general care is very similar for all illnesses. The infant should be allowed to lie quietly in bed, and the feedings, treatments, etc., should be spaced at as long intervals as possible. There is often a strong tendency to keep doing things to and for the patient, with the result that little of the much needed rest is obtained, and the baby becomes exhausted. Excitement should be avoided and unnecessary entertainment reduced to a minimum.

An effort should be made to have the air of the sick-room fresh at all times, but this does not mean that it need be raw, cold winter air. No illness of infancy requires any special type of clothing. The clothing should be that to which the infant is accustomed during sleep in health. Except in the case of premature and very delicate infants, the patient should have a cleansing bath (at least one) daily. There is no acute illness in which bathing is harmful. The feeding of the sick infant is discussed subsequently.

Infants have higher body temperature from the same or less important causes than do adults. A temperature of 104 or 105 degrees in an infant does not demand any measures for relief unless it is of considerable duration or unless it is associated with such nervous symptoms as restlessness and inability to sleep.

A common and effective method of reducing high temperature is bathing. A bath of the type designated as a sponge bath is satisfactory.

At times definite indications for the use of drugs are encountered in infancy, but in general, drug treatment plays a relatively minor rôle. The measures which assume greater importance are diet, hygiene, and general nursing care.

COMMON ILLNESSES AND ABNORMALITIES

JAUNDICE IN THE NEWBORN

Icterus or jaundice occurs in newly born babies with considerable frequency and in the vast majority of instances is without significance for the health of the infant. When jaundice is present the white part of the eyeball is yellow, and in the more marked cases the skin also has a definitely yellow color. It appears in the first two or three days of life, and its persistence varies from a few days to several weeks. No treatment is indicated.

HERNIA OR "RUPTURE"

The most frequently encountered hernia in infancy is at the navel or umbilicus. At this point the usual finding is a weak place in the abdominal wall, which upon finger pressure is felt as a hole, usually smaller than the end of the finger. With the intra-abdominal pressure produced by crying a protrusion is to be observed at the site of the hernia. Umbilical hernia usually causes no discomfort or other difficulty. With the wearing of some device which effectively prevents protrusion of the hernia, the defect nearly always disappears in the course of some months. The simplest method of controlling the hernia is to cover it with a tightly drawn strip of adhesive tape. No device should be used which keeps the defect open by pushing inward through it.

The inguinal hernia occurs with considerably less frequency. In this condition the protrusion is on one or both sides of the lower abdomen (the groin) immediately above and to either side of the genitalia. The general principles of management are the same as for umbilical hernia. Adhesive tape cannot be applied effectively, and the simplest truss is made from a skein of yarn.

COMMON COLDS

The symptoms of the common cold are well known to everyone, and it is unnecessary to enumerate them. Some of the consequences of this infection are very important for the infant. An infant cannot nurse satisfactorily when the nose is obstructed. Difficulty will be encountered in the feeding, with the possible result of marked underfeeding. In infancy some vomiting and looseness of the stools frequently accompany a cold. In general, colds affect infants much more seriously than older individuals, not only by producing more marked symptoms, but also by having a greater frequency of complications. Secondary inflammations in the ears, bronchi, and lungs are not infrequent.

In the endeavor to prevent colds it is important to realize that they are infectious and contagious. They are readily contracted from others. Exposure to drafts and low temperatures can be of no significance unless infectious material is present also. The difference between those who are subject to frequent colds and those who seem relatively immune is not known with exactness, but in general those who have good hygienic care, receive a complete diet, and are in a good state of nutrition, have fewer colds than those who are lacking in these factors. Deficiency of vitamin A very definitely leads to nasal infections, but when the amount of this vitamin is already adequate, additional amounts probably have little effect. Cod-liver oil is desirable as a part of the diet of every infant.

A measure important in the management of a cold in an infant is an endeavor to keep the nose open sufficiently for breathing and for drainage. Sometimes this may be accomplished by the regular installation of a few drops of mineral oil. Oil preparations containing such substances as camphor or menthol should be used in infancy with the greatest caution, since they sometimes cause a spasmodic closure of the larynx with consequent obstruction to breathing. Frequently physicians prescribe a drug, such as a solution of ephedrin, to be sprayed or dropped into the nose for the purpose of reducing the swelling and thus producing a larger breathing space. Often free drainage from the nose is a great aid in the prevention of a complicating ear infection.

OTITIS MEDIA

Otitis media is inflammation within the cavity of the ear immediately behind the eardrum. This cavity is connected directly with the throat by what is called the eustachian tube. Thus infections in the nose and throat have a more or less direct path to the ear. It is the rule in infants that otitis media produces a relatively high fever, pain, restlessness, and often general constitutional symptoms among which may be vomiting and diarrhea. A few babies sometimes have otitis media with only a part of these symptoms or even none of them, and the otitis is diagnosed only by examination of the ears.

Otitis media occurs in varying degrees of severity and may be seen first by the physician in different stages of development or subsidence. The treatment to be instituted depends upon these various factors. With a severe inflammation and bulging of the eardrum, the drum should be incised to permit drainage of the pus lying within. In cases of moderate or early inflammation the proper treatment may be to let it alone and observe its progress. If there seems to be pain, the physician often advises the dropping into the ears of certain oily preparations.

The bony cavity of the mastoid connects directly with the middle ear and consequently is inflamed in every case of otitis media. In most instances the products of inflammation drain by way of the middle ear, and the mastoid inflammation subsides along with that of the ear. In a few instances the mastoid inflammation causes sufficient swelling about the opening into the ear that drainage is not possible. The mastoid inflammation then assumes increased importance and is designated mastoiditis. In many of these cases it becomes necessary to make a surgical opening into the mastoid from the exterior. Mastoiditis is even more likely than otitis media to produce constitutional symptoms, and sometimes in infancy the resulting vomiting and diarrhea constitute a grave menace to life. Often the gastro-intestinal symptoms completely overshadow the slight or even negative external evidences of mastoiditis.

CROUP

The term croup has been used to designate inflammations in the larynx which give rise to difficulty in breathing. The term "membranous croup," now being used decreasingly in the interest of more exact diagnosis, has been applied to the obstruction of the larynx produced by inflammations associated with exudates in a form resembling membrane. Membranous croup is practically synonymous with diphtheria of the larynx.

The less serious form of croup, and the form which is usually implied in the term croup, is known also as spasmodic or catarrhal croup. In this condition a relatively mild inflammation of the larynx leads reflexly to a spasm of the muscles of the larynx. During a period of spasm the opening through the larynx is almost completely closed, and air is drawn into the lungs with considerable difficulty and with a plainly audible noise. No difficulty exists in expiration. The attacks of spasm, which are often alarming but rarely serious, tend to recur for a period of about three days, when the inflammation and its symptoms usually subside. The attacks are more frequent at night, the days often being entirely free from them.

The attacks may be relieved by breathing air containing warm-water vapor (steam), and for this purpose croup bottles have been devised. A less troublesome effective method is the administration of certain antispasmodic drugs, with which the attacks may be forestalled and prevented as well as relieved.

PNEUMONIA

Pneumonia may be classified as of two kinds, viz., primary and secondary. By secondary is meant that the pneumonia occurs as a complication or an extension of some other disease, such as a common cold, bronchitis, measles, influenza, etc. Primary pneumonia occurs in a manner similar to other contagious diseases, being contracted from one who has the disease or a carrier, and not ordinarily secondary to or complicating some other disease. In many respects the general nature of the illness is much the same in these two types of pneumonia. On the other hand there are certain essential differences. Both types of pneumonia are serious, but the primary type is much less so. The primary type tends to appear suddenly, run a fairly stormy course, and disappear in a week or possibly two. The secondary type develops gradually, may shift from one place to another in the lungs, and last four to six weeks or longer. The fact that it complicates some disease also increases its seriousness.

The treatment in infancy is much the same in the two types of pneumonia, viz., what is known as symptomatic treatment. Treatment is applied according to the symptoms present which require relief. Sedatives are indicated for severe or constant cough; hydrotherapy (bathing) for high fever accompanied by nervous symptoms; oxygen for breathing if the patient should become blue; stimulation in case of failing vital functions. In the early stages of pneumonia sometimes counterirritants such as mustard paste seem of benefit. In cases of primary pneumonia, often the breathing of cold air is of benefit, though in infancy this measure should be carried out with caution. Babies with secondary pneumonia, babies with any considerable degree of bronchitis, and delicate infants should not be placed in cold air, but should be given warm moist fresh air. Babies with pneumonia should have their position changed frequently. Pneumonia is one illness in which it is of advantage to hold the infant in arms, because of the frequent change of position that this causes. The administration of considerable amounts of water or fluid is especially advantageous in pneumonia.

THRUSH

Thrush is the result of the growth of a specific fungus on the mucous membrance of the mouth. The fungus in its growth forms small slightly elevated white plaques which are difficult to remove. Thrush, as it usually occurs, causes no symptoms. The treatment consists of local applications made gently by means of cotton on the end of an applicator. Roughness in treatment tends to spread the infection. The preparation to be used as a local application depends upon the preference of the individual physician. Several preparations are about equally effective.

INTUSSUSCEPTION

Intussusception is a condition almost exclusively of infancy, in which one part of the bowel enters and becomes invaginated in the part of the bowel in immediate continuity to it. The blood supply of the invaginated bowel becomes cut off and in the course of a short time that part of the bowel dies and becomes gangrenous. The condition is characterized by an abrupt onset, associated with vomiting, sharp pain, and increasing prostration. At the onset there may be one or two small bowel movements, usually with some evidences of blood. After this time nothing is passed by the bowel. If an enema is returned it will usually contain blood.

Intussusception demands immediate operation for its relief. Early operation has a low mortality, while delay increases the seriousness of the condition.

RECTAL PROLAPSE

Rectal or anal prolapse is a protrusion of the mucous membrane of the anus or anus and lower rectum which occurs usually only at stool. It is possible for this to occur occasionally in a normal infant when the stool is large and hard and is passed with much straining. However, it is more frequent in babies who are poorly nourished and as a consequence have relaxed muscles about the anus. In these prolapse may occur either with constipation or with diarrhea; occasionally when the prolapse has recurred over a long period, it may occur with more or less normal stools.

Three factors should be considered in the treatment. The prolapse should be replaced whenever it occurs and some means should be used in an endeavor to hold it in at all times. For this purpose the buttocks can be strapped tightly together with adhesive tape or a pad should be worn which makes pressure at the anus. If either constipation or diarrhea is present it should be corrected by appropriate means. The stools should be made of such a consistency that they are passed with a minimum of effort and without straining. The general nutrition should be improved, thus improving general muscular tone. It is seldom that the proper application of these measures fails to be effective.

PYELITIS

Pyelitis is an inflammation of the pelvis of the kidney. It may occur at any age, but is much more common in infants and young children, and more frequent in girls than in boys. The infection may ascend the urinary tract to the kidney from the exterior, or perhaps more frequently the bacteria causing the inflammation are carried to the kidney by the blood. The bacteria most often responsible are normal inhabitants of the intestinal tract. The intestinal wall seems more permeable to these bacteria in the presence of diarrhea or marked constipation. In infancy the tendency to intestinal disturbances as a result of colds and respiratory infections increases the frequency of pyelitis during the existence of these head infections.

The symptoms of pyelitis in infancy are usually general rather than local. Fever is the most constant symptom, and this tends to be very irregular. Sometimes fever is the only definite symptom, or perhaps fever and irritability. Because of the lack of localizing symptoms, the diagnosis is not made except by examination of the urine. The urine shows evidence of inflammation, chiefly pus cells and bacteria.

In the great majority of cases the inflammation disappears spontaneously or responds well to simple treatment. The outlook therefore is usually very good. In the very few cases in which the inflammation becomes chronic, usually some anatomical or functional partial urinary obstruction is present.

Free urinary excretion produced by the administration of considerable quantities of water is always beneficial. The giving of alkaline medication to the point of altering the urine from acid to alkaline is frequently effective. Certain drugs are used which are antiseptic when excreted in the urine. Sometimes vaccines are employed in the obstinate cases. The physician will combine these various measures according to the indications in the individual case.

VAGINITIS

Inflammation of the vagina or of the vulva and vagina as it occurs in infancy and childhood is chiefly of two varieties. The most frequent of these is due to lack of cleanliness. In general mothers seem very hesitant about the detailed cleansing of the external genitalia of their children, and later about teaching the children to cleanse themselves. Secretions accumulate, decompose, and not only give rise to an unpleasant odor, but actually set up inflammatory processes. Usually these are of mild degree, but they can be severe enough to cause an active discharge. This variety of vaginitis can be prevented and usually cured by ordinary cleansing measures. Sometimes in the more severe cases medicated douches are indicated to bring about a cure.

Less frequently is encountered vaginitis due to a specific bacterium, the gonococcus. Among adults this variety of infection is looked upon as a social disease. Among girls, however, it is contagious, and it is nearly always innocently contracted. It is distinguished from other varieties of vaginitis chiefly and definitely by identification of the specific bacterium in the discharges. Bacteriological examination of the discharge is usually the first measure undertaken by the physician. The treatment is chiefly by medicated douches and local applications. Cure is obtained only after prolonged treatment.

CONVULSIONS

The common type of convulsion is a condition in which the child loses consciousness, becomes rigid and then has spasmodic jerking movements of the face and extremities. They may be very brief, may last several minutes, or occasionally a longer time. They may be repeated, the child having a series of short convulsions.

A convulsion is merely a symptom and the possible disease causes are many. Infants have convulsions more readily than do adults. Sometimes convulsions usher in some acute infection such as pneumonia. In fact, the onset of some acute infection with rapid rise in body temperature is perhaps the most frequent cause of convulsions. A convulsion is

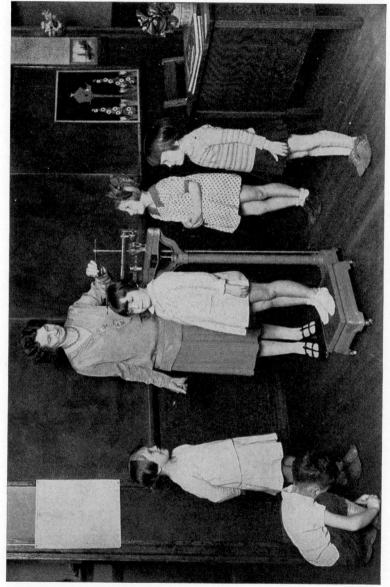

Fig. 23.   A weekly weighing of the child indicates state of nutrition.

very alarming to the parents, but in itself it is not serious except as the underlying cause may be serious. Sometimes the underlying cause is not readily found. In the case of pneumonia, for example, several days may elapse before the diagnosis can be made with certainty. Whether or not the diagnosis can be made at once, the indication is to bring the convulsions under control and take measures to prevent their recurrence. The most effective remedies are sedative drugs, and these must be administered or prescribed by the physician according to the individual indications. A hot bath is often used in an endeavor to control a convulsion. Wrapping the baby in blankets and applying a hot-water bottle or electric pad to the feet is equally effective and considerably less disturbing.

The foregoing discussion concerns chiefly those convulsions associated with fever. Those occurring in infancy without fever are most frequently a symptom of tetany, an occasional complication of rickets. The relief of convulsions of this type is most readily and advantageously brought about by the use of certain mineral salts. These and the method of their administration would be chosen according to the preferences of the physician.

Convulsions which occur without fever and which recur from time to time and for which no definite cause can be found are usually classified under the term epilepsy.

FEEDING IN ACUTE ILLNESS

It has been mentioned previously that any acute illness lowers the digestive capacity of the infant and consequently may be a cause of vomiting, or diarrhea, especially when the usual type of feeding is continued. It has been mentioned also that the underlying infection may be obscure, and the difficulty erroneously attributed entirely to the gastro-intestinal tract. Because the continuance of the usual diet is so likely to lead to disturbance in the presence of acute illness, it is desirable to make certain alterations in the diet.

It is often beneficial to remove some or most of the fat from the milk and to discontinue the more solid and less easily digestible foods. If the illness is prolonged it will be found necessary to continue to give fair amounts of food, even though a certain amount of digestive disturbance is present, for otherwise the general nutrition will suffer greatly. The baby must be given enough food to keep up his resistance in order that he may be aided in overcoming the disease.

VOMITING

Vomiting may occur in infancy from many causes. The most frequent cause in the otherwise normal baby is some factor which produces distention of the stomach. This may be produced by too large a feeding or by feeding at such frequent intervals that the stomach is only partially empty when the next feeding is given. The stomach may be distended by the presence of a large amount of swallowed air in addition to the usual feedings. The effects of distention are obtained with tight clothing or abdominal bands. Occasionally the infant has a small stomach capacity, and the feeding of the usual volume of food causes distention. The remedy for all of these distention-producing factors is obvious, once the cause is determined.

The next most frequent cause of vomiting is illness. Almost any acute infection in the infant will produce this event. Vomiting in the acute infections is largely the direct result of irritation of the stomach by the fermentation of food which lies in the stomach unusually long because of the impaired emptying power of the stomach. An excess of fat in the diet may act in this same manner, by delaying the emptying of the stomach. Other less common causes of vomiting depend upon stomach irritation or the ingestion of spoiled foods or inappropriate foods.

A few babies vomit merely because of an apparent desire on their part to do so. This is spoken of as "rumination" in certain instances in which the food is voluntarily brought up for no good reason. In occasional cases babies seem to vomit as a defense reaction against certain foods or against forced feeding. In cases of voluntary vomiting a change in the method of management is indicated. A temporary complete change in environment including caretaker often is all that is necessary.

Any obstruction in the intestinal tract leads to vomiting. The varieties of obstruction are numerous, and all are serious. Some of these seem to have a gradual beginning, as in the obstruction at the lower end (pylorus) of the stomach, which is noticed in the first six weeks after birth; and some may have a sudden onset associated subsequently with evidence of great prostration, as in cases in which one part of the bowel becomes looped into the part immediately next to it.

This is not a complete enumeration of the causes of vomiting, but, the discussion includes the most important causes from the standpoint of frequency.

Thus, vomiting may be produced by such simple and easily remedied conditions as overfilling of the stomach, or it may be a symptom of some very serious condition which demands immediate medical attention.

COLIC

In practically all instances intestinal colic in infancy is associated with the presence of gas in the intestines. This gas may have either one of two sources. It may be air which has been swallowed and which has passed beyond the stomach, or the gas may be the result of fermentation of sugar within the intestinal tract. For permanent relief of colic the cause must be abolished. Swallowed air should be made to pass upward after each feeding. Since underfed babies are more likely to swallow air, one should make certain that the food supply is ample. Fermentation may be the result of overfeeding or of the presence of a large quantity of sugar. The correction of overfeeding at the breast has been discussed. When colic occurs in the breast-fed baby in the absence of overfeeding, often the giving of an ounce of boiled skimmed cow's milk before each breast feeding will bring relief. In the artificially fed baby the sugar may be reduced in quantity or altered as to variety, and it should be made certain that the baby is receiving sufficient food.

Effective simple measures for temporary relief are enemas or hot applications to the abdomen. In the more severe cases sometimes an opiate (paregoric) in suitable doses is required to give relief.

CONSTIPATION

With the rare exception of certain congenital defects, the causes of constipation in infancy can be classified chiefly into two groups. One group includes those instances in which the residue of food left for excretion is too small to constitute sufficient stimulus to intestinal movement. A small residue is usually the result of underfeeding, though it may also be due to the giving of a type of food which is absorbed to an unusually high degree. The other group includes those instances in which the fecal mass becomes so firm or putty-like that it is moved along with difficulty. This type of constipation is not seen in the naturally fed infant. In the artificially fed infant it is dependent chiefly upon the relative proportion of milk to sugar. A high-milk, low-sugar diet tends to produce the dry type of stool, and thus this kind of constipation; whereas a low-milk, high-sugar formula is laxative.

In the treatment of constipation in infancy drugs ordinarily should not be used except as a temporary measure, pending dietary adjustment. When a drug cathartic is considered necessary, milk of magnesia is usually satisfactory in doses of one to two teaspoonfuls. Instead of drugs it may be preferable to use enemas or suppositories also as temporary measures. In practically every case it will be found that constipation can be relieved by appropriate alteration in the diet, and an earnest attempt to establish a regular habit.

In cases in which the food residue is small it is desirable first to make certain that the food intake is adequate. Additional measures are the feeding of fruits and vegetables somewhat earlier than the customary age, or if these are already being given, to increase the amount. Strained orange juice is not laxative.

In cases in which it is desirable to alter the nature of the fecal mass a favorable result often may be achieved by increasing the amount of sugar in the formula. If moderate and reasonable increase in the sugar does not give relief, a change in the type of sugar is advisable. Certain sugars are more laxative than others. Milk sugar is more laxative than some of the malt sugars, though the syrupy malt sugars (malt soup extract) are the most laxative of all the sugars. Though constipation may be relieved by decreasing the amount of milk, this should not be done unless the quantity taken is well above the requirements which have been stated previously.

DIARRHEA

In general it may be considered that diarrhea is the result of irritation or abnormal stimulation of the intestinal tract. Because of the unusual stimulus the intestinal movements are increased in intensity, and food material is passed along at a rapid rate. Because of this rapid rate of passage some of the food and much of the water are not absorbed, and as a consequence the stools are fluid and often contain a fair proportion of undigested food.

The increased stimulus may be caused by actual inflammation of the intestinal wall. Such inflammation is quite often caused by the dysentery bacillus, and the disease is known as "dysentery." Dysentery is not rare in infants who are fed raw milk. In cases of dysentery usually pus and some blood are evident in the stool. In infancy dysentery is a serious disease, and recovery requires close medical and nursing attention. The most difficult and at the same time most important part of the treatment is the maintenance of an adequate food and fluid intake. Usually the appetite is more or less completely lost. Often it becomes necessary to feed by means of a tube passed into the stomach. Though the type of food should be that which is less likely to aggravate diarrhea, food should nevertheless be given. The illness may be of several weeks' duration, and much emaciation or even worse can occur in such a period if food is withheld either because of the child's appetite or because of fear that it will make the diarrhea worse.

In the majority of cases of diarrhea in infancy the cause is not an inflammation in the intestine, but is an irritation produced by substances formed when bacteria grow in the food. Bacteria may grow in food outside the body as happens in occasional instances when diarrhea results from the feeding of "spoiled" food. More often the bacterial growth takes place in the food after it has entered the intestinal tract. Any food which is not readily digested may be subject to bacterial action. Even perfectly proper foods may also be a cause if they are given in excess of the infant's ability to digest and absorb them. For example, almost any infant can be made to have diarrhea by increasing sufficiently the amount of sugar in the diet. Probably the most common of all of the causes of diarrhea is some infection or inflammation elsewhere than in the intestinal tract. Particularly is this true of infections in the nose and ears, ordinary colds and their complications. These infections in some manner lower the infant's ability to digest food, and when food is given in the usual quantity and variety, some of it is subject to bacterial action in the intestine. Thus an ordinary head cold may give rise to diarrhea even though the previous feeding has been entirely suitable and proper.

The serious effects of diarrhea are chiefly food and water loss. Great emaciation and dehydration may result, either of which may be a cause of death. In the most severe cases water loss may be so rapid that death occurs within a day or two of the beginning of the difficulty. Fortunately these severe cases are infrequent. In the usual case the patient is not particularly ill.

Even though the diarrhea may not be primarily dependent upon the diet, certain alterations in the diet are desirable when the diarrhea has occurred. First, it is desirable to allow the intestinal tract to empty. It is customary for some physicians to give a cathartic to hasten the emptying, but this is not necessary. During a brief period, when the tract is emptying, water but no food should be given. The fasting period need not be more than a few hours, though its duration depends upon the severity of the diarrhea and the general condition of the infant. The first food after the fast may advantageously be one which is high in protein and low in sugar and fat. Boiled skimmed milk, acidified, is a customary means for fulfilling these requirements. As the diarrhea improves, sugar and fat are gradually replaced in the diet.

MALNUTRITION

Malnutrition may be due to a low food intake, or to failure of absorption. A common cause of malnutrition is failure to offer the infant sufficient food. The body continues to burn food materials whether or not sufficient food is given. If the ingestion and absorption of food are inadequate, the body burns its own tissues. It is thus possible for extreme malnutrition to occur even to the extent of causing death of the individual. Malnourished infants are more susceptible to infection than are the better nourished. These infections only add to the difficulties in improving the nutrition.

Another common cause of severe malnutrition is loss of food by chronic or frequently recurring diarrhea together with the underfeeding so often employed in the treatment of diarrhea. Chronic infection anywhere in the body tends to decrease the appetite and to increase the tendency to diarrhea and increase the food requirement.

When malnutrition is caused solely by underfeeding, the remedy is obvious. When it is caused by diarrhea, which in turn is dependent upon infection, the management is more difficult, but even so, careful treatment will usually bring about recovery.

RICKETS

Rickets is a disease of nutrition in which the chief fault lies either in a deficiency of calcium and phosphorus in the diet, or an inability on the part of the body to make proper use of these materials. If the infant receives sufficient milk, the amount of calcium and phosphorus will be adequate. The proportion of these two substances relative to

each other affects their absorption. However, when the intake of vitamin D is adequate or with a sufficient amount of sunshine or ultraviolet energy, calcium and phosphorus are well utilized regardless of
their proportion. The high incidence of rickets in late winter and
spring is explained by the small amount of available sunshine.

The most striking effects of rickets are seen in the bones because
bones have such a large proportion of calcium and phosphorus in
their structure. The mineral deficiency associated with rickets causes
them to be softer than normal and more easily bent and deformed.
When the minerals are not being laid down in the bones, the softer
tissues (cartilage) continue to grow at the ends of the long bones;
this enlargement develops at the wrists, ankles, and at the points of
growth of the ribs. As a result of rickets the skull is often late in
closing, the teeth delayed in eruption.

The effects of rickets are seen also in the muscles, which become
more lax and weakened. Infants with rickets are likely to be delayed
in such muscular acts as sitting, standing, and walking. Infants with
rickets are subject to profuse sweating and often to restlessness.

The symptoms which have been enumerated are chiefly those of
well advanced cases. The milder cases greatly outnumber the more
severe ones. The same changes take place in the milder cases, but these
changes are more difficult to detect. The accurate diagnosis of rickets
in these mild cases is made easier by X-ray examination of the bones.

In a few cases of rickets very marked and alarming symptoms appear which are associated with a decrease in the amount of calcium in
the blood. When these symptoms occur, the condition is termed
"tetany," or "spasmophilia." Tetany may exhibit itself in the form
of convulsions or as a spasm of the larynx which causes obstruction
and difficult breathing; or as a peculiar spasmodic state of the hands
and feet. All of these symptoms subside promptly with suitable medical treatment and their return is made impossible by the effective
application of the same measures as bring about the cure of rickets.

Rickets is a disease which is easily prevented and easily cured.
Prevention is preferable. Any infant who receives the amount of milk
that he should is thereby receiving sufficient calcium and phosphorus.
If he receives one or more teaspoons of cod-liver oil daily, the chances
are that no rickets of any significance will develop. The same factors
that are effective in prevention are equally effective in bringing about
the cure of this disease.

CHAPTER VIII

Infant Hygiene
FREDERICK F. TISDALL, M.D.

EVERY GROWING CHILD should be examined by its physician at least every six months, as defects may be present which can produce serious results, if they are allowed to persist. Infants, because of the more rapid changes which take place in their bodies, should be seen more frequently. Immunization against smallpox and diphtheria can now be carried out by the doctor so that the child, even if exposed to these diseases, will probably not contract them.

EXERCISE FOR BABY

Lack of exercise results in flabbiness of the muscles and other evidences of poor health. Exercise starts at birth when the infant cries. It is surprising how soon a newborn baby squirms and kicks about. The infant obtains exercise when he is picked up or moved about as he invariably tries to move himself. In addition, every infant under five months of age should be placed on a bed, dressed only in his shirt, diaper, and stockings, and allowed to kick for fifteen minutes or more every morning before his bath. One can note his obvious enjoyment as he kicks his legs and waves his arms about. After five months of age regular exercises may be instituted, such as grasping the baby's hands and pulling him up into a sitting position. A second exercise is to lay him on his back, grasp both his feet and gently resist any movement that he may make, which stimulates further kicking. Another exercise is to grasp the baby's legs near the ankle with the closed fingers around the outer side of his legs and towards his face. The baby's feet are then brought towards his nose, keeping his knees straight until his thighs are in contact with his abdomen. This tends to strengthen not only the legs but also the abdominal muscles, and is of particular benefit to babies with constipation or a distended abdomen. Each of these exercises should be repeated three or four times each day.

For the runabout child, two hours' exercise in the open air, preferably playing with other children, should be regarded as the average daily requirement.

Fresh Air for Baby

Baby should be placed outside every day. This may be started even at two weeks of age during the summer months. If the weather is not cold or windy, he should be outside practically all day, being brought in only for the feedings. During the winter months, starting at three to four weeks of age, the baby should be dressed for outdoors and placed a few feet from a wide-open window in a room with the door closed in order to prevent a draft. Fifteen minutes is long enough for the first day. If the baby reacts well, that is, if his face develops a healthy red color, and his hands and feet do not become cold, the exposure may be increased fifteen minutes daily up to one hour a day. By this time he may be put outside for a short period and the time lengthened each day until he is outside from two to four hours. Of course, our winter weather is so variable that common sense must be used in following these directions. Naturally, if a blizzard is blowing, it is not advisable to put the baby out. The real criterion is his reaction to the cold, for if his face becomes pale and blue and his hands and feet cold, he should not be left outside.

Exposure of Baby to Sunshine

Although sunshine was used as a curative agent by the ancients, it is only recently that scientific proof of its great importance to the human system has been developed. Sunshine includes not only the rays which are felt as heat and perceived as light, but also invisible ultra-violet rays. During the past fifteen years it has been shown that the shortest of these invisible ultra-violet rays act on a substance in the skin which they activate or change into the sunshine vitamin D. Cod-liver oil and viosterol provide this vitamin. When the body is in the sun, this vitamin is being actually formed in the skin, whence it is carried by the blood stream to all parts of the body. The human race is largely dependent for its supply of this vitamin on this effect of sunshine. One must not think, however, that the beneficial action of the sun's rays is limited to these invisible rays. The longer light and heat rays are also of importance for the maintenance of health. Recent investigations have shown that exposure to these rays along with fresh air increases resistance against disease. For these, and other reasons, a child should be out in the sun for some time every day if possible. Even if the sun is not shining, a beneficial effect is obtained from skyshine, that is, from the reflected rays from the sky.

The best time of day to expose the baby to the sun's rays during the winter and spring months is from 11 A.M. to 1 P.M., when the sun is at its height. In spite of an almost universal belief to the contrary, the sun's rays will not hurt the baby's eyes. During the hot summer months the sun bath should be given before ten o'clock in the morning, as at that hour the heat of the sun is not so intense. However, on very hot days it is advisable to omit the sun bath entirely. When this is done, the baby should be allowed to stay on the shady side of the house. If he is not under cover, he will then get the reflected rays from the sky which have been found to be of considerable value.

The age at which the baby may be given his first sun bath varies with the time of the year. As a general rule, if the baby is born in the summer months the sun baths should be started at two weeks of age, but if he is born in the winter, they should not be given until he is five or six weeks old.

During the winter months, because of the cold, it is impossible to expose more than the face of the baby to the sun's rays. The first sun bath should not exceed ten minutes in length, the baby being turned first on one side and then on the other so that both cheeks may be exposed. The baby should be placed in such a way that he is not looking directly at the sun, as that makes him uncomfortable. The duration of the sun bath may be increased three to five minutes daily until he receives a daily exposure of one to two hours. Care must be taken during the late winter and early spring months not to sunburn the baby's delicate skin. When the winter days become warmer, the bonnet should be pushed back to expose more of the face and head. Later on the mitts should be removed and, as the warmth increases, the arms, legs, and finally the whole body should be bare, with the exception of the area covered by the diaper. The heat of the sun must be watched, however, as it is possible to cause sunstroke from the excessive heat. A good practical guide is for the mother to sit beside the child for a time, and if she is uncomfortably warm she will know it is too hot for the child. The older infant or child, when the weather is suitable, should play in a sun suit which allows the greater portion of the body to be exposed.

SLEEP FOR BABY

Sleep is one of the prime requisites for the health of an infant or child. No matter how fine a body he may have, no matter how carefully his food may be selected, no matter how much exercise, fresh air, and sunshine he may receive, if he does not get sufficient sleep he soon becomes hollow-eyed, restless, and irritable; his appetite diminishes; he loses weight, and his muscles become flabby. In order to establish good sleeping habits certain general rules should be observed. Regularity of sleeping hours is most essential. Children should be put to bed at the same hour each night and nothing should be allowed to interfere with this routine. After being put to bed the child should go to sleep in fifteen to twenty minutes. Frequently a child attempts to get further attention by calling out, "I want a glass of water," or, "I want to go to the toilet." As these needs have been attended to just before he was put to bed, such requests should be ignored. No effort should be made to keep the house quiet for his benefit, and he will soon form the habit of sleeping in spite of the noise. The average hours of sleep required during twenty-four hours at different ages are as follows:

1st month	22 hours
1 to 3 months	20 hours
3 to 6 months	18 to 16 hours
6 to 12 months	16 to 14 hours
1 to 3 years	14 to 12½ hours
3 to 6 years	12½ to 11½ hours
6 to 10 years	11½ to 10½ hours
10 to 15 years	10½ to 10 hours

The very minimum requirements are about one hour less than the average figures. Every infant up to one year of age should have a morning and an afternoon nap of one and a half hour each. Every child up to five years of age should have an afternoon nap of one half to two hours as enough energy cannot be stored during the night's sleep to last the whole day. The hours of sleep during the day time are included in the total hours given in the above table.

Diet

There are five essential groups of substances which go to make up the child's diet, namely, fats, carbohydrates, proteins, minerals, and vitamins. The fats are usually well supplied by milk, butter, eggs, and the fat of meats. Due to the ease with which we can get highly refined carbohydrates such as sugars, jams, white flour, and most breakfast cereals, many diets contain too much of these substances. When we realize that nearly 50 per cent of the food value of the average diet today consists of sugar and white flour, both of which are practically devoid of both vitamins and minerals, we see the very definite strain that is placed on the rest of the diet to supply the necessary amount of these other substances. In addition, cooking destroys some of the vitamins, and there is a very definite loss of both vitamins and minerals in the discarded cooking water. For these reasons, it is advisable in planning a diet to include first those articles of food which will supply the minerals, vitamins, proteins, and fats, and after they have been supplied in sufficient quantities, to add any more calories that are needed as sugars and starches. At first glance this might seem to be a complicated and difficult task, but it is really very simple if the following rule is observed.

Build up the meals around the following five groups of foods:

1. Milk, which supplies minerals, particularly calcium and phosphorus, proteins, fats, and some of the vitamins.

2. Meat, which supplies proteins and some of the vitamins.

3. Eggs, which supply proteins, vitamins, fats, and minerals such as phosphorus and iron.

4. Vegetables, which supply minerals and vitamins.

5. Fruits, which supply minerals and vitamins.

The above five groups of foods of course supply other materials than the ones enumerated, but they are of particular value as an adequate source of minerals, vitamins, proteins, and fats.

Certain canned sieved vegetables are available which are particularly valuable for the infant and small child. When properly canned, the vitamin and mineral content of these vegetables is not impaired. A number of these products have been approved by the Committee on Foods of the American Medical Association, and this approval is an indication that the advertising claims are correct.

There are also certain cereals which have been specially prepared for infants and children so that they contain not only the purified carbohydrates but also considerable amounts of minerals and vitamins. The names of these can be obtained from your physician.

The scarcest of all vitamins in foods is the sunshine vitamin **D**. This vitamin is obtained in cod-liver oil, other fish oils, and in viosterol. Again, standardized products which have been approved by the Committee on Foods of the American Medical Association should be used. In order to make vitamin **D** more widely available, it is now being produced by the irradiation of milk, and it also has been directly incorporated in both bread and milk.

Toilet Habits

Training of the bowels should be begun at one to two months of age, and good control should be established by the eighth month. The mother should try to have the baby's bowels move just before the

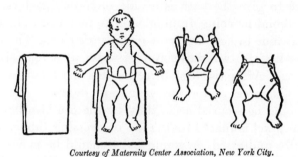

Courtesy of Maternity Center Association, New York City.

Fig. 24. Applying the square diaper.

morning bath. In training the child, absolute regularity in carrying out the following procedures is essential. A soap stick is first made by whittling down a piece of white soap until it is in the form of a pencil about one third of an inch thick and two inches long. The baby is then laid on his back on the mother's lap and the soap stick, moistened with water, inserted into the rectum. A small chamber is then held against the baby's buttocks, and usually, in the course of four or five minutes the stool will be passed. The soap stick should be used for the first few days only, until the baby understands what is desired of him. At three months of age the chamber may be placed in the mother's lap, and the baby can be held on it with his back against the mother.

Control of the bladder during the daytime is usually possible by two years of age. If it is not established by two and a half years of age the condition should be regarded as abnormal. The child should have bladder control at night by three years of age. It is well to start training the infant at ten months. He should be made to sit on the chamber two or three times a day at a regular hour, and an attempt should be made to associate the act with some word in order that he may make known his wants in the future. By the use of these methods, results can be obtained in a very short time, although naturally the development of complete control requires many months. The proper method of applying the square diaper is shown in illustration on page 225.

BATHING

Tub baths are not given until the cord separates, and this usually occurs between the fourth and seventh days after birth. A very convenient time to give the bath is a half to three quarters of an hour before the second morning feeding. A soft face cloth should be used, as it is impossible to keep an ordinary sponge clean. The bath should be filled one half to two thirds full of water at a temperature of 98 to 100 degrees. After the first three months the temperature may be reduced to 95 degrees and at one year to 90 degrees. The proper temperature should be secured accurately by the use of a bath thermometer. A bath towel is placed on the lap or dressing table and the baby then partially undressed. A young baby should be moved as little as possible and the clothes taken off over the feet and not over the head. With the diaper and shirt on, the face and head are soaped with the face cloth and then rinsed and thoroughly dried. The shirt and diaper are now removed, and the baby is soaped over the body and extremities and then placed in the tub. The left hand of the mother should support the baby's head out of the water, while the right hand should be used to wash the soap off gently. The baby should not be in the water more than three or four minutes. On removal from the tub the baby is wrapped in the towel on the mother's lap or table and gently dried by patting. The baby must be thoroughly dried, particularly where two skin surfaces come together, as in the armpits, groins, etc., as otherwise the moisture will irritate the skin. After drying, the baby is powdered and then dressed. There is no need to bathe the eyes each day with boracic solution. The eyes keep themselves clean, and ex-

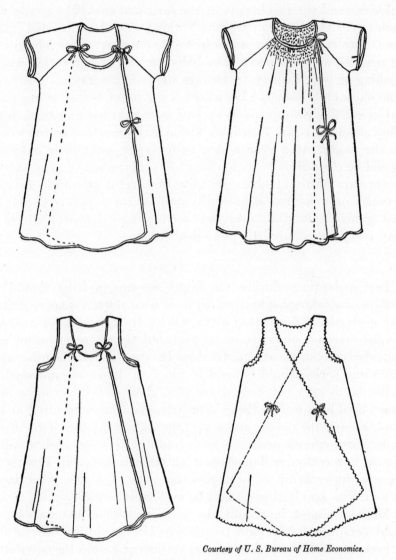

Courtesy of U. S. Bureau of Home Economics.

FIG. 25.   New clothes for the baby, avoiding pins and buttons.

cept for the removal of any small crusts which may form at the inner corner of the eyes, no attempt should be made to wash them. The outer ear and the visible part of the ear canal should be gently wiped each day with absorbent cotton. Nothing should be inserted into the nose. Any crusts or secretions in the lower part of the nostrils may be removed with absorbent. The baby's mouth should be left alone as washing it out is likely to irritate the delicate mucous membranes. The older child should have a bath each night before going to bed.

Care of the teeth should be started as soon as the first teeth appear. They should be cleaned each day with a little absorbent cotton wrapped on the finger. At a year and a half of age, or a little older, they should be cleaned daily with a small toothbrush and a good standard toothpaste. Many children, in spite of careful attention, develop a greenish or sometimes a brownish stain at the junction of the teeth and gums. This stain does not produce any harmful effects and may easily be removed by your dentist.

CLOTHING

In the daytime, during the winter months, a baby should wear bootees or stockings, a knitted rayon or wool shirt, a diaper, a flannelette gertrude, and a cotton dress. Under three months of age, knee-shaped woolen bootees should be used, but for the older infant rayon and wool stockings are preferable. In the summer months, cotton shirts and socks should be used in place of the rayon and wool, and if the day is very hot, only a sleeveless shirt and diaper, or a diaper alone, need be worn. In the cold months, the clothes required at night are the shirt, the diaper and a nightgown, and bootees if the child is under three months or if it is very cold. On very hot nights a diaper pinned to a cotton or flannelette nightgown is sufficient. For the first six or eight weeks the night clothes should be used during the daytime as well. Pins and buttons should be avoided if possible.

Mothers almost invariably dress their children too warmly. The child perspires freely, and the skin and underclothes become damp or even wet. The child then becomes restless and kicks the outer clothes off, with the result that he gets a chill. Time and again we see infants so warmly dressed that they are restless and cross and sleep poorly. When the excess clothes are removed and the skin is dried and powdered, the child usually goes off into a quiet, restful sleep. The skin should never be moist with perspiration. The outdoor clothes required vary, of course, with the season. In the winter time a warm coat or sleeping bag is necessary. If it is very cold, a knitted sweater may be used in addition. The infant should also wear a bonnet made of flannel covered with silk, or a tightly knit woolen bonnet and woolen mitts. He should then be tucked in his carriage with one or two flannel blankets, and if it is very cold an eiderdown comforter should be added as well. It is essential to see that the baby's feet are warm, and extra stockings may be necessary. A hot-water bottle should never be used unless great care is taken, for one is liable to burn the baby, if the water is too hot.

Mental Development of the Child

One important phase of child hygiene which is neglected by many parents is the mental development of the child. Often parents do not realize that it is during the first five years of the child's life that the foundations of his future character are laid. This aspect of child hygiene cannot be discussed in detail here. However, the importance of playmates for the child should be emphasized. Many children are brought for medical treatment with various symptoms such as poor appetite, sleeplessness, and irritability, and on inquiry it is found that the child has no playmates and spends all his time in the company of adults. This is obviously an unnatural surrounding for the child, and in many cases surprising results are obtained when playmates of his own age are provided for most of the day.

CHAPTER IX

The Prevention and Treatment of Infectious Disease

MORRIS FISHBEIN, M.D.

A<small>BOUT</small> <small>FIFTY</small> <small>YEARS</small> have passed since it was first shown that germs actually cause disease. In the intervening period hundreds of germs have been identified definitely as associated with certain diseases that attack human beings. In 1880 the germ associated with typhoid was isolated. Since that time such important diseases as tuberculosis, diphtheria, glanders, pneumonia, cholera, lockjaw, undulant fever, meningitis, dysentery, plague, syphilis, whooping cough, gonorrhea, leprosy, and many other specific infections, have been definitely related to invasion of the human body by specific germs.

ABOUT GERMS

Few people really know what a germ looks like or how it invades the human body. Germs are so small that it takes three hundred billions of an average germ to weigh a pound. They multiply rapidly under favorable conditions. One germ can produce two new ones in twenty minutes. Anyone who has tried to estimate how much money he would have by beginning with a penny and doubling his fortune every hour can realize how rapidly germs multiply. If a germ divided and made two new ones every hour it would, at the end of a day, have sixteen and a half billion descendants.

Doctors identify the germs that cause disease in various ways. First they take some of the material from the infected saliva or from the discharges or from the blood of the person who is infected. They examine this under a microscope. The germs are seen as little round dots, or as rod-shaped organisms, or even as long, slender filaments when they are greatly magnified under the microscope. Like human beings, the germs tend to live preferably in certain forms, sometimes two together, sometimes a group of many, sometimes a chain. Some germs are surrounded by capsules, usually a sort of fatty envelope that enables the germ to resist attacks in the body or in the blood of the animal it invades. Other germs have little tails like fins which enable them to move about.

There are still people foolish enough to talk about the germ theory. Germs are no more a theory than are plants, birds, and other living things that live and reproduce. The power of most germs to cause disease can be tested on animals. When the germs are injected into animals they produce changes in the tissues of the animal which are specific for the germs concerned. A pneumococcus in the lung of a man produces pneumonia; first a consolidation of the lung due to invasion by red blood cells and other material and later a softening of this mass and a clearing up of the lung if the patient lives.

When the typhoid germ gets into the human body it produces ulcers in the intestines, and germs are found in the ulcers. When the meningococcus gets into the linings of the spinal cord and brain it sets up an inflammation of these linings, which are called meninges; then the person has meningitis, an inflammation of the meninges. When the spinal fluid is examined the germs can be found in the fluid.

These tests which were developed by the great Robert Koch, with Louis Pasteur, a founder of modern bacteriology, constitute the acid tests for determining with certainty that any germ is associated with the production of a certain disease. If the germ can be found in the infected tissues, if the germ can be artificially grown outside the human body, if the germ can then be injected into an animal like the monkey and produce in that animal a condition like that in the human being from whom the germ was originally taken, it is the cause of that particular disease. Anyone with a reasoning mind should be willing to grant that the germ actually causes the disease.

INCUBATION PERIODS

The common contagious diseases include measles, scarlet fever, diphtheria, whooping cough, mumps, chicken pox, and German measles. The best way to avoid these diseases is to keep away from people who have them. However, this is not so easily done, since many parents do not feel their responsibilities greatly and do not see to it that their children, when ill, are kept away from other children.

Really the chief responsibility rests on the parents of the sick child for the prevention of infectious diseases rather than on the parents of the well child.

Most of the common infectious diseases are caused by organisms which get into the body and then begin their action. A certain amount of time elapses between the period when the germ first gets in and when its visible manifestations appear. This is known as the incubation period, and it varies with different diseases. For instance, in meningitis it is from two to four days, in erysipelas from one half to three days, in measles from ten days to two weeks, in German measles from five days to twenty-one days, in scarlet fever from a few hours to a week, in smallpox from ten days to two weeks, in typhoid fever from six days to twenty-five days, and in chicken pox from four days to sixteen days.

In most of these diseases an eruption occurs on the surface of the body. These eruptions have characteristic distribution on the skin, so the physician asks particularly as to whether the redness first began on the face, the neck, the hands and feet, the abdomen, or the chest. The eruptions also differ greatly in their appearance: from tiny red spots to large red patches, from tiny pimples to crops of blisters.

Practically all of these conditions are likely to begin with a mild cold. In some of them the sore throat is severe; in most of them there is fever, slight headache, dizziness, nausea or vomiting. Obviously it is not safe to disregard any of these symptoms, particularly when they appear in a child.

It is important to remember that the excretions which carry disease include the material that is coughed from the throat, that is spread by spitting, by sneezing, or that may pass from the body in the form of discharges of one kind or another. Therefore, mothers should guard particularly against contact of a well child with one that is coughing, sneezing, spitting, or that manifests any of the other signs of infectious disease that have been mentioned.

RESISTANCE TO INFECTIOUS DISEASE

Four factors are chiefly responsible for infection of the human body: First, the presence of a germ with sufficient toxic power to grow in the body; second, a sufficient number of these germs to overcome attacks by the body against the germ; third, some special condition in the body that makes it possible for the germ to live and grow; and fourth, some method of getting the germ into the body.

Were it not for the fact that human beings develop within their bodies conditions which make it difficult for germs to live and grow, the human race would long since have been destroyed by the bacteria. However, the resistance which the human being has is not absolute. The constitution of the human body changes from time to time. Resistance is decreased when the body is greatly undernourished, when a person is exceedingly fatigued, when he has been exposed to sudden severe changes of temperature, or in several other ways.

Therefore, the line of defense varies in its intensity from time to time. When the enemy is sufficiently numerous, or sufficiently strong, it breaks through. For this reason, even in the most severe epidemics, some people escape, although there are conditions in which practically everyone attacked is unable to resist. Such conditions occur, for example, when a population among whom a disease has never previously appeared suddenly comes in contact with it. This occurred in the Faroe Islands when measles was brought by a ship carrying white men; at that time more than half the population of the islands died of that disease.

Sometimes the resistance of the body to one disease is broken down by a mild attack of another previous disease. For instance, a person who has had influenza, diabetes, tuberculosis, or some other chronic disorder, may thereafter develop pneumonia, typhoid fever, rheumatic fever, or tuberculosis much more easily than he would have previously.

CARRIERS OF DISEASE

Frequently people who are healthy carry about in their bodies germs which do not attack them but which have sufficient virulence, toxicity, strength, or poison to invade the body of another person and in that person to cause disease. A person who carries the germs about is called a "carrier." Should the carrier suddenly have his own resistance lowered by any of the factors that have been mentioned he might suddenly be invaded by these germs, although previously they had not been able to set up infection in his body.

There is no doubt that all of us are constantly being invaded by germs in contaminated food and water, in breathing, in touching infected items with our hands, which are then conveyed to the mouth and nose. Germs occur on money, in clothing, and on various other objects. However, the dosage of germs received through such contacts, or the virulence of the germs, may not be sufficient to bring about disease. The exposure of the germ to fresh air and sunlight, and the fact that it is trying to live on a substance not suitable to it as a habitation, may prevent its multiplying and may cause the germ itself to lose its strength.

Under other circumstances, germs multiply in tremendous numbers, so that the human being who comes in contact with them sustains a massive assault. For instance, an infected fruit peddler may use saliva to polish the fruit, and the germs might grow well on the fruit thus polished. Germs may be deposited with sewage in running water and multiply tremendously in the sewage. When the water from the contaminated stream is drunk by a human being he gets in enough germs to cause prompt infection. Sometimes an infected food handler is employed to mix a potato salad, to bake a custard, or to make a pie which is then kept under insanitary conditions before being eaten, so that the germs multiply profusely. When this occurs anybody who eats the infected food may become seriously infected, as occurred recently at a picnic when eight hundred people became sick from eating infected potato salad.

Paths by Which Germs Invade

Germs can get into the body in all sorts of ways: with food and water, by inhaling, through open wounds on the skin, by the bite of an insect, as occurs with mosquitoes in malaria and yellow fever, ticks in Texas fever, fleas in plague, and tsetse flies in African sleeping sickness.

Obviously, when the means by which the germs get into the body is understood, scientific medicine develops methods for keeping them out. When the means are not understood, as occurs, for instance, in infantile paralysis, prevention is difficult.

Often the germs produce disease by developing a poison which is then absorbed by the body. After absorption, the poison acts on the nerves or the muscles or the blood vessels. Sometimes the germs themselves gradually break up, and the products of their disintegration are poisonous. Again clumps of germs float around in the blood and cause death by developing in overwhelming numbers in the blood. On other occasions the germs may attack certain organs of the body and so injure these organs that death ensues.

It has been said that the germs like to pick out certain places in which to live under the conditions which suit them best. This happens, for instance, with a germ called the pneumococcus which settles in the lungs and produces pneumonia, but which also may infect the eye or the spine. It occurs with the germs of meningitis, which practically always settle on the coverings of the spinal cord and of the brain, the typhoid germ which settles in the intestines, the germs of lockjaw and of hydrophobia and of epidemic encephalitis which attack the nervous system. On the other hand, there are some germs, like those of tuberculosis, which may affect any tissue in the human body although preferably entering by way of the lungs. There is tuberculosis of bones, of joints, of the eye, and of the nervous system. The organism that causes syphilis actually attacks every organ and tissue in the human body.

RESPONSE OF THE BODY TO GERM INVASION

When germs get into the body and release their poisons the tissues react usually in definite ways. One of the reactions of the body is fever. This is apparently due to the effects of the poisons of the germs on the nervous mechanism of the body which controls the body temperature. Associated with the fever there is speeding up of the chemical changes that go on in the body so that there may be perspiration and, as a result of the increased activity, a loss of weight. For this reason it has become customary to feed fevers rather than to starve them.

Associated with the disturbance of the nervous system there may be dizziness and loss of appetite, also vomiting and an increased activity of the motion of the bowels. This helps to cause loss of material from the body. Due to accumulations of fluid or swelling of tissue there may be aches and pains in the joints and in the muscles. The interference with the action of the kidney may cause fluid to be retained in the body. The blood usually responds by an increase in the number of the white blood cells, but there are some conditions in which the number is decreased, notably influenza and typhoid fever.

Because the fever is considered to be one of the mechanisms of the body in defense against the attack of germs, scientific medicine does not always attempt to reduce the fever too suddenly or too rapidly by the use of drugs. A fever that is not exceedingly high or prolonged for any length of time is not especially harmful to the body, particularly if the amount of fluid in the body is watched and enough of the right type of food is put into the body to prevent too great a wastage of the tissues.

A normal temperature is 98.6 degrees F. A great many investigations indicate that temperatures over 100 degrees F. are unfavorable to the growth of bacteria and may inhibit the action of some of the poison developed by the bacteria. As will be shown later in the discussion of many of the individual infections which attack human beings, it is much better to prevent infections than to endeavor to treat them after they have been established.

STAMPING OUT DISEASE

By scientific methods applied since the nature of the germs and their methods of attack on the body have been discovered, certain diseases are now practically eliminated as of exceeding danger to mankind. Yellow fever occurs now in only a few isolated spots throughout the world. In the United States the number of cases of typhoid fever has been so greatly reduced that many young physicians never see a case even in the hospitals where they take their training. Cholera and plague are limited to the remoter areas of China and India and are seldom if ever seen in the United States.

Mankind has undergone progressive changes from the beginning of time, and there is reason to believe that the diseases of man, particularly such as are caused by living organisms, likewise undergo such changes. True, some diseases have been overcome and eliminated, but new diseases constantly appear and demand consideration. The development of new methods of transportation and conveyance, such as the airplane and the ease of intercommunication between various portions of the earth, have brought into the temperate zone the diseases of the tropics which were formerly limited to such areas.

There is much evidence that many a great civilization has fallen because of the development, endemically or epidemically, of diseases that were previously under control, or because of the introduction of some new disease that had previously been considered a rarity. It has been urged that the great civilizations of Greece and Rome fell because of epidemics of malaria. In the United States today certain forms of infections of the glands, certain forms of infestation by tape-

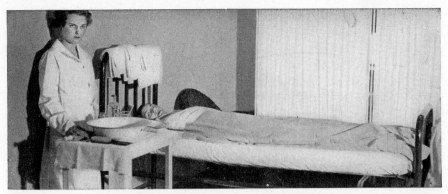

FIG. 26.   Patient ready for bed bath.

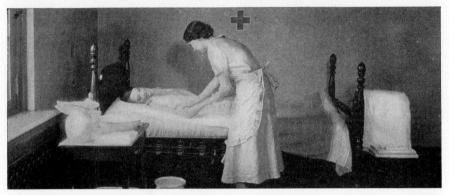

FIG. 27.   Bathing the patient.

Place a towel lengthwise beneath the patient's arm, and bathe gently with the wash cloth wrapped around your right hand.   Notice the orderly arrangement of bathing necessities on the stand and the linen on the chair. The bed is raised upon blocks in order to prevent back-strain.

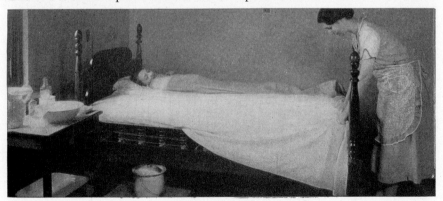

FIG. 28.   Making the patient's bed.

The bed linen is changed after the bath. Have the patient roll to the side opposite you. Loosen the soiled bottom sheet and roll it up against the patient's back. Spread the clean sheet over the vacated area.

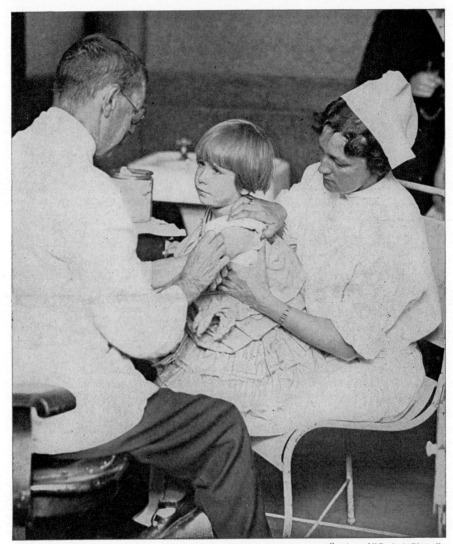

FIG. 29.   Vaccination against smallpox.

worms, and similar disorders, are seen with comparative frequency, whereas formerly they were practically unknown.

The time will never come when man will be free entirely from the fear of disease. The battle is unending, but more and more mankind can celebrate the fruits of victory. As diseases change and as new diseases appear, scientists observe them in their earliest stages, determine their causes and their modes of transmission, and prevent their development.

PREVENTION OF INFECTION

The prevention of disease must, as has previously been mentioned, be related to our knowledge of the way in which infectious disease gains entrance into the body. In the first place, everything possible must be done to see to it that the germs in the person who is infected do not get out and thus get into contact with other people. If this could be done in every case, many infectious diseases would probably disappear.

If everything possible is to be done, all of the sheets, pillow cases, clothing, handkerchiefs, and, in fact, everything touched by a person who is infected, will have to be sterilized by boiling or by steam under pressure before being permitted in contact with other people. All of the excretions from the body of the infected person must be disinfected by proper antiseptics or by burning. The person with a discharge from the nose, such as occurs in the common cold, might at all times wear a face mask. To carry out completely these procedures would mean such an obstruction and hampering of the usual routine of existence that it is not likely to be generally adopted.

The next step is, of course, to do everything possible to prevent infected material from being passed from one person to another. This means complete control of food, drink, and air, also the earliest possible detection of human beings, animals, or insects which carry disease, the control of such carriers and their possible elimination.

It can be seen at once that a human being who is carrying typhoid cannot be eliminated but must be controlled. Since there are millions of persons who carry disease constantly, it is not likely that this source of infection will ever be brought completely under control. Moreover, there are some diseases of which the cause is not definitely known, and it is unlikely that healthy carriers of such diseases will ever be controlled until the cause of the disease is known.

PERSONAL HYGIENE

The best step that the average person can take to prevent infectious disease is first of all to raise his individual resistance by practising the best possible personal hygiene. This means the eating of a suitable diet, the securing of sufficient exercise and sunlight, and enough rest to give the tissues of the body opportunity to recuperate from fatigue.

Moreover, in the presence of certain infectious diseases it is possible to aid resistance by injecting the human being either with blood that has resistance, such as the blood from a person who has recovered from the disease, or by injecting serums from an animal which has been infected with the disease and which has in its serum substances opposed to the disease. There are available today a considerable number of such specific preventive serums and vaccines which will be discussed under each of the infectious diseases as it is considered.

INCIDENCE OF INFECTIOUS DISEASE

The number of cases of the various infectious diseases varies from time to time, as everyone knows. There have been great epidemics of influenza such as the epidemic of 1918, in which tremendous numbers of people were involved, whereas there have been minor epidemics in which relatively few people were concerned. Cases of influenza are difficult to differentiate from the common cold. The reports of the United States Public Health Service indicate about 700,000 cases of influenza in 1929, but if all of the conditions resembling influenza were included, the number would be many millions.

The figures for such conditions as measles (about 366,000), chicken pox (216,000), scarlet fever (182,000), mumps (103,000), and whooping cough (197,000) are relatively accurate, since the large majority of such cases are reported. Everyone knows that the rate of incidence of tuberculosis has dropped greatly. The number of deaths from this disease has dropped from 275 per hundred thousand people in the United States to around 75 or 80 in most communities.

Notwithstanding the fact that typhoid fever can be completely controlled by proper measures, there are still more than 20,000 cases of typhoid fever annually in the United States. Notwithstanding the fact that we have in vaccination and in isolation certain methods of controlling smallpox, there are still a considerable number of cases and deaths from this disease.

Cleanliness and Infection

If infectious disease is to be prevented and brought under control, people must learn to know the nature of disease, the method of its spread, and the methods of prevention. They must, however, do everything possible to keep themselves in such fit condition that infectious disease will not readily attack them.

Much infectious disease can be prevented by keeping as clean as possible, including frequent bathing with plenty of soap and water. Thorough washing of the hands with plenty of soap, particularly before eating, will destroy millions of germs which may otherwise infect human bodies. Vaccination against smallpox is important for everybody. Children should be protected against diphtheria by the use of diphtheria toxoid or toxin-antitoxin. When there are epidemics of typhoid or of other infectious diseases, physicians should be consulted as to the desirability of using other specific vaccines, serums, or antitoxins. Remember that most infectious diseases are spread by contact with persons who have the disease or who may be recovering.

Treatment of Infectious Diseases

In the treatment of most of the common infectious diseases, rest in bed is absolutely necessary. The diet should invariably be mild and bland, depending largely on milk, but supplemented with well-macerated vegetables and occasionally with enough thoroughly macerated liver or lamb's kidney to supply the necessary iron and vitamins that are needed in the diet.

For many of the specific infectious diseases there are now specific methods of treatment. For example, there are serums, vaccines, or antitoxins available in scarlet fever, measles, diphtheria, whooping cough, tetanus, meningitis, erysipelas, and undulant fever. In some of the conditions, moreover, the blood serum taken from a person who is convalescing from the disease has been found to have virtues in certain instances.

Typical of the treatment of most of the infectious diseases is the usual method of handling measles. Every child with this disease should be put to bed and kept there, with light covers, as long as it has any fever and for a few days thereafter. If the eyes are irritated, they may be treated with iced cloths soaked in a cold solution of boric acid. The doctor may prescribe the application of an ointment which will keep the lids from getting sticky. The itching and burning of the skin which frequently occurs in the infectious diseases is often relieved by bathing with a simple solution of bicarbonate of soda or a calamine lotion.

The doctor will treat the cough, if it is distressing, by small doses of sedative drugs. The restlessness, headache, and general discomfort may also be relieved by small doses of aspirin or similar remedies, as the doctor prescribes. When, however, any patient develops serious complications or symptoms, such as dullness, stupor, or convulsions, whenever he breathes rapidly or turns blue, it is well to have the physician in immediate attendance. Under such circumstances, the application of a bath, a pack, or a proper remedy may mean a turning between the tendency toward recovery or the tendency toward a more serious condition leading to death.

The details of the treatment of infectious diseases are discussed much more fully in the chapters dealing with individual diseases.

CHAPTER X

Infectious Diseases of Childhood
MORRIS FISHBEIN, M.D.

DIPHTHERIA

In A NOVEL, *The Marriage of Simon Harper*, by Neil Bell, appears an account of a diphtheria epidemic in a small town in England in the period just preceding the discovery of diphtheria antitoxin. The author depicts graphically the child who is severely infected by this disease. Tchekhov also depicts the horror of this deadly disease in an earlier day. Its conquest has been as dramatic as any struggle known to man.

The condition begins with a sore throat and with repeated attempts to expel, by spitting, the membrane that forms in the throat. If the disease continues, severe paralyses prevent swallowing and injure the heart. There comes a period when breathing becomes impossible, and finally, death. No one who has read such a description or who has actually seen a child with this condition, and who has then seen the marvelous effects of a suitable dose of antitoxin given early in the disease, can fail to appreciate what a great blessing this conquest has been for mankind.

In an earlier day, the physician would frequently be called in the middle of the night to the bedside of a gasping child. Then he would either suck the membrane from the throat by mouth-to-mouth suction or through a tube, if one was available. In severe cases he sometimes opened the windpipe with a knife to permit the child to breathe through the throat beneath the membrane.

Then came the great discovery by the German, Von Behring, and by Roux, a pupil of Pasteur, that an antitoxin could be prepared which would overcome the poisons of this disease. Since that time, there have been developed preparations called toxin-antitoxin and toxoid which can be injected into children early in life and which will give them immunity, or protection, against being infected with diphtheria.

In 1883, shortly after Pasteur had announced his discovery of the germ causation of disease, Klebs and Löffler isolated the germs that cause diphtheria. These germs are known as diphtheria bacilli. They are found in the membrane which appears in the throat of a person infected with diphtheria.

In order to determine whether or not infection is present the physician takes a smear from the throat and sends it to the health department, which then studies the germs to see if they are the germs of diphtheria. By taking a smear one means merely the introduction into the throat of some cotton on the end of a stick, which collects a small portion of the infected material. This is deposited on a preparation which permits the germs to remain alive until they can be studied.

There are various ways in which diphtheria may be spread from an infected person to a well one. The germs have been found on the bedclothing, on handkerchiefs, candy, shoes, hair, pencils, and drinking cups used by infected children. They are, of course, found in any discharges coming from the noses or throats of children who have the disease or who are recovering from it. There are, moreover, healthful carriers of diphtheria who, although they have recovered from the disease, still carry the germs about and distribute them to people who have not had the disease.

It is not safe for anyone to gamble on the possibility that a child infected with this disease does not really have diphtheria but simply some mild throat infection. Most of the serious results can be avoided if the child is seen early in the course of the disease and if proper treatment is given immediately.

If a child complains of sickness, and particularly of sore throat of the type mentioned, a physician should examine it promptly. A physician should be summoned immediately if the child complains of swelling of the neck or of any croupy condition with hoarseness. Early attention is particularly important in small children, because 85 per cent of the deaths from this disease usually occur in the first five years of life. Children are much more likely to catch diphtheria than are grown people. Moreover, the disease is likely to get a better start in a child, before it is properly diagnosed and treated, than in the case of a grown-up person.

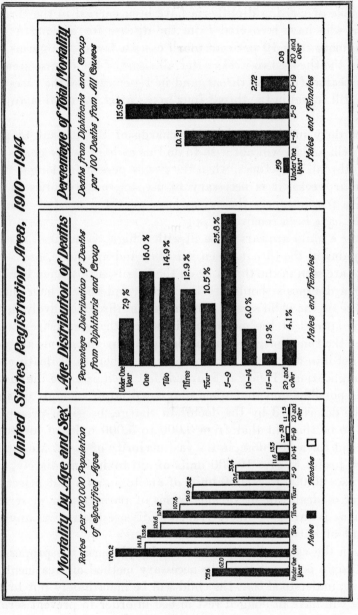

Original Tabulation, Statistician's Dept., The Prudential Insurance Co. of America.

FIG. 30.   Mortality from diphtheria and croup.

The child should not be released to play with other children until it has been pronounced free from the germs. Cases are known in which germs capable of causing diphtheria have been carried in the throats of children who have recovered from the disease for as long as ten months. In more than 10 per cent of all cases a few of the germs can be found in the throat two weeks after all signs of the disease seem to have disappeared from the throat, and in 1 per cent of the cases the germs are still found in the throat four weeks after the child is apparently well.

It is the duty of the physician in charge of the patient to pronounce it well, and he will not wish to do this as long as the germs are still in the throat. Sometimes, when the germs persist for longer than three or four weeks, it is necessary to use active antiseptics in the throat; in a few instances the germs have persisted until the tonsils of the child have been removed.

Whenever a child appears to be ill with a high fever, when it complains of pains in the throat, when it is dull and apathetic, and when white spots are seen in the throat or on the tonsils, a physician capable of making a diagnosis should see the throat and should have immediate charge of the child's care. The more the throat is involved, the greater the spread of the membrane in which the germs are found. The longer the time that the poisons developed by the germs are permitted to get into the system, the more danger there is of death or of serious complications. Hence it is urged that such cases be diagnosed as early as possible, and that when diagnosed large amounts of antitoxin, to be determined by the doctor in charge, be given promptly.

It used to be thought that from 3,000 to 5,000 units of antitoxin were sufficient for a first dose, in the vast majority of cases. Most physicians now prefer to give 10,000 units of antitoxin immediately, and in severe cases 20,000 to 30,000 units of antitoxin as a first injection. The danger of death, or of various forms of paralysis, or of serious complications is far more likely from the disease than from any excess amount of antitoxin.

Indeed, in the vast majority of cases of diphtheria the proper use of the antitoxin is almost the only necessary method of treatment. It is, of course, understood that the child will be immediately put to bed and that it will have prolonged rest in bed in order to prevent serious complications. It is the development of such complications that demands particularly the constant care of a physician.

Years ago, a physician named O'Dwyer developed a method for permitting persons with diphtheria to breathe when the membrane had developed to such a point that it obstructed the throat. This method includes the use of gold tubes, called intubation tubes, which an expert can pass through the throat and from the throat into the larynx, or breathing tube, thus permitting the child to breathe. The use of such tubes requires expert knowledge; they are a most valuable method in certain types of cases.

As the condition improves under the use of suitable doses of antitoxin, the membrane disappears, and the child usually coughs up the tube and gets rid of it. In other instances the physician easily removes the tube when it is no longer needed.

During the first few days of diphtheria the child should have a liquid diet as nourishing as possible, including plenty of milk and eggnog and cereals. Thereafter its diet may be gradually improved, particularly with substances that will aid the rebuilding of blood which may have been injured by the infection.

In the prevention of diphtheria in recent years chief reliance has been placed on the use of the Schick test, on toxin-antitoxin and on toxoid. The Schick test is simply a method of injecting a very small amount of the toxin of diphtheria into the skin. Those people who have in their blood antitoxin against the diphtheria poison will have a negative test. On the other hand, those who do not have antitoxin or who cannot develop it will have a positive Schick test.

In a positive Schick test the spot at which the toxin was injected becomes red and slightly raised within twenty-four to forty-eight hours. The application of Schick tests in thousands of cases has shown that about 8 per cent of newly born and young infants are susceptible to diphtheria, which means that they are likely to become infected if exposed to the disease. The remainder are not likely to have the disease at this early age because they have from their mothers a certain amount of resistance to the disease. This is gradually lost, however, so that from 30 to 40 per cent of children will be susceptible at one year of age, and about 65 per cent at five years of age. Apparently, through mild infections, this susceptibility then begins to decrease so that approximately 30 per cent are susceptible at ten years, and 18 per cent at fifteen years.

In the presence of an epidemic it is, of course, desirable that Schick tests be performed on all of the children exposed so as to know which ones are to be especially watched and which ones are to be immediately immunized against the disease by the use of toxin-antitoxin or toxoid. Millions of children have been given toxin-antitoxin and toxoid without the slightest harmful reactions, so that it has become customary in most large cities where there are competent health departments to recommend immunization of all children against diphtheria. Your family doctor will inoculate all the children against diphtheria. You should have this done as soon as possible.

Few people understand the difference between toxin, antitoxin, and toxin-antitoxin. When a horse is injected with the poison which diphtheria germs develop, he develops in his blood a substance which opposes the poison of the diphtheria germ. The poison is called toxin.

The material in the blood which opposes the poison of diphtheria is antitoxin. If a child does not have enough of this antitoxin in its blood to overcome diphtheria infection, the physician gives it antitoxin to help it. If a child has been exposed to diphtheria, and it is necessary very promptly to give it something to help it ward off the disease, antitoxin may be injected.

However, this antitoxin does not protect for a long period of time. It must be remembered that it has been elaborated in animals and not in the patient's own body, and that therefore its effects wear off in about three weeks. Of course, if a person has diphtheria, the antitoxin, when injected, helps to overcome the disease, and when the person recovers he has developed in his own body his own antitoxin, which is one reason why no one seems to have this disease twice.

If one is injected with small doses of toxin or poison, he builds up resistance to diphtheria in his own body. If it is desirable to stimulate his resistance-building factor still more, it is necessary to give him larger doses of toxin. However, such a procedure would be unsafe. Therefore, it is customary to add antitoxin to the toxin, which prevents it from working harm but does not prevent the body from responding to the injection of the toxin by building up more resistance. Toxoid is merely toxin detoxified by the addition of formaldehyde.

Few people realize the background of the way in which the body opposes disease. The process is called immunization. The terms vaccination, inoculation, injection, and similar terms refer to the fact that the substance is being put into the body in order that the body build the materials to oppose it.

Quite recently the preparation called toxoid has been developed for use in protecting children against diphtheria. Toxoid does not contain any horse serum, but is merely toxin detoxified by the addition of formaldehyde. It is used in the same way that toxin-antitoxin is used and serves to stimulate the development of immunity, or of resistance to diphtheria.

There are some people who react unfavorably to injections of antitoxin because they are sensitive to horse serum. Hypersensitivity of this kind is the same type of hypersensitivity that produces asthma, or hay fever, or eruptions of blisters, or similar manifestations. When there is a possibility that a child is going to be especially sensitive to antitoxin, the physician can find out by injecting under the skin a small amount—one or two drops—of the antitoxin and then waiting for an hour to see if there is going to be a reaction. Whenever a reaction appears it can be combated by giving suitable preparations of drugs which serve to control the reaction.

TREATMENT OF DIPHTHERIA

In the treatment of diphtheria, the antitoxin, as has already been mentioned, is of the utmost importance. A delay of two, three, or four days in giving antitoxin may mean damage to vital organs in such manner that they can never recover completely. Moreover, the first dose of antitoxin that is given should be large enough to control the disease. This antitoxin is usually injected by the doctor in the back below the shoulder blade, but sometimes into the thigh or under the breast. In very severe cases the antitoxin is injected directly into a vein; in less sever cases, into the muscles, and in the milder cases, under the skin.

In the vast majority of cases a striking improvement is seen shortly after the antitoxin is injected. The improvement is demonstrated by a fall in the fever and a favorable change in the general condition of the patient. Usually within twenty-four hours after a sufficient dose has been injected, the membrane in the throat stops spreading, becomes softened and loosens up, and the swelling goes down.

There are, of course, patients with diphtheria who come to treatment so late that the antitoxin seems to be of little help, but even in these cases it exercises a tremendously beneficial influence in comparison with the effects when no antitoxin is given. In an occasional case of diphtheria there is sensitivity to the antitoxin, so that the patient may have a severe eruption or a reaction. These are exceedingly rare, developing perhaps in one out of every one thousand people. So far as is known, death from severe reaction to the serum occurs in only one in about seventy thousand people. These reactions occur more often in people who have had severe asthma or who have developed sensitivity to horse serum following a previous injection.

The heart is usually subjected to a severe strain in diphtheria, so that the patient should always be at rest in bed. Moreover, the heart must be watched carefully for several weeks after the patient recovers to make certain that it has not been damaged in any way.

There was a time when it was customary to wash the nose and throat of a patient with diphtheria with all sorts of gargles and sprays, usually of some alkaline solution. Nowadays it is customary to leave the nose and throat alone. In most instances when there is a foul odor in the throat, a mild wash or gargle may be desirable.

In the very severe cases of diphtheria, when the patient seems to be strangling because of lack of air, it may be necessary, as previously mentioned, to pass an O'Dwyer tube into the larynx so as to permit breathing. In the still more severe cases, an emergency operation is sometimes done, the physician opening the tube that leads to the lungs so that the patient is able to breathe. These cases are, however, exceedingly rare, since a powerful diphtheria antitoxin has been introduced, and since the vast majority of doctors give a large dose of antitoxin as soon as the diagnosis is made.

Diphtheria is one of the diseases about which scientific medicine has the most information. Yet the condition is still far from being under complete control. Some years ago an eminent epidemiologist said that if all the knowledge now available were to be applied practically, diphtheria would disappear from the world. Nevertheless, human beings, because of their unwillingness to learn to put into effect the knowledge that they have, continue to suffer from this disease.

In several communities in this country, notably, Auburn, N. Y., and New Haven, Conn., where almost the entire population of children has been immunized against diphtheria, the disease has been practically eliminated. The prevention of this disease by application of the various methods that have been described represents one of the greatest contributions of modern medical science to the welfare of humanity. Recent tests show that 80 per cent of the children who have been immunized by the use of toxin-antitoxin or of toxoid remain immune for at least ten years after the injections. It is reasonable to be-

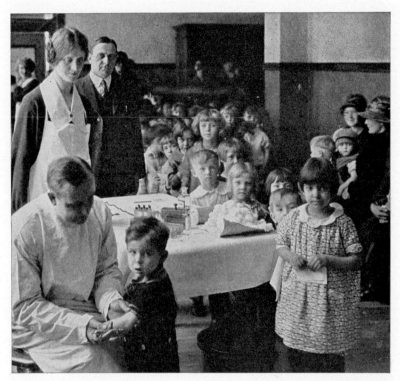

FIG. 31. Injection of toxin-antitoxin for prevention of diphtheria.

lieve that we may yet see the time when diphtheria is no longer a menace to any civilized child.

In the meantime, medical scientists continue to study the germ of diphtheria, its nature, its method of transmission, the way in which it changes its own capacity to infect from time to time, and similar facts that are necessary in controlling this disease.

Measles

Measles is one of the oldest diseases known to modern medicine. There is some evidence that it may have existed in the early Christian Era. It is even described in the writings of physicians of the seventh and ninth centuries. However, it was for a long time confused with scarlet fever, and it was not until the seventeenth century that it was clearly distinguished from scarlet fever. Moreover, it was occasionally confused with smallpox, and it was not definitely distinguished from smallpox until the eighteenth century.

Two of the greatest names in English medicine are associated with these two observations. Thomas Sydenham distinguished measles from scarlet fever, and William Withering, who introduced the use of digitalis, distinguished measles clearly from smallpox. The English word measles resembles a word in Sanskrit, *masura*, and the German word is *masern*.

For a long time it was generally believed that every child had to have measles. In fact, mothers used to expose their children to the disease with the idea of getting it over. Now it is known that the disease is definitely transmitted from one person to another, and that it is possible, by exercising precautions, to avoid the disease in most instances.

Measles is essentially a disease of childhood. More than half the cases occur in children under five years of age, and more than 90 per cent occur in children under ten years of age. There are occasional epidemics of measles in which considerable numbers of people are affected, even people of advanced years. In such cases it is usually found that the people concerned have come from rural areas and that they have not previously been exposed. For example, there were severe outbreaks of measles among the soldiers in the training camps in 1917 and 1918, because large numbers of recruits came from farms, ranches, and remote districts and had never had measles before.

Measles among a people who do not have anything resembling resistance through heredity may be a most serious and fatal disease. A terrific epidemic of measles occurred in the Faroe Islands in 1846. There were 7,800 people on the Islands and 6,000 of them had the disease in a few months. There was also a great epidemic in the Fiji Islands in 1875. A British ship carrying measles brought the disease to the Islands. Out of a population of 150,000 there were 40,000 deaths in a few months. Part of this was due to the great virulence with which the disease attacked a community without resistance. Much of the fatality is ascribed to the fact that so many people were sick at the same time that there were not enough well people left to take care of the sick. Some people died of starvation, and many died from lack of care.

As with diphtheria, measles is spread mostly through direct contact with those who have the disease. Apparently, the virus or poison that causes the disease is present in the secretions of the nose and throat. Hence it is spread by coughing and sneezing. Fortunately, the virus which carries the disease is injured by exposure to air and sunlight, so that it is seldom likely that measles is carried from one person to another through the medium of a third person or an animal. For this reason it is quite safe for doctors and nurses who see cases of measles to go in the open air to visit other patients.

However, it is well for those who take care of patients with measles to observe all of the precautions that are associated with the care of infectious disease generally. This means thorough washing of the hands after visiting a patient, the wearing of a clean gown on entering the room, and removal of the gown on leaving. Moreover, the dishes, bedding, and other materials associated with the child sick with measles must be boiled before they are used again.

[Two new methods have been developed for prevention of measles; one involves the injection of serum from a child who has recovered; another includes the use of a protein substance called immune globulin taken from the placenta or afterbirth, which contains anti-substances against infectious diseases. These methods are applied particularly when there is an epidemic.—Ed.]

Before any discovery is accepted as certainly established in relationship to the cause of an infectious disease, as has previously been mentioned, it is necessary to grow the germ outside the body and to reproduce the disease in animals by injecting the germ and to find the germ invariably associated with the disease. None of the discoveries thus far made meets these conditions. In a few instances the investigators claimed that they had the organism, but others were not able to duplicate the work. Scientific medicine is jealous of its science and does not readily accept new announcements until they are fully confirmed and well established. This is fortunate for the public, since it has here a protection against early exploitation of unestablished work.

From the time when the child first comes in contact with a case of measles, and thereby develops the likelihood of catching the disease, until the disease appears, is usually thirteen or fourteen days. This is known as the incubation period. Authorities give the shortest incubation period as eight days and the longest as seventeen days. During this period the patient does not have symptoms. However, he does develop early three definite signs which permit a physician to diagnose the disease in its earliest stages. These signs include fever, running nose and watering of the eyes, and an eruption on the mucous membranes lining the mouth.

The inflammation of the eyes differentiates measles from other infectious diseases, in which this symptom is not common. The child avoids the light and, as has been mentioned, the eyes are moist and full of tears. Particularly interesting are the little spots which appear on the sides of the mouth and on the palate and which resemble the rash that is later to appear on the skin. These little bluish white spots, surrounded with an area of red inflammation, were described by a New York physician named Koplik and are commonly called Koplik's spots. A Dutch physician on an isolated island described them earlier, but his report did not circulate; hence Koplik's name goes with the spots.

Three or four days after the running nose and the slight fever appear comes the rash. The child breaks out on the face, the mouth and chin, and then over the trunk, arms, thighs, and legs with red spots which enlarge and join together. The color is purplish red. During this period the child is likely to be sicker than at any other time in the course of the disease. He may have lack of appetite, a coated tongue, even looseness of the bowels; there may be a slight cough and other disturbances related to the lungs.

The child with measles should be placed in a room alone and not permitted to come in contact with other children. Particular attention must be given to the prevention of chilling, because this is especially harmful in measles. The secondary complications affecting the lungs are far more serious than the disease itself. The room should be well ventilated, but care must be taken to avoid drafts by placing screens properly before open windows. This does not mean that the room is to be kept stuffy or hot. It is the draft that should be avoided.

For years it was customary to keep darkened the room used by a child with measles because of the trouble with the eyes. Now it is realized that strong sunlight should be excluded because glare will cause pain in the eyes. The child should not be permitted to read nor should there be a brilliant artificial light. If the child complains particularly of the light, colored glasses may be worn. If the eyelids tend to stick because of the slight inflammation they may be bathed with boric acid solution or with plain warm water, which removes the crusts and prevents pain and irritation.

During the period of restlessness the child will sleep better if it is given a warm sponge bath just before going to sleep. This serves to cool the child and to bring down the fever slightly. It also avoids chilling. After the sponge bath the skin may be powdered with any light, clean talcum. This helps to avoid irritation.

It is not necessary to cover the child with heavy woolen blankets or to use flannel sleeping garments. The child should be kept warm but not made uncomfortable.

The food to be taken by the child with measles should be chiefly light and fluid as long as there is any fever. Just as soon as the fever disappears and the child begins to convalesce, plenty of nutritious food should be supplied, particularly foods containing iron and vitamins, as these will help to build up the depleted blood. Laxatives and cathartics should be given only on the order of a physician. It is much better to keep the bowels regular by the use of proper foods. It is also well in these conditions to give plenty of fluids, including drinks tending toward alkalinity, such as orange juice and lemon juice.

When a person has an infectious disease he builds up in his blood materials for opposing the disease. When he recovers, the material remains. For this reason the person who has measles, scarlet fever, or another infectious disease, usually has the disease only once. For this reason also it has been found helpful, in the presence of severe epidemics of measles, to inject into those who are exposed small amounts of the blood of those who are getting over the disease. This procedure has been found to be safe. It seems to minimize the severity of the disturbance if it does not prevent it.

It is the contagious material from the patient with measles that spreads the disease. This contagious material is found chiefly in the excretions from the nose and throat. Every possible step must be taken to prevent other children from coming in contact with these excretions. Occasionally also there are infections of the ear with discharges. The discharges from the ear may also contain the infectious substances, although quite frequently the ear is infected secondarily with other germs, such as the streptococci, which are always present in the throat.

When the resistance of the body is broken down by any one disease a human being becomes susceptible to infections from others. Measles is particularly important in this regard. It has been noticed that epidemics of measles are frequently followed by invasion of other contagious diseases, such as whooping cough, chicken pox, diphtheria, and scarlet fever. Measles is noted also for lowering resistance to tuberculosis so that children who have quiescent infections from tuberculosis in the glands, the bones, the joints, or the lungs may develop activity in these foci when they become infected with measles.

It is a mistake to consider measles a trivial disease. Perhaps many children do not die of measles, the number approximating in this country seven thousand per year. Diphtheria causes twice as many deaths, scarlet fever half as many, and whooping cough about the same number. However, there are many complications which cause serious conditions that are carried through life. Of all the deaths from measles, 75 per cent occur in children under five years of age. If a child gets measles before it is one year old, the chance of its dying is fifty times greater than in measles in a child between five and fifteen years of age.

Whenever a case appears in a school, the parents of other children should be warned that a case has occurred and that they should be on the lookout for symptoms of infection in their own children. Parents should be warned particularly to keep their children who have measles, or who are just recovering, away from other children who may not have had the disease.

A few years ago a Christmas party was held in a Sunday school. One mother, who did not want to disappoint her child, a little girl seven years old, who was just recovering from measles, sent her to the party. Following that Christmas party thirteen other children came down with measles.

When a child with measles is put to bed promptly and given satisfactory care of the type that has previously been mentioned, it tends to get well. The prevention of the complications in measles is largely due to the kind of attention that is given. Careful management, skillful nursing, and early control of complications by competent medical attention make all the difference between prompt recovery and the possibility of permanent complications or death.

GERMAN MEASLES

German measles brings on one of the reddest eruptions of any disease that affects mankind. Its scientific name is *rubella*, and in German it is called *Rötheln*. Because of its red eruption it is frequently confused with scarlet fever or with measles. Fortunately, it is not nearly so severe a disease, although it is highly contagious.

From fourteen to twenty-one days after a child comes in contact with another who has had German measles it will begin to feel ill and break out with the eruption, which occurs first on the chest and face and then gradually spreads over the body. There is not much fever in most cases. However, the lymph glands, particularly those at the back of the neck, swell up and get hard, a condition that seldom occurs in other infectious diseases. Associated with this swelling and hardness of the glands at the back of the neck there will be tenderness and even stiffness.

It is important to make sure about the cause of such tenderness or such stiffness of the neck because many of the conditions of infection which concern the nervous system, such as meningitis, brain fever, and infantile paralysis, also develop stiffness and pain on motion of the neck. There are conditions in which lymph glands are infected in which the glands later soften and develop pus which has to be released by an opening. In German measles, however, the glands gradually soften and disappear without developing pus or matter.

The doctor tells the difference between German measles and ordinary measles by the absence of the spots in the mouth and by the slightness of the condition, by the nature of the eruption and by the absence in measles, in most cases, of the hard spots at the back of the neck.

Few, if any, people die of German measles. The disease usually proceeds toward prompt recovery. The chief trouble with it is that it causes loss of time from school. Seldom is anything required in its treatment except good care, a mild diet, cleansing of the throat by proper gargles, and the early care of any secondary complications. It is well to handle every case of German measles as if it were scarlet fever, because sometimes a diagnosis may be wrong. If the condition turns out to be scarlet fever, as is apparent from the preceding descriptions of that disease, much more serious attention is required.

SCARLET FEVER

No doubt scarlet fever was known to the ancients, but it is only within the last ten years that its nature has actually been thoroughly elucidated. It is an acute infectious disease that comes on suddenly, with a red rash which disappears gradually and is followed by peeling of the skin.

For many years it was known that a germ called the streptococcus was associated with scarlet fever, but it is only recently that the definite relationship of this germ to the cause of the disease has been established. The proof is in the fact that the germ can be found in the throat, the blood, and other tissues of people who have the disease, that the disease can be produced in human beings by putting the germs into their bodies, and that there is a reaction in the skin of a human being who does not have the disease when the toxin or poison taken from the germs is inoculated into the skin.

Scarlet fever usually comes on in epidemics that are worst in the winter or fall. The chief factor necessary is contact, usually of a child, with someone who has the disease. Most of the cases develop in children between five and twelve years of age. There is probably something that the child gets in its blood from the mother which in most cases prevents children below one year of age from catching the disease.

Scarlet fever does not spread nearly as rapidly as measles; apparently only about one in ten people who come in contact with cases of the disease later develop it. It is, of course, possible that people are infected with mild attacks of scarlet fever which are overlooked, and that as a result they are later protected against the disease. Scarlet fever is one of those diseases which happen once in a person's lifetime and then are not likely to happen again. In other words, one attack of the disease protects.

Occasionally scarlet fever is spread through milk or through the excretions or secretions of persons who are infected, but the spread through food is far less frequent than the spread directly from person to person. Most people are interested to know whether or not the scales or the skin that peels off after scarlet fever will transmit the disease. Apparently the scales will not spread scarlet fever unless contaminated with the secretions of the nose and throat.

From two to four days after a person has been in contact with someone who has had scarlet fever he will have a chill and complain of severe sore throat. If the person affected is a child, he is likely to be nauseated and vomit. Promptly the pulse becomes rapid as the fever goes up. The fever may rise as high as 102 to 104 degrees. There is severe headache. Then bright red spots about the size of a pin point appear, usually first on the neck and chest, then rapidly spreading over the rest of the body. The face is flushed because of the fever, but the eruption on the face is seldom severe.

After two or three days the rash or eruption begins to fade, and in about a week the skin appears to be normal in color. Then ten days to two weeks after the disease first appears the skin begins to peel. Great patches of skin may come off the hands and feet, but over the rest of the body the skin comes off in small scales. Occasionally the teeth, the hair, and the fingernails also are affected by the destructive process. An interesting symptom of scarlet fever is the appearance of the tongue. Because of its bright red appearance and because the tissues of the surface of the tongue swell so as to show tiny pits, the tongue of scarlet fever is called a strawberry tongue.

Scarlet fever in many instances is a fairly mild disease. When, however, it is complicated by certain forms of invasion of the kidneys, the ears, the glands or the joints, it may be most serious and destructive.

Until recently there was no certain method of confirming the diagnosis of scarlet fever, no certain method of determining whether or not a person who had not had the disease was likely to be infected on exposure, no method certainly useful in treatment except to put the patient to bed and to protect him against complications, such as is the general method of treatment of all infectious diseases.

Then Drs. George F. and Gladys Henry Dick in Chicago, and Drs. Dochez and Avery in New York, developed information relative to the germ and to the poison that it produces, which led to knowledge of a specific character. They found that a germ of the type called the streptococcus is responsible for scarlet fever; that it produces a poison or toxin which can be found in the material in which the germs grow;

that this toxin, when injected into the skin of a person who has not previously had the disease, would produce a severe reaction, whereas in those who were protected against the disease it would not produce a reaction. They found, furthermore, that the injection of a small amount of this toxin or poison in a human being, after it had been made harmless, would cause the person to develop resistance against scarlet fever. Also a horse may be injected with this poison or toxin. The horse will then develop in its blood an antitoxin which is valuable in overcoming scarlet fever.

Since these discoveries were announced, many thousands of persons throughout the world have been tested with the Dick test. Many thousands of persons have been injected or inoculated with the toxin so as to free them relatively from the danger of contracting scarlet fever.

Because scarlet fever is not an extremely widespread disease, it does not appear to be worth while to inject every child with the preventive toxin. However, when a child has been definitely exposed to the disease, or when a girl is going to work as a nurse in a hospital where there are frequently cases of scarlet fever, it is probably advisable to give them the benefit of the preventive inoculations against scarlet fever. There are few, if any, records of severe accidents or injuries following the use of these preventive methods.

Scarlet fever varies in its severity from time to time, from epidemic to epidemic. In the presence of a severe epidemic with numerous serious complications, it is more advisable to inoculate against the disease than under other circumstances.

Because of the danger to other children from a child or an adult who has scarlet fever, the patient should be promptly put to bed and kept separate from other people for about six weeks. If there are discharges from the nose and throat or from the ears the patient should be isolated until all discharges have ceased. These discharges are extremely dangerous in spreading the disease.

Beyond this placing of the patient in a separate room, attention must be given to protecting the kidneys and the heart from the special strains associated with activity at a time when they are exposed to the actions of the poisons that come from the germs. Therefore, every patient with scarlet fever should remain in bed for at least three weeks. It is customary to give a light, soft diet consisting mostly of liquids until the fever has disappeared, and then gradually to add cereals and similar soft foods until the peeling has begun. Then it becomes necessary to build up the tissues and the blood again. This can be done by feeding plenty of milk, fresh vegetables, foods rich in vitamins, mineral salts like calcium and iron, and more protein than is allowed in the active stages of the disease.

It is important to avoid exposure to cold. Therefore, the patient should be bathed with sponges of lukewarm water. Sometimes the skin may be oiled, which aids the peeling and prevents irritation.

In most cases the throat can be let alone because the initial soreness and swelling soon disappear. If, however, there is severe pain from the sore throat, the usual mild gargles may be used. It is well, however, that only persons who have already had the disease should be in contact with the patient and help him with these procedures.

There is no certain method of preventing the complications that affect the kidneys in so many cases of scarlet fever. All that one can do is to make sure that the patient is quiet and that the diet does not throw an undue burden on the kidneys. For this reason it is customary, during at least the first two or three weeks, to eliminate meat and eggs from the diet.

In treating scarlet fever doctors usually prescribe remedies that will prevent headache and pain, giving small doses to avoid irritation of the kidneys. If earache occurs, the ears are closely watched so that the eardrum may be punctured and the infectious material allowed to escape before there is danger to the internal ear from pressure of the poison and danger of mastoiditis. If the infection is virulent, these complications may develop in spite of every precaution.

It was found long ago that the blood of those who have recovered from scarlet fever contained substances which oppose the disease. Therefore, in this disease, as in measles, small amounts of such blood taken from the patients who are recovering from scarlet fever may be injected into those with serious and complicated cases.

Later, Drs. Dick developed their antitoxin. It has been found that in serious cases this antitoxin is valuable as an aid in preventing the complications of the disease. Because some people are sensitive to the serum of the horse, it is customary before injecting large doses of antitoxin to try the effects of a very small dose. When this is done dangerous reactions are prevented, and the patient may have the benefit of the specific antitoxin.

WHOOPING COUGH

At least four hundred years ago diseases were described which resemble what is called whooping cough today. This condition is one of the most difficult with which health officials and physicians have to deal. A few cases appearing in any group of children spread rapidly to include all who have not had the disease previously.

Whooping cough causes more deaths than do most of the other infectious diseases of childhood. It is fatal chiefly to the very young, and the immediate cause of death is nearly always some secondary infection. In older children whooping cough is quite frequently followed by pneumonia or tuberculosis and is especially menacing from the point of view of these complications.

A germ has been found in connection with the disease by two Belgian investigators, Bordet and Gengou, but possibly this is not the exclusive cause, and other factors may also be present.

The chief epidemics of this disease occur in winter. Whooping cough is transmitted, of course, by the material coughed out from the lungs. It has been shown that the explosive cough which occurs in this condition can throw droplets of infected saliva six feet or farther. Far too frequently parents permit children to begin playing with other children just as soon as they are without fever. Yet these children, if they continue to cough, may be active in spreading the disease to children who have not had it. Moreover, there is evidence that whooping cough is infectious in its earliest stages, so that children who are not put to bed and kept isolated until after they have been coughing for some time may also actively spread the disease.

It is the duty of parents not only to their own children, but also to others, to put a coughing child to bed as soon as possible. Moreover, they ought to keep him in bed until a physician says that it is safe for him to be up and around.

What is called the incubation period in whooping cough is the period from two to ten days before the patient begins coughing. During this period the child is infected but not sick. Therefore, the child exposed to whooping cough must be watched carefully for at least ten days after its contact for the signs of whooping cough. During this period there may be symptoms resembling those of a common cold. After the characteristic whoop and the paroxysm of coughing appear, the child is likely to be able to spread the disease for at least three weeks longer. Therefore, doctors advise that children be kept alone as long as the cough continues and for two weeks after it ends.

The doctor diagnoses whooping cough not only by the typical coughing spells, which are usually accompanied with redness of the face and the development of a thick, sticky mucus in the mouth, but also by changes which occur in the blood in this disease. Not only do the white blood cells increase in number, but a particular form of the white blood cells, known as the lymphocytes, mononuclear or single nucleus cells, increases even more than do the others.

As has been said, the chief danger from whooping cough is not from the disease itself, but from the secondary pneumonia and changes which may affect the heart and lungs.

The total period of quarantine may be as long as six weeks. In attempting to control whooping cough all sorts of methods of prevention have been tried, including inoculation of the blood from people who are recovering from the disease, the injection of germs that have been killed, with the idea that these injections will stimulate the body to form anti-substances against the germs of the disease, and many similar measures. The use of the vaccines, which means a mixture of killed germs, is thought by many specialists in diseases of children to have value in preventing whooping cough in children who are exposed, and also in diminishing the severity of the symptoms. However, there are other physicians who have had little success with the use of such vaccines, and they do not employ them.

As soon as the child who has had whooping cough is free from fever and any other serious symptoms, it is customary to permit him to be about, particularly where there are sunlight, warmth, and fresh air, but the child should not be exposed to air that is too cold.

Because the coughing spells are frequently accompanied by vomiting, such children sometimes lose weight and may suffer from a lack of water in the body. Hence, the parents must aid the physician in seeing to it that the child has sufficient water and also that it eats between meals, if necessary, or in fact whenever it can retain food, so as to keep up its nutrition.

Because coughing may bring undue pressure into the abdominal cavity and thereby cause rupture or hernia by pushing the abdominal contents through the wall, it is advisable in some cases to put an abdominal binder on the child, which helps to support the abdominal wall and, at the same time, gives the child comfort during severe coughing.

Although the use of various drugs does not cure whooping cough, there are many things that a physician can prescribe which will lessen the severity of the coughing and will sometimes permit the child to sleep. Practically every remedy that is known to have a sedative effect has been tried in this condition, and physicians prescribe those with which they are most familiar and which they themselves have found to be most useful. One of the simplest methods of relieving a cough is to inhale warm steam perhaps medicated with a little tincture of benzoin. Fill a cup with boiling water, drop in a teaspoonful of the tincture of benzoin, and inhale the hot steam for five or ten minutes. Such medication is more useful for an ordinary cough than for whooping cough, however. In this condition, frequently, the only way to get relief is by taking sedative remedies that are so strong they can be taken only with a doctor's prescription.

As in other types of infectious disease, all drops from the nose and throat should be disinfected, and all articles contaminated by such discharges, if they are without value, should be disinfected or burned.

In keeping up the nutrition of the child, it is well to rely primarily on milk and the use of vegetables containing plenty of vitamins and mineral salts.

In preventing the spread of whooping cough everyone must coöperate. If parents know of other children in the neighborhood who have whooping cough and who are being permitted to play outdoors with children who have not had the disease, the health department should be notified. In most communities the parents who have children with whooping cough are permitted themselves to go to work and to go outdoors, although the children are kept under isolation. However, a sign on the door to the effect that whooping cough is present in the household will inform other parents of the fact and will enable them to take suitable precaution so that their children may not undergo any unusual likelihood of catching the disease.

Chicken Pox

All sorts of names have been applied to chicken pox, not only by the public, but also by physicians. In some parts of the country it is known as water pock, glass pock, sheep pock, and crystal pock. These names obviously are related either to some resemblance of the blisters to similar conditions occurring in animals, or, in fact, to the resemblance of the blisters to water or crystal. Scientifically, the condition is called *varicella*, but it was also called *variola spuria*, or spurious smallpox, because it was so frequently mistaken for smallpox.

The cause of chicken pox is still a mystery. The condition occurs most often in children and, because it is so highly contagious, spreads rapidly. Usually a person who has had the disease once does not develop it again.

Even though the cause is not known, it is realized that the infectious agent is present in the blisters. The blisters appear early and break almost as soon as they appear. It is probable, therefore, that the disease may be spread before the eruption is visible in the form of blisters. About two weeks after a child has been in contact with children who have chicken pox, it will probably come down with this disease.

The blisters on the skin appear in groups, usually first on the back, the chest, and the face, but most profusely on those parts of the skin that are covered by clothing.

As has been mentioned, the condition may be spread not only from contact with infectious material that is in the blisters, but far more frequently through some infection that may be inhaled.

Dr. J. F. Schamberg recites an instance in which a physician's daughter sixteen years old developed a slight sore throat and was immediately isolated in a room in the upper story of her home. On the following day she was found to have the eruption of chicken pox. An eight-year-old brother who was with her on the previous day was kept in a distant part of the house, but sixteen days later he also came down with chicken pox. His only possible contact with the disease was through his sister.

Nobody knows how long a person who has chicken pox remains infectious for others, but it is safe to keep the person who is recovering away from other people until the skin is entirely free of the original crusts.

Chicken pox is not a particularly serious disease, since it is seldom associated with high fever or with much depression. Usually the fever disappears in from one to three days, although it may last four or five days. With the exception of German measles, chicken pox is probably the mildest of all the infectious diseases that attack children.

Usually all that is necessary in such cases is to make certain that the child does not scratch the spots with the likelihood of secondary infection. The finger nails of children should be closely trimmed to prevent such scratching. If it cannot be stopped in any other way, the hands may be enclosed in mittens of cloth or celluloid, or tubes may be put about the elbows which will prevent bending the elbow and scratching.

Ordinarily, the blisters, if let alone, will last a few hours, break, dry up, and form a crust. This crust disappears in from two to four days.

The diet is mild and soft. Mild, warm baths are used, and it may be desirable for the physician to prescribe powder to prevent itching, or ointments and antiseptic solutions to prevent secondary infection.

Chicken pox seldom concerns older people. Most children have had it by the time they grow up. If, however, they have not had it, they may get the disease later. Chicken pox can be exceedingly inconvenient for a grown-up person, but the most important step for a grown-up person is to make certain that he really has chicken pox and not small-pox.

After a patient recovers, it is merely necessary to wash the bedding thoroughly with hot water and soap and to clean and air the room in which the patient has been while sick.

It is also well for everyone who is in contact with the child to wash the hands thoroughly after leaving the room and preferably to wear a gown or covering while in the room.

MUMPS

Of all the annoying diseases that afflict the child, and which also occasionally attack the adult, mumps is the one most likely to arouse the risibilities of those in the vicinity. Swelling at the sides of the face gives the person who is infected a distinctly comical appearance. There is a current superstition that the person with the disease cannot eat pickles and that anything sour will pucker up his face like the phenomena that follow the eating of a green persimmon.

There is no doubt that the condition is infectious, because it spreads rapidly wherever it gets a start among a group of young people. Cases have been described as long ago as one hundred fifty years, and there is reason to believe that something resembling mumps was described by the famous father of scientific medicine, Hippocrates, 300 years before the Christian Era.

Since the time when Pasteur first proved definitely that germs can cause disease, the experts have been trying to find the germ that causes mumps. They have taken material from the glands, from the saliva, and from various other parts of the body, and on several occasions investigators have claimed that the germ was isolated. The evidence thus far in support of any one of these claims is not sufficient to convince other experts that the real germ has been discovered.

Most often mumps appear in a child from five to fifteen years of age. Because the glands most commonly concerned are the parotid glands, just in front of the ear, the disease is called scientifically epidemic parotitis. The Germans fondly call it *Ziegenpeter,* which perhaps has some reference to a goat.

In most cases, mumps is a mild condition. It occurs usually during the cold season of the year. Out of 150 epidemics, only 21 occurred in the warm months. In the World War something resembling an epidemic of mumps occurred among the soldiers in the American army. In 1918, there were almost 170,000 cases among the soldiers. For some reason, the colored soldiers seemed to be more easily affected than were the white.

As has been said, mumps is primarily a disease of adolescence, but cases have been observed in a woman eighty-four years of age, and in a man ninety-nine years of age—no doubt, both in their second childhood.

Mumps is probably spread from one person to another by the saliva. Occasionally a third person may become contaminated with this infectious saliva and, although himself not infected by the disease, carry it from a sick person to a healthy one. Study of the disease shows that it is most contagious during the early days, and that once convalescence begins it is not nearly so dangerous. For this reason it is not customary to quarantine or isolate cases with mumps for more than two weeks.

Beyond the stiffness of the jaw and the pain on opening the mouth, which are associated with the swelling of the glands, the person with mumps usually has little trouble. There are, however, cases in which the mumps seem to spread particularly to the glands of sex. When this occurs, it is a serious complication. There are instances in which the ability of the human being to have children has been irreparably damaged by this secondary complication. Incidentally, the complication is more likely to occur in grown people than in children. With the complication of this character there may be fever that is fairly high.

There is not much that can be done about mumps, except to make certain that the person is absolutely quiet and that there is no secondary complication in the form of pus infection. When this occurs either in the glands in front of the ear or in the sex glands, only the most judicious and careful attention of a competent physician can be of much service. Fortunately, such secondary infection is rare.

In the majority of cases the condition gets well without any complications. Usually it is mild. In the army of 1918, there was about one death for every seven hundred cases.

The usual treatment of infectious diseases, already described, is ordinarily applied by good physicians in cases of mumps. The attention of the physician is necessary so that he may detect possible complications at the earliest moment in order to prevent their spread or extension or to prevent an increase in their severity.

People who have had mumps should be kept under observation for at least three weeks, to make sure that the condition is fully healed and that no further complications are likely.

INFANTILE PARALYSIS

Of all the diseases that strike dread to mankind, none is more feared by mothers than acute poliomyelitis, or, as it is more commonly known, infantile paralysis. This is an acute infection in which the inflammation attacks the tissues in the front part of the spinal cord. Possibly it has occurred throughout the centuries, but it was first widely recognized as an epidemic disorder around 1887. No doubt, previous to that time, cases of this disease were confused with meningitis and paralysis due to other disorders.

The majority of cases of this condition occur in young children, afflicting boys and girls in about equal proportions. There are, however, numerous cases in which the condition attacks older persons, among the most conspicuous examples being Franklin D. Roosevelt, who was infected late in life.

From time to time investigators have claimed the isolation of the germ causing infantile paralysis, but not yet has any one of the germs thus far isolated been accepted as the cause of this disease. Nevertheless, its infectious character is certainly established through transmission from one animal to another. There seems to be reason to believe that the disease is spread principally in the secretions of the nose and throat, possibly by direct contact with those having the disease, and possibly also by healthy carriers of the infection. The appearance of the paralysis usually follows three or four days of fever and disturbances of digestion. In some cases the preliminary symptoms are so slight that the paralysis is the first symptom noted. In other cases, the paralysis may be so slight that the condition is unrecognized except for the fact that the child happens to be sick at a time when infantile paralysis is prevalent in the community.

Infantile paralysis usually begins to appear in June, increases during July and August, diminishes in October, and disappears by November. In the northern part of the United States it reaches its highest point in August and September; in the southern half, between December and May. While the condition occurs usually in warm weather, it is not especially a disease of tropical countries. It is most frequent in the temperate zone. By far the vast majority of the cases have occurred in northern Europe and in the northern part of the United States.

The disease attacks rich and poor alike and appears equally in good and bad sanitary situations. Whereas 95 per cent of those attacked are children, the condition seldom occurs during the first year of life. This may be due to the fact that the infant, during this period, is separated from the community generally. It is also due, however, in some part, to the fact that the mother transmits to the infant at birth a certain amount of resistance against this as well as other infectious diseases, and that perhaps a year is required for the immunity of this character to wear off.

In any event, when infantile paralysis is present in a community, any child with the slightest symptoms of a cold or a fever should be given most careful study by a physician.

Those who have been exposed to infantile paralysis should have temperatures taken regularly for a period of at least three weeks so as to detect the onset of fever and symptoms at the earliest possible moment. During times when there are epidemics in the community, children should not be allowed to mingle with crowds, and travel should be discouraged. The occurrence of fever, headache with vomiting, drowsiness, and irritability when disturbed, flushing, congestion of the throat, and notable sweating during a period when infantile paralysis is prevalent in a community should be looked on with suspicion. Any evidence on the part of the child of stiffness of the back and resistance to movement of the neck is to be considered as a suspicious symptom, demanding the most careful medical investigation.

[In the prevention of infantile paralysis, all sorts of experiments have been attempted to develop methods of inoculation against the disease. Thus far none of these methods has been proved to be of value. Indeed, the only technic which has really been established as of value in the prevention of infantile paralysis is to avoid contact with anyone who has the disease in its early stages.

The virus of infantile paralysis is spread not only by secretions from the nose and throat but also by that from the bowels. Bowel excretions must not come in contact with anyone who is well. The secretions and excretions from the patient with infantile paralysis should, therefore, be handled exactly like we handle the material from the patient with typhoid. Particularly dangerous is hand-to-mouth infection. Everyone associated in the care of a patient with infantile paralysis in its early stages should wash the hands thoroughly with soap and water each time he is near the patient.

A serious outbreak of infantile paralysis coming at the end of 1940 established no new facts regarding the method by which the disease is disseminated. In order to give the widest possible opportunity for recovery to those patients who had paralysis affecting the breathing apparatus, the National Foundation for Infantile Paralysis has made available a complete list of all respirators that exist in the United States with the places where they are kept. Thus any community which is overwhelmed with an excess of cases of infantile paralysis may borrow respirators from neighboring communities. The National Foundation for Infantile Paralysis, Inc., 120 Broadway, N. Y. C., is ready to help any community with advice regarding the handling of outbreaks.

The blood of a person with infantile paralysis contains antisubstances against the disease. However, the disease is so rapid in its onset that there does not seem to be any reason to believe that the injection of such blood will, with certainty, prevent the disease or control it once the diagnosis has been made.—Ed.]

EARLY DIAGNOSIS OF INFANTILE PARALYSIS

As soon as infantile paralysis is well established it becomes important to have a careful examination of the muscles in order to find out which are permanently involved so that plans may be outlined for treatment leading to recovery of the power of motion.

Among the remedies used in the treatment of infantile paralysis it is necessary to mention first absolute rest in bed. This is important in avoiding any unnecessary irritation to the affected tissues. A considerable number of investigators are convinced of the value of injections of blood serum, which is the fluid matter of the blood, taken from patients who recently have recovered from infantile paralysis. In the absence of ability to get such blood serum, materials are used obtained from animals which have been injected with the poison of infantile paralysis and which have developed in their blood "anti" substances against the poison.

Among the most important factors in giving relief from serious pain and depression in this condition good nursing is especially to be emphasized. Good nursing in infantile paralysis must be exceedingly gentle. It must minimize as much as possible any movement of the patient and avoid any unnecessary output of energy. The physician can prescribe various drugs which tend to keep such patients quiet. The nurse may aid in giving warm baths which help in bringing about relief.

One of the recent discoveries which already has saved many lives in infantile paralysis is the artificial respirator. In the past any child who developed a paralysis of the muscles of breathing during the course of infantile paralysis was likely to die. Nowadays machines have been developed into which the child's whole body may be put and its breathing motions kept up automatically. Then, as the infectious condition subsides, it is possible, through good training and care, to bring about a restoration of the breathing function.

Once the active disease has passed, it is necessary to make a complete examination of all the muscles to find out which have become weakened and which have lost their functions entirely; then the weakened muscles may be benefited. In cases in which some functions have been lost entirely, reëducation of the muscles may be used to enable children to walk and to carry on other activities. Throughout all treatments it is necessary to guard against too much fatigue. Children should not be encouraged to walk too soon. They should never be allowed to stand in a deformed position. If the legs are too weak, splints may be applied, and corsets, jackets, and braces may be worn in order to aid in supporting the weakened tissues.

Exercise in water has developed a great vogue, particularly through the encouragement of the Georgia Warm Springs Foundation by

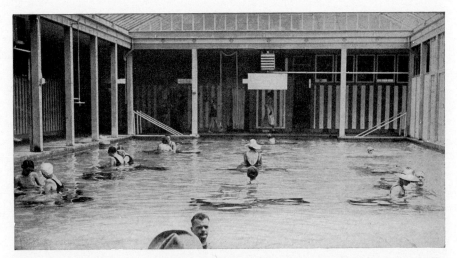

FIG. 32. Pool at Warm Springs Foundation for Treatment of Infantile Paralysis.

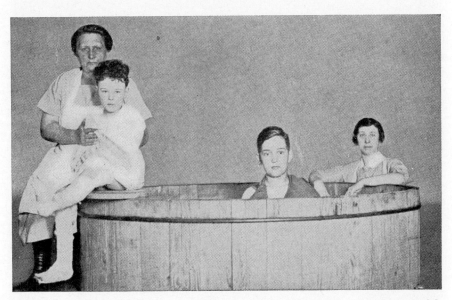

FIG. 33. Home constructed pool for giving treatment to children with infantile paralysis.

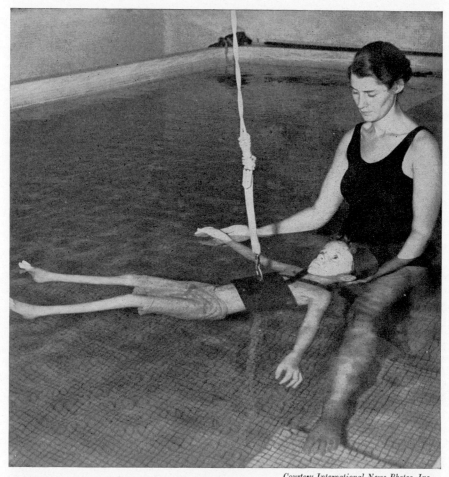

FIG. 34. Physical therapy technician treating child in pool for infantile
paralysis.

President Roosevelt. The chief advantages of the use of the swimming-pool method are the aid derived from supporting the limbs by the buoyancy of the water. Even under the best of conditions, however, the swimming pool itself is not a cure for paralyzed muscles. It is the training given in the swimming pool by competent teachers that brings about restoration.

The number of deaths from infantile paralysis varies greatly in different epidemics. In the great epidemic which occurred in New York in 1916, 27 per cent of those attacked died.

Of the greatest importance in the care of such patients is the proper handling of all their normal functions. They should be moved sufficiently often to prevent the occurrence of bed sores. There is danger of pneumonia. The patient should not be allowed to lie continually on the back. If he cannot swallow the mucus and saliva which develop in the mouth, he must be turned so that these will be drained out. More recently the development of mechanical devices to aid normal breathing during the period when the lungs are paralyzed has saved many lives.

The majority of children who have had infantile paralysis still retain the ability to perform certain movements but lack the power to make other movements. For this reason general exercises which are good for normal people are not suited to the unequal movements of these patients. A distinguished committee of the American Medical Association, realizing that the assistance of another person is necessary to insure that the exercises are given correctly, outlined some suggestions for the mother who is to aid with daily treatment:

1. The patient must know what movement he is to do and must try to do it, after which he relaxes and lets the mother put the arm or leg back in the starting position ready for him to try again.

2. The mother should understand that it does not strengthen the muscles if she moves the leg back and forth. The patient must try and should not be helped until he has done as much of the movement as his strength allows; then the rest of the movement should be finished for him while he still tries.

3. The mother may make any of these exercises harder by resisting the movement with her hand. This resistance should not be given until the movement can be performed strongly and correctly, without help, ten times. When resistance is given, it should be smoothly graduated to the movement throughout, being great enough to make the muscle

work hard to perform the movement, but never great enough to stop it or make it jerky.

4. The patient should never be allowed to turn or twist his body in order to get the part to the desired position, since this will entail the use of muscles other than the ones it is desired to strengthen. If he is unable to do the movement correctly, the mother must guide the limb with her hands, being careful not to help unless it is necessary.

5. The exercises must be done every day to obtain benefit—in the morning, before the muscles become tired, is the best time. Each exercise should be done about five to ten times, with a stop to rest whenever the movement is done less well than the time before. Fatigue should be strenuously avoided and is to be judged better by the relative success in the performance of consecutive movements than by the expressed feelings of the patient. Weakened muscles may be tired by overactivity so that they cannot work as well, without the patient's being conscious of fatigue.

6. As a general rule, it is better not to give as exercises the movements which the child can do pretty well, for fear of producing a deformity from the pull of the stronger muscles, but instead to have him try to do the movement which he finds difficult. For instance, if a parent says that the child can pull the leg up but can't put it down, or can turn the foot out but can't turn it in, that child should have exercises of pushing the leg down and of turning the foot in, the mother being very careful not to allow him to do the stronger movements.

A physician selects exercises which are graded according to the amount of the deficiency of the muscle, and gradually increases the scope of the exercises to be performed as the weakened muscles straighten. No exercises of any kind are recommended for use during periods of active inflammation in this disease.

As an example of how a handicapped person can overcome his disability of this type, it is well to recall the story of Sir Walter Scott, who lived one hundred years ago. He was one of twelve children, the first six of whom all died in infancy. In the period in which he lived deaths among babies were frequent. Indeed, the infant mortality rate was in many places as high as four hundred per thousand, which means that two out of every five infants that were born died before they were one year of age. Today the rates vary from fifty to one hundred per thousand.

In fact, Scott himself almost succumbed because his parents employed for him a nurse who was tuberculous and who concealed this fact. Fortunately the famous professor of chemistry, Dr. Black, discovered it and notified the parents, who then dismissed the nurse. Even at that time the risk to the child of being nursed by a tuberculous woman was understood.

When Sir Walter Scott was eighteen months old his first serious illness overtook him. Apparently he suffered with the cutting of teeth and a fever. On the fourth day thereafter he was found to have lost the power of his right leg. His parents consulted every possible type of medical practitioner, both scientific and unscientific, and, all of this being without success, he was finally sent to the country to recuperate. This was, of course, an attack of infantile paralysis, not sufficient to cause death but sufficient to produce permanent crippling, for Sir Walter Scott was thereafter lame for the rest of his life. It was probably excellent advice to send the young boy to the country to recuperate.

As Scott himself said, "The impatience of a child soon inclined me to struggle with my infirmity, and I began by degrees to stand, to walk, and to run. Although the limb affected was much shrunk and contracted, my general health, which was of more importance, was much strengthened by being frequently in the open air, and, in a word, I who in a city had probably been condemned to hopeless and helpless decrepitude, was now a healthy, high-spirited, and my lameness apart, a sturdy child."

CHAPTER XI

Transmissible Diseases
MORRIS FISHBEIN, M.D.

TYPHOID FEVER

IF THE CASE RATES and death rates for typhoid fever that existed in 1890 prevailed today, the city of Chicago would have this year 60,000 cases of typhoid fever and approximately 6,000 deaths. Instead, the city of Chicago has had in recent years regularly less than 200 cases and seldom as many as 10 deaths. In Chicago from April 1, 1890, to April 1, 1892, there were 2,372 deaths from typhoid fever representing approximately 24,000 cases. Compare that figure with the population of that day to the great population of Chicago at present and the low incidence of typhoid. What a tremendous benefit modern scientific preventive medicine has been for all of mankind.

In an earlier day, the family doctor claimed that he could smell typhoid fever. His guess was likely to be accurate, since one out of five seriously sick people whom he saw was likely to have typhoid fever. There was a time when any doctor could definitely count on the financial returns from typhoid fever, and they were usually sufficient in amount to permit him to send all his children to college.

Typhoid fever is an acute infection caused by a germ known as the typhoid bacillus. The germ can be found in the blood of a person seriously sick with the disease, and in 80 per cent of the cases is found in the stools or excretions of the sick. The germ is spread from the sick person to those who are well by means of the excretions, by soiled food and clothing, particularly by contaminated water and milk, and to a large extent by people who carry the disease; that is to say, they themselves have been sick and have recovered, but they still have in their bodies germs which reside frequently in the intestinal tract and also in the gallbladder, and which may get out of those places and infect other people.

There was a time when cases of typhoid fever occurred from the use of ice made from water in polluted streams. Today the vast majority of ice used in this country is made artificially from clean water, and there is no danger of typhoid. Milk used to be a common source of typhoid germs; and milk products such as ice cream, butter, buttermilk, and cheese were also known on occasion to carry the germs. Once the eating of infected oysters was a prominent cause, because the oysters were developed in contaminated water. In fact, the best fattening grounds for oysters were known to be in and around sewers. Now the control of oyster breeding in uncontaminated water, and suitable methods of storage and transmission for oysters, have largely eliminated the shellfish as a source of contagion. Cases have been reported due to the eating of raw vegetables which had been fertilized

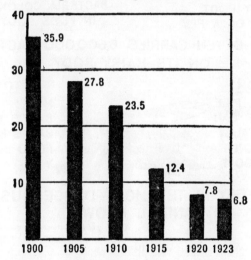

FIG. 35. Typhoid is in retreat in the Registration Area of the United States.

with contaminated materials or watered with contaminated water.

It was thought for a while that flies were more responsible for spreading typhoid fever than any other cause, but today it is not believed that transmission by flies is an important item. However, the fly does feed filthily and may transmit any condition associated with the filth on which it feeds.

Typhoid fever follows a long and serious course once a person becomes infected with it. After a person gets the germs in his body, from three to twenty-one days elapse, known as the incubation period, during which the germs develop and liberate their poisons. The average length of time is ten and a half days. The condition begins with the usual symptoms of infection, such as headache, pains in the body generally, a feeling of exhaustion and loss of appetite. Sometimes there are chills. Quite frequently there is nosebleed, and almost inva-

FLIES CARRY FILTH

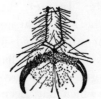

BECAUSE
BRED IN
FILTH

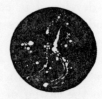

HAIRY FOOT
OF A FLY

BACTERIA COLONY
IN FLY'S FOOTPRINT

A FLY OFTEN CARRIES 6,600,000 BACTERIA
ON ITS HAIRY BODY

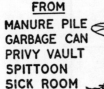 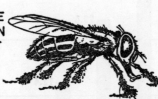

FROM
MANURE PILE
GARBAGE CAN
PRIVY VAULT
SPITTOON
SICK ROOM

TO
MILK
BABY'S LIPS
BABY'S BOTTLE
FOOD
YOU

A FLY IS THE MOST DANGEROUS
ANIMAL KNOWN

Courtesy of International Harvester Company.

Fig. 36.

riably there is disturbance of the action of the bowels in the form of constipation or diarrhea.

As the disease goes on, the person becomes sicker and sicker, developing occasionally not only a high fever with a stepladder rise, but also occasionally severe chills. There is a tendency for involvement of the blood vessels and the formation of clots. Rose spots appear on the skin at the end of the first week or at the beginning of the second week. In addition to the loss of appetite, there is a tendency to the formation of gas with bloating of the body; and sometimes, because of the ulcers in the bowels and the bloating, sudden severe hemorrhages from the bowel. Sometimes the infection and the poisoning affect the nervous system so that there is delirium and even the appearance of mental disturbance during the course of the disease.

The physician who examines a patient with typhoid fever makes his diagnosis from the history of the case and from the appearance of the symptoms, and also by careful studies of the blood. It is possible

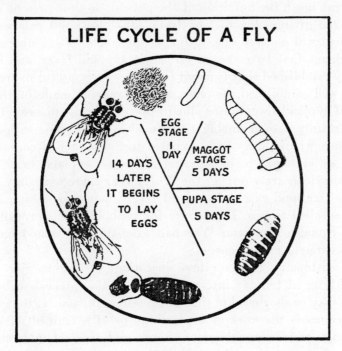

Fig. 37.

to examine specimens of the blood and to determine by the use of a test, called the Widal test, after the Frenchman who discovered it, whether or not the condition is quite certainly typhoid fever. Any serious complications such as hemorrhage, perforation of the bowel, and changes in the heart action and in the nervous system, demand prompt and careful attention by a competent physician.

A person who has typhoid fever must be kept alone and preferably cared for by an experienced nurse. The room should be screened if the condition occurs during the summer, when flies are a common pest. Because the person with typhoid is likely to remain long in bed he should have a bed with a firm mattress, and arrangements must be made to change the bed linen any time it is soiled. The patient must be bathed at least once a day and the back and buttocks kept clean in order to prevent secondary infections. It is also important to see that the mouth is kept clean and rinsed each time after food is taken.

There was a time when it was thought advisable to starve patients with typhoid fever. It is now known that the condition is so serious as to break down the nutrition of the patient, so that present methods involve the giving of a diet of from 3,000 to 3,500 calories. Then the patient will not lose weight during the course of the illness. There are no drugs that have special virtues in typhoid fever, and it is not certainly established that typhoid fever vaccine is useful in treatment.

It is well established, however, that a vaccine made of the killed germs of typhoid fever is of value in preventing the disease. This was quite certainly proved during the World War. Anyone with average intelligence who is likely to be exposed to the taking of contaminated food or water ought to be vaccinated against typhoid fever. In the entire American army during the World War there were only slightly over one thousand cases of typhoid fever among something like five million enrolled troops. If the rate for typhoid which prevailed during the Spanish-American War had existed, there would have been approximately a million cases.

It is customary to give three injections of the vaccine against typhoid fever at ten-day intervals, although the intervals between injections may be shortened in time of necessity. Obviously, the giving of such vaccines is the work of a physician or of a trained nurse, since the average person cannot inject himself and does not understand the technic of preparation. Only rarely indeed are there reactions of a serious character following the injection of ordinary doses of anti-typhoid vaccine.

It is reasonable to believe that persistent attention to water supplies and disposal of sewage, pasteurization of milk, education of the public in hygiene, and the control of typhoid carriers will eventually eliminate typhoid fever entirely throughout the civilized world. Means are now available in most states for proper control of carriers when they are discovered, but the discovery of a carrier demands expert bacteriological investigation.

The rates for typhoid fever have been falling steadily. Six deaths for each one hundred thousand population is not a great many. As was said before, the control of this condition represents one of the greatest accomplishments of preventive medicine.

Erysipelas

The condition called St. Anthony's fire is an acute inflammation of the skin caused by the streptococcus, an organism of the same type as that which causes scarlet fever and many other infections. Apparently, the condition was known in the time of the ancient Greeks and Romans. In fact, the greatest writers of those days, Hippocrates, Galen, and Celsus, all described this condition and credited it to living under unhygienic conditions. Finally, in 1882, a German investigator proved the specific character of the disease by isolating the germs and injecting them into animals.

Erysipelas occurs most often during the months from October to March, and in fact reaches its highest frequency in March. The disease is not so common in children as in persons between the ages of twenty and sixty. Men apparently have erysipelas more often than do women, perhaps because men are more frequently exposed to physical injuries and bad weather conditions during the winter months.

Erysipelas starts most often in a wound, abrasion, or rubbed place on the skin, and particularly in those places where the mucous membranes, such as those which line the nose and the mouth, join the outer skin. In hospitals, in the past, there were frequently epidemics of erysipelas because the infection was carried from one patient to another by attendants. Nowadays the great danger of erysipelas in a surgical ward has been recognized, and a person with erysipelas is promptly put in a room by himself and attended by a single individual who is not attending other people. In cases which occur in homes under ordinary conditions it is merely necessary to make certain that the other people in the family do not come in too close contact with the patient. The spread of this disease is almost always by the hands of the person who is taking care of the patient.

Erysipelas usually begins with a severe fever and a chill and associated with this all of the usual symptoms of an acute poisoning of the body such as headache, loss of appetite, vomiting, and, in the case of a high fever, perhaps some delirium.

The disease usually lasts from five to ten days, the average being eight days. When the erysipelas affects large areas of the body it may continue for as long as fifteen days.

Usually erysipelas begins on the face and extends from day to day, so that it eventually covers the entire side of the face, including the eyelids, which become enormously swollen and filled with fluid. Sometimes the swelling is sufficient to close the eye completely. Then the disease spreads onto the ear, which thickens tremendously, and finally reaches the line of the hair, where it stops abruptly. In other cases it may spread down the back. In many instances the condition begins on the bridge of the nose and spreads rapidly to each side so that it forms what is called a "butterfly" pattern.

Often any natural boundary such as the hair line, the nape of the neck, and places where the skin is tight over the cheek bones, will stop the spread of the disease.

When the inflammation of the skin stops, the fever begins to drop. Sometimes the skin peels where it has been greatly swollen. If the disease occurs again and again, almost a permanent thickening may develop, which is, of course, exceedingly unsightly.

The doctor is able to diagnose erysipelas certainly by studying its general character and also by examining the blood in which the white cells are found to have been increased tremendously.

The most serious complication in erysipelas is a secondary infection with germs that cause pus. Under such circumstances the swelling changes to abscess. These abscesses, if they occur in important areas, may even reach the brain or the spinal fluid and thereby bring about death. In the vast majority of cases, however, erysipelas is not a fatal disease. In young infants and in old and sickly people it may be exceedingly serious, but in general it causes a death rate per year of about three people for each hundred thousand in the community.

[Numerous remedies have been developed for the treatment of erysipelas, including the use of ultraviolet and X rays, antiseptics, antitoxins, and all sorts of chemicals, particularly the newer derivatives of sulfanilamide. Doctors used to attempt to control the disease by painting on iodine, silver nitrate, and similar preparations, but modern authorities feel that these accomplish little, and besides may so hide the spread of the disease as to interfere with its control. Sulfanilamide, sulfapyridine and sulfathiazole prevent the growth in the blood of the germs that cause erysipelas. These should be prescribed by the doctor. If the eyelids are involved, it is customary to drop some mild antiseptic solution, which the doctor will supply, directly into the eyes.—Ed.]

Dr. Konrad Birkhaug recommends the use of compresses soaked in an ice-cold solution of magnesium sulphate (or Epsom salts). If these cloths are kept cold and applied repeatedly, they offer great relief by lessening the tightness of the skin and diminishing the burning pain and swelling. This will not, however, stop the spread of the erysipelas.

In 1926, Dr. Birkhaug developed a specific antitoxin to be used in erysipelas. It is given in small dosage but, of course, can be given only by a physician. When this antitoxin is injected, there is usually a prompt improvement in the toxic depression, a lessening of the fever and a slowing of the rapid pulse rate within twelve to eighteen hours. Moreover, there is a quicker control of the spread of the swelling and infection of the skin. By this time thousands of cases have been treated with this antitoxin, and it is generally recognized as an important measure for the control of erysipelas. In the vast majority of the cases it is considered to be an exceedingly valuable measure.

Because erysipelas, like other infectious diseases, tends to break down the blood and weaken the patients generally, it is well to give people who are sick with erysipelas plenty of fluids, actually forcing them to drink not less than ten and as many as sixteen glasses of water daily. It is also well to have the food easy to digest and nourishing, in fact, what is ordinarily called a nutritious soft diet. There is danger in using too much cathartic because of irritation of the bowels during the presence of a serious infection.

A person who has once had erysipelas is likely to have it again and again. It is recommended that such people be exceedingly careful about picking the nose or scratching the ear. If these parts of the skin are exceedingly irritated, they should be kept covered with mild ointments or cold cream.

TETANUS OR LOCKJAW

The ancient Greeks knew about lockjaw. Indeed, the father of modern medicine, Hippocrates, described it and made some statements about the likelihood of recovery which are still good. It was not, however, until 1865 that it was thought to be infectious. The germ was not described until 1886. Today it is possible to isolate the germ, to grow it artificially, and to produce lockjaw in animals by injecting the germs into their bodies.

The poison produced by these germs is one of the most powerful poisons known. It is especially interesting to have all of this information when it is remembered that most people used to think that tetanus, or lockjaw, was always caused by scratching the skin with a rusty nail. Today it is known that the rusty nail produces the disease because it is contaminated with material containing the germ of tetanus.

When this germ gets into the body by any means whatever, it sets up inflammation of nerve tissue. Because these germs have a special predilection for certain nerves, the condition called lockjaw is produced.

It is now well established that certain types of wounds are more likely to cause tetanus than others. The most important are wounds which are deep, penetrating, lacerating, or crushing and which, because of that fact, permit particles of foreign matter containing the germs of tetanus to go deeply into the tissues and to remain there. This germ lives much better in the absence of oxygen. When it is pushed deep into a wound it is without oxygen and therefore is under the best possible conditions for its growth. The effects are produced more by the poisons produced by the germs than by the germs themselves. Indeed, it is believed that the poison, or toxin, is transported by the lymphatics and that in this way it reaches the nerve tissues.

The germs of tetanus seem to live preferably in the intestinal tracts of cattle, horses, and man. Because the germs are fairly widespread it is remarkable that the disease is not more common. Apparently, however, it is necessary for the germs to get deep into the tissue through a wound in order to multiply and produce the disease.

During the World War small epidemics of tetanus frequently broke out after battles because the soil was heavily contaminated owing to the rich fertilization.

In the United States somewhere around one thousand to thirteen hundred deaths occur each year from tetanus. The number is less now than formerly because of the disappearance of horses and manure from city streets, because of the diminution of Fourth of July accidents associated with explosives, and because of the use of new methods of prevention which were not formerly generally available.

Tetanus usually begins about seven days after the wound which permits the germs to get into the tissues. It may, however, come on somewhat later or, rather rarely, earlier. The first signs are a sense of drawing pain in a wound with the twitching of muscles near by; also the usual signs of infection such as irritability, headache, chilliness, and fever. Then comes the stiffness of the muscles of the jaw and neck which gives the disease its name.

It becomes more and more difficult to open the mouth, and finally the jaws may be clamped shut and the neck rigid. Attempts to open the mouth intensify the spasm. Due to the fact that the muscles of the face are contracted, the corners of the mouth are drawn back and the eyebrows raised. This gives the person a typical grinning appear-ance which is described by the scientists as *risus sardonicus*—in other words, a sardonic expression.

Eventually, of course, other muscles and nerves are involved so that there are serious spasms and convulsions. In fact, there may be from three to forty spasms in an hour. The whole body may be involved, in-cluding even the muscles of the bowels and of the bladder. Of course, when the heart and the breathing muscles are involved, the condition is fatal.

Even under the best of treatment, patients with lockjaw may die because of the potency of this poison. Much depends on the time at which the antitoxin is given and on the amount. Of greatest impor-tance is the prevention of lockjaw through the proper treatment of people who have been wounded, at the earliest possible moment. It should be taken for granted that a wound acquired in localities where the soil is likely to be contaminated, such as wounds acquired in fields, stables, and farmyards, or such as gunshot and powder wounds, are infected.

A physician who treats such a case will probably open the wound widely, removing any clothing, soil, or other visible contamination that may be present, and then treat the wound with proper anti-septics such as tincture of iodine or hydrogen peroxide to destroy the germs that can be reached. The opening of the wound is especially important, because this germ multiplies in the absence of air. Opening of the wound permits air to be present. It also permits removal of contamination, and it allows the antiseptics to reach the infectious material.

It is also important at this time to inject under the skin the specific antitoxin against tetanus, and perhaps to give another injection one week later.

If the disease develops in spite of preventive treatment, the patient should be placed in a quiet room, preferably in a hospital. The room must be kept darkened, and all noises or vibrations prevented, be-cause they may serve to stimulate spasms. It may be necessary even to use an anesthetic to prevent these spasms. In order to feed the patient it is sometimes necessary to pass a narrow tube through the nose and down into the stomach, because the jaws may be so tightly clamped as to make it impossible to get food into the body otherwise. Someone must be constantly with the patient to prevent injury from convulsions and to guard against sudden death from paralysis of the breathing.

In no condition is the constant and immediate attention of a competent physician, and at the same time good nursing, so important. This makes the difference frequently between life and death. The antitoxin which opposes the poison must be given early in the disease and in large doses. Because of the great irritability of the patient it is sometimes necessary to put him to sleep in order that the antitoxin may be given. Under the best of treatment it is possible to save the lives of from one half to two thirds of the people who are infected.

Rabies or Hydrophobia

The word *"rabies"* is Latin for madness. "Hydrophobia" means fear of water and thus defines what seemed to be the most significant symptom of the disease. Many ancient writers described this condition. It is one of the oldest of the diseases definitely classified by man. As early as 1804, long before the nature of the disease was discovered by Pasteur, it was known that the saliva of a person or of a dog that had the disease would transmit it. Since, however, no means was known for preventing its spread, sufferers at that time were sometimes put to death by strangulation or smothering because people so greatly feared the disease. Until the time when Pasteur made the great discovery which freed mankind from fear of hydrophobia it was customary, as a means of treatment, to burn with a redhot iron the flesh of a person who had been bitten by any mad animal.

There are some strange superstitions about hydrophobia still remaining. One is that it commonly occurs in the "dog days." It has been believed that the danger from mad dogs was greater at that time than at any other. There is no evidence to support this view, because the bites of mad dogs occur at any time. They are likely to be more frequent from April to September than from October to March because dogs run loose more often and more generally in the spring and summer than they do in winter.

When a mad dog bites another animal or a human being the disease is transmitted by the saliva, which contains the poisonous virus or germ. It is called a virus because it is so small that it will pass through the pores of a clay filter. The time when the disease attacks is from fourteen days on. The shorter the distance from the bite to the brain, other factors being equal, the shorter the period before the disease sets in. There are wide variations in the period of incubation, in fact from twelve days to twelve months, but in the vast majority of cases the onset follows the bite in from twenty to ninety days.

During this period of incubation the person may show only signs of restlessness and apprehension, sometimes of irritation or tingling and pain at the site of the bite. However, when the disease begins, the horrible symptoms which give it its name reach their peak. A slight huskiness of the voice and a sense of choking are followed by severe spasms of the muscles of swallowing and breathing. There is shortness of breath. So severe are the symptoms following any attempt to swallow that the affected person will refuse to take water. This, of course, gave rise to the name hydrophobia, or fear of water. Eventually the convulsions and spasms may affect almost the whole body, and the nervous system is so sensitive that the slamming of a door or a sudden draft of wind will bring on an attack. Finally, the spine may stiffen and bend and death result from paralysis of the apparatus of breathing.

Because the affected person or animal is unable to swallow, thick saliva accumulates and drips from the mouth. Because of the paralysis of the muscles of breathing the breath comes in harsh gasps. The person who is infected does not necessarily foam at the mouth or bark like a dog, but the nature of the symptoms is such as to give people this impression.

Because of the great danger associated with this disease, everything possible should be done to prevent its spread. At times when hydrophobia, or rabies, is prevalent in any community the lives of both dogs and children may be freed from menace by protecting them from exposure to the bite of a mad animal. Homeless animals should be picked up and disposed of by the usual methods. A failure to enforce the laws regulating the control of homeless animals represents nothing in the way of friendship for the animal and exposes innumerable human beings to the danger of one of the most serious of diseases.

The dog that is kept in a good home is usually watched carefully, kept from contact with savage dogs, and is not so likely to be involved as the one that runs free. However, any dog may suddenly bite a human being, under provocation or sometimes without provocation.

Because of the terrible possibilities of rabies, there is only one course to follow after a dog bite. The animal should be penned up or kept secured for at least ten days, during which time it will either die or develop the symptoms of hydrophobia, if it has that disease.

Far too often, when police are called to kill a dog suspected of hydrophobia, the dog is shot in the head or the head crushed with a club. This should not be done, because it is difficult for a laboratory to examine the brain of the dog when it is too severely injured.

The diagnosis of hydrophobia is made by examination of the brain of the animal under the microscope. When this disease is present the brain contains certain substances known as Negri bodies, which can be seen by the investigator. If there is the slightest suspicion that the dog which has bitten a person was mad, the Pasteur treatment for the prevention of hydrophobia should be begun immediately. If there are bites on the face or even on the hands it is wise to commence immediate treatment because of the short time which usually elapses when bites occur in these places. Otherwise it may be safe to delay for a few days to make sure that the animal was rabid or mad.

The wounds should be immediately cauterized with carbolic or fuming nitric acid. The Pasteur treatment is administered by any private or state laboratory. Moreover, it is available to physicians in any village or town through material that can be supplied by pharmaceutical houses. In the Pasteur treatment a special vaccine is used which is prepared from the spinal cords of rabbits that have been injected with the disease. In these spinal cords the virus has been attenuated by passage through many animals and by other treatment, such as drying. There are no contra-indications to the use of this treatment.

The success of the Pasteur treatment for preventing hydrophobia is almost certain. Failures occur in less than one half of one per cent of the cases in which it is used. Notwithstanding the fact that information concerning this disease has been widespread for many years, there are still more than one hundred deaths annually from the disease in the United States. These are preventable deaths. Once the disease has developed, the physician can do much to relieve suffering and should be in constant attendance for this purpose.

VINCENT'S ANGINA

In 1898 a French physician named Vincent described an infection of the mouth and throat due to a peculiar spiral organism. Apparently the disease occurred only in man, was accompanied by slight general disturbances with but a small increase in temperature, but there was pain on swallowing, enlargement of the glands, and a yellowish gray membrane in the mouth and throat. Because of this membrane, the disease was often mistaken for diphtheria until the differences were clearly established.

Sometimes the germs responsible for Vincent's angina were found in mouths that were not infected, but which were in bad condition. Occasionally also the disease appeared to be especially favored by fatigue, chill, exposure, improper food, or the excessive use of alcohol or tobacco. During the war the disease spread widely among the soldiers and was given the common name of trench mouth.

Many physicians are convinced that the disease is increasing in extent because of the general complexity of civilization. Much of the prevention of this disease lies in proper care of the mouth and of the general nutrition.

When the disease is once established, it may be controlled by the repeated use of solutions of hydrogen peroxide or by the application of a paste of sodium perborate, as the physician or dentist may advise. In severe cases internal treatment may be necessary, as well as the local application of drugs. For the prevention of the infection, it is also advisable to have the teeth clean and smooth and to discontinue tobacco in all forms as long as any evidence of the disease remains.

Undulant Fever

Years ago, British soldiers quartered on the island of Malta developed a disease in epidemic form which was called Malta fever. Later, as the disease spread about the world it became known as Mediterranean fever. Finally, it was called undulant fever because of its intermittent character; that is, the fever went up and down in waves.

The menace of undulant fever is not the menace of epidemics of yellow fever or even of influenza. It is a disease which insidiously creeps into a population and gradually affects increasing numbers of people. Fortunately, it is likely to spread slowly, if at all, in American communities, because milk is the most important medium in transmitting the disease. Since 1900, milk supplies in the United States have been controlled through suitable public health laws and measures. Milk is made safe for human consumption by pasteurization, in which the milk is heated for a sufficient length of time to destroy dangerous germs.

Before 1927, undulant fever was regarded as a curiosity when it occurred in a human being in the United States. Since that time cases have appeared in practically every state of the union. In the great majority of cases the taking of raw milk containing the germ, which is identified also as the one which causes contagious abortion of cattle, was demonstrated to be the source of the infection. Apparently the condition is more likely to be spread by goat's milk than by that from cattle, particularly since the goat's milk is not usually as well controlled in its assembling and distribution as is the milk of cows. Moreover, the infection is more generalized among goats than among cattle.

From ten to fifteen days after the person becomes infected with this disease he has the usual symptoms associated with an infectious disorder—weakness, tiredness, chilliness, loss of appetite, general aching, chills and fever. The condition develops slowly, so that frequently weeks may pass before the person who is infected considers himself sick enough to call a physician. He is inclined to believe that he has something like a persistent cold or rheumatic condition and that it is hard to break up.

Eventually, the symptoms of a person who has contracted undulant fever develop with sufficient fullness and persistence to make him realize that he is subject to a serious complaint. The physician who examines the blood of a patient with this disease finds that changes have taken place in the blood, and it is possible for a laboratory to make the kind of test that is made on the blood in typhoid fever and to determine with certainty that the patient is infected with undulant fever.

The disease resembles many other infectious diseases, such as typhoid, tuberculosis, malaria, or almost any other infectious disorder. In a few instances, perhaps two out of every one hundred cases, death may occur as a result of the seriousness of the infection or from secondary complications.

Of course, the way to avoid undulant fever is to avoid milk that has not been properly pasteurized. Men who work in packing houses where they come constantly in contact with infected animals should, of course, take the necessary precautions in their work. Men with wounds or abrasions on their hands should be certain to wear gloves and perhaps to clean their hands thoroughly at frequent intervals.

The real control of this disease will rest on the ability of government bureaus and of the veterinary industry to eliminate the condition from domestic animals.

The patient who has undulant fever must be handled in much the same way as one who has had typhoid. He must be put into a separate room; the health authorities must be notified; all of the excretions and secretions must be sterilized before they are disposed of in any way. This means either burning, boiling, or the use of proper antiseptic solutions. The patient, of course, must remain in bed and be properly fed to overcome the loss of weight, the anemia, and the weakness that are due to constant chills and fever. The wearing effects of such conditions on the body are extremely serious in producing changes in the nature of degeneration of important organs.

[Thus far no specific method of treatment has been discovered which will quite certainly overcome the infection with the germ of undulant fever. However, the new derivatives of sulfanilamide are reported to be useful in this condition. There is also a vaccine which is occasionally helpful. Artificial fever treatment is now especially recommended.— Ed.]

Amebiasis and Dysentery

Since the outbreak of amebic dysentery, from a source in two Chicago hotels, the whole country has become aware of this disorder, which was formerly considered a tropical disease. Instead of being caused by an ordinary germ, this condition is caused by a large type of organism known as the *entameba histolytica*. This organism gets into the large bowel, and once there sets up symptoms that are exceedingly serious. Moreover, the organism may spread to the liver particularly, or to other organs of the body, and there set up secondary places of infection which are also a menace to health and life. Although this condition was formerly unheard of in the northern portions of the United States, more recent evidence indicates that from five to ten per cent of all the people of this country are infected.

The organism which causes this disease multiplies in the bowel and gives off daughter cysts. These cysts are passed out of the body with the excretions, and if they reach food or drink in any way are naturally swallowed. They pass through the stomach and small intestines and then get into the upper portions of the large intestines. Here they divide up and multiply organisms which invade the walls of the bowels.

Ordinarily, the entameba histolytica which infects mankind comes in food or drink that has been contaminated in the manner suggested. After a person has had the disease and recovered, he may carry the organisms in his bowel for long periods of time, and as a carrier of the disease is constantly able to transmit it to other people. These carriers, who apparently are healthy or who have mild symptoms of the infection, are the ones most concerned in transmitting the disease.

Occasionally, however, the disease is transmitted by impure water supply. It has been shown that the cysts of the entameba histolytica may live for days and several weeks in water, depending on the temperature of the water and the number of bacteria in the water. It was thought in the past that these methods of transmission were of comparatively little importance in this country, except in the rural districts where people deposit their excretions on the soil, and where wells and springs are the chief sources of the water supply.

More recently, it has been found that any severe contamination of the water supply in a large building may result in the spread of amebic dysentery. This is what occurred in the Chicago outbreak. It occurred recently when an engineer permitted river water, ordinarily used to fill the boilers in a manufacturing plant, to get into the drinking water supply of that building.

In China and Japan human excretions are frequently used as fertilizing material for vegetables. This is a serious menace to health, because it has been shown that the cysts of this parasite will remain alive in the moist excretions for as long as two weeks, and when they contaminate the vegetables, they may in this way transmit the disease.

It has also been shown that it is possible for the fly, which feeds on excretions, to carry the organism and deposit it on food. The most common method of transmission of this disease, however, is through the contamination of food and drink by food handlers who happen to be carriers of the entameba histolytica. The food handlers concerned may be waiters, cooks, dish washers, or any other kitchen personnel in a family or in a large hotel.

Inasmuch as the organism may live in the intestines for months or years without producing serious symptoms, it is not possible to say just how long a time is required for infection to develop. However, there is some good evidence that the swallowing of the cysts of entameba histolytica is followed in from ten to ninety-five days, with an average period of 64.8 days, by the beginning of the symptoms which are characteristic in this disease. Usually the disease comes on suddenly, but most often it begins with mild diarrhea which gradually becomes worse. When the disease begins suddenly, there is severe abdominal pain with nausea and vomiting and a chilly sensation. The irritation of the bowel becomes acute, and the patient tries to evacuate the bowels repeatedly. This irritation may be so constant that the number of actions of the bowels will vary from six to eight in twenty-four hours to as many as thirty to forty actions of the bowels in twenty-four hours in severe cases.

As a result, the patient becomes exhausted, complains of aching in the back and great weakness in the legs, and is likely to be mentally depressed. There may be little or no fever; even in severe cases the temperature reaches at most from 100 to 102 degrees, but in very severe cases may go higher.

As a result of the extensive action of the bowels, such patients have tenderness in the abdomen, the skin appears sallow and jaundiced, and the patient loses weight rapidly. The doctor will want to examine the blood to find out how much the red cells of the blood have been injured and also whether or not there is any significant rise in the number of white blood cells. Frequently the distinction between this condition, appendicitis, and peritonitis will depend on a careful examination of the blood.

In times when amebic dysentery is prevalent and physicians are naturally on the lookout for it, they are likely to check up the cases. However, in the past physicians have not been particularly aware of this disease; certainly not in the northern parts of the United States. Since the diagnosis is made with certainty only after the excretions have been examined under the microscope in order to determine whether or not entameba histolytica is present, it is not safe to make a diagnosis until such a microscopic study has been made. At the same time, the man who makes the laboratory study must make certain that the ameba is the real entameba histolytica and not a form of the other amebas that live in the bowels without causing symptoms. He must also distinguish between the dysentery that is caused by the ameba and the dysentery which follows infection with some bacteria.

There are certain ways in which the community may protect itself against amebiasis. Much depends on having a properly guarded water supply, on the proper disposal of sewage, the protection of food from flies, and on suitable examinations and treatment of waiters, cooks, dish washers, and other food handlers in public eating places.

Chlorination of water will sterilize it so far as bacteria are concerned, but it takes one hundred times as much chlorine to kill the cysts of the entameba histolytica as it does to kill bacteria in water. In fact, the addition of this amount of chlorine to water would make the water unfit for drinking. Therefore, whenever water is heavily contaminated with entameba histolytica, the only way to make it safe is to boil it: obviously a difficult matter for any city water supply.

In controlling food handlers, it is necessary that they be examined at fairly frequent intervals, and that their excretions be examined in the laboratory to rule out the presence of the organism. Following the outbreak which occurred in Chicago, most large cities developed a series of rules regarding the examination of food handlers.

Fortunately, there are now available several methods of treatment which have been established as useful in controlling amebic dysentery. All of the remedies concerned are potent. Since they are powerful remedies, they are dangerous if taken in excessive dosage and should never be taken except under the advice and control of a physician. Among the remedies most commonly used today, and proved to be valuable, are chiniofon, carbarsone, and vioform. These remedies will control the entameba and eliminate it from the body. The drug called emetin, which is much used in this condition, is especially valuable in controlling the symptoms of the disease and is usually given early in order to bring about prompt recovery of the patient.

TULAREMIA

For the last thirty years market men have known about a condition called "rabbit fever." About 1907 certain cases were described in medical literature, and about 1911 other cases of the same type were described under the name of deer fly fever. Finally, in 1912, investigators of the United States Public Health Service found a plague-like disease among the squirrels in one of the counties of California and discovered that this disease was caused by a germ which they named in honor of Tulare County, Calif., the *bacterium tularense*. Finally, Francis, another investigator from the United States Public Health Service, found in 1919 that this germ which caused both the plague-like disease of rodents and deer fly fever could infect human beings with a condition which was named tularemia. Francis later examined the livers of a thousand rabbits offered for sale in the markets of Washington, D. C., and found at least one hundred seventy of these rabbits infected with the same germ.

While the disease caused by the bacterium tularense is not an especially serious disease, seventeen out of four hundred twenty people who had it died. The human being who becomes infected with this germ usually does so in the handling or dressing of rabbits sick with the disease. The rabbit sick with tularemia is not likely to be active. Health authorities warn particularly against eating rabbits that can be knocked over with a stick. If the rabbit gives a good chase and has to be shot with a gun he is probably not a sick rabbit.

The person who has tularemia develops swellings of the skin with the formation of abscesses, swelling of the lymph glands and nodules, and small spots of infection in the internal organs. The typical history of such a case is that the man in question or the woman in question dressed wild rabbits, that he or she had at the time a sore on the finger, and that shortly thereafter the sore developed into an ulcer; then the glands became involved, and finally other organs of the body.

Rabbit meat, even from rabbits infected with this condition, is harmless as a food if it is thoroughly cooked, since a temperature of 133 degrees F. will kill the germ. It is safer, however, for everyone who is dressing rabbits for use as food to wear rubber gloves during the process.

It has now been found that this condition can be transmitted from one animal to another, including the human being, by means of deer flies, wood ticks, rabbit ticks, and lice; and that such creatures as the sheep, the coyote, the cat, the quail, and the grouse may be infected, as well as rabbits and squirrels. However, as far as is known, the horse, cattle, dogs, and chickens have not been infected with this disease. In the Eastern states it is most likely to occur during November, December, and January.

Most people who become infected with tularemia have to go to bed from ten days to three weeks, and sometimes recovery is slow. There is no specific serum, nor any special treatment for the condition other than that which a competent physician can give by prescribing remedies to relieve pain and by controlling secondary abscesses. Sometimes it is necessary to put hot packs on the spots of infection and then to open the abscesses in order to relieve the pressure of the broken-down material. In this infectious condition, as in every other, it is wise to convalesce slowly, since any disease with considerable fever and infection throws a strain on the heart and the circulation.

MALARIA

Authorities in medicine have attributed the fall of the Roman and Greek civilizations to the development of malaria among the population. Certainly, a constant incidence of this disease will devitalize any individual.

Today enough is known about malaria to make it possible for any community that is willing to spend sufficient money to stamp out the disease. Because of this fact malaria is becoming less prevalent in the United States each year. It has been argued that a million people in the United States constantly suffer from malaria, but most authorities believe that this statement is an exaggeration. Local surveys indicate that the amount of sickness and the number of deaths from this disease are constantly falling.

The physician diagnoses malaria by the characteristic symptoms, which include regularly recurring attacks of chills and fever, the presence of an enlarged spleen, and the presence of the malarial parasite in the blood of the sick person.

The plasmodium, as the organism which causes malaria is called, was discovered by the famous scientist Laveran, who received the Nobel Prize for this discovery. Ross and Grassi, a British and an Italian investigator, proved that the organism of malaria is transmitted from one human being to another through the bite of the anopheles mosquito.

Although malaria has practically disappeared as one of the great medical problems in large cities, the disease is still to be found in many rural communities, particularly in the southern portions of the United States. Dr. J. Lyell Clarke, one of the sanitary engineers of the Illinois Department of Public Health, finds much work still necessary to stamp out the mosquito breeding places surrounding the villages of the southern part of that state.

In the hill territory of southern Illinois there were about three cases of malaria for every one hundred persons. In the river valleys and creek bottoms malaria was found to be highly endemic, averaging fifteen cases for every one hundred persons. The worst infection was always found in the immediate vicinity of some lake, pond, or marsh which could be the natural habitat of the malaria mosquito. The dis'

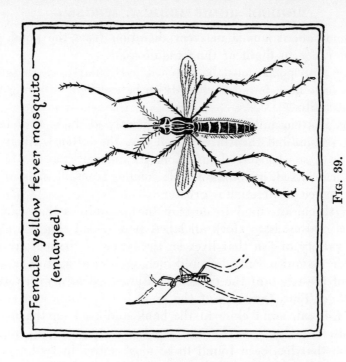

Female yellow fever mosquito
(enlarged)

FIG. 39.

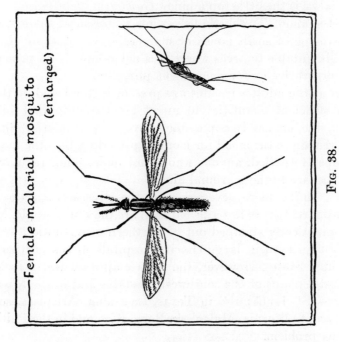

Female malarial mosquito
(enlarged)

FIG. 38.

293

trict extends about a mile in every direction from the pond, which marks the range of flight of the mosquitoes.

Country club ponds must be watched particularly, as these artificial pools have been found frequently to be excellent breeding places for the mosquito.

The malaria mosquito bites most frequently at dusk. If it has fed on a sick person and then bites a well one, the latter is likely to be supplied with some malarial infection. In summer resorts where the population is mixed, including people coming from all sorts of localities, the chance of infection is greater.

One of the means used to destroy the mosquitoes that carry the malaria organisms is to stock all lakes, ponds, and sluggish streams with the variety of fish that lives on the larvæ of the mosquito. The routine for mosquito control should include, according to Clarke, the clearing of the edges of the ponds of willows, cattails, water grasses, and floatage. Thus the bank of the pond is left sharp and clean, so that the fish can swim close to the bank and feed on the mosquito wiggletails.

The fish that has been found to be most active in feeding on the mosquito larvæ is the little top minnow *Gambusia affinis*, also called the pot-bellied minnow. This little fish swims in the most shallow waters.

The drainage of small ponds or marshes and the use of oil sprays are methods suitable to areas where it is not necessary to preserve the pond for decorative or for amusement purposes.

As long as the adult parasites are present in the blood of the individual in sufficient quantities to infect the mosquito that bites the individual, the person is a possible conveyor of malaria. Since the parasites remain in the blood for months, providing that the individual is not properly treated, anyone who is not undergoing regular treatment is a menace to those around him.

Children suffer more severely with the disease than do adults. Negroes apparently are less affected than are the white people. Malaria has been practically stamped out of northern communities, and cases are rarely seen even in large charity hospitals in the northern part of the United States. However, the disease appears fairly frequently on the coastal plains of the southwestern states and in the Mississippi Valley below St. Louis; also in Texas, Louisiana, Arkansas, southern Missouri, and California. Malaria in Porto Rico and in the Philippines is a serious problem.

In the more serious types of malaria not properly treated, anywhere from 10 to 30 per cent of the people die. The milder forms of the disease become chronic, and the fatality rate may be less than 5 per cent.

In controlling malaria, patients who are sick with the disease are protected from the bites of the mosquito. It has been established that the regular use of sufficient doses of quinine will control the condition. [Special forms of quinine, called plasmochin and atabrine, have recently been found to be most efficient, since they practically sterilize the blood of those who carry the adult sexual form of the parasite.—Ed.]

The real control of malaria comes through proper handling of the breeding places of the mosquitoes that carry the disease. Oil poured on the water that cannot be removed by draining or by other sanitary measures will prevent the development of the mosquito.

Rat–Bite Fever

When human beings are bitten by animals of the rodent type, including incidentally not only the rat but the weasel and the pig and occasionally, as will be seen later, even the cat, they are sometimes infected with a peculiar organism which produces a disease of the whole body. This disease is characterized by short attacks of fever alternating with periods without the fever, and also an eruption on the skin. Such cases have been known in the United States for a century, and medical journals have reported approximately one hundred.

The usual course of such a case is as follows: After the person has been bitten, the wound heals promptly unless a secondary infection occurs. From one to three weeks after the date on which the patient was bitten, the spot of the bite becomes red and swollen, and the person who is infected develops the usual symptoms of infections in general: namely, headache, general pains and fever, sometimes a chill and a general feeling of sickness. Finally an eruption appears, at first most prominent in the region of the wound, but later spreading over the body.

From this time on, attacks of fever will occur every five or six days, sometimes less frequently. Gradually the person loses weight and may become exceedingly sick due to the loss of nutrition and general health. Somewhere between 6 and 7 per cent of the people who are infected eventually die of the disorder, but the tendency is for the majority to recover.

There have been instances reported in medical periodicals of children who have been bitten by rats when left alone by their parents, particularly when they live in basement homes or poverty-stricken tenements. Of course, a cat may become contaminated through its hunting of the rats.

The doctor makes his diagnosis of this condition not only by the symptoms that have been mentioned, but also by finding the germ which causes the disease in the wound, and sometimes in material taken directly from lymph glands near the wound. There are also cases in which people have been bitten by rats and become infected, and with this organism but with the usual germs that cause infection, such as the staphylococcus and streptococcus.

Because the germ which causes this disease is of the same general type as the one which causes the major venereal disease, it is customary to treat the condition with salvarsan or arsphenamine or, as it was more popularly known, "606." This has been found to be specific in controlling this condition so that most patients are quite cured after two injections of this remedy.

ROCKY MOUNTAIN SPOTTED FEVER

As was shown years ago in investigations made by Dr. Theobald Smith, many diseases of man are transmitted by the bite of a tick. Among the most serious of these is the condition called Rocky Mountain spotted fever, an infectious disease seen frequently in eastern Idaho and the Bitter Root Valley of Montana, but also occurring in most western states and occasionally in eastern portions of the United States.

This condition, as is pointed out by Dr. George Blumer, occurs most commonly in men because of their occupations as surveyors, foresters, hunters, fishermen, sheep herders, or cowboys. These occupations expose them to the bite of the tick. If bitten, women and children are just as likely to become affected.

The tick is found on the rodents in the areas mentioned, and from these rodents picks up the organisms which it then transfers to man when it bites. From four to seven days after he is bitten, the man comes down with the disease. At first there are loss of appetite, general aches and pains, and slight fever. Then suddenly there is a chill followed by a high fever. This may reach 104 or 105 degrees. At first there are severe headache and backache with pains in the muscles.

Even the skin may be tender. Eventually the nervous system may be involved, with restlessness and lack of sleep and even disturbance of the action of the bowels.

About the third to the seventh day, the infected person breaks out with tiny pinkish spots which generally appear first on the wrists and ankles, and which give the disease its name—spotted fever. In serious cases the spots run together. Since they are due to blood, they gradually turn purple. The fever remains high for a week to ten days and, if recovery occurs, falls gradually. In the fatal cases death occurs from the seventh to the tenth day, with high fever.

The physician is able to make his diagnosis certain by examining the blood, in which he finds not only changes in the blood cells but also specific reactions which are certain evidence of the presence of the disease. This condition resembles the old typhus fever, or jail fever, as it was called, which is transmitted by the bite of a louse.

In some epidemics the condition is fairly mild, so that only 5 per cent of the patients die, but in one Montana epidemic 76 per cent of the patients died. Children apparently withstand infection with this condition much better than do grown people.

The obvious method of preventing this disease is to avoid the bite of the tick which causes it. This has been attempted in some places through eliminating rodents and through dipping cattle. As a method of prevention this has not, however, been extremely successful.

Investigators of the United States Public Health Service have developed a vaccine made of the ground-up bodies of the ticks. This is found to be a protection against infection with this disorder.

GLANDERS

Most farmers think of glanders as a disease affecting horses and mules, but occasionally it attacks human beings. It has been reported also in cats, rabbits, sheep, mice, and various wild animals of the cat tribe.

Because the disease is commonly transmitted by horses and affects horses more frequently than any other animal, it is now rarely seen in large cities, from which horses have practically disappeared.

In the first twenty years of the present century there were seven cases of glanders in the wards of the Bellevue Hospital, New York City, but in the last ten years, according to Dr. Douglas Symmers, not a single case has been seen.

Glanders is caused by a germ known as the bacillus of glanders. From three to five days after the germ gets into the body, the symptoms first appear. There are the usual symptoms of infection, such as nausea, headache, vomiting, chills, and some fever. Quite soon, however, nodules appear on the skin, associated with inflammation of the lymphatic ducts and glands near the places where the abscesses are located. Sometimes a hard nodule develops which ulcerates and breaks down, discharging a profuse, sticky substance. If the disease attacks the lungs it gives symptoms like those of pneumonia.

Nowadays, a diagnosis of glanders is hardly likely to be made unless the condition described happens to occur in someone who is constantly working around horses. The acute infection is very serious in the human being, and most of the patients die.

In the control of a disease like glanders, everything depends on stamping out the source of the infection in the animal which transmits it. Hence, it is recommended that practically every animal with glanders should be promptly destroyed and the stables thoroughly disinfected, including all harness and watering buckets. All animals that have been exposed should be examined for the infection and kept under observation until well past the time when there is any likelihood that the infection may develop in them.

A doctor who takes charge of such cases treats them usually by the surgical method of opening the abscesses and draining away the infectious material.

Psittacosis or Parrot Disease

In 1904, three cases of psittacosis or "parrot disease" were reported in Boston. In the fall of 1929 an outbreak of this disease was reported in Buenos Aires, and more outbreaks have since been reported in the United States. In Hamburg, Germany, twenty-eight cases, with five deaths, occurred in the fall of 1929. In the epidemic of psittacosis which occurred in Paris in 1892 there were forty-nine cases and sixteen deaths, and it was reported that the infection had been caused by parrots brought from South America.

When psittacosis occurs it begins with a chill and fever, with a good deal of weakness and depression, and usually some inflammation of the lungs. The extent of the inflammation of the lungs determines whether or not the patient will live.

When the records of a considerable number of cases are assembled it is found that from thirty to forty per cent of the patients die. When the disease was first described in Paris, a germ was isolated from the parrots, and it was found to be of the type of the same family as the typhoid germ. This germ is now called bacillus psittacosis.

"Parrot disease" is essentially a medical curiosity and need occasion little alarm among the people of the United States. The symptoms resemble those of other infectious diseases, and one should be certain that the disease is actually psittacosis and not pneumonia or other infection of the lungs.

Obviously, the first step is to get the suspected parrot and to find out whether or not he contains the germs which are responsible.

The United States government has prohibited the importation of South American parrots until we know more about the way in which parrots transmit to humans the disease called psittacosis.

The occurrence of this condition is another demonstration of the fact that we are likely to contract diseases from all sorts of contacts and that it is not safe to demonstrate too much fondness for our animal neighbors.

Psittacosis, as pointed out by Dr. T. G. Hull, has been known for a long time as a disease of parrots, but the first cases of pneumonic infection traced directly from parrots to man were described in 1879 in Germany. Similar conditions also occurred in 1882 and in 1886, and the first epidemic sufficient to attract attention occurred in Paris in 1892 and was traced definitely to parakeets imported from Buenos Aires.

The proof of the fact that human infection has come from the parrot depends on isolation of the germ from both the parrot and the affected human being. This was done in five human cases in one family in Florence, Italy, in 1895, and since that time in other cases throughout the world.

In parrots, psittacosis is highly fatal, killing from 50 to 95 per cent of the infected birds. The disease can be transmitted from one parrot to another by infected feathers, food, water, dishes, or the soiled hands of attendants. Mice or insects may carry the infection from one cage to another. When a parrot becomes infected it gets weak, loses its appetite, has diarrhea, and is likely to die in a few days. Then the germs will be found in practically all of its organs.

As might be expected, a disease that can pass from parrot to man may also infect chickens, rabbits, mice, and guinea-pigs. It is interesting that this disease which chiefly infects the intestinal tracts of birds strikes the lungs in man. In many instances the infection is due to the fact that the parrot is fed by the mouth-to-mouth method. Not infrequently, however, it occurs merely from handling the sick birds, and not infrequently the person in a family who becomes sick passes the disease on with infected hands to other members of the family.

Fortunately, this disease is rare in civilized communities, probably because parrots are not nearly so frequent as pets as are other animals and birds, and probably also because the disease kills the parrots so rapidly that the likelihood of infection is lessened.

The occurrence of cases of psittacosis in the United States is new evidence of the fact that methods of transportation, exchange of products among various nations, and the complete abolishing of boundary lines between peoples make it impossible any longer for a nation to be isolated. The disease of one people will sooner or late: appear among others.

Already cases of many of the tropical diseases have been found among the sick in the United States. It is probable that more and more cases are likely to appear in the future, notwithstanding the fact that the United States Public Health Service and all of the health organizations of various nations are concerning themselves with the prevention of such transmission.

Epidemic Encephalitis

No one knows when the first epidemic of lethargy associated with fever and destruction of brain tissue first afflicted mankind, but several observers have pointed out that Hippocrates, the famous father of modern scientific medicine, himself described an epidemic of this character which appeared in the spring and continued on into the autumn, at which time it was more fatal. It was suggested that there were similar epidemics in the sixteenth century in various parts of Europe. At the end of 1890, such an epidemic occurred in southern Europe and was described under the name of *nona*. However, the modern condition called epidemic encephalitis was described in Vienna in 1917, during the World War, and was given the name *encephalitis lethargica* because it is an inflammation of the brain associated with drowsiness and somnolence. The disease spread to England and to the United States and Canada; it seems possible, however, that there were individual cases in the United States before 1915.

Epidemic encephalitis occurs most frequently in February and March but may occur at any time of the year. Special attention is being paid to it in the newspapers of the United States at this time because of the case of Patricia Maguire of Oak Park, Ill., who has apparently been somnolent, or partially somnolent, for several years following infection with this disorder. The disease seems to have been more common in the United States and in Europe than on other continents. It is quite mildly contagious, but outbreaks have been reported in schools, asylums, and barracks in which large numbers of people are housed.

The cause of this condition is not known. There has been much research in an attempt to find a definite germ and a definite serum or vaccine based on the discovery of the germ. While much of this has been of interest and perhaps leads to the eventual solution of the problem, the exact organism has not yet been found.

In most cases of encephalitis the disease occurs in three stages: first, the beginning, which is sudden; second, a milder condition following the first acute condition; and, finally, a sort of chronic condition in those who recover. In the acute stage there are the usual symptoms of infection, such as fever, weakness, headache, and running of the nose, but in addition in these cases there are quite frequently double vision and emotional disturbances indicating that the brain has been affected. Most of the patients become lethargic or sleepy at the beginning of the disease and remain in this condition until the recovery from the acute stage has taken place. There are, however, other cases which actually have insomnia, and there are some who are lethargic in the daytime and awake at night.

While these patients seem to be completely unconscious, there are recorded instances in which the patient who apparently slept was aware of everything that went on in the room. The brain was affected in such a manner that the patient could not speak or let other people know that he heard what was being said. In association with the somnolence or lethargy in many of these cases there is a delirium in which the patient may have emotional outbursts, delusions, or periods of depression. An exceedingly interesting phenomenon is the development of what is called occupational delirium, in which the person who is affected dwells constantly on the occupation; the orator continually makes speeches, the teacher lectures, the accountant adds figures. Dr. W. B. Stewart has described the case of a child who became infected while studying in a French school. This child spoke French for three days and then became unconscious.

In association with the primary symptoms that have been mentioned there are many other symptoms indicating that the nervous system has been involved, such as paralyses, convulsions, tremors, and similar disorders.

After the patient has recovered from the first stage, which may have been slight—in fact, so slight as hardly to have had medical attention—comes the second stage of this disease, in which the patients are weak and say that they have been sick since an attack of influenza. They remember that they were drowsy, but they never feel well, and they are likely to be called neurasthenic or hysterical or simply plain lazy by their families. However, the condition is likely to go on to the time when anyone can realize that these patients are seriously sick, since they begin to develop symptoms like those of Parkinson's disease, or the shaking palsy. In this condition the face is mask-like, the arms and legs are held rigid, the movements are slow, the speech monotonous, and the thumb and forefinger move rather constantly in a pill-rolling movement.

In association with this there may be an apparent oversupply of saliva with some drooling from the mouth because of the changes in the muscles of the face.

There develop frequently in the later stages difficulties of behavior in children who tend to become moral imbeciles. These children are cruel, disobedient, destructive, abusive, rather filthy in their habits, and may actually become a menace from the point of view of their lack of sanity. Without a recognition of the disease which is involved such children are frequently brought before the courts and treated as criminals rather than as invalids. In the same way adults occasionally develop strange mental conditions following encephalitis and constitute a problem for those responsible for their care.

It should be borne in mind that none of these patients are actually sleeping over months or years, but that the mentality is seriously disturbed, and that the rhythm of sleep may be changed. They are not to be considered as curiosities for the delectation of the public, but as sick people entitled to a reasonable amount of privacy.

Unfortunately, scientific medicine has not yet developed any specific method of treatment that will prevent this disease or arrest its progress. It does, however, attempt to aid these patients by what is called symptomatic treatment, treating each of the symptoms as it develops by well established methods. A number of serums and vaccines have been tried. These patients have been injected with non-specific proteins in the form of typhoid vaccine; malaria germs have been injected to produce shock and artificial fever; and artificial heat has been tried, but thus far the results are quite inconclusive, and no one can say definitely that any of these methods of treatment actually stops the progress of this disorder.

During 1938 outbreaks of a form of sleeping sickness or unconsciousness called epidemic encephalitis broke out in North Dakota, Minnesota, Vermont and Massachusetts. In the same area at the same time there were numerous cases of a form of inflammation of the brain among horses called equine encephalomyelitis. The investigators proved that both conditions were caused by a virus of a certain type and that this virus is also to be found in a disease that affects the field mouse and other rodents, as well as partridges and pigeons. With an understanding of the nature of the disease which has thus been made available it only remains to find the chain of communication from the animals to man. Then it will be possible to prevent the further appearance of the disease among human beings.

[Quite recently another form of epidemic encephalitis has appeared in the United States, known as equine encephalomyelitis. This condition is apparently due to a virus and occurred, first on a large scale, in horses. Later it has been found that this condition could be transferred to human beings. Mediums of the transference may be the field mouse or other types of rodents. Investigators have found a serum which they believe may be useful, but the condition is still under careful investigation.—Ed.]

CHAPTER XII

The Respiratory Diseases
MORRIS FISHBEIN, M.D.

THE COMMON COLD

WHEN WILLIAM OSLER wrote his *Principles and Practice of Medicine,* the most popular textbook of medicine ever published, he began with typhoid fever, probably because typhoid was one of the most serious and incapacitating diseases affecting a vast number of people. Students learned to study diseases according to the way in which William Osler systematized knowledge of typhoid. Today typhoid is definitely under control and really disturbs but few people.

Now one of the most widely used textbooks of medicine begins with the common cold—and rightly. Infections of the nose, throat, and sinuses are responsible for more than one half the time lost by wage earners due to sickness. Everybody knows how to cure a cold, and, even if he does not, will tell *you.* You can put your feet in a mustard bath, drink several glasses of hot lemonade, carry a buckeye in your right rear pocket, wear an iron ring, indulge freely in many of the widely advertised remedies, and even take some of the beverages that once required a doctor's prescription and about which the government expressed considerable doubt as to curative value—and at the end of three days you will probably begin to get well almost regardless of the treatment.

The common cold is essentially a self-limited disease. Unfortunately, however, it does not, like an attack of measles or scarlet fever, induce in the person who has it a resistance or immunity which will prevent him from having a cold soon again. People who have colds seem to have them often. Those who are easily susceptible constitute about 23 per cent; they have colds four or more times a year. Sixty per cent of people have colds two or three times a year and 17 per cent once a year or not at all.

There is a great difference between the common cold and epidemic influenza of the type that devastated the world in 1918. That was a definite infectious disease, highly contagious, affecting vast numbers of people and causing a terrific number of deaths. The history of medicine shows that at least eight great pandemics of influenza had previously swept the world, beginning with one in 1580, the seventh occurring in 1889–1892. The common cold is something quite different.

CAUSES OF COLDS

Changes in the weather have been incriminated as a cause of colds from the time of Hippocrates. Geologists, geographists, physiographers, and biometricians have tried to find certain relationships between changes in the weather and the occurrence of colds; as a result, some definite knowledge is now available. Most colds occur in October; then comes a slight drop in the incidence, with a new peak in January and in February, working up to a rather high point in March; then another gradual drop with a low rate in summer, the rate rising gradually to the October maximum. From October to April, whenever the maximum temperature, the average temperature, or the dry bulb temperature falls below the ordinary figures, there is a slight tendency of the incidence of colds to rise. It has not been found, however, that there is any relationship between the maximum temperature, humidity, rainfall, wind velocity, sunshine, or atmospheric pressure. In the warm period, from April to October, whenever the maximum temperature, the average temperature range, the dry bulb temperature, the vapor pressure, or the percentage of sunshine falls below the ordinary level, there is likely to be a rise in the number of colds. Apparently there is a great deal in the general effect of atmosphere on the human being, but it is rather difficult to determine just how these effects are brought about.

Some time ago investigators in a large clinic proved that the ability of a person with rheumatism to predict a change in the weather is an actual ability, and that it is based on changes that take place in the body before the change in weather occurs. The opinion of at least twenty centuries that there is a definite relationship between sudden changes in the weather and catching cold tends to be borne out by modern scientific investigations but is not absolutely established. A professor of hygiene in the University of Amsterdam found a definite relationship between changes in temperature and the occurrence of the common cold in seven thousand people who kept a careful record of their colds while he kept a record of the weather. If it can be shown that difficulties with the heat regulation of the human body are fundamental to catching cold, the obvious way to prevent colds will be to develop methods for keeping the heat of the body constant.

The noted British physiologist, A. V. Hill, believes that cold weather brings about a large number of colds because people shut themselves up in warm, stuffy rooms and perspire; then submit themselves to the outdoor air without proper protection. The statistician for our largest insurance company found that a sudden drop of 10 degrees in the temperature brought an increase of eighteen colds per week among 6,700 employees in his office. Moreover, Prof. E. O. Jordan of the University of Chicago discovered that 90 per cent of colds occur at a time when there is less ventilation in both public and private dwellings. Here certainly is well established evidence that changes in the weather are associated with colds.

Everybody has experienced the development of a cold following a night in a sleeping car, a swim in the pool, or a shower bath immediately after being overheated by exercise. Investigators are convinced that the overheated and dehydrated air in the homes and in offices in the United States lowers the resistance of the membranes of the nose; then germs, which are almost constantly present among human beings, begin their work of infection.

There are several ways of emphasizing this fact. Extreme cold does not cause colds. Eskimos seldom have colds. A group of explorers found on visiting one Eskimo settlement that there was not one cold among the Eskimos from the tiniest infant to the most ancient patriarch of the tribe. Seventy-two hours after the expedition, which included several people who had colds, arrived in the settlement, practically every one of the Eskimos developed the characteristic symptoms. That ought to be sufficient proof that there is some transmissible agent which produces the infection. It correlates with the fact that germs do well on new soil.

Obviously, therefore, some search must be made for the germ cause of the common cold. When the germ cause is isolated, specific measures of prevention may follow. It is conceivable, indeed, that not one but several different germs may produce the symptoms.

Granted that the cold is caused by an infectious organism, there must apparently be other factors or all of us would have colds all the time. These factors constitute what are called predisposing causes. Tobacco, dust, gas, the amount of sleep, sitting in a draft, constipation, perspiration, and footwear have all been suggested as possible predisposing elements. A research made by investigators at Cornell University failed to incriminate definitely any one of them. Changes in the weight and quality of underwear that is worn have been suggested. Enough evidence is available to indicate that the wearing of woolen underwear is not a panacea; besides, it itches!

Experts in diseases of the nose and throat feel that obstruction in the nose and enlarged tonsils are important in relationship to the number of colds. Numerous studies recently made failed to prove that either one of them is a certain factor. Obstructions in the nose ought to be taken care of because they interfere with breathing and perhaps bring about congestion. Enlarged and infected tonsils are a menace to health and should be removed. But the person concerned may have just as many colds, if not more, after these factors are attended to than he had previously.

Our modern methods of living are probably largely responsible for the increased incidence of colds. We are crowded together in offices, in motion-picture houses, at football and basketball games. We are packed into elevators and subway cars. We breathe constantly, cough frequently, and sneeze unexpectedly in one another's faces. Moreover, our hands are constantly in contact with door knobs, pencils, dishes, and other utensils, also handled by other people. We carry our hands to our mouths and to our noses and thus transmit by what is called hand-to-mouth infection.

SYMPTOMS OF COLDS

Because of its symptoms and its rather poorly understood character in relationship to other diseases, the common cold is variously called by a number of high-sounding scientific titles, in most instances related to the part of the body particularly affected. What is known as a head cold is called coryza. Because of the increase in the temperature and the outpouring of fluid from the nose, the cold has been called acute catarrhal fever. Because the running is principally from the nose, it has been called acute catarrhal rhinitis. If the throat is hoarse, the portion affected may give the title to the disease so that it becomes acute pharyngitis, acute laryngitis, or acute tracheitis.

These anatomical designations nevertheless hardly convey the stuffiness, the chills, the irritability, the loss of appetite, and the other symptoms that are commonly associated with this disorder. The chief changes in the tissues involved are those which affect the mucous membranes of the nose and throat. The lining of the nose is red and swollen, and from it pours continuously the fluid that causes much sniffling and blowing. With the sniffling and blowing comes irritation of the skin around the nose and mouth, and, if the trouble extends down far enough, there is coughing without much discharge from the throat. The mouth is held open during sleep so that the tongue becomes thick and coated.

PREVENTION OF COLDS

What everyone wants to know is how to prevent a cold, how to stop a cold, and how to cure one. In every infection of the human body three factors are concerned: First, contact with the infecting substance; second, sufficient virulence in the infecting germ to overcome the resistance of the body, and third, sufficient resistance in the body to overcome the infecting germ.

The human family, particularly in large cities, is so crowded that it is practically impossible to avoid contact with those who have respiratory infections. Our modern apartment dwellings are simply great barracks into which families are packed, and individual dwellings are like cans into which the individual members of the family are crowded closely together.

If a single organism is responsible for the common cold, it may, of course, vary in virulence from time to time exactly as diphtheria, scarlet fever, and similar infections vary in their potency. However, what is called a variation in virulence may really be the reflection of lessening of resistance or the development of a new generation that has not the resistance of a previous generation. One conception of epidemic influenza emphasizes the fact that it occurs in cycles of some thirty years which permit the development of new generations of human beings not capable of resisting the infection. Since the germs are living organisms, it is conceivable that they may vary in their power from one occasion to another exactly as human beings vary.

Germs may be affected exactly as human beings are affected by the atmosphere in which they live, the soil on which they rest, the diet on which they thrive. The organism of the common cold may die readily on the surface of the skin but grow happily on a mucous membrane. It may die readily on a normal mucous membrane, but multiply exceedingly on a mucous membrane that has been vitiated by the continuous residence of its possessor in a hot, dry, stuffy, dusty room. Here then comes the question of proper ventilation as a factor in the onset and in the prevention of the common cold. Investigators from the United States Public Health Service studied various ventilation systems in their relationship to catching cold by children in seven schools in Connecticut. In three schools ventilation was controlled by windows, in three by fans, and in one by a special ventilating system. About thirty-six hundred pupils attended the schools. Records were kept of their absences, the daily temperature of the rooms, and the occurrence of coughs and colds among the children. The total number of absences on account of coughs and colds among the children in rooms with artificial ventilation was much larger than among those in rooms ventilated by the open-window method—indeed, almost twice as much. Of course, the children were in school only eight hours of the day. This need not be taken, therefore, as a general condemnation of all mechanical systems of air conditioning. Assembly rooms, theaters, motion-picture houses, and places seating great crowds of people simply cannot be properly ventilated by the open-window method. In general, however, authorities on ventilation are agreed that window ventilation provides the best system for changing the air and keeping it healthful.

The most serious problem is the question of proper heating and the provision of sufficient moisture in the air. Private homes should be heated to 68 or 70 degrees, and large halls to 60 or 65 degrees F. The large halls require less heat because human beings will provide from their own bodies enough extra heat to make up the deficiency. Equally important with heat is moisture. A sufficient amount of humidity prevents chilling. Moisture can be obtained either by special devices built into furnaces which are now widely advertised and which have been proved to be efficient, or by special electric devices which have been developed for moistening the air.

The common impression that chilling, dampness, and fatigue are predisposing factors in catching cold is, as has been shown, supported by much good scientific evidence. The theory is that chilling and dampness induce a cold through disturbing the heat-regulating mechanism of the body by sudden evaporation of moisture from the surface of the body. For example, one who is quite well may sit in front of an electric fan and get up after fifteen minutes with the nose congested and with all of the beginning symptoms of a cold. The draft from the electric fan brings about chilling of the surface of the body and disturbs the circulation of the blood in the mucous membranes of the nose.

Conditioning against colds has behind it the acceptance of many hygienic authorities. The technic of conditioning involves the building of resistance through proper hygiene and a few special measures directed specifically against the predisposing causes. One of these technics is the cold-bath technic. A cold shower is all right for anyone who wants it, provided he rubs himself thoroughly thereafter with towels so as to restore a brisk circulation to the congealed surface. The majority of people probably do better with a lukewarm bath taken primarily for purposes of cleanliness and only secondarily with the idea of benefiting resistance to disease.

There is also the conception that children may have their resistance increased by wrapping their throats and chests with towels wrung out of cold water. There is no good evidence in favor of this notion. Then there are the mothers who believe that they help the health of the child by baring to the wintry blasts the portion of the leg from the calf to the upper third of the thigh. It remains to be shown that any child had its resistance to colds increased by this exposure.

Certainly the biometricians have not credited such statistics as are available in favor of conditioning to cold by subjecting one's self unnecessarily to it. The reasoning in favor of the procedure is only symbolical, like the suggestion that the proper treatment of smallpox is to put the patient in a room with red velours hangings.

Germs in general succumb to sunlight. For human beings it is a pleasant measure. Hence the argument early advanced that exposure to the rays of the sun or to the rays of ultraviolet from the artificial sun lamp, using either the carbon arc or the quartz mercury vapor burner, would aid in building resistance to colds. The Council on Physical Therapy of the American Medical Association, after examining all of the evidence that could be offered in support of such measures, has withdrawn its approval from sources of ultraviolet that are advertised as beneficial in the prevention of colds. Perhaps the ultraviolet does enhance the power of the body in some generally beneficial way, but certainly it has not been proved that its effects are specific against respiratory diseases. Indeed, the exact words of the council are, "As far as normal persons are concerned, the claim that exposure to ultraviolet rays increases or improves the tone of the tissues or of the body as a whole, stimulates metabolism, or tends to prevent colds, has not been conclusively substantiated."

Vaccines Against Colds

Another measure of which much is heard in these advanced times, when people are beginning to understand medical progress and medical methods, is the use of the vaccine for the prevention of colds. The hoi-polloi refer to the use of vaccines or of any other substances administered by injection as "shots." Physicians build resistance against typhoid fever by injecting the patient with vaccine made of killed typhoid and paratyphoid germs. The injection of these killed germs stirs up the tissues of the body to resistance against the constituents of the typhoid organism. Some physicians inject mixtures of the killed bodies of germs frequently found in the noses and throats of people with colds, with the idea of building resistance to infection by these germs. There are two reasons, however, why many scientists do not approve the use of the "shots" in the cases of people with frequent colds. First, it has not been shown that any of these germs are specifically the cause of or definitely related to the colds; second, it has not been shown that the injection of these germs will stimulate resistance. If an attack of the cold itself does not produce immunity from a second attack, as does an attack of scarlet fever or measles or typhoid, there seems to be little reason why an injection of dead germs should produce such an immunity.

TREATMENT OF COLDS

First, everybody who knows advises rest in bed until the temperature is normal, with the head of the bed elevated in order to make breathing easier. Actually, only hygienists or people who are quite serious in medical affairs go to bed when they have a cold.

The skin is usually so uncomfortable that a sponge bath with water of a temperature about 98 degrees F. is desirable, and the skin may be fairly well rubbed with a rough towel after the bath. If the bowels are inactive, it is advisable to clear them of their digested and undigested contents. The clearing may be accomplished either by washing out from below or by the usual laxatives administered above.

Fever burns tissue. Hence the diet during a cold should consist of nourishing food. Since appetite is lost in most instances anyway, food should be appetizing and enjoyable. A child should not be forced to eat what is repulsive, particularly in the presence of disturbed appetite. Let the child have what it wants. Many physicians administer sugar and fruit juices with a view to providing calories and to preventing the acid reaction which is believed to be favorable to the persistence of the cold.

The common home remedies, such as bathing the feet in mustard baths, perspiring freely under hot blankets, drinking quantities of hot lemonade and orange juice, are time-tried helps to comfort. Of a similar character are the home remedies employed to lower fever and to diminish pain. Of this type is aspirin, a widely used home remedy. Any good aspirin will do, and fifteen or twenty different pharmaceutical houses now make it available. Aspirin, like every other remedy, is a two-edged sword, capable of damage when employed improperly as well as of good when given in proper dosage at the right time. A new remedy is a mixture of codeine and papaverine that must be prescribed by a doctor.

Diets for Colds

Then there is the specific diet. Rats which have had in their food an insufficient amount of vitamin A begin to develop a breakdown of the mucous membranes of the nose and throat. Rats that are fed sufficient amounts of vitamin A do not develop such changes. From this it has been argued that human beings who eat proper amounts of vitamin A or even excess amounts should be able to preserve the integrity of their mucous membranes and thereby avoid colds. Such experiments as have been done over short periods of time not only on chimpanzees but also on human beings do not support the idea strongly. These experiments, of course, cover but a few months, whereas the entire life of the rat is but ninety days, and a week in its life may be approximately equivalent to seven years of human existence. Whether or not excess vitamin A taken over a period of seven years eventually produces an immunity to colds remains to be studied and probably will not be. Human beings do not lend themselves readily to seven-year experiments. Even presidents get only four-year terms and eight seems to be the limit. Russia seems to be satisfied with a five-year plan.

Nose Sprays for Colds

A man with an eruption wants something to put on it. A man or woman with a running nose wants something to put in it. Hence the development of innumerable antiseptics, sprays, ointments, and lotions for administration in the common cold. There are drugs which dry up the secretions, but apparently that is not the road to cure. There are other drugs which increase the secretions, but the duration of the cold still seems to average three or four days. The experts in diseases of the nose and throat feel that the discomfort when too great should be relieved by one of the sprays which diminish secretions, and which include either the old adrenalin or the modern ephedrine. For years camphor-menthol solutions and preparations of oil, camphor, menthol, and eucalyptus have been used to give relief in nasal irritation. The actual worth of such preparations in curing the cold is doubtful. Their value in securing comfort is considerable.

GENERAL TREATMENT

When the chest seems tight, a mustard poultice is sometimes helpful. This may be bought ready made in the drug store. If it is to be made at home, a paste is made by mixing ordinary household mustard and flour stirred together with warm water as described in the package; it is then spread between two layers of thin muslin. This plaster is put over the upper chest of the patient until the skin becomes quite red. It usually requires from fifteen to thirty minutes.

When the cough is relieved, the discomfort in the chest usually becomes less. Many remedies are used to loosen the cough, most of them being what are called expectorant remedies, containing ammonium chloride. The dose of ammonium chloride usually prescribed is eight grains to each teaspoonful. This is given every two hours. The ammonium chloride is put up with some pleasant syrup. Sometimes sodium citrate, taken in ten-grain tablets mixed with lemonade or warm water, will help to loosen the cough. It is usually taken every three hours and has the double advantage of being alkaline and of stimulating the kidneys at the same time.

If, however, a patient is sick enough with a common cold to be disturbed about his cough or about any of the other symptoms, he should be in the hands of a doctor.

Most important in this condition is taking plenty of water. A person with a cold should take a half tumblerful every hour while awake. The water can be as is, or as lemonade or orangeade. If a more alkaline drink is desired, a little baking soda or sodium bicarbonate—usually about 10 grains—may be added to the lemonade.

There are lots of people who think they want a cathartic every time they have a cold, to clean out the system. Really the cathartic, when the cold begins, does not seem to make a great deal of difference. Sometimes it is so irritating as to induce a condition much more discomforting and worse than the cold itself.

SUMMER COLDS

Beyond the common cold there comes with the beginning of spring another type—the allergic cold, rose cold, summer cold, or hay-fever. The spring or rose cold is due to sensitivity to various protein substances derived in the spring primarily from the dandelion, the daisy, maple, and poplar, and also from various other pollens of weeds and grasses. The season and the nature of the sensitizing agent depend on the location in which the person lives and the kinds of grasses and flowers in his vicinity. The symptoms of onset are much the same as those of the common cold, but with most of the emphasis on the redness of the eyes and on the sneezing. That type of cold is a special condition prevented and treated by proper diagnosis and attempts at desensitization.

If you must blow your nose, be careful not to blow it in such a manner as to force the infected secretions from the nose through the eustachian tube into the ears. Always keep one nostril open as a safety valve. Be careful to protect yourself so as not to develop the secondary complications of bronchitis and pneumonia. The cold itself is not a fatal disorder. The complications of colds in the form of infected ears, bronchitis, pneumonia, cause long maladies and many fatalities. Try going to bed for a day, give yourself a fair chance, and get well soon!

PNEUMONIA

At those seasons, with increasing cold and exposure, and when epidemics of influenza strike in various parts of the country, the number of cases of pneumonia increases rapidly and also the number of deaths. Pneumonia today is the most serious acute disease which confronts the physician. The number of deaths varies from year to year, apparently related to the severity of the climatic conditions and also perhaps to changes in the nature of the germ that causes the disease.

This germ is known as the pneumococcus, a round germ which passes with the discharges from the mouth and nose of the infected person to others, and which may occasionally be carried by a healthful person who is not himself infected, and thus is distributed to others. There seems to be reason to believe that the overcrowding and the innumerable human contacts associated with modern life aid in the dissemination particularly of diseases of the mouth, nose, throat, and lungs.

It has been found that the germs causing pneumonia may be divided into thirty types. The germs of Types 1, 2, and 3, as they are called —which are classified according to the methods of bacteriology and immunology, not easily understandable by one untrained in these subjects—cause about 80 per cent of pneumonia. Type 4 causes about 20 per cent. Incidentally, the organisms of Type 4 are those found most frequently in the secretions in the mouths, noses, and throats of normal people.

Since normal persons may have the germs in their breathing tracts without having the disease, it is obvious that there may be factors related to the person himself which are concerned with the question of whether or not he will develop the disease. It has long been known that any factor which will break down the resistance of an individual will tend to cause him to become more easily infected.

A direct injury to the tissue of the lung, such as might occur from inhaling a poison gas, or such as might occur from inhaling some foreign body which would cause an irritation, will open the way for infection by the germ of pneumonia.

It is well known that the disease occurs in people of all ages but that it is rather rare during the first year of life. It is also very well established that the disease is much more serious during the earlier and later years of life than it is during the middle period. The rate of incidence and death is very high during infancy, decreasing up to the age of ten, and then very gradually increasing up to the age of forty, when it again begins to become exceedingly high.

For some reason pneumonia is much more serious in the colored race than in the white. It also follows frequently after such conditions as measles, smallpox, scarlet fever, and even after typhoid. There seems to be good evidence that exposure to severe fatigue, bad weather, and to malnutrition gives the germs of pneumonia greater opportunity to attack. For some years it has been believed that hard drinkers were more likely to suffer with pneumonia than others, but this has also been related to the fact that hard drinkers occasionally lie out in the open and are exposed to rain and freezing temperatures for long periods of time.

Modern evidence points to the fact that crowding is an important factor in the occurrence of pneumonia. The disease is more frequently found in the city than in the country and is probably more fatal in the city than in the country. The chance for infection from one person to another is much greater where people are crowded together. In trains, street cars, theaters, motion-picture houses, in tenements and under similar conditions, human beings come into contacts that are intimate for fairly long periods of time. Under such conditions germs pass directly from the mouth, nose, and throat of one to another.

When the germs of pneumonia attack the lung it becomes filled with blood, so that quite soon the person begins coughing and spitting material which contains the red streaks showing the presence of blood in the lung. This lung is, moreover, rather solid because of the presence of the material in it. The physician, therefore, fails to hear the air passing because of the obstruction in the air spaces. Moreover, when he thumps the chest over the lungs it gives forth the dull sound of a solid object rather than the resonant reverberation of one which is full of air.

After a period of time, depending on the severity of the condition, the lung begins to clear up, the breathing takes place with less difficulty. At the same time the fever goes down.

Pneumonia sometimes begins suddenly with a chill, pain in the chest, vomiting and coughing and difficulty in breathing. In other cases there may be fainting and weakness. In the serious stages of pneumonia the fever may vary from 104 to 106 degrees. Because of the difficulty in getting the blood through the lung there is great stress on the heart. Furthermore, the obstruction to the circulation causes the patient to develop a blue color which indicates that the blood passing through the lung is not receiving enough oxygen.

Most people know that the usual case of uncomplicated pneumonia lasts from a week to ten days and that it then may clear up by what is called a crisis; or more slowly by what physicians call lysis, or a gradual dissolving of the disease. In those cases that clear up by crisis the patient suddenly begins to get better and within a few hours is without high fever. He feels much better, his pulse is better, his breathing is slower, and in every way he is improved. Unfortunately, the majority of cases do not clear up in this manner. One expert reports that only about one sixth of all the cases seen recovered by crisis. In most instances the recovery is gradual. It is the belief that recovery is due to the fact that the blood of the patient has developed the power to overcome the germ of the disease.

In preventing pneumonia it is well to bear in mind again that contact with those who are infected is the chief source of its spread. Certainly, a baby should not be taken into a room in which someone is suffering from pneumonia. Mothers must do everything possible to prevent their children from coming in contact with other children who have running noses, coughs, colds, and sore throats. It is especially important to protect children against sharp falls in temperatures which, through centuries of experience, have been associated with the onset of fall and winter colds.

In some cities people with pneumonia are isolated, as with other serious infectious diseases. This has not yet been done on sufficiently large a scale to permit accurate estimation of the worth of the procedure, but there is reason to believe that its effect may be definitely for good.

The person attending a patient with pneumonia should wear a clean gown which is changed before contact with other people. The hands should be thoroughly cleaned with soap and water after attending the patient. The room of the patient should be kept as clean as possible and thoroughly aired, washed, and sunned after the patient's recovery.

When a person is isolated for an infectious disease the utensils, bedclothing, personal clothing, handkerchiefs, and other material in close contact with him should be sterilized. They should be kept separate from similar materials used by other members of the family.

It is recognized by physicians that one of the most important steps in the care of the patient with pneumonia is to keep him as quiet as possible, both mentally and physically, and to give him the best possible nursing care. It is believed by many physicians that the difference between good and bad nursing may mean the difference between life and death.

Because of the importance of proper care and nursing in such a case, most physicians feel that a patient with pneumonia is better off in a hospital than at home. Moreover, it is better to get the patient under good care early and not to wait until he has reached a critical stage before transferring him to a hospital. "By this time," says Dr. Rufus Cole, "it is usually too late, and any extra care possible in the hospital is more than offset by the injury done the patient by the excitement and effort of the change."

The patient with pneumonia should have a large, well-ventilated room with plenty of access to good fresh air. This does not mean that a patient with pneumonia is to be exposed to storm and stress. In inclement weather it is much better to prevent such additional exposure. The patient himself is frequently the best judge as to when he is breathing with most ease and least distress.

The number of visitors must be kept to a minimum. The patient should not have to worry about troubles in the family or business affairs and must be kept flat on his back for at least a week after recovery has begun. Only gradually is he allowed to assume a sitting posture.

The diet in this condition, as in any serious infection, must be chiefly liquids such as soups, gruels, milk, and soft-boiled eggs. Occasionally it is well to add milk sugar to keep up the energy. Rest and quiet are more important even than nourishment in the serious stages of pneumonia. When recovery has begun, feeding is gradually extended so as to aid the improvement of the blood and the broken-down tissues.

It is well for patients with pneumonia to have plenty of water. This does not mean, however, much more than two to three quarts a day. The patient will not drink unless the water is given to him when he is quite sick. Under such circumstances it is perhaps best to give water with a teaspoon, giving small amounts frequently, or to have the patient suck small pieces of ice.

Of greatest importance in the treatment of pneumonia is the care of a competent physician. He himself must direct the nursing and determine its value. He himself must administer proper remedies at the proper time in order to support the extra work of the heart, in order to relieve stress from the circulation, in order to permit the patient to sleep, and in order to control the actions of the bowels, the skin, and of all the other organs. There is no substitute of any kind for the type of care that a well-trained physician can give in this disease.

The use of oxygen in the treatment of pneumonia has been elaborated of late and is found to be exceedingly valuable. Tents have been developed which may be placed over the patients as they lie in bed, and many large hospitals have oxygen rooms into which the entire bed may be moved and in which the nurse may remain and attend the patient. Oxygen is not to be considered an emergency measure to be applied when the patient is at the point of death, but instead one which is to be used promptly when the physician feels that it is required.

In its attack on pneumonia medicine has, of late, developed specific serums which are shown definitely to attack the organisms causing the disease and to overcome their toxins. The physician in attendance must be responsible for selecting the serum suitable to the case concerned. This he does most efficiently when he is able to determine promptly the type of organism causing the disease. This typing is done in the laboratory of the hospital or in other laboratories where materials are available for the purpose. In many institutions, as, for example, the hospital of the Rockefeller Institute, where the serums are used under properly controlled conditions, there seems to be good evidence that they are valuable in lowering the number of fatal cases.

[Most recent in the control of pneumonia is the use of sulfapyridine. With this product, during 1939, the death rate from this disease was reduced by at least 25 per cent. The patient is given immediately large doses, approximately four grams of this remedy, and later one gram every four hours. This method is now so well established that it will be routine in the care of patients in the military services, along with the use of oxygen and antiserums.—Ed.]

TUBERCULOSIS

The protection of mankind against tuberculosis is based on two principles which were formulated by the famous Pasteur and Robert Koch. The first is to preserve the child against infection with the germ of tuberculosis by removing it from contaminated surroundings; the second is the isolation of the sick and the education of the sick in the prevention of the disease.

Tuberculosis is a social disease in the sense that it affects groups of mankind as well as individuals. Second, it is involved with the economic status of those who are infected. For example, in Vienna in 1913 deaths from tuberculosis were five times higher in the poorer quarters than in the better class quarters.

Tuberculosis attacks all races, all ages of mankind, and indeed all classes of human society, but it is largely a disease of poverty and malnutrition. All of the available evidence indicates that the number of deaths from tuberculosis per hundred thousand of population is steadily decreasing throughout the world. There seems to be some question as to just why this trend has taken place. The decline in the death rate from tuberculosis began long before the era of bacteriologic discoveries and of modern hygiene based on such discoveries. The reason may be not only a change that has taken place in the germ of tuberculosis, but probably also a change has taken place in the nature of man.

The death rate drops among people who have had tuberculosis for many decades. The death rate rises when tuberculosis comes into a country area or into a district in which the population has previously been relatively free from tuberculosis. There seems to be evidence that the coming of the industrial era with crowding and long hours of labor produced a higher death rate for this disease. Then came the protection of labor, particularly of child labor, social hygiene, improved nutrition and improved housing, with a lowering of the rates for tuberculosis.

With the truly extensive knowledge of tuberculosis which we have, its complete prevention ultimately should be a possibility. However, perfect success in a problem of this kind is not likely in a day, a month, or even a generation.

The path to prevention seems to be clear. Young children must not be exposed to infection, or, in any event, the possibility of infection in young children must be reduced to a minimum.

Let us consider what this means in our modern civilization. Human contacts have been multiplied enormously. Today the home has largely disappeared in our great cities; instead, we have the apartment house, housing from three to fifty families. Obviously under such circumstances children are exposed not only to their own parents and relatives, but to vast numbers of other children and other families.

The child of an earlier day played in its own backyard at least until the age of six. Today it goes early to nursery school and thereafter to kindergarten. Moreover, human beings now assemble in crowds of thousands in motion-picture houses and of tens and hundreds of thousands at baseball and football games.

It is easy enough to suggest that young children be not admitted to the presence of known consumptives. It is far more difficult to establish the principle that they be kept out of all gatherings where they may be exposed to infection from unknown sources.

There are, of course, still some differences of opinion as to the proper procedure for eliminating tuberculosis. We are not at this time prepared to isolate all carriers of the germs of this disease or to exterminate them. The fact is emphasized when it is realized that practically everyone has had the disease by the time he is fifteen. Were this not the case, the mortality among adults would be terrific. The earlier infection establishes a resistance against the severe infection of later years.

The only regions in the world thus far free from tuberculosis are those in which primitive savages live completely away from all human civilization.

The savage and barbarian races of Central Africa and Asia have no tuberculosis until white people bring it to them. The tuberculin test applied to one group of natives in the interior of Africa brought only 20 per cent of positive results, and in one village far inland only 2 per cent reacted. The danger to such native races on first admixture with the whites is tremendous.

The Negroes in the crowded districts in northern cities have the highest tuberculosis rate of any group in the community. The Mexican population of Chicago has eleven times the average rate of the rest of the population.

The attack on tuberculosis has been thus far an economic attack. Realizing that it is primarily a disease associated with bad hygiene, great importance has been placed on physical well being.

The treatment consisted largely of good diet, sufficient rest and fresh air. Special attention was paid to housing and types of employment, to the prices of food and wages, since it has been shown that a drop in wages is usually related to an increase in tuberculosis.

In the United States the number of beds available for patients with this disease increased from 10,000 in 1904 to 60,000 in 1932. Moreover, there has been a tremendous growth in open-air schools, preventoriums, clinics, and dispensaries.

An investigation made by Linsly Williams and Kendall Emerson revealed, however, that only 17 per cent of patients in sanatoriums are in the early stages of the disease, and that 97 per cent of patients who come to physicians have symptoms that are severe. In other words, they come as people sick with tuberculosis rather than for the prevention of tuberculosis.

If the vast majority of people were to be examined regularly, much more tuberculosis could be detected in the earliest stages, better hygiene could be practised, and the rate thereby could be greatly reduced. Nevertheless, the complete control of the disease will not come from such procedures, except over a long period of time.

It was possible to stamp out yellow fever just as soon as it became apparent that the disease was transmitted by the mosquito, even though the exact organism of the disease was not known.

In tuberculosis, we know the cause of the disease: namely, the germ of bacillus of tuberculosis. We know the method of transmission, which is from the patient with the disease to the person who does not have it, particularly the child, and occasionally through infected milk and food.

We know that the disease could be prevented by complete isolation or extermination of those who have it, but we cannot apply such procedures on a suitable scale, simply because social conditions do not permit the application of such stringent procedures.

The attack on tuberculosis has, therefore, in recent years continued along the lines of hygiene and epidemiology, but has, at the same time, been expanded into other methods that seem more likely to offer possibilities for a dramatic extermination of the disease in a single generation.

There are companies in New York which specialize in raising money for needy educational and philanthropic institutions. These specialists first locate some individual with sufficient money to give part of it away—a task not so difficult in 1929—but considerable of an effort in 1935.

Then they make a study of the history, the desires, and the habits of the person concerned. They find out the day of his birth, the number of persons in his family, the dates of any deaths that may have occurred. They look into the type of car that he drives, his favorite amusements, and indeed everything that can be known concerning him.

They then take advantage of every one of his little weaknesses in their solicitation of funds. He is likely to be asked for money on his birthday; he is likely to be asked for a donation to commemorate the life of his favorite relations. He is provided with occasions that will put him into a genial humor and then solicited for his contributions while in a "giving" mood.

It is somewhat similar to the type of study the scientists are now making of the germ of tuberculosis. They are looking into the natural history of this extraordinary bug. They are taking it apart and studying it chemically. They are finding out what it will do under various circumstances and in various environments.

They are breeding it into numerous generations, and they are studying the effects on these various generations of different types of diet and air and similar conditions. They are studying not only the effects of the germ as a whole, but the effects of its protein, its fat and its sugars.

Obviously this type of study must yield information of great value in controlling the growth and development of the germ in relationship to human disease.

The next step has been to determine the way in which the germ gets into the body, and then what happens to it after it is in the human body. Once in the tissue of the lung, the germ produces definite changes. It has been found that its growth and the progress of these changes can be prevented by various procedures which will put the lung at rest.

These procedures involve not only actual rest of the entire individual in bed, but specific rest of the lung brought about by the weight of sandbags applied to various portions of the body, and the use of pneumothorax, which is the injection of air around the lung forcing it to collapse.

They involve also the use of various surgical procedures, which bring about a complete and permanent collapse of the diseased lung, and finally the cutting of nerves which control the movements of the diaphragm and thereby bring about rest of the lung.

The mechanical methods of treating tuberculosis are, of course, aided by the use of suitable preparations for inducing rest, as well as by attempts to attack the germ and its effects with drugs, in the same way that arsphenamine attacks the germ of syphilis or that diphtheria antitoxin attacks the poisons of that disease.

MEDICAL TREATMENT OF TUBERCULOSIS

Out of this type of research came such preparations as sanocrysin, the gold cure; cyancuprol, the copper cyanourate-potassium cyanide cure; and the biologic preparations known as the Dreyer antigen, the Spahlinger vaccine and the Calmette inoculations or B. C. G. Some of these already have been abandoned; the value of the others is doubtful or at best unestablished.

With every discovery in the field of science, medicine has gained. The development of the microscope, of artificial ultraviolet rays, of the X-ray, of various drugs and anesthetics, has come in fields correlated with medicine and has been applied to the benefit of the human being.

It is quite conceivable that progress in the control of tuberculosis may depend not only on discoveries made in the field of medicine as such, but also on discoveries made in allied fields.

The chemists, the physicists, the bacteriologists, the workers in the field of plant and animal husbandry are all engaged in research which may, in the end, lead to the type of dramatic control of tuberculosis that has been mentioned. In the meantime, there is plenty for idle hands to do.

DIET IN TUBERCULOSIS

There seems to be no doubt but what the diet, particularly the diet of invalids, has long been important in the treatment of tuberculosis. The incidence of tuberculosis is closely related to the general level of civilization. Some people simply do not get enough food. Many people are badly fed because they do not know how to select the right foods and to make the best use of what food they have. There seems to be not the slightest question but that malnutrition has an extremely unfavorable effect on the death rate from tuberculosis. In England, associated with the war and the post-war period, the increase in the tuberculosis death rate was 13 per cent, in Germany and Austria the figure associated with malnutrition increased by 70 per cent. In France the tuberculosis death rate in 1916 for persons under nineteen years of age was double that of 1912. Incidentally, in 1916, the ration was greatly reduced to a bare maintenance diet in the section of France studied, and there was a complete dearth of milk and an almost complete dearth of suitable protein.

Human beings may contract and transmit tuberculosis at all ages. Young people are more particularly susceptible than are older ones. The two most dangerous periods are early infancy and adolescence. The charts of deaths from tuberculosis show a high peak in earliest

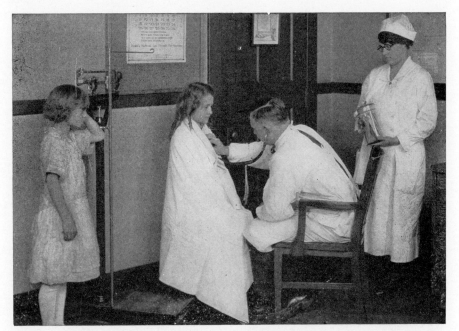

Fig. 40.   Chest examinations of suspected tuberculous children.

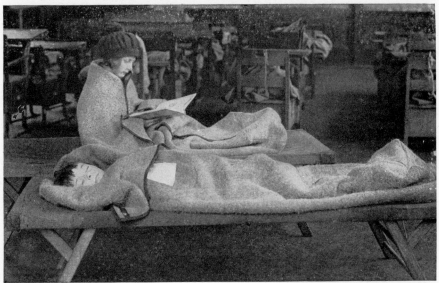

Fig. 41.   Children suitably dressed for outdoor study and sleep.

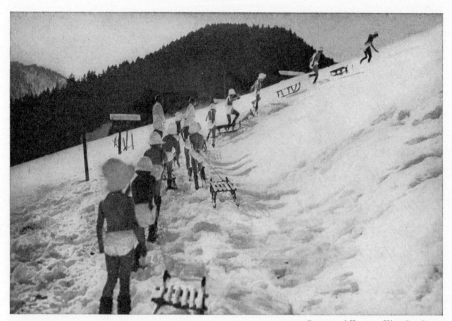

FIG. 42.   Outdoor sun bath.

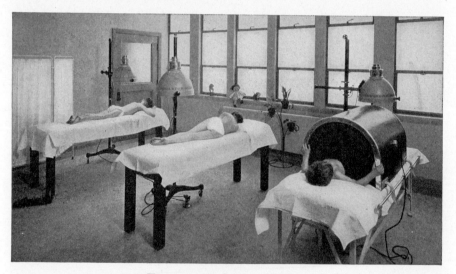

FIG. 43.   Indoor sun bath.

infancy, then a definite drop in the rate during later infancy and school age, and a rise at the beginning of adolescence. This points definitely to the periods when children must be most closely watched for the development of symptoms and when everything possible must be done to keep up their nutrition and to see to it that they have plenty of rest and good hygiene.

CONTROL OF TUBERCULOUS CATTLE

Of special importance in the prevention of tuberculosis is the control of tuberculous cattle. The germ of tuberculosis of the type which lives in cattle is rather rare as a cause of tuberculosis of the abdomen, the glands, the bones, and the joints. There are certain methods for controlling tuberculosis in cattle which are now subject to legislation in this country.

In the first place, milk for children, unless coming from cattle free from tuberculosis, must invariably be pasteurized, and in fact it is probably better to pasteurize all milk for children—at least there is more certainty of safety. Second, it is desirable to stamp out tuberculosis among cattle. This is commonly done by testing cattle for the presence of the disease and then destroying all that are infected, at the same time compensating the owners for the loss of the animals.

CLIMATE IN PREVENTION AND TREATMENT OF TUBERCULOSIS

It is generally recognized that while it is possible for a person to recover from tuberculosis in almost any climate, climatic factors nevertheless play a considerable part in the speed of the recovery.

In considering climate one is concerned not only with temperature and humidity, but also with wind, dust, and storms, with rain, the character of the soil, the sunshine, and many other factors.

Heat or cold in great excess are dangerous to health and may be fatal to life. The effects of temperature on the body are dependent to a great degree on humidity.

Warm moist climates are generally believed to have a depressing effect. Cold, dry air is stimulating, but as pointed out by Dr. James A. Miller, demands a capacity for response from the individual.

If the body is not able to respond properly to cold, dry air, as is the case with persons who have been greatly weakened by long continued illness or by old age, the effects of cold, dry air may be harmful.

Excessive moisture has a relaxing effect which may predispose to

infection. The movement of the air materially influences the temperature and the humidity.

If the air is hot and moist, movement of the air will aid in elimination of heat. If the air is very cold, there will be an increased demand
for heat produced from the body. If the air is both moist and cold, conditions are extremely uncomfortable and may be harmful.

In selecting a climate for the invalid, Dr. Miller suggests that there
is no one best climate for tuberculosis. In other words, proper treatment under scientific conditions is more important than climate alone.

Some types of patients never should be moved in search of climate.
This includes patients who are severely ill in the early stages of the
disease or in the late stage of the disease. In such cases, complete rest
in bed either at home or in an institution in the home city is the first
step in treatment and should be continued until the patient is able
to travel without risk.

Not long ago the United States government, through the Public
Health Service, protes'ed against the shipping of patients to certain
states when such patie.ts did not have the means to provide for the
necessities of life after their travel.

The cost of invalid care almost anywhere is from $25 to $50 per
week. Therefore, at least $1,200 to $1,800 per year must be available
for the care of the invalid if he is to go to any health resort.

When the burden of providing for one's self in a strange land is
added to those of the disease itself, the invalid has a handicap to overcome which may result in the difference between life and death. Good
food and lodging are just as necessary as plenty of sunlight and fresh
air.

The satisfaction of the patient's mind is of the utmost importance.
A mother will not get well if she is constantly worried about the condition of the children that she has left at home.

A business man will not recover as well in a strange climate as at
home if he is constantly worried about his business. It is for this reason
that many institutions have grown up near all of the large cities in our
country.

The routine of treatment in such instances is of greater advantage
than any possible advantages to be derived from climate. The biggest
advantage of an institution is the fact that the patient can be educated in the proper routine of life leading to recovery.

The second reason for treating a patient in an institution rather than at home is the advantage of a change. As pointed out by Dr. James Alexander Miller in his complete consideration of the subject in the *American Review of Tuberculosis*, healthy people, when tired, experience a tremendous improvement in their general physical and mental tone by a complete change of environment.

This is all the more true of those with tuberculosis. People who live in apartments or tenement houses frequently do better merely by transfer to a day camp near the seashore or in the country.

The advantages of open-air life and open-air sleeping are now recognized by common experience. These increase the general tone of the body, quiet the nervous system, and favor relaxation and sleep.

Dr. Miller made a complete survey of various resorts for the care of the tuberculous in this country, as a result of which he has drawn up certain definite conclusions relative to the importance of climate in this disease.

The eminent authority in tuberculosis, Dr. Francis Trudeau, once said that patients with that disease did well in the desert, upon the mountain, or in the middle of the ocean.

However, perpetual sunshine will not prevent tuberculosis, and excessive sunshine is exceedingly irksome to many people.

In order to establish the current view of this problem, Dr. James Alexander Miller surveyed the available medical literature and studied the records of patients in various portions of the United States.

As a result of his study he has drawn certain conclusions which should be borne in mind by every person with tuberculosis who may contemplate a change of climate.

Here they are:

1. The regimen of regulated rest and exercise, proper food and open-air life, is the fundamental essential in the treatment of tuberculosis. Suitable climatic environment makes this open-air life more easy, enjoyable, and beneficial.

2. When these essentials are assured, a change of climate is of definite value in a considerable number, probably the majority, of cases, but with the proper regimen many cases will do well in any climate.

3. Any change of climate involving the fatigue of travel is contraindicated in acute cases with fever or hemorrhage, or in very far advanced and markedly debilitated cases. Absolute bed rest is the one essential here.

4. No patient should be sent away in search of climate who cannot

afford to stay the reasonably to be expected time and to have the necessary food, lodging and care.

5. Competent medical advice and supervision are essential.

6. One of the most valuable assets of change is the education of the patient. This may, of course, be obtained in a suitable environment without reference to climate, as in a sanatorium near home.

7. Selection of a suitable locality is an individual problem for every patient, depending upon his temperament, tastes, and individual reaction to environment, as well as the character of his disease. The advising physician should have an appreciation of these as well as a knowledge of the particular environment to which the patient is being sent. Contentment and reasonable comfort are essential.

8. There is no universally ideal climate. For each patient there may well be a most favorable environment, if we are wise enough to find it.

9. There is a reasonable amount of evidence that certain medical types of cases are more favorably influenced by certain conditions of climate, everything else being equal. For example, reasonably cold, dry, variable climate, such as is found in the mountains, for young or vigorous constitutions which will react well. Dry, sunny climates for laryngeal cases and those with marked catarrhal secretions. Equable mild climates at low altitudes for the elderly and those of nervous temperaments, as well as for those with arteriosclerosis, weak hearts, or marked tendency to dyspnœa.

10. Successful selection of climate and environment for cases of tuberculosis requires wide knowledge of human nature, of places, and of the disease. This can only be acquired by patience, skill, and experience.

SKIN TESTS FOR TUBERCULOSIS

Many years ago it was proved that almost every human being has tuberculosis before he dies.

Indeed, the vast majority of people become infected with the disease in childhood and recover. However, a considerable number do not recover, and these represent the constant mortality from this disease. The death rate from tuberculosis has been cut tremendously through the advancement of modern medical science and modern hygiene.

In order to detect cases as early as possible and to apply as soon as possible suitable methods leading toward recovery, several systems have been established. The first, as pointed out by Dr. F. M. Mc-Phedran of the University of Pennsylvania, is to examine all school children physically and by means of the X-ray and to give all of them the tuberculin test. The tuberculin test is a simple skin test, less painful than a pin scratch and much less dangerous.

One of the advantages of such a procedure is the fact that during the physical examination for tuberculosis, it is also possible to detect any other disease which may happen to be attacking the child.

Another method is to select from among school children those who seem particularly likely to have tuberculosis and to limit the examination to them. When a child is found to be positive to the tuberculin test, a thorough study is made of its physical conditions, then the X-ray examination is made. The X-ray reveals even small changes which may have taken place in the lungs.

If a child is found to be susceptible to tuberculosis or in a very early stage, it can be put under a course of hygiene which will aid its prompt recovery in the vast majority of cases.

One of the modern developments in the care of tuberculosis is the establishment of the preventorium to which children are taken who have very mild degrees of tuberculosis or who come of families in which tuberculosis is prevalent. There they have opportunity to recover under the best conditions.

REST IN TUBERCULOSIS

According to the medical director of the Municipal Tuberculosis Sanatorium in Chicago, it would require five times as many sanatoriums as are now available if every person with active tuberculosis were to be taken care of in such an institution.

In 1927 there were almost 100,000 deaths from tuberculosis in the United States, and on the basis of five active cases for each death there would be about a half-million active cases of the disease always among us. The number of beds available in sanatoriums for the tuberculous, according to a recent study, is 69,152. It is obvious, therefore, that the vast majority of people with this disease cannot be taken care of in institutions and that the chief purpose of the institution may be to instruct a considerable number of people how to take care of themselves at home.

Rest, fresh air, and food, Dr. Goldberg emphasizes again, constitute the important trilogy by which the person with tuberculosis must regulate his life. The sanatorium teaches the person how to follow this trilogy automatically and as an everyday procedure.

The person with active symptoms must have absolute rest. As symptoms quiet down the competent physician is able to tell the patient how much exercise is to be taken along with the rest to secure the best results. To most people fresh air means a lusty breeze pouring through a window or below-zero weather on an outdoor sleeping porch. It is important to realize that fresh air does not demand physical discomfort. Windows may be kept open, but the temperature should be equable, and drafts are unnecessary.

One of the chief values of the sanatorium is to teach the patient the routine facts regarding such matters as rest, exercise, diet, and fresh air. It will teach him also how to prevent the contamination of clothing, dishes, and other human beings with the organisms that are in his body. It will teach him his limitations in work and help to find work that he can do.

Thus will it have fulfilled a most useful function and when he is improved sufficiently to be on his way, the place he occupied will be filled by another pupil, and he will go out to help educate the public.

TREATMENT OF TUBERCULOSIS

For many years all sorts of specific remedies have been tried on the tuberculous, and millions of dollars have been mulcted from these people for patent medicines.

Among the first of the new scientific remedies to be announced was Koch's tuberculin, which was developed in 1890. This is not a specific remedy, and there are many experts who feel that it is worthless. However, some doctors who use it very carefully and who study their patients, find it useful in some cases.

A number of remedies have been introduced, consisting of combinations of copper, of gold, and of other metals. All of these remedies are experimental, and although they have been reported as useful in some cases, the vast majority of the evidence does not seem to indicate any special value for any of them.

Because the lesions of tuberculosis heal by calcification, it has been customary with many physicians to use a great deal of calcium in the condition. In fact, it is commonly believed that workers in lime dust do not have tuberculosis, yet the evidence for this fact is not particularly convincing. The more recent studies seem to indicate that some change must take place in the tuberculosis itself before calcification can begin, and that in the vast majority of cases there is plenty of calcium in the body for the needs of the situation when the mechanism of healing starts.

Cod-liver oil has been used in tuberculosis for several centuries. It has the advantage of furnishing a large amount of fat and also provides vitamins which are of great importance to the body. If cod-liver oil is to be taken, it is usually best in doses of one to three ounces after a meal. In the case of tuberculosis, the whole cod liver is believed to be preferable to any of the extracts of the vitamins.

For years creosote and guaiacol were considered to be specific remedies in tuberculosis, and they are still used in some cases to produce expectoration, lessening of tightness in the throat, and for the relief of coughing.

Among the most recent discoveries for use in tuberculosis are the so-called Sauerbruch and Herrmannsdorfer, and Gerson diets. These were developed in Germany in 1933, and it was believed that by the use of these diets it was possible to change the soil on which the tuberculous germ grows. The essential of these diets is the practical exclusion of table salt and the substitution for it of a salt rich in calcium. The diet also includes large selections of uncooked fresh vegetables or salads with added fruit juices. Other vegetables are cooked in their own juices in waterless cookers. The meats in the diet are cut down, as are also the sugars. The water intake is also cut down, but is substituted with fairly liberal amounts of fresh fruit juices and vegetable juices. Dr. Harry Beckman has prepared a table indicating the chief facts of these two diets.

These diets are still experimental, and their exact value has not yet been determined.

People with tuberculosis suffer frequently with fever and sweating at night. When these symptoms become oppressive, the doctor can prescribe drugs which will control them. An alcohol rub at bedtime or a sponge bath with lukewarm water containing about one gram of alum to the ounce is helpful in preventing night sweats.

One of the most severe symptoms that may occur in a patient with tuberculosis is bleeding from the lungs. The appearance of this symptom is a danger signal which should cause the patient to lie down immediately and to get medical attention at once.

In the sanatorium in which the patients are treated for tuberculosis, one of the most useful remedies thus far developed is artificial pneumothorax. This involves the injection of air into the chest cavity, which serves to put the lung at rest. The same effect is also brought about by cutting the nerve which leads to the diaphragm, or by performing surgical operation on the ribs.

COMPARISON OF SUGGESTED DIETS FOR TUBERCULOSIS PATIENTS

	Gerson diet	Herrmannsdorfer-Sauerbruch diet
Proteins	About 55 to 67 gm. daily.	About 90 to 120 gm. daily.
80 per cent Animal	Meat............ 100 gm. weekly.	600 gm. weekly
20 per cent Vegetable	Fish............ 70 gm. weekly.	About the same
	Viscera......None (sweetbreads, etc.)	Rather freely permitted
	Legumes................ None	Permitted
Fats	About 170 gm. daily.	About 170 gm. daily
	Cream.................... None	About 250 cc.
	Eggs............ Yolks only.	Whole egg
Carbohydrates	Total—250 gm. carbohydrates given daily.	About the same amount
	Sugar................ 20 gm. weekly.	About the same amount
	Honey............ 50 gm. weekly.	
Fluids	1,400 cc. vegetable juices; fruit juices 600 cc.	Restricted vegetable and fruit juices; about 2½ pints in form of milk, cream, soup, juices, etc.
	Milk.................. 250 cc.	About 1,000 cc.
	Soup.................... None.	
Sodium Chloride	About 1.56 gm. in food. About 1.15 gm. in juices. About 2.7 gm. of sodium chloride intake daily.	
Aim	Ratio of protein to fat to carbohydrate is about 1 to 5.6 to 3.4	Ratio of protein to fat to carbohydrate is about 1.5 to 2.7 to 3.7

Dehydration of tissues and altering body's mineral metabolism. Poor in salt and carbohydrate. Vegetables steamed; much raw food given, with cod-liver oil with phosphorus, and mineral compound (chiefly calcium). Calories: 21 to 22 calories per pound of body weight; 2,770 or 3,030 if patient weighs 182 pounds (60 kg.). In Herrmannsdorfer diet, calories furnished are 15 per cent by protein, 53 per cent by fat, and 32 per cent by carbohydrates.

Rich in fat, vitamins, and minerals (perhaps protein).

MENTAL ASPECTS IN TUBERCULOSIS

One of the most important factors in the care of the tuberculous is the coöperation of the patient in the handling of his disease.

In a thesis prepared in the University of Minnesota, Blanche Peterson insists that the most important single factor in the cure of tuberculosis is an intelligent attitude of the patient.

Doctors, nurses, and social workers endeavor, therefore, in every possible way to influence the patient to assume an intelligent and constructive outlook.

A questionnaire sent to a score of leading physicians who have specialized in this subject resulted in the almost universal response that reasonable and courageous attitudes are highly constructive. The worst states are those of fear, anxiety, and depression.

The patient with tuberculosis who becomes discouraged, hopeless, pessimistic, or rebellious is difficult to treat and aids in his downfall.

When a person first learns that he has this disease, he is likely to be upset and depressed. Knowing nothing of modern care, he is likely to feel that the disease will be promptly fatal.

If, however, the physician who makes the diagnosis will tell the patient that help is possible, that the disease is curable if treated sufficiently early and sufficiently long; that dozens of persons have achieved world-wide fame even though suffering from this disease, he is likely to have a different attitude and to coöperate fully in treatment.

Courage and reasonableness can come only with complete understanding of the situation. For this reason the health education of the tuberculous has come to be one of the most important factors in the control of this condition, and a vast literature has been developed for the purpose.

Practically every tuberculosis sanatorium and tuberculosis society now publishes books and pamphlets which are helpful in informing the tuberculous of the important facts relative to their condition.

The National Tuberculosis Association, 50 West 50th Street, New York City, publishes much material that is useful. Such books as the guides and calendars for the tuberculous, edited by Lawrason Brown, are exceedingly helpful.[1]

Above all, the persons living with and surrounding the tuberculous

[1] *Laws for Recovery from Pulmonary Tuberculosis.* Lawrason Brown, Saranac Lake, N. Y.

must realize that it is their duty to keep the patient in a hopeful frame of mind and not treat him as a helpless invalid from the moment the diagnosis is made.

HEALTH HINTS FOR THE TUBERCULOUS

Several years ago Dr. Charles L. Minor of Asheville, N. C., wrote some hints for people with tuberculosis which were so successful that they have recently been republished by another authority on this disease who has brought them up to date and modified them to meet modern conditions.

Many of these hints constitute excellent advice regarding hygiene for everyone who is slightly run down, whether tuberculous or not. It is impossible to reprint all of the suggestions here, but a selection is made of some of the most important.

1. Never exercise to the point of fatigue. If you find yourself tired, you have done yourself harm.

2. Remember that rest comes before exercise. By resting a surplus of strength and energy is built up and stored in the body.

3. Aim to spend as much of each day outdoors or in absolutely fresh air as possible. Remember that the air, to be fresh, need not necessarily be cold.

4. Ideal food should be appetizing, nutritious, and not too bulky. If appetizing and not nutritious, it will not nourish you; if nutritious and not appetizing, you will not eat it; if too bulky, however appetizing, it upsets your stomach.

5. Eat up to the limit of your digestion. It is the food which is digested and absorbed, and not what is put into your mouth, which will do you good. A glass of milk with each meal is advisable. Raw eggs are not so digestible as cooked eggs. Take nothing between meals unless ordered by your doctor.

6. If your digestion is poor, tell your doctor.

7. Eat your meals at regular hours. Do not take reading matter to the table. Smiles and laughter are the best possible aids to digestion.

8. Approach and leave each meal in a rested condition. Never eat when tired. Never exercise immediately after eating.

9. In winter, warm, light, or medium wool underwear; in summer, ordinary summer cotton underwear.

10. Never wear very heavy underclothing or chest protectors.

11. Let your shoes be stout and warm in winter and wear warm woolen socks, by all means. Woolen socks at night are often a great

comfort. In winter, a flannel shirt is much more comfortable than anything else. When sitting out in winter, have an extra wrap near by.

12. If you get overheated and perspire, change your clothing and rub dry.

13. A healthy condition of the skin is most important. A warm bath once or twice a week if ordered by your physician is advisable, and a cool sponge bath or a tub bath in the morning if your doctor permits it. Remember that the water should be cool but not ice cold. If you do not have a proper reaction after your bath, if you feel chilly or are blue, the water is too cold. Ask your doctor about it. See that your room or bathroom or wherever you take your bath is warm.

ULTRAVIOLET RAY IN TUBERCULOSIS OF THE LARYNX

Tuberculosis of the larynx has been considered, until recent years, one of the most dangerous forms of the disease, leading usually to fatality.

All sorts of remedies have been tried in an endeavor to control the condition, but without exceedingly good results. As far back as 1898, attempts were made to treat tuberculosis of the larynx with sunlight, but due to lack of proper apparatus the results were not as good as they might have been.

With the discovery of the apparatus which yielded ultraviolet rays, in the form of the carbon arc and the quartz mercury vapor lamps, it became possible to apply concentrated sun's rays directly to the larynx. In order to get the rays directly to the laryngeal cords, various systems of mirrors have been devised, and also quartz stems along which the ultraviolet rays pass.

It has been found that people who are very frail, those with advanced tuberculosis of the lung, and those who have very severe lesions in the throat are treated better by means of the mirror reflection than by other methods.

A steel mirror will reflect about 44 per cent of the valuable rays into the larynx, according to Dr. Joseph W. Miller, whereas ordinary glass mirrors absorb these rays and reflect only about 9 per cent. It has been found that practically all of the patients treated by direct sunlight to the cords tend to heal. Dr. Miller reports fifty-nine out of seventy-two patients who showed complete healing of the tuberculous lesions in the larynx. The symptoms improved in the other patients even though the healing was partial.

In many of these cases, because it was impossible for the patient to stay in a sanatorium, it became necessary for the patient to treat himself. The apparatus has now been developed so that the patient can actually see his larynx and treat himself by means of the reflecting mirrors.

CONCLUSIONS

Particularly of importance in controlling the spread of tuberculosis is the use of dispensaries in which the disease can be diagnosed in its earliest stages and properly controlled. Experimentation with the method of vaccination against tuberculosis by Calmette has not yet gone sufficiently far to warrant its general adoption in this country.

The most powerful social factors in controlling the disease are housing, nutrition, and education. In educating people it is desirable to educate them not only in general hygiene but also especially as regards the prevention of tuberculosis. The regular examination of school children and teachers, studies of the nutrition of the school child, and education of those who are infected in methods of preventing the spread of the disease are significant factors.

The preventive institutions against tuberculosis today include holiday camps, open-air schools, preventoriums for children who are perhaps not certainly infected with tuberculosis but in such poor state of nutrition and general health that they offer easy prey to the disease, and certainly removal of children as soon as possible from contact with adults who are infected.

CHAPTER XIII

Rheumatism, Arthritis, and Gout
MORRIS FISHBEIN, M.D.

RHEUMATISM AND ARTHRITIS

ANY CONDITION involving an inflammation of the bones and joints is called arthritis. Arthritis is not the same as rheumatism. Rheumatism is a condition of inflammation which may affect nerves, muscles, fibrous tissue, or any other tissues of the human body. When it affects bones and joints the condition is called arthritis.

Not all arthritis is the same. There may be sudden inflammations or chronic conditions lasting many years. There may be forms of arthritis in which there is simply collection of fluid in the tissues, others in which there is overdevelopment of the membranes. Furthermore, inflammations of bones and joints may vary according to the kind of germ associated with the inflammation or with the manner in which the inflammation comes about.

In cases in which there is a sudden inflammation of a joint the first signs are usually pain with limitation of movement, swelling, redness and a feeling of heat in the joint. Moreover, the muscles around the joint may be affected by spasm because they endeavor to limit the movement of the joint. All sorts of germs may be involved in such inflammations, including the typhoid germ, the germ that causes pneumonia, the general pus-forming germs, and even those associated with venereal diseases.

Just as soon as the cause of the condition is definitely determined, the condition may be attacked through the cause. Thus for certain forms of germs, vaccines or serums may be of value. In other cases it may be necessary to remove the infectious material from the joint by surgical procedures. Associated with such measures it may be desirable to apply heat, massage, and similar physical procedures to encourage the blood supply of the tissues which will result in bringing the forces of the body to bear in overcoming the condition.

As the healing occurs, the joint may be gradually moved, and suitable manipulation will eventually result in a complete restoration of function provided the damage to the tissues as a result of the infection has not been too great.

Much more serious than the ordinary acute inflammation of a joint are those forms in which infection persists over a long period of time and in which it may be associated with changes in the blood and in the tissues of a more permanent and damaging character.

CAUSES OF CHRONIC ARTHRITIS

Scientifically the chronic forms of joint inflammation are classified according to their causes and to the changes that take place in the tissues. Doctors recognize many possible causes, including changes in the glandular mechanism of the body, errors of diet, poisoning by alcohol, tobacco, or lead, disturbances of the circulation of the blood, changes in the nervous system and deformities like knock-knees, bow-legs, and poor posture. Furthermore, there are forms of sensitivity to various substances in which reactions occur in the joints. These reactions disappear when the sensitivities are discovered and the possible exposure of the patient to the protein substances prevented. Moreover, there may actually be inflammation of a joint following a sudden straining or twisting or a blow on a joint such as may occur during athletic sports. In many instances the injury following a blow or a strain gives opportunity for invasion by germs which are always present in the body.

Most inflammations of the joints appear in people past forty years of age, but of course young people are also occasionally affected. Interestingly enough, people who live in hot climates suffer much less with arthritis than do those in the temperate zone.

SYMPTOMS OF INFLAMMATION OF JOINTS

The symptoms of a chronic inflammation of a joint are much like those of the acute types. There may be pain, stiffness, swelling, limitation of motion, fatigue on action, and sometimes deformity. Another exceedingly interesting symptom is the rustling sound or cracking which is likely to be heard in an inflamed joint. This sound is like that of two pieces of leather being rubbed together or like the crackling associated with the crushing of some stiff paper. Sometimes it may be heard by other people in the room when the patient sits down and in other cases may be so light and delicate that it becomes perceptible to the hand and ear of the doctor when he examines it, but is otherwise not heard.

People with arthritis feel the stiffness of their joints more particularly when they get up in the morning—the reason being that the tissues have had a chance to become set during the long-continued quiet. When the condition becomes worse, this stiffness may appear even when the patient rests for just a moment during the day. The afflicted person finds that he has difficulty in getting up after he has been sitting down a while, and that after bending down he is forced to get up slowly. The explanation of this is, of course, that the tissues shorten during the relaxation and that sudden attempts to lengthen them are accompanied by certain discomforts. If the person remains long ill in bed as a result of a considerable amount of pain, movement on getting up is even more difficult.

Because of the many types of inflammations of joints and of the varying severity of the symptoms in different cases, many forms of treatment have been developed both to bring about relief from the symptoms and in many instances to bring about a cure.

It has been well established by many years of experience that the person with a rheumatic or arthritic condition passes through periods in which he is worse and in which he is better and that he is likely to credit each period of improvement to the latest treatment followed. For this reason quacks and charlatans are likely particularly to exploit the rheumatic individual.

Since it has been shown that inflammations of the joints are frequently associated with infections in the teeth and tonsils, persons who suffer with chronic inflammations of the joints should have such infections attended to as soon as possible. In some instances difficulties of digestion and an accumulation of food in the bowels seem to be a factor, and the condition of the stomach and intestinal tract should always be most carefully surveyed in connection with any inflammation of a rheumatic character. When such people become fatigued, the condition is likely to be worse. As these conditions develop, there are tendencies toward crippling because of fixing of the joints in certain positions. Such crippling may be prevented if competent attention is given early to the condition by a qualified physician. Such specialists will arrange to protect the joint by holding the tissues in proper position through the use of plaster of Paris casts, splints, or braces. In general relief may be secured through the application of heat, by the use of liniments and lotions and baths, by devices which pull the tissues so that the swelling does not bring about pain and by the direct application of various healing measures.

It must be realized first, however, that the general care of a person with a chronic inflammation of the joints is of the utmost importance. In order to secure such care, it may be necessary to put the patient into a hospital or institution where he will be under definite medical control. If the person is depressed through his condition, a cheerful environment and an optimistic attitude in those around him may mean a great deal in obtaining suitable coöperation in treatment and in eventual success.

Various authorities estimate that inflammations of the joints and rheumatic conditions are due to intestinal causes in from 20 to 40 per cent of cases. One group of authorities insists that the taking of sugars is largely responsible, and they cut down on such substances. Another group claims that overeating of protein foods, like meat, eggs, and fish, may be harmful. It may be taken for granted that people who regularly overeat ought to eat less, and those who are overweight must certainly take smaller amounts of carbohydrates. The sick person is likely to suffer in the nutrition of his tissues, and it may be hazardous to cut down too greatly on the protein foods such as meat, eggs, cheese, fish, and similar products.

DIETS IN ARTHRITIS

In a recent survey of this topic Dr. Walter Bauer has outlined the present point of view regarding diets prescribed by various cults and faddists and has considered in connection with these diets their advantages and disadvantages.

There are some who insist on the omission of all acid fruits and vegetables. The foods that are commonly called acid fruits include tomatoes, oranges, grapefruit, and lemons. Actually these foods contain weak acids which are oxidized in the body and the end result of which is alkaline. It must be remembered, however, that such foods represent the primary contribution to the diet of vitamin C and that they also provide a goodly amount of vitamin A. They are really essential to any well balanced diet, and there is no real contra-indication to their inclusion in the diet of a person with arthritis.

Quite recently some faddists have insisted that the person with a rheumatic condition should not eat a mixed diet and that the presence of protein in the stomach interferes with the digestion of starches. This is another indication of the lack of knowledge of physiology. Meat and potatoes, which are two foods especially rich in protein and starch, have been eaten for thousands of years. The digestion of starch begins in the mouth, because the saliva is important in digestion. The digestion of starch may be temporarily interrupted in the stomach, because starches are not digested in the presence of acid from the gastric juice. However, the digestion of starch is again resumed when the food passes from the stomach into the intestines, where the juices are alkaline. There seems to be no reason to believe that there is any actual basis for refusing to mix proteins and starches.

It has been pointed out that such animals as the dog, the cat, and the cow do not have ferments in their saliva for digesting starches, and that in such animals which live chiefly on foods containing starches all of the digestion of starch takes place after the food has left the stomach.

Another group of faddists says that people with arthritis should eat foods tending to alkalinity. The human body is a self-regulating mechanism which must always incline toward alkalinity, and it is rather silly for most people to attempt to make any special effort to keep the body on the alkaline side.

In gout it may be particularly desirable to have a diet low in proteins, but this does not apply to the diet in most forms of arthritis. Therefore, the one important principle would seem to be restriction of the carbohydrate foods, principally because patients with arthritis have difficulty with carbohydrates due to abnormalities in their intestinal tract, and because the records show that some of these patients improve with the lessening of the carbohydrate intake.

A careful study of the various diets that have been developed has led Dr. Walter Bauer, however, to the view that the best diet for any arthritic or rheumatic person is a well balanced diet. Moreover, one should be certain that such a diet is adequate in vitamins and in the mineral salts and contains sufficient amounts of calories to keep up the nutrition. An example of such a diet is the following:

Breakfast:
Fresh fruit—average serving.
Orange or grapefruit juice—1 glass.
Eggs—2.
Bacon—3 slices.
Rye bread toast—1 slice.
Butter—2 squares.
Coffee with 40 per cent cream.

Dinner:
Clear soup or broth.
Meat or fish—average serving.
Vegetable—average serving.
Fruit or vegetable salad with mayonnaise.
Extra vegetable—average serving.
Milk or buttermilk—1 glass.
Rye bread—1 slice.
Butter—2 squares.
Fruit dessert.

Supper:
Tomato juice—6 ounces.
Liver, chicken, or lamb chop—average serving.
Vegetable, cooked—average serving.
Fresh vegetable, as lettuce, tomatoes, celery, etc.
Rye bread—1 slice.
Milk or buttermilk—1 glass.
Fruit dessert.

1. Sugar, bread, and other desserts would be allowed in this dietary if the patient were not overweight.

2. In addition to the above, we usually prescribe cod-liver oil or one of the cod-liver oil concentrates, as well as some one of the vitamin B concentrate preparations.

This diet gives protein, calcium, phosphorus, iron, and vitamins and may be still further supplemented in its vitamin content by small amounts of cod-liver oil.

The person with a rheumatic condition should of course observe the maximum quantity of personal hygiene. This means enough fresh air and sunshine, enough bathing, clothing that is adequate to the weather, and a job which will minimize exposure to heat and cold and particularly to sudden alteration of temperature. The teeth should have regular attention by a competent dentist and the toothbrush must be used regularly.

A great deal has been said about the use of various vaccines and serums or so-called "shots" in the treatment of rheumatic disorders. Unfortunately, no single germ has been incriminated as the cause of rheumatic conditions in all cases. Therefore two types of vaccines are used: one involving germs taken from infections in various parts of the body including occasionally the joints themselves, and the other mixtures of germs taken from various cases of arthritis and cultivated in the usual way in which germs are cultivated. Thereafter the germs are destroyed by heat and injected into the body. Since many patients react severely to such injections, it is customary to begin with a small dose to test the effect of the treatment and then to regulate the dosage according to the patient's response. There are many specialists in the treatment of arthritis who feel that a considerable number of patients are relieved by such methods.

Another group of authorities insists that the use of specific germs is not necessary and that it is primarily the reaction in the body of the patient that brings about benefit. Such reactions are produced by the injection of any protein substances as, for example, heated milk or nonspecific vaccines.

In an endeavor to attack the disease, attempts have also been made to use transfusions of blood from other people and to use injections of the patient's own blood into his body. This latter method of treatment is a mild form of nonspecific protein therapy, bringing about a reaction in the patient's body.

The drugs that have been used in the treatment of arthritis are legion, most of them being employed because they relieve pain. There is no reason why a patient should suffer pain while undergoing treatments such as have been mentioned. The right drugs properly administered will do much to keep the patient in comfort.

Many forms of physical treatment are applied. These include alternate hot and cold baths, heat applied through hot-water bottles, electric pads, baking devices, and various forms of light. In the great spas in which rheumatic disorders are treated, hot mud packs and the waters from hot springs are frequently used. A more recent method includes the application of hot paraffin baths with a temperature from 118 to 130 degrees sustained from five to twenty minutes. Moreover, it is possible to obtain generalized heating by the passing of electrical currents through the tissues against resistance. Massage is useful when done by a person who is skilled in its performance and who understands the danger of too much motion to a sensitive and painful joint. The slightest bruising or injury to the tissues may result in much more harm than good.

Thus the treatment of chronic rheumatic conditions today involves a wide series of measures based on multiple causes. Again it should be emphasized, however, that the frame of mind of the patient is of the utmost significance. This accounts for the cures said to be brought about by laying on the hands, by twisting the feet, by prayer, by changing the shoes, and by all sorts of similar measures. A well-known authority has said that hopefulness and patience, physical treatment, sunlight, fresh air, good hygiene, massage, and good food will bring about benefit in the vast majority of patients, and that the removal of mental and physical overactivity, freedom from worry, and the building up of general resistance will take care of a good many more.

Gout

Gout is a disease of ancient lineage. It was first definitely described by the famous physician Sydenham in England during the eighteenth century—Sydenham himself being a sufferer from this disorder. In his description of the disease he was so graphic that every sufferer from the condition reads it with special sympathy:

The victim goes to bed and sleeps in good health. About 2 o'clock in the morning he is awakened by a severe pain in the great toe; more rarely in the heel, ankle or instep. This pain is like that of a dislocation, and yet the parts feel as if cold water were poured over them. Then follow chills and shivers, and a little fever. The pain, which was at first moderate, becomes more intense. With its intensity the chills and shivers increase. After a time this comes to its height, accommodating itself to the bones and ligaments of the tarsus and metatarsus. Now it is a violent stretching and tearing of the ligaments—now it is a gnawing pain and now a pressure and tightening. So exquisite and lively meanwhile is the feeling of the part affected, that it cannot bear the weight of the bedclothes nor the jar of a person walking in the room. The night is passed in torture, sleeplessness, turning of the part affected, and perpetual change of posture; the tossing about of the body being as incessant as the pain of the tortured joint, being worse as the fit comes on. Hence the vain effort, by change of posture, both in the body and the limb affected, to obtain

an abatement of the pain. This comes on only towards the morning of
the next day. . . . The patient has a sudden and slight respite, which
he falsely attributes to the last change of position. A general perspiration is succeeded by sleep. He wakes freer from pain, and finds the part
recently swollen.

Gout is today an exceedingly rare disease in this country. It is
believed to be associated with the abnormal production within the body
of the products of uric acid. Apparently something is wrong in the
way in which such people take care of their protein foods. The disease
seems to run in families and to be associated with overindulgence in
eating and drinking and with a lack of exercise. However, some people
get the condition who do not suffer from these habits.

Gout is treated successfully by carefully supervising the activity
of the person concerned, by taking suitable measures for the relief of
pain, and by eliminating from the diet foods that are rich in nucleins,
such as liver, thymus, kidney, brain, and pancreas. Such substances
as caviar, fish roe, and meat extracts are also believed to be harmful.
The best diet for a person with this condition includes milk, cream,
cheese, fruits, fresh vegetables, and water. Liquors, wines, and alcoholics are generally forbidden.

Some drugs seem to be particularly helpful in bringing about relief
from pain. The pain may also be avoided by the application of heat
and by fixing the affected parts in such a way with sand bags, hot-
water bottles, and similar devices, as to keep the bedclothing and other
pressure away from the affected parts.

CHAPTER XIV

Diseases of the Heart and Circulation
NEWELL C. GILBERT, M.D.

INTRODUCTION

THE HEART OF A CHILD *at birth weighs less than an ounce; that of an adult, a half pound. The energy which causes the heart to contract develops in some nervous tissue called the pace-maker of the heart. Apparently its energy is the equivalent of a thousandth of a volt. The heart beats one hundred times a minute in a small child, and on an average of seventy-two times a minute in an adult.*

This pump, because the heart is a pump which circulates the blood throughout the body, moves five hundred gallons of blood a day. During a lifetime the heart beats two and a half billion times and pumps a total of nearly thirty-five million gallons. The heart begins working before a child is born and is never quiet until death. The only rest it gets is when its beat is slowed a little or decreased somewhat in its force. The heart never gets a complete rest. This vital organ must therefore be protected in every possible way against damage. It would be far better if more people knew the importance of a reasonable amount of rest for the heart.

There is one disease of the heart which has thus far baffled medical science. It is known as rheumatic fever. This disease is responsible for a vast amount of crippling and handicapping of young children. Because of its great importance, it is given more than usual consideration in the pages that follow.

Almost two hundred and twenty-five thousand people die in the United States each year from heart disease. The condition is more expensive in cost of human lives than cancer, but somewhat less expensive than tuberculosis. On those who live, however, the burden of heart disease falls heavily.

Because of the greater realization of the importance of heart disease in relationship to the cause of death, and since today it leads all other causes, and since it is estimated that there are at any time at least two million people in the United States suffering from heart disease, this section of any modern home medical book is important.

From the earliest times the heart has aroused the curiosity and interest of man to an extent not equaled by any other organ in the human body except the brain. Most people who get sick are inclined to refer unusual symptoms to the heart. This organ has often been associated with the idea of courage, as in the phrase "faint heart,"

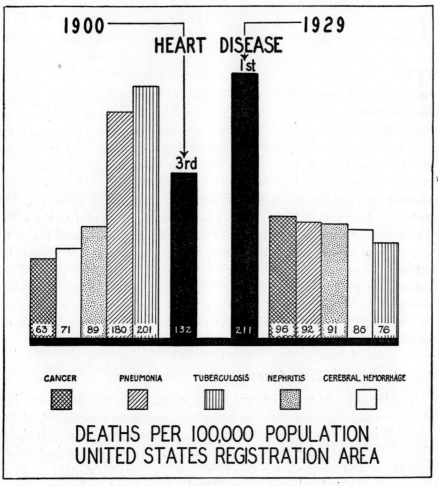

FIG. 44.

and the average man is likely to speak of the other person as either "weak-hearted" or "strong-hearted." It was once believed that the heart was the seat of the soul. It is still referred to as the seat of one of life's most interesting emotions.

The heart is one of the involuntary muscles of the body. There are but few instances recorded in medicine in which people were able voluntarily to control the heartbeats. Nevertheless, there is plenty of evidence to indicate that the speed of modern life and the stress of modern emotions modify greatly the work of the heart. There is also evidence that a suitable hygiene in relationship to this organ will lead to longer life.

M. F.

THE CIRCULATORY SYSTEM is in reality the transportation system for the body. It carries to the cells, of which every organ and tissue of the body is built, essential materials for construction, reconstruction, and replacement of the tissues broken down by wear and tear. The blood carries fuel, and oxygen to burn the fuel, so that the necessary energy for repair and rebuilding may be obtained; each cell is thus enabled to perform its special function. Many other products, for instance, the secretions of certain glands, must be carried to the cells. The waste products from the cells must be carried away and taken to organs whose duty it is to excrete the waste or the waste may be utilized elsewhere, and made over for certain needs of the body. This system acts perfectly under normal conditions and automatically takes care of the changing needs of each part of the body. When an organ or tissue is doing active work, that part receives an increased flow of blood, while parts at rest receive a reduced amount.

THE ANATOMY OF THE HEART

The heart is the great central pump which moves the fluid carrying the necessary supplies through the blood vessels to every part of the body. It is a hollow organ with strong muscular walls. Its size is about that of the clenched right fist of its owner. The heart lies just below and to the left of the lower two thirds of the breastbone. Its shape is similar to that of a large pear with the broadened end upward and under the breast bone, and the pointed end downward and to the left, where one may feel the impulse as the heart beats.

THE PERICARDIUM

The heart lies inside a fibrous sac, called the *pericardium*, which is a resistant membrane and which forms a chamber, separating the heart

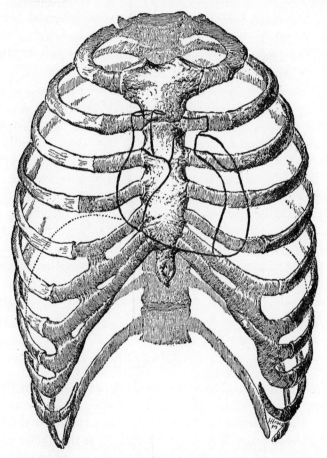

FIG. 45.   Position of the heart in the chest cavity.

from the other organs of the chest and holding it in position. In case of necessity this sac prevents the heart from dilating or stretching beyond a certain point. The surface of the heart itself is enclosed in a second fold of the same membrane. The two surfaces of the peri-cardium which lie against each other are covered by a smooth glistening layer of tissue, kept moist by a thin layer of fluid. This fluid prevents any friction between the layers as the heart beats.

CONSTRUCTION OF THE HEART

When the heart is opened it is seen to be separated into two halves with no communication between them. The halves are right and left in position and similar in arrangement. They act in unison. Each of the halves is also divided into two chambers. Above, on either side, is a thin-walled chamber which acts as a receiving reservoir for the blood returned to the heart. This chamber is called the *auricle*. Below the auricle is a chamber with thick, strong muscular walls, called the *ventricle*. This connects with the upper chamber by means of an opening provided with *valves*, which admit the blood freely into the ventricle when it relaxes, but close tight when the ventricle contracts, and thus prevent the return flow of blood back into the auricle during the contraction of the ventricle. The only essential difference between the right and left sides of the heart is that the muscle walls on the left side are thicker; for the left side must propel the blood through the entire body, while the right side needs to pump the blood only through the lungs. Leading from each ventricle is a large artery or blood vessel which carries away the blood forced out of the ventricle when it contracts. At the point where the blood leaves the ventricle and enters the artery there are other valves to prevent the reflow of blood into the ventricle, when its muscular walls relax again after contraction.

THE HEART MUSCLE: THE MYOCARDIUM

The muscle wall of the heart is referred to as the *myocardium*. The entire hollow interior of the heart is lined with a thick smooth membrane called the *endocardium*. This is continuous with a similar membrane lining the arteries. From these terms come the names of diseases in which these tissues are inflamed, such as myocarditis and endocarditis.

The heart muscle itself is supplied with a system of arteries and veins for its own fuel and repair requirements. This is called the *coronary system*. The coronary arteries open from the interior of the *aorta* (the large artery leading off from the left side of the heart). They begin just below the valves which separate the aorta from the ventricle. The flow through these arteries, then, will be greater or less as the blood pressure in the aorta is greater or less.

The Function of the Heart

The blood returning from every part of the body is brought back to the right auricle by two large veins, one coming from the upper, the other from the lower, part of the body, called respectively the superior and inferior *vena cava*. From the right auricle, the blood enters the right ventricle, which forces the blood through the lungs. There it gives up its carbon-dioxide, carried from all parts of the body, and takes on a fresh supply of oxygen. The blood returning from the circuit through the lungs is returned to the left auricle by the pulmonary vein. The auricles act as receiving reservoirs for the blood. Between the beats of the heart, their muscle walls relax and become distended with the returned blood. The period between each contraction or beat is referred to as the *diastole*, and is a period of rest and recuperation for the heart.

When the walls of the ventricles relax in their turn, after each contraction, the blood from the distended auricles flows into the ventricles during the relaxation or diastole of the ventricle. Just before the end of the ventricular diastole or period of relaxation of the walls of the ventricle, the muscle walls of the auricle contract, further emptying the auricle and more completely filling the ventricle. A fraction of a second later, the ventricle begins to contract. As the walls of the chamber contract and draw together, the pressure of the contained blood increases; the valves leading back into the auricle are closed and held firmly shut by the blood in the ventricle pushing against them. When the pressure in the contracting ventricle becomes greater than the pressure in the artery, the valves leading into the artery are opened and the contents of the ventricle forced into the artery. At the end of the ventricular contraction or systole, the ventricle in its turn relaxes. As it does so the valves leading back into the ventricle from the aorta are closed by the pressure of the blood, thus preventing a reflow of blood back into the ventricle. During the period of ventricular systole the relaxed auricle has again been filling with blood, whereupon the now relaxed ventricle is again filled. This cycle is repeated, many times a minute, hour after hour, and year after year during life. The heart works constantly, but the amount and speed of its work may be varied.

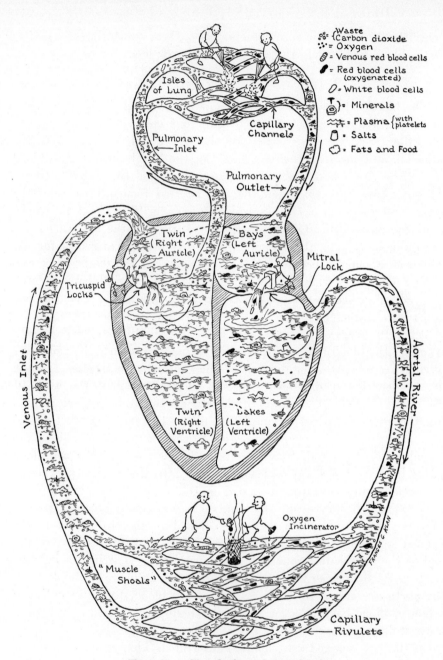

The following labels appear in the figure:

Waste
Carbon dioxide
= Oxygen
= Venous red blood cells
= Red blood cells (oxygenated)
= White blood cells
= Minerals
= Plasma { with platelets
= Salts
= Fats and Food

Isles of Lung

Capillary Channels

Pulmonary Inlet

Pulmonary Outlet

Twin (Right Auricle)

Bays (Left Auricle)

Mitral Lock

Tricuspid Locks

Venous Inlet

Aortal River

Twin (Right Ventricle)

Lakes (Left Ventricle)

Oxygen Incinerator

"Muscle Shoals"

Capillary Rivulets

FRANCES G. KEAN

FIG. 46. Circulation of the blood.
(*See opposite page for caption.*)

352

Circulation of the Blood

The blood, composed mainly of red blood cells, white blood cells, platelets and plasma, enters the heart by way of the superior and inferior vena cava (Venous Inlet). From the right auricle it passes through the tricuspid valves into the right ventricle and flows into the pulmonary artery which carries it to the lung capillaries. It is replenished with oxygen and started back to the heart through the pulmonary veins. When the blood reaches the left auricle it passes by way of the mitral valve into the left ventricle, where it is distributed by the aorta to all the arteries of the body (except the pulmonary artery). In this way the blood furnishes the tissues of the body ("Muscle Shoals") with oxygen and food, and carries away carbon dioxide and waste by means of the veins to the vena cava and hence to the heart, where the whole process is repeated.

The heart and the blood and lymph vessels which make up the circulatory system of the body constitute a mechanism equipped to meet every need of the body under normal conditions. This mechanism automatically adjusts itself to changing and varying needs in every part of the body. Provision has been made for almost every contingency that may arise. In addition, nature has given this mechanism a wide margin of safety so that it may still continue to do its work, even after a considerable amount of damage to the heart has been sustained.

Except in the rare instances in which the structure of the heart is defective from birth, it continues to do its work day after day and year after year without its possessor being conscious of its activity.

Certain factors, while they may produce symptoms which make us conscious of the heart, probably never cause any impairment of function in a normal heart. Such factors are most frequently disturbances of the automatic nervous mechanism regulating all of the activities of the body. Such simple conditions as fatigue, worry, excitement, or digestive disturbances may alter the heart's action. Many of the unusual responses of the circulatory mechanism represent reactions which were purposeful in lower animal ancestors of mankind and should perhaps be interpreted as purposeful now. They disappear, however, when normal conditions are restored.

CHANGES IN THE HEART

Structural changes in the heart are largely permanent. They may be compensated for in many ways by the body, and there is such a wide margin of safety that the heart may continue to do its work for a normal lifetime in the presence of extensive damage. But such changes are never to be ignored. Such structural changes are due to two causes: infection or disease, and the degenerative changes which come with age. Possibly much of what is considered to be due to the degenerative changes in later life may also be the result of infection.

Overexertion does not injure a normal heart. Uncomfortable symptoms, or if these are not heeded, unconsciousness, stop the overexertion long before the heart is damaged. But overexertion can cause great and perhaps irreparable damage in a heart in which an active infection is present or in a heart previously damaged by infection.

Except, then, for the small group of hearts which are defective at birth, permanent changes in the structure of the heart which interfere with its function as a pump, and which are crippling, are due almost without exception to infection. If a heart is not able to perform its functions, either structural defects present at birth or structural changes acquired as the result of disease may be responsible.

CONGENITALLY DEFECTIVE HEARTS

A small number of children are born with hearts which are structurally defective. The defect may consist in a narrowing of one of the two large arteries leaving the heart, or there may be a defect in the structure of the heart itself which interferes with its function. This defect may so seriously interfere with the ability of the heart to do its work that the child may die at birth or shortly after. In other cases, when the defect is less serious, or when its presence is compensated for by other abnormal conditions, the child may survive for varying periods, or may even lead a normal life, with the heart doing its work well in spite of its handicaps.

A certain proportion of children who survive may suffer during childhood or later in life from shortness of breath on exertion and may have occasional fainting spells. They may appear blue, and the fingers may be "clubbed," that is, the ends may be broader and flatter than normal. Most of them are below normal in growth and development. The majority of children with such outward symptoms do not survive.

A few suffer little, if at all, and show no outward evidence of congenital heart disease. The condition may be discovered only incidentally in the course of a physical examination of the child for some other cause.

Children with hearts which are congenitally defective do not require any medical treatment for their condition. They do require attentive care of their general health and hygiene. They should be allowed to lead the lives of normal children as far as possible, always keeping within the limits of exertion which their defect has imposed. Exertion should not be allowed to produce more than a moderate shortness of breath.

One point of especial importance should always be kept in mind, that is, the increased likelihood of infection. Particularly to be guarded against is the predisposition to tuberculosis and to those infections which cause additional heart damage, as infective endocarditis. The child must be carefully guarded against exposure to infection, or to conditions which predispose to infection; and the general health must be kept at the highest possible level. Such children should receive the same care as those whose hearts have been previously damaged by rheumatic fever, and the same precautions should be taken. They should be examined at frequent and regular intervals, and any possible question of doubt should be referred at once to the physician for advice.

Hearts Defective because of Disease

The illness responsible for more heart disease than any other, and for almost all the heart disease of childhood and early life, is known variously as rheumatic fever, acute rheumatic fever, or inflammatory rheumatism. Chorea, or St. Vitus's dance, is only a manifestation of rheumatic fever.

The name "rheumatic fever" is not apt! The name "rheumatism" calls to mind symptoms of disease of the bones and joints, and rheumatic fever may exist and cause severe damage to the heart without any such symptoms or with symptoms so slight that they do not attract attention.

Fever, while it is doubtless present in some degree at times during the disease, may be a minor symptom or may remain undiscovered. However, the name "rheumatic fever" has been in general use for so long that it would be confusing and inadvisable to attempt to change it.

Manifestations of Rheumatic Fever in Childhood

Rheumatic fever is a generalized disease, not confined to any one part of the body. It is essentially chronic, and its course, in one form or another, covers a period of years. It should never be regarded as cured or as a closed incident, no matter how complete the apparent recovery after an acute attack may seem.

It may come on abruptly, or the onset may be insidious. There may never be any acute symptoms. It is, however, usually characterized by intervals of varying duration which come on more or less suddenly and sharply, and by much longer intervals of apparent quiescence, when but slight symptoms or none at all are apparent.

Most of the damage done to the heart occurs during the acute stages, but damage may also be going on slowly, though none the less certainly, during the periods when the disease is apparently inactive.

Rheumatic fever may exist and cause structural damage to the heart without any recognizable symptoms. Frequently unquestionable evidence of heart damage due to rheumatic disease is found in patients whose record, after the closest questioning, furnishes no clue to the time when the damage might have occurred.

The earlier and milder manifestations of rheumatic fever, unless accompanied by some more definite sign, such as rheumatic nodules on the bones, or the so-called growing pains, are difficult to differentiate from symptoms occurring in other conditions.

The child may only appear to be below what would be considered the normal health level. Colds and sore throats may appear with more than usual frequency. The weight may be below the normal average, or a loss of weight may occur rather conspicuously and suddenly. Fatigue is present out of all proportion to the play or exertion which brought it on. There may be loss of appetite, symptoms of stomach or intestinal disturbance, headache, nervous instability, or many other symptoms which are not characteristic of rheumatic fever particularly, but which are indicative of mild illness. There may be pallor, and a blood examination may reveal mild anemia, although sometimes the pallor is out of proportion to the anemia actually present. Blood examination may also show an increase in the number of white cells, indicating the presence of an infection, even during these mild and doubtful stages. The pulse may be more rapid than normal. Careful and repeated trials may indicate the presence of fever. A reliable temperature record, especially when only a slight rise is present, requires that even the best thermometer be held under the tongue for fully five minutes. Rectal temperatures are more reliable in children and require less time.

There is nothing characteristic of any one disease in the symptoms described. These cases do, however, demand careful examination and reëxamination by the family doctor. It is significant that there is a period of a few months up to three to five years of such indefinite symptoms, which have been called "toxic debility," in the majority of cases, before there is definite evidence of rheumatic fever. It is also significant that in many of these cases of toxic debility some evidence of rheumatic fever may occasionally be found on examination.

"Growing pains" are usually an important symptom and may occur during the doubtful stages. Many such indefinite pains are not significant, but there should always be careful questioning to determine their true nature. If there is any doubt, careful and repeated physical examination by the physician is of the greatest importance. About three fourths of all cases of rheumatic fever have had such pains. They are rather indefinite nagging muscle or joint pains, occurring anywhere, but most often in the legs, in front of the thighs, or behind the knees, or in the so-called "hamstring muscles." Sometimes the child complains of neck pains. Similar pains may occur from many natural causes. But no matter how mild they may be, they constitute an early danger signal. The watchful mother should listen to the child's story in order that the true nature of the pains may be determined.

Another minor manifestation which occurs with variable frequency is the "rheumatic nodule." It is a small round nodule, visible under the skin and movable. It is not tender. The size varies with the location, but on the average is about the size of a small pea. These nodules are most easily found where the tendons join the muscles with the bones, as close to the elbows or wrists, the knees, or the nape of the neck, or over the shoulder or hips, and less frequently over the shoulder blade or the collar bone. The presence of these nodules may be presumed to indicate rheumatic fever, although they have been observed in apparently healthy children, in cases in which rheumatic fever could not be definitely proved.

More frequently the actual onset of rheumatic fever occurs abruptly. It begins with the immediate appearance of joint symptoms or sometimes heart symptoms. There may be a short premonitory stage of fever. Some infection of the upper respiratory passages, such as a cold or sore throat, usually precedes the attack, and there may have been exposure to cold or dampness. In more than half the cases, the attacks begin with an inflammation of one or more joints. There is pain in the joint, which is swollen, tender, reddened, and feels hot to the touch. The symptoms may be severe or mild. The joints may be tender with little or no swelling, or slightly swollen with little or no tenderness. Characteristically the symptoms migrate from joint to joint, with a duration of one to eight days or more for each joint. At a given time, one or several joints may be involved. Fever is present from the start during these stages, and its height varies with each case. Its severity or lack of severity must never be taken as an index of the involvement of the heart.

Pleurisy or inflammation of the membrane lining the chest cavity may be the first symptom of the onset of rheumatic fever. Severe pain on breathing may occur suddenly, without any previous warning, or may follow after a few days of what is apparently only a "cold." The symptom of pain may disappear, and the pleura, or lining membrane of the chest, escape further trouble. Sometimes the pain may be followed by a collection of fluid in the chest cavity. Occasionally the fluid may appear silently without any preceding pain. A form of pneumonia, peculiar to rheumatic fever, may appear at the onset, but is more likely to occur later in the disease.

CHOREA

Chorea, or St. Vitus's dance, is another condition which occurs in rheumatic fever, much more frequently in girls, and is limited usually to the early school age. Most cases occur between the ages of five and ten, and most frequently independently of the joint symptoms. The child who has had choreic twitchings will probably have chorea when rheumatic fever recurs, just as the one with symptoms affecting the joints most frequently has joint symptoms when there is a recurrence. In a part of the cases chorea and joint symptoms are present at the same time, or the child may show chorea at one time and joint symptoms at another.

Heart disease probably ensues in the children with choreic manifestations just as frequently as it follows with other signs and symptoms. It does not always follow so promptly, however. Children with the joint symptoms usually develop the heart disease while they are still under observation because of the acute attack, or shortly after, although the appearance of heart disease is often delayed in them also. In chorea the heart disease most frequently appears later, after the symptoms of chorea have subsided, or even after a period of years. Chorea is less disabling and is often mild, and does not always attract the attention it should. Occasionally it occurs without being noticed. Sometimes there are only minor symptoms, such as fidgeting, restlessness, or lack of attention and concentration. The lack of concentration may be noticed only at school, or the nervousness may show in the handwriting. There may be loss of appetite, headache, and general nervous instability. The child may be forgetful, irritable, emotional, and may have crying spells. In the less mild cases the nervousness is more evident. There are spasmodic involuntary movements of the face and hands. The child may drop things that he is carrying and be unable to sit still. The more severe cases cannot escape attention. The spasmodic movements are more extreme and pronounced; the face is distorted, and there are uncontrollable grimaces. The tongue may be involuntarily thrust out; the speech may be interfered with.

Choreic manifestations are always worse during excitement or when attention is attracted to them. The choreic movements disappear during sleep. A child with chorea requires rest and quiet surroundings and should never be sent to school. Chorea should be considered as active rheumatic fever and treated as such.

Rheumatic Inflammation of the Heart (Carditis)

Inflammation of the heart and its consequences are as much a manifestation of rheumatic fever as are the joint symptoms or the nodules. It is not to be regarded as a complication or as an aftermath of rheumatic fever, but as an essential part. Rheumatic fever is a generalized chronic infection, doing similar damage to similar tissue in many parts of the body. The damage may be much greater in one part of the body than in another, or it may be more evident, because it may interfere with functions, as in the heart, or cause pain, as in the joints; or it may occur where it produces no symptoms and be silent. The heart may escape, or apparently escape, or the joints may escape, or both may escape and the infection manifest itself in some other way.

The infection may seem to expend all of its energy on the heart, and the effects of rheumatic fever on the heart may appear without previous evidence of rheumatic fever. Occasionally when a child is examined because of an acute attack of rheumatic fever with joint symptoms, or other manifestations, the heart is found to have been already involved at some previous time. In such cases there is always the probability that minor manifestations of rheumatic fever had occurred and were unobserved.

Such cases are not the common rule; more frequently involvement of the heart is associated with one or more of the other manifestations of rheumatic fever. Unless there are symptoms of pericarditis or inflammation of the heart sac, the inflammation of the heart may not be noticed at the onset and for a long period give no indication of its presence.

Pericarditis is an inflammation of the walls of the sac in which the heart is inclosed. As these inflamed walls rub past each other with each beat of the heart, they may cause intense pain. In some cases the pain is absent. Frequently fluid appears between the two walls of the pericardium, separating them, and sometimes causing great distention of the pericardial sac, even to the point of interfering with the work of the heart. This is referred to as *pericarditis with effusion.*

Pericarditis may be the first manifestation of rheumatic fever and may come on suddenly. It more frequently occurs in the course of the disease and in the presence of other manifestations. It always means that an inflammation of the heart is present. Rheumatic inflammation of the heart is to be considered as an inflammation involving all of the tissues of the heart. While one tissue, as the pericardium or the endocardium, may give more evidence of involvement than the other tissues, or may be more extensively involved than the other tissues, the other tissues do not escape.

Except when pericarditis makes an inflammation of the heart evident, signs of heart involvement, or changes in the heart which interfere with its function, may not appear for a long period after the actual involvement of the heart in the rheumatic inflammation. Indeed, such changes may not appear until long after all the other symptoms of rheumatic fever have subsided and the patient is apparently well.

Usually in such cases there is evidence that an inflammatory process is still active somewhere. A slight fever is found on careful examination, the pulse is more rapid than normal, and an increase in the number of white cells in the blood may be found on examination. Such a child should be kept in bed under the supervision of a doctor until all possible chance of an active infection of the heart has been ruled out.

The absence of signs of damage to the heart does not mean that an active inflammation of the heart is not present. Such signs of damage are the results of the inflammation, and not signs of the inflammation itself. No child in whom rheumatic fever is ever suspected should be allowed out of bed while there remains any elevation of temperature or until after the temperature has been normal for at least two weeks or more.

The heart may be found to be damaged three or four years after an attack of rheumatic fever without any evidence of an intervening attack having been noted, or, in the case of chorea, as long as seven years after the attack and with apparent good health in the intervening period. Probably in such cases a mild infection has recurred at intervals, or has been present all of the time, and careful examination and watching would have revealed its presence. Because of this it is essential that after any of the signs or symptoms of rheumatic fever the child should be carefully watched by its parents and frequently reëxamined by the physician.

Rheumatic fever causes what is essentially an inflammation of the whole heart, the enveloping membrane or the pericardium, the heart muscle or the myocardium, and its lining membrane or the endocardium. Because of the inflammation of the endocardium, deformities of the valves develop so that they cannot close properly. This may affect any of the valves, but most frequently the mitral valve, between the left auricle and ventricle, and the aortic valve are involved. Less frequently the tricuspid valve, between the right auricle and ventricle, and rarely the pulmonic valve are concerned. The mitral valves may have a deformity which is especially characteristic of rheumatic fever, a narrowing of the valve due to scar contraction following the inflammation, referred to as *mitral stenosis*. Such a deformity also prevents the valve from closing properly when the ventricle contracts. This makes an *"insufficiency"* of the valve (*valvular insufficiency*). so that the blood flows back into the auricle during contraction of the ventricle. This insufficiency of the mitral valve also occurs without the narrowing, and is what people refer to when they say they have a "leaky valve" or a "heart leak."

The heart muscle is invariably involved in the inflammation to some degree, perhaps slightly, or perhaps to a degree which interferes with its efficiency.

Permanent changes may also persist in the pericardium, increasing the work of the heart. The two layers, the one covering the heart and the one forming the sac in which the heart is suspended, may adhere together, so that at each beat the heart not only has to pull against the normal attachments of the pericardium, but frequently against new and abnormal attachments due to inflammation of the outer sac and its attachment to surrounding tissue.

In order to compensate for damage done to the heart, nature causes the heart to enlarge and the muscular walls to become stronger and thicker. In this way it can pump more blood at each stroke and make up for reflow of blood through the damaged valves, or it can pull against the adhesions of the pericardium to adjacent structures. A heart that has been damaged is almost always enlarged and in rheumatic fever may become greatly enlarged.

The Attack on Rheumatic Fever

Because of the increasing prevalence of heart disease, and especially because of the realization that rheumatic fever is productive of almost all of the heart disease which cripples in early life, much organized effort has been expended in an endeavor to discover exactly what conditions predispose to rheumatic fever and what is the causative infective agent. While this coördinated effort has taught much about rheumatic fever, it has not yielded the discovery of one or two definite underlying factors or any simple, specific treatment. However, knowledge has been systematized, and thus the way is prepared for future advance. The most important result has been the undertaking of an educational campaign, similar to that which has been so effective in the fight against tuberculosis.

Many acute infectious diseases are produced by one variety of germ, which always produces the disease when it enters the body under conditions favorable for its growth. In rheumatic fever the actual bacterial agent is not known. It is one of the streptococcus family, but there is some reason for thinking that it is not always the same one. Perhaps different streptococci produce similar bodily changes and responses in different people who offer a favorable soil for their growth. Or it may be that identical bacteria grow differently and show different characteristics under differing conditions. No one knows why, in a family in which all are infected by the same organism in an epidemic of sore throats or colds, one should develop rheumatic fever and the others escape. Rheumatic fever does not appear to be the result of one or two factors only. This is true of many chronic diseases which are caused by organisms with which all men are in frequent contact, but which find favorable conditions for growth only occasionally in certain predisposed people.

Rheumatic fever is probably the resultant of many factors in addition to the invading organism. The effects of many different environments on the growth of the germ and of different responses by different bodies to the growth of the organism must be considered. Some of these differences in environment or response may be determined by hereditary predisposition, by the effect of fatigue or exercise, by the effect of previous infections or ill health, or by many factors not accurately known.

There are several general conditions which seem to influence the incidence of rheumatic fever. In the first place it is much more frequent in the Caucasian or white race, although it does occur among all races. While it occurs all over the world, it is much more frequent in the temperate zones. When it does occur in the tropics, it is likely to run a milder course.

Damp climates have been considered an important factor; but apparently a damp climate does not necessarily predispose to rheumatic fever, nor does a dry or warm high climate prevent its occurrence. Rheumatic fever is not especially common in Holland, and is much less frequent there than in England or the northern United States. It is more common on the Mexican plateau than on the Mexican seaboard. In the West Indies it is infrequent. In Puerto Rico, in spite of poor living conditions, it is uncommon among the native population. It does occur in Egypt, but is unknown in the Malay peninsula. Much remains to be learned in regard to the influence of climate as a single factor in the incidence of rheumatic fever. This much can be said, however: that it is less frequent in warm climates and less common where there are no abrupt or sudden changes in temperature.

Bad housing, cold, damp surroundings, or proximity to water courses have been considered important causative factors. There is much to indicate that such conditions may be a determining influence in the occurrence of rheumatic fever, but again there is the low incidence in Holland, and there was a low incidence in the late war among the troops in the trenches.

There is much evidence to indicate that rheumatic fever is less common among the well-to-do. Life insurance data in this country show a definitely lower incidence among the more favored classes. Yet in England, while it is less frequent among the wealthy it is again less frequent among the very poor than among the moderately comfortable working classes. In Chicago an examination of all the children in three schools, representing different sections of society, showed no significant difference. While it is probable that social status is a factor, it is probably not as important a factor as would appear at first glance. Perhaps among the well-to-do predisposing ill health and minor infections are better cared for than among the poor. When rheumatic fever does occur it is recognized earlier and managed more adequately, so that there is less probability of serious consequence. Among the well-to-do classes there is less crowding and less frequenting of crowded places of amusement and crowded conveyances. There is much greater chance of transmitting minor infections of the nose and throat from one to another in crowded surroundings.

Probably there is a family predisposition to rheumatic fever. It is also difficult to be sure just how to evaluate the importance of contagion. Rheumatic fever is not contagious in the sense that it is transmissible from one developed case to another. Local epidemics have been reported and ward epidemics have occurred in hospitals. Epidemics of recurrences have been reported in convalescent homes for rheumatic fever patients. These may be explained as epidemics of colds or sore throats, referred to as "upper respiratory infections," which resulted in rheumatic fever in a part of those affected. When such an epidemic occurs among rheumatic fever patients, a "flare up" or recurrence of the original process takes place as a result of the epidemic of "upper respiratory infections."

Rheumatic fever does show annual variation, in which there are years of increased incidence and years of lower incidence. This would suggest some epidemic influence, although it may be that these variations are due to climatic or other causes.

There are seasonal changes also. In the United States rheumatic fever is more frequent in late winter and early spring than in March, April, and May. In England it is more frequent in the fall months.

Rheumatic fever is much more common in childhood; indeed, it is largely a disease of childhood. There are a few cases from three to five years of age, but after five the frequency steadily increases until the twelfth year. After twelve the frequency of the initial attacks decreases, and they are much less frequent after twenty, but do occur with constantly diminishing frequency through old age.

Rheumatic fever, generally considered, is somewhat more frequent in girls, and the choreic manifestations are much more frequent in girls.

The debilitated child seems to have what has been termed the pre-rheumatic state. This may be a definite constitutional state, due to inherited tendencies, or to repeated minor infections, or deficiencies in diet and general care; or perhaps it is actually a stage of the disease itself. The truth probably includes both views: that it is a definite predisposing constitutional state, and that among the group are many who already show the minor manifestations of rheumatic fever. Such conditions either predispose to rheumatic fever or actually may be a part of it.

Some children are under the standard of weight for their age, are prone to listlessness, and tire more easily than a normal child. Such children have poor appetites, constipation, and other minor and indefinite symptoms. These children are especially liable to recurrent upper respiratory infections, or colds. By the upper respiratory tract is meant the upper air passages, the membrane of the nose and pharynx and the lymphoid tissue of the tonsils, adenoids, and walls of the pharynx. It is a question as to whether these recurring infections are a cause or a result of the subnormal condition of the health. The same question applies to the gastro-intestinal symptoms.

However indefinite may be the effect of these factors on the incidence of rheumatic fever, there can be no doubt of the importance of infections of the upper respiratory tract as a whole. Such infections are almost always associated with the occurrence and recurrence of the different manifestations of rheumatic fever, with the single exception that there is a less close relationship with the occurrence of chorea.

This of course brings up the question of the relation of the tonsils to rheumatic fever. The tonsils are frequently the portion of the upper respiratory tract most obviously infected, although similar infection may be and usually is present in other portions. The tonsils are only a part of the tissue which may be involved in such infections. Their normal function is to act as a barrier to infection.

The fact that the tonsils are only a part of the tissues which may serve as a point of entrance for the infection must be borne in mind in considering the prevention of rheumatic fever and the prevention of its recurrence and progress. Normal tonsils serve as a barrier to infection and should not be removed under any circumstances, even if they are larger than normal. The same applies to tonsils which have recurring attacks of infection but are normal between the attacks. The inflammation at such times is due to the fact that the tonsils are acting as a barrier to infection. Not infrequently, when tonsils of this type are removed, the attacks still recur, involving the walls of the pharynx, and are not only just as frequent, but more resistant to treatment.

If the tonsils, however, have constant, chronic infection, they should be removed. Such chronically infected tonsils need not be large. Small

tonsils which show signs of chronic infection, associated with enlargement of the glands of the neck and large, ragged chronically infected
tonsils, should be removed. Adenoids which are infected or are an
obstruction to breathing should of course always be removed. Such a
procedure will at least aid in conserving the health of the child and
will tend to make attacks or recurrences less likely.

PREVENTION

The prevention of rheumatic fever is largely a matter of attention
to the many details which go to insure the best possible general
health. Absolute rules for this care cannot be put in detail, for just
what are the best conditions vary with the individual child. In general
they may be summarized in the words "good maternal care." This will
mean first of all a quiet, restful home life, free from the disturbing
influences which make a "nervous child," with the attendant disturbance of digestion and sleep. It will mean well-ordered and adequate
rest periods and supervised recreation. Overfatigue interferes with
digestion and rest and predisposes to infection. A rest period of a half
hour before and after meals will aid in digestion and nutrition.

The clothing should be warm and adequate. Damp, wet clothing
should be changed at once. Fresh air in the home and sleeping quarters
is essential, but quest for it may be carried to an extreme. Fresh air
need not be damp, irritating air. Certainly infections of the nose and
throat have been made worse by overenthusiasm in the matter of fresh
air. Here again individual judgment must be applied to each child.

The diet should be a sensible, easily digested, nutritious general
diet, without extremes in any direction. Vitamin deficiency is not apt
to play a part in the diet of an ordinary American home. It may be,
and usually is, advisable to give cod-liver oil in some form during the
dark months of the year. That is a matter for the physician to decide.
Vitamin B is probably the vitamin most likely to be deficient in the
ordinary diet.

Colds and sore throats are more apt to be contracted from the
"droplet infection" of crowds, or crowded places of amusement or
public conveyances. Minor colds and sore throats should be watched
and treated carefully, and the child should be kept in the house for a
period after all temperature has subsided.

Children with chronic throat, nose, and sinus infections should receive especially watchful care at home and be under the observation

of a physician. When possible they should be given the benefit of a warm, equable climate, if only for a time, where such infections are at least less frequent. The treatment of rheumatic fever when it has once occurred is a matter for the best judgment of a good physician. There is no specific cure or drug or serum. There are just two factors of known and certain value: Absolute Rest and Time.

On the part of the family the physician can best be helped by patience and by not trying to hurry him. The child should be in bed for at least two weeks or for even a longer time, after the fever has completely subsided. He should be allowed out of bed only gradually and with very careful watching. Reëxamination by the physician should be frequent.

After the infection is over, if the amount of damage done is not so great but that the heart is able to do its work adequately, no treatment is necessary. The heart damage is done and cannot be undone. If the heart is able to do its work now, it can always continue to do it, provided that no further infection occurs to do further damage. Nature has provided so wide a margin of safety that even after repeated infections the heart may still perform its daily work adequately.

Prevention of further infection and the resultant damage is again a matter of daily care as to health as considered briefly under the section entitled "Prevention."

If the damage done to the heart has been such as to prevent the adequate performance of its duties as a pump, this will be evidenced by discomfort after exertion, as by shortness of breath, or swelling of the feet after the patient has been on his feet for a variable period. Such a condition always calls for constant medical attention and will demand further complete and prolonged rest and usually medication. Any child or grown-up who has ever had any of the manifestations of rheumatic fever should have frequent examinations by the family physician, even in the absence of any symptoms.

ENDOCARDITIS

While rheumatic fever is the one largest single factor in the production of heart disease, other illnesses arise later in life which are also causatives. Just at the time when rheumatic fever is becoming less frequent, endocarditis, or inflammation of the interior of the heart, begins to appear. It may occur in childhood but is uncommon until after puberty, when its frequency increases until some time in the early twenties, at which time it gradually decreases, although it may persist through all ages.

Endocarditis occurs much more frequently in those who have previously had rheumatic fever, and this is especially true of the less acute forms.

The acute, sudden, sharp form may occur at any age, and usually occurs in the course of some severe illness such as pneumonia, childbirth fever, multiple abscesses with pyemia, severe gonorrheal infection, influenza, severe tonsillitis, or recurrences of rheumatic fever. The causative germ is in each case the causative germ of the original infection. This condition is always more prone to occur in hearts previously damaged by rheumatic fever, or in those with congenital defects. Unlike rheumatic carditis, it is limited largely to the lining membrane, or endocardium of the heart.

The symptoms of the acute endocarditis are those of a severe acute infection with high fever, chills, and prostration. Recovery is infrequent; indeed, it occurs only in rare instances.

The milder, subacute form is of more concern because some cases of this form do actually recover, and others might recover if recognized more promptly. This form is much more closely related to rheumatic fever, and at least 80 to 90 per cent of cases follow rheumatic fever infection. The connection is so close that in many cases there is some doubt as to the separate identity. In the acute form only a little over half are due to the streptococcus, while in the subacute form about 95 per cent are due not only to the streptococcus, but to one type of streptococcus, the *S. viridans*, and the remaining 5 per cent are divided between other forms of streptococci, the influenza bacillus and the gonococcus.

As in the acute form, the infection is practically confined to the endocardium, especially to the valves, where it results in a productive inflammation, causing vegetation upon the valves, with underlying ulceration of the tissue.

The symptoms may be mild indeed at the onset, so mild as to attract little or no attention for a long time. The condition is frequently similar to mild, incipient tuberculosis. There may be only fatigue on slight effort, weakness, feeling of malaise, or slight digestive disturbance, or loss of weight and strength. There may be some pallor, and an actual anemia is often present.

Fever is invariably present, although there may be periods of days when it is absent. It varies, from a rise of only a fraction of a degree in the milder cases to higher temperatures in the more sharp types. In the cases associated with the higher temperatures, chills may occur. The pulse rate is usually faster than normal.

The fingers may show clubbing, the spleen is usually enlarged, and the symptoms of the preëxisting heart disease may be accentuated. At some time during the disease what are known as petechiæ, or spots, always occur. They should be watched for constantly, as they occur in crops with sometimes long intervals between them, and last only for a day or two or three days. They are small round red dots, not appreciably raised, and differing in size, rarely larger than a pinhead in diameter, and do not disappear on pressure. They occur most frequently above and below the collar bone and over the chest, but may extend over the abdomen, down the arms, or to the back. They are frequently seen in the white of the eye, where they cannot be confused with minor blemishes of the skin.

Still another sign of the disease is the occurrence of emboli in various parts of the body. These are small fragments which have become detached from the growths on the valves of the heart, and are carried by the blood stream through the arteries to lodge in some distant part. The symptoms and signs will vary with the site of the artery which is occluded by the embolus. Occasionally the lodgment of such an embolus in the brain, with consequent paralysis, or in the spleen, with intense pain, or in the kidney with pain and the appearance of blood in the urine, or in one of the arteries of the extremity, is the first symptom which brings the disease to the attention of the patient and his physician.

There is every gradation between the mild type of the disease and the severe. In the milder cases there is always at least some chance of recovery, and the chance is greater the earlier it is recognized that the infection is present and treatment started. Treatment, again, consists primarily of just two factors: absolute rest in bed and time. [Recently doctors have been testing sulfanilamide derivatives in these cases. Transfusion of blood from persons who have had the disease and recovered, who are rare indeed, are also frequently tried in these cases.—Ed.]

Syphilis of the Heart

Syphilis of the heart and aorta may occur in the twenties but is more common in middle and in later middle life; it is the causative factor in much heart disease first appearing at this time, and especially among certain elements of the population.

Syphilis of the heart may exist silently until extensive or irreparable damage has been done. For this reason repeated blood examinations, like Wassermann or Kahn tests, should be made on those in whom there is any reason to suspect the disease to have occurred, no matter how well it has been treated. The heart should be carefully watched, and the observations checked by X-ray examination, for the infection does not always show in the blood examination. A physician's examination may not always be conclusive, even with the X-ray as a check.

When syphilitic disease of the heart is known to be present, treatment should be directed primarily at the heart condition, and the underlying syphilis may be treated secondarily and with great caution.

Heart Changes in Hyperthyroidism

In the cases known as toxic thyroid, or exophthalmic goiter, or more popularly known by the misleading name "inward goiter," there is an oversecretion of thyroid material or a secretion which is in some way abnormal.

In these cases there is almost invariably one symptom referable to the heart: the rapid pulse rate. Occasionally there may be an abnormal rhythm, or some shortness of breath, or even pain. The presence of a definite increase in the metabolic rate will confirm the diagnosis.

Such symptoms subside when the abnormal condition of the gland is remedied, by operation or otherwise. It is doubtful just how much, if any, permanent damage is done by the toxic thyroid itself, or how much if any damage persists after the symptoms of thyroid disease are relieved.

Angina Pectoris and Coronary Thrombosis

In later life, in addition to the degenerative changes which must eventually occur in the heart as elsewhere, there are two conditions associated with the heart which are of especial importance. These are *angina pectoris*, and *coronary thrombosis*. Each has pain of the same character, which is usually the outstanding symptom, but the significance is different in each case. Coronary thrombosis is a single incident with prolonged pain, and with permanent damage done to the heart during the attack, which may be great or may be slight indeed. In angina pectoris identical pain occurs but is of short duration and recurs in attacks at varying intervals, without symptoms between attacks, and often with perfect health in other regards. Only within recent years has it been learned how distinct the two are when they occur typically.

Each of the two conditions has as its basis an interference with the blood supply to the heart muscle; in the one case prolonged, and in the other momentary.

The heart muscle is supplied with the blood necessary for its activity and life by means of vessels which run through the heart muscle itself, dividing and subdividing, to furnish an abundant supply of blood to every part of the heart muscle.

These arteries have their origin in the aorta, the large vessel leading from the heart, at its beginning, just as it leaves the left ventricle or chamber of the heart, and just above the valves which separate the aorta from the ventricle. The flow through these arteries will be greater or less as the pressure in the aorta is greater or less, and vary also somewhat with the rate of the heart, the flow becoming greater as the rate increases. Any changes in the lining of the aorta which would narrow the opening of the arteries as they leave the aorta might interfere with the flow of blood through them. As the walls of the arteries become thickened and the arteries narrowed with age, their ability to furnish an adequate blood supply is obviously subject to interference. Nature has furnished some safeguards, by increasing the connection between the different arteries as age increases, so that if one artery in one locality is insufficient, blood may be detoured through the other pathways. There are nerves going to the walls of these arteries also from the central regulating nervous system of the body so that their caliber may be increased or decreased by impulses from other parts.

Any factor which interferes with the flow of blood through these arteries interferes with the supply of blood essential for the heart muscle. Symptoms develop, the severity and duration of which depend on how seriously the blood supply is interfered with. When a muscle

anywhere in the body is obliged to contract, and when it has not a
supply of blood sufficient for its needs, there is always pain. This is
the cause of the pain occurring in coronary thrombosis and in angina
pectoris.

ANGINA PECTORIS

In angina pectoris symptoms are of short duration, because the
blood supply is only temporarily diminished, or because it is insufficient for the work of the heart just at that time, as when some extra

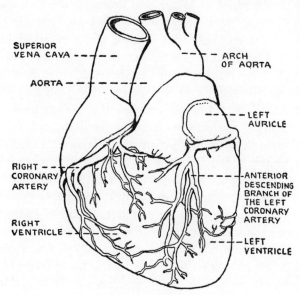

FIG. 47. Circulation and blood supply of the
heart.

demand is made on the heart. Such a decrease in the blood supply of
the heart might be due to a temporary and transient narrowing of
the vessels supplying the heart with blood, due to nervous impulses
having their origin elsewhere. Since the flow through these arteries
rises and falls with the blood pressure in the aorta, a fall in blood
pressure, as occurs during sleep, or as occurs during the day from
many causes, might decrease the flow to a point at which it would
cause pain. This is particularly the case in a heart whose arteries
show the hardening which comes with age, but would probably not
cause any symptoms in a more normal heart. Whatever may cause the

temporary decrease in the flow of blood in the vessels of the heart itself, it is this decrease and the consequent transient inadequacy of the blood supply to the heart which causes the symptoms.

Pain is the one most important symptom in angina pectoris. The pain is usually under the breast bone, and more frequently under the upper portion of the breast bone, or just to the left of the upper portion. It may remain in that position, or it may radiate to the shoulder, or down the left arm, perhaps only as far as the elbow, or the wrist, or it may extend to the tips of the fingers. Occasionally it may radiate to the right shoulder and down the right arm, or it may radiate to both shoulders, and down both arms. In other persons it may radiate to the left side of the neck or be referred to the lower back teeth. In others it may radiate to the pit of the stomach and be considered as having its origin in the stomach, or it may be felt just below the ribs on the right side. Frequently the pain may never be felt in the chest at all, and be felt only at the points to which it may radiate, as the left shoulder, the elbow, or the little and the ring finger, or the left lower jaw, or the pit of the stomach. The pain is often severe and agonizing, but it is not necessarily so, and may be mild.

Except for these symptoms, associated or appearing singly, there is nothing which characterizes an attack, except that it is of short duration, a matter of seconds or minutes. Attacks lasting hours, or with other symptoms, are not merely angina pectoris.

There are no certain signs which enable the physician to recognize the presence of an attack or to judge of the probability of the future occurrence of such an attack. Nothing characteristic can be found by examination of the heart, or the pulse or blood pressure, or by laboratory methods. The physician must be guided altogether by the story of the attack and such characteristics as the patient tells him.

Attacks are most frequently brought on by exertion. In some persons they are brought on by moderate exertion at any time; in others by moderate exertion only under certain conditions; and in others the attacks may accompany only unusual exertion. Attacks are especially apt to accompany exertion soon after a meal. With an empty stomach a man may be able to walk briskly for a long distance without distress and find himself unable to walk a hundred feet after a meal without symptoms of pain. In some the attacks may follow exertion after any meal, or may follow especially some one meal, as in the evening or in the morning. Attacks are likely to follow a meal which is too hastily eaten, or one which is indigestible, or too full a meal, or one eaten when too tired.

For these reasons, it is best not to eat when tired, nor to eat heavily at such a time. It is well to take a rest period before and after each meal and to eat leisurely. The diet should be chosen so as to avoid those foods which are indigestible or which in the patient's experience cause gas.

Attacks are more likely to occur also when walking facing a cold wind, or walking up an incline, or when there is a sense of being hurried, even though the pace is no more rapid than usual.

Exertion does not necessarily bring on an attack. An attack may come when sitting quietly, especially after a meal. An attack may occur in the early morning hours in the midst of a normal sleep.

When Heberden first described angina pectoris in 1785 he spoke of the effect of what he referred to as "passionate affections of the mind" and of "hypochondriac languors" in producing the attack. This was a true observation. Attacks are more frequent in the emotionally and nervously unstable. Any emotion may bring on an attack, but especially anger, grief, or worry. It is not unusual for the attack to begin with the onset of business reverses. Attacks are more frequent also in the presence of fatigue, and especially of nervous or mental fatigue.

While angina pectoris may occur in people in any walk of life, it is much more common in those whose work demands an undue proportion of strain and energy and worry, and who are obliged to do their work under tension, or what is especially true, those who are so constituted that they do any work under tension, and with an undue amount of nervous energy. This is probably one reason why angina pectoris is more frequent in cities and why it is much less frequent in the more leisurely tropics. It is always less frequent in the more placid and tranquil, and in those who do their work easily and quietly, and who provide themselves with adequate recreation which relaxes and rests.

Much could be said in favor of quiet evenings at home, in favor of leisurely week-ends instead of those spent in long and tiresome motor trips, and in favor of quiet and restful vacations of adequate length.

Angina pectoris is by no means the hopeless disease which is often pictured. It may be serious, but it is possible in many cases for patients to go on for years with recurring attacks, or the attacks may cease to occur and the patient lead a normal life with only moderate restrictions.

CORONARY THROMBOSIS

In coronary thrombosis the pain is identical with the pain of angina pectoris, and occurs for the same reason: some part of the heart muscle is deprived of its necessary blood supply. In angina pectoris the insufficient supply of blood is only transient, the pain quickly passes away, and actual damage is not done to the heart muscle. In coronary thrombosis a clot forms in one of the coronary arteries, or more frequently in one of the branches, and a portion of the heart muscle is deprived of blood for a length of time sufficient to do damage, and frequently a great deal of damage. The seriousness of the accident depends on the size and location of the branch which is stopped up by the clot, and on how successfully the heart is able to detour blood through the other arteries to the heart muscle beyond the clot.

In coronary thrombosis, the pain, instead of being a matter of minutes, as in angina pectoris, is a matter of hours or days. Often it is relieved only with difficulty. Here, also, other symptoms are in evidence. There is almost always shortness of breath, even when lying quietly, and the patient may be obliged to recline propped up in bed and may not be able to lie down flat. There may be some cough, because of water accumulating in the lungs as a result of the impaired circulation. The patient may become blue and the hands and feet cold and pulseless. The pulse is usually rapid, or rapid and irregular, and characteristic changes may show in electrocardia graphic tracings taken in the laboratory. The blood pressure almost invariably falls to a low level.

Just as in angina pectoris, the symptoms are not always typical and show many variations. The pain may be slight, transient, or even absent. But the shortness of breath, the rapid, or rapid and irregular, pulse and the fall in blood pressure are sufficient to establish the probability of what has happened. There is more than has been enumerated here: the patient is usually obviously ill, and the general condition affords little doubt that something serious has taken place.

The patient with recurring attacks of angina pectoris is in most cases better if allowed to go about his daily duties with moderate restrictions. The patient with a coronary thrombosis must have absolute rest in bed, quiet, and careful medical supervision and nursing for weeks. His future activities will depend on how much damage has been done and the nature of the damage.

Disordered Action of the Heart

In a large group of cases, especially in early life, there are symptoms regarded often as due to the heart, especially by the patient, but in whom the heart and the circulatory system are perfectly normal structurally. What is abnormal is the automatic nervous mechanism controlling the heart and controlling all of the activities of the body. This automatic nervous system temporarily responds to smaller stimuli than normal, and when it does respond, overresponds. An exertion which would make the pulse of a normal individual beat only a little more rapidly than normal causes the pulse of such a person to beat exceedingly rapidly. An exertion which would hardly affect the rate of breathing in a normal person would cause rapid breathing in such a person.

During sleep, or when resting quietly or unobserved, the pulse and the respiration are normal. On exertion, and in some cases on slight exertion, the pulse becomes rapid, and there is severe shortness of breath. The hands and feet, and sometimes the entire body, may appear blue. The hands are cold and wet, even in a warm room. Such patients often complain of what they refer to as dizziness; this is not a real dizziness, when there is a sense of rapid rotation, but is rather a giddiness, a sense of unsteadiness; surrounding objects may appear to sway or turn slowly. Fainting attacks are frequent among such patients and rare in actual cases of heart disease. Some of these patients complain of pain in the heart region.

When they are examined, the heart is always normal in size and normal in every determinable way. If it is not normal, the case does not belong to this group. To add to the difficulties, what is called a heart murmur is often heard. It is the kind of murmur which, although it is heard in heart disease, is also heard in normal hearts, and is not of significance in a heart of normal size. In those belonging to this group, the murmur is rarely constant. It may be heard at one time and a few moments later may have completely disappeared.

Such patients often complain of various other symptoms, which are on a nervous basis. They will in addition show a lack of initiative, an unwillingness to go about their normal duties, and be subject to worry, and fear, and apprehension. Others may lead a normal life, be energetic in their work, but still show the symptoms referable to the heart.

These cases may suffer real disability, but a disability that is not based on actual abnormal changes in the body structure; the disability is not permanent.

There is always a certain proportion of such people in any population. They are frequently classified as having real heart disease or as having thyroid disease, or early tuberculosis, or as being simply neurotic. Such hearts have been a source of disability in every war, for many decades past. In the Civil War they were known as "soldiers' hearts." In the late World War, when armies of such large size were mobilized, the number of men incapacitated in this way was so great that an especial study was necessary.

The condition is little more than a group of symptoms which might occur in any of us if he were overtired, or with what might be termed chronic fatigue, or if some mild infection were present, or after a too brief and inadequate convalescent period following an illness or an operation, or with the undue mental strain of prolonged worry or apprehension. In those more robust, much fatigue or physical or mental disturbance is necessary. In those not so well equipped constitutionally, the symptoms might follow on minor causes. One aviator or one broker or one worker might develop the symptoms after a few hours in the air or in the market, and another only after many more hours; another might never develop them.

In the army a period of rest and recreation always restored the soldier to normal. Of the large number who showed the symptoms on entrance into the army from civil life, or who developed the symptoms in the army, more than half were restored to normal in camps where they were given special care and put on gradually increased exercise.

Care should be taken that there is no underlying minor infection in such cases. An adequate period for convalescence should always be allowed after illness or even a minor operation. When these symptoms are present, rest, recreation, exercise increased gradually and carefully, and attention to the general health should restore the patient to normal.

It is unfortunate that there are no facilities available for general use such as those which the army offered, where the patient could be put on a carefully supervised routine, with supervised graduated exercise, and where he would not be associated with the group of nervous and near-mental cases found in the ordinary sanatorium. What are greatly needed are convalescent centers for such cases, located in the country, with special facilities for rest, recreation, and exercise.

CHAPTER XV

Digestion and Digestive Diseases
DRS. MILTON M. AND SIDNEY A. PORTIS

INTRODUCTION

THE TERM "INDIGESTION" *is an unscientific word like dyspepsia, but almost everyone knows what it means. It merely means that the person who suffers with this symptom is having trouble with the digesting of his food or in absorbing it. Some years ago the word "dyspepsia" was one to conjure with. It described the great American disease, now transformed into the possibly more scientific term "nervous indigestion." However, as will be seen in the following pages, there is far more to a consideration of the disturbance of the gastro-intestinal tract than merely indigestion or dyspepsia.*

As will be seen from the illustrations accompanying these articles, the gastro-intestinal tract extends from the mouth, through the pharynx, the esophagus, the stomach, the small intestines, including the duodenum, the jejunum, and the ileum. The large intestines include the cecum, the ascending, transverse, and descending colon, the sigmoid and the rectum, to the point of excretion of undigested material and wastage known as the anus. Moreover, this central tube for digesting and absorbing food is in intimate contact with most of the organs of the body which are concerned with aiding the process of digestion and absorption.

The glands empty into the gastro-intestinal tract at various points and provide the secretions that are necessary for digestion. Blood vessels and tubes of various kinds carry away the digested materials and distriubte the basic substances for tissue building and repair throughout the body. In the debates that are frequently held as to what are the important tissues of the body, the gastro-intestinal tract will take a very high place.

In the articles which follow, an attempt has been made to discuss the diseases of the gastro-intestinal tract and the organs associated therewith, and at the same time to explain something of the mechanisms involved in the development of these diseases. It might be taken for granted that the control of dietary diseases is practically always dietetic. While diet is important, there are many other factors which are probably even more important in relationship to controlling such diseases. Mechanical, glandular, and infectious causes are probably more frequently responsible for diseases of the stomach and intestines than are merely irregularities of the diet. For this reason the articles which are here included do not provide corrective diets for some of the gastro-intestinal diseases. The subject is, however, discussed in the chapter on diet, and special diets used in some of the gastro-intestinal diseases are there provided.

M. F.

THE MOUTH is the first organ in which digestion begins. The tongue, with its taste-buds, distinguishes between types and varieties of foods. There is the sense of sweet, sour, salt, and bitter and the feel of the food upon the tongue. The nose with its sense of smell helps to give piquancy to the sense of taste. With the aid of the teeth, the food is chewed; then, emulsified by saliva from the glands on each side of the jaw, it is made easy to swallow. In addition, the saliva begins partial digestion of starches. The more completely the food is chewed, the easier it is to swallow, and later the more readily is it digested.

The esophagus is just a tube that conveys the food from the mouth to the stomach. It is controlled by nerves from the central nervous system in the spine and brain. At its bottom end it is closed by a sphincter (a muscle surrounding the outlet) to prevent too rapid entrance of food or liquid into the stomach. The mucus from the glands of the esophagus is supplied purely for lubrication.

As the food and water enter the stomach, the first really important digestion begins. Here the food is mixed with gastric (stomach) juice. This juice is ordinarily a thin, colorless, or nearly colorless liquid with strong acid reaction. Belching of sour fluid is a reflection of this acidity. The essential constituents of the gastric juice are an acid (hydrochloric) and two or possibly three enzymes (digestive ferments) called pepsin, rennin, and lipase. There are many patent medicines based on these substances. They will be discussed later. The stomach itself consists of an outer layer, called the peritoneum; a muscle layer, in which the blood vessels and nerves lie; a submucous membrane; and an inner lining called the mucosa. The glands of secretion are in the mucosa, and the absorption of material goes on through its tissues.

The acid of the gastric juice is a mineral acid and is present in considerable strength. It is secreted by acid cells situated in the glands of the mucous lining. The other constituents of gastric juice are secreted normally at the same time as the acid. The pouring out of gastric juice is first started by the sensations of taste and smell; i.e., it is a psychical secretion. Stimuli from the nose and mouth call forth, reflexly, a secretion in the stomach. Secretion in the mouth and stomach may begin by the sight or at thought of food. This is the reason that the mouth waters under such conditions.

Certain foods contain substances designated as secretagogues, which are able to cause a secretion of gastric juice when taken into the stomach. Thus, meat extracts, meat juices, and soups are particularly effective in this respect, while milk and water cause less secretion. In other foods, these ready-formed secretagogues are present in smaller amount or may be lacking. Certain common articles of food, such as bread and white of egg, have no effect of this kind at all.

Of the enzymes or digestive ferments, pepsin is the most important. Peculiarly pepsin acts only in an acid medium. If acid is absent, pepsin remains inactive. The result of digestion in the stomach is to convert the protein of the food into a simpler and more soluble form. Thus proteins are only partially digested in the stomach. Rennin is another enzyme, whose main purpose is to coagulate milk. It is rapid in its action, especially in an acid medium. The fats are not digested in the stomach but are liquefied owing to the body heat. The starches or carbohydrates are acted on not by stomach secretion properly but by an enzyme called ptyalin which is present in saliva and continues to exert its action in the stomach. In this way food is prepared for intestinal digestion.

There is some absorption in the stomach. Little water is absorbed, while alcohol is readily absorbed. Some salts and sugar and the soluble proteins are absorbed slowly, while fats are probably not absorbed at all. The food and the products of the changes in the stomach undergo most complete digestion in the intestinal tract. Here also the final products of digestion are mainly absorbed.

Intestinal digestion begins in the duodenum, the first portion of the small bowel attached to the stomach. It is called duodenum from the Greek words meaning two and ten, because it is twelve fingers long. Digestion is largely completed by the time the food arrives at the end of the small intestine. This is effected through the combined action of three secretions: the pancreatic juice, the secretion from the intestinal glands (*succus entericus*), and the bile. These secretions are mixed with the food beginning in the duodenum, and their action proceeds simultaneously.

The pancreas is a long, narrow gland situated in the back wall of the abdomen. Its secretion into the intestine is composed of three enzymes: trypsin, which splits up proteins; lipase, which splits up fats; and amylase, which digests starch. The direct secretion is distinctly alkaline, in contradistinction to the acid of the stomach. Besides, it has an internal secretion into the blood called insulin, the secretion necessary to prevent diabetes. Thus the food proteins are completely broken down into their finer components—amino-acids— and when absorbed as such, the body constructs its own peculiar type of protein from these split products.

The tissue cells reconstruct from these pieces—or building stones— a form of protein adaptable to their needs and more or less characteristic for the needs of a particular organ. Just as letters of the alphabet may be combined in different ways to make different words, so various amino-acids may be combined to make proteins of different kinds.

Starchy food that escapes digestion in the mouth and stomach is digested in the duodenum, where it is split up into absorbable sugars. The fats are split up into fatty acids, and when the latter are combined with alkaline salts they form soaps. The digestion of fats is materially aided by the presence of bile. The mixture of bile and pancreatic juice digests neutral fats more rapidly. There are certain enzymes secreted by the small intestine. These effect the final stage in preparation of the food for absorption. There is, in addition, a hormone or excitant of gland secretion in the small intestine, called secretin, which stimulates the flow of pancreatic juice.

Absorption takes place readily in the small intestine. Carbohydrates are absorbed for the most part as simple sugars. From the intestines these pass into the liver, where some are stored as glycogen —the material used for muscle action—so that the amount of sugar

in the blood is kept quite constant. When a large amount is taken and
the liver is not able to take care of it readily, it increases in the blood,
and later the excess may appear in the urine, provided the kidneys
are normal. Those carbohydrates which escape digestion undergo
bacterial fermentation with the formation of acids.

Fats are absorbed with the aid of the bile, especially the bile salts.
They, for the most part, do not pass through the liver but get into
the general circulation by way of the lymph stream. They are picked
up in the lymph directly from the intestine. From the general circulation they are taken to the cells of the body for their use.

Proteins are split up or absorbed in the intestinal wall, and, as explained, pass through the liver for the most part, later to build up the
protein of the tissues. Some proteins escape and pass into the large
intestine, where they are acted on by bacteria.

The secretion of the large intestine, while it contains much mucus
and has an alkaline reaction, does not seem to have any distinctive
enzymes. Water is readily absorbed from the colon or large intestine.
The alkaline reaction makes the colon a favorable environment for
bacteria. Putrefaction is a normal occurrence in the large intestine.
The splitting of the protein which escaped small intestinal digestion
is completed here. Many of the products are given off in the stool,
while others are absorbed in part and excreted subsequently in the
urine. It is well known that excessive bacterial action may lead to
intestinal troubles, such as diarrhea, or possibly to more serious interference with general nutrition, owing to the formation of poisonous
products.

The Feces or "Stool"

The end products of digestion are excreted, for the most part, by
the bowel as the stool; the composition of the excretion from the bowel
depends on the character of the food eaten. If the diet is composed
exclusively of meats, the stool is small in amount and dark in color;
with an ordinary mixed diet, the amount is increased, and it is largest
with an exclusively vegetable diet, especially vegetables containing
cellulose of much crude fiber. When the processes of digestion and
absorption are entirely normal, the stool should be well formed and
devoid of offensive odor. If it is soft or liquid with a disagreeable
odor, there have been indiscretions in diet or some distinctly abnormal
causes. In other words, such excretions are an indication of some

abnormality in the digestive mechanism. The bad odor is usually due to excessive putrefaction.

When the excretion of the bowel is studied with a microscope the following constituents may be seen or found chemically: (1) Undigested material, such as ligaments of meat or cellulose from vegetables; (2) undigested material, such as fragments of meat, starch, or fats which have in some way escaped digestion; naturally, the quantity of this material present is slight under normal conditions; (3) unabsorbable material; (4) products of bacterial decomposition; (5) mucus and cells thrown off from the lining of the intestinal tract; (6) color or pigment, especially from the bile; (7) salts—inorganic salts, salts of sodium, potassium, calcium, magnesium and iron with phosphoric acid; (8) bacteria—these may make up two thirds of the weight of the material, and, (9) the gases, which arise mainly from bacterial action, especially on protein, although some of it may be due to swallowed air.

The liver has an important part in the general nutrition of the body. Its functions are manifold. Most of the absorbable material, except fats, passes through it. In addition to being the defense mechanism against poisonous products manufactured in the intestine, it also possesses a secretion called bile which plays an important part in digestion, especially of fats. Sugars have an important rôle in the normal activities of the liver, and depletion of sugars at times leads to serious damage to the organ. The liver has a great deal to do with almost every function of the body. The coagulation or clotting of blood is dependent on its proper functioning. The liver is the largest organ in the body. It has been estimated that it is seven times as large as necessary, this constituting a factor of safety.

Bile is composed of bile pigment, bile acids, salts, water, mucus, etc. It is formed in the liver cells and passes into small ducts or tubes which lead to larger channels; then some passes into the gall bladder, for purposes of storage, and some goes directly into the small intestine. Bile is usually of a golden color, but when exposed to the air it may become green. It is secreted normally, but the amount may be increased by such foods as fats or salts similar to the cathartics, or by taking laxatives like citrate of magnesia, Epsom salts, or effervescent sodium phosphate. As a digestive secretion, the most important function of bile is attributed to the part it takes in the digestion and absorption of fats.

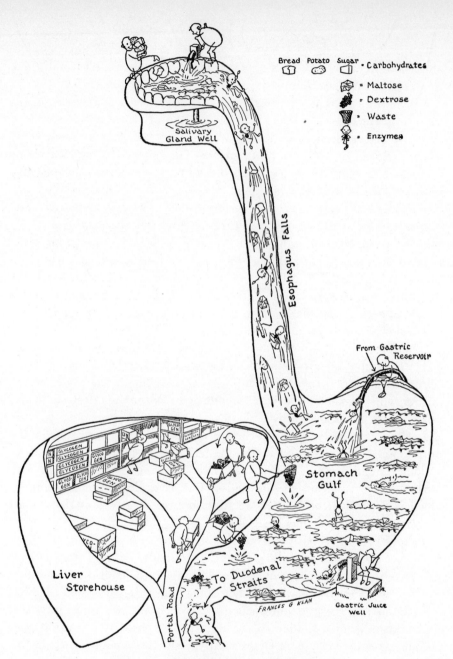

Fig. 48. The journey of carbohydrate.

In the form of sugars and starches, carbohydrate is taken into the mouth where the action of the enzymes in the saliva converts some of the starches to sugar (maltose). The action of the saliva continues down the esophagus to the stomach, where some absorption of the simpler sugar products (dextrose) takes place. Most of the carbohydrate is carried to the duodenum to

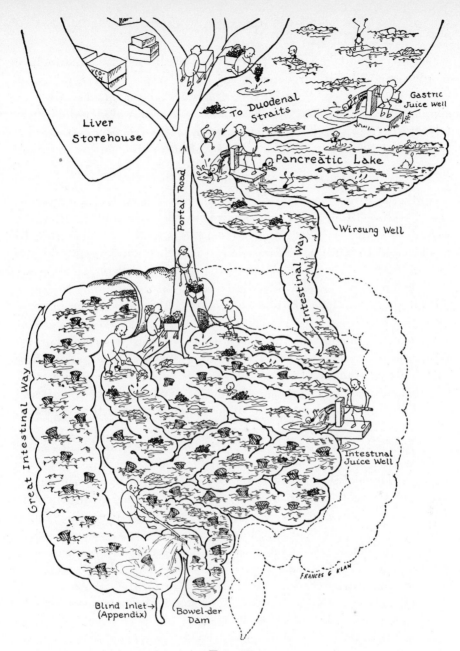

Liver Storehouse

To Duodenal Straits

Gastric Juice Well

Pancreatic Lake

Portal Road

Wirsung Well

Intestinal Way

Great Intestinal Way

Intestinal Juice Well

FRANCES G KLAW

Blind Inlet→ (Appendix)

Bowel-der Dam

FIG. 49.

undergo further digestion by the pancreatic juices which enter by way of the duct of Wirsung. Throughout the duodenum and small intestine digestion and absorption continue until all the carbohydrate has been assimilated by the time the ileocecal valve ("Bowel-der Dam") has been reached. The portal vein carries it in the form of dextrose to the liver where the excess of sugar **is** withdrawn and stored as glycogen for future use by the body tissues.

One of the most important functions of the liver is the manufacture of glycogen. This sugar depends for the most part on the intake of sugars and starches. The bulk of the starches reaches the liver as simple sugar and is there converted into glycogen and stored as such. Glycogen is also stored in the body muscles. It is from these two store-houses that the sugar necessary for function of the body is supplied.

METHODS OF STUDYING DIGESTION

With the foregoing knowledge of the physiology and anatomy of the digestive tract, numerous analytical methods and instruments were devised to recognize changes from the normal. The stomach tube has brought to light many facts that were hitherto unknown. When it became feasible to remove a part of the stomach contents and subject it to a laboratory study physicians began to understand, to better advantage, the nature of stomach troubles. The decrease or increase of hydrochloric acid, or its complete absence, and the presence of pepsin are important in the diagnosis of various ailments. For in-stance, a German physician, Ewald, suggested that the patient first eat a definite standard test breakfast. This consists of a cup of weak tea, without cream or sugar, and a slice of dry toast or an unbuttered roll. This is given on an empty stomach and a part is then removed, in an hour, with a stomach tube and tested.

As was noted in the physiological considerations, acid and pepsin are present in normal stomach juice. If the acid is absent and pepsin is present, the condition is called achlorhydria, which means absence of hydrochloric acid. If both are absent, the condition is called achylia (or absence of chyle or stomach juice). Each of these conditions may be found in different disorders. For instance, in pernicious anemia just the acid is absent early in the disease, but as the disease becomes more severe, both the acid and pepsin are noticeably absent from the stomach juice. As hydrochloric acid and pepsin are secreted accord-ing to the needs of the stomach for digestion, there must necessarily be some variation in the amount and character of the stomach juice from time to time. Therefore, during the day the secretion is low or even absent. Because of this, the ordinary test meal as described may not be a true measure of the cycle of secretion of stomach juice. With this in mind, a test called the fractional test was devised. This is carried out by the use of a small soft rubber tube, swallowed, kept in the stomach, and then through this tube small amounts of stomach juice are withdrawn every fifteen minutes for a period of two or three hours. Occasionally even this test does not reveal the presence of acid. Then the doctor gives a weak alcohol solution instead of the ordinary test meal. Sometimes special drugs are used to determine the presence or absence of acid. For instance, a substance called histamine may be given by hypodermic injection to provoke secretion. Finally, certain dyes when given to an individual by means of a hypodermic needle may be secreted by the stomach. If acid is able to be formed, the acid cells then secrete the dye.

Likewise, the motor power of the stomach may vary in disease. The stomach may empty too soon, or emptying may be delayed, especially if there is any obstruction at the outlet of the stomach. A full meal is given, and the stomach tube is introduced in seven hours. The stomach should be found empty of food, if its action is normal.

If pus or blood or bile are found in the stomach contents, they are evidences of a diseased condition. Sometimes in cases of obstruction at the stomach outlet, in the absence of hydrochloric acid, lactic acid may be found. This may indicate the beginning of a cancer.

By filling the stomach with a substance that is opaque to the X-ray, the size, shape, and motility of the stomach may be readily demonstrated. Barium sulphate is commonly used; it is added to any palatable liquid, such as buttermilk or malted milk. Lots of times the mere taking of this mixture may cause people to think they are better. By looking with the fluoroscopic X-ray screen, the doctor can detect changes in the peristaltic waves or contractions of the stomach, and any abnormal appearance in the outline of the silhouette or changes in the density of the normal shadows. The fact that the stomach can be manipulated during the X-ray examination under the screen is of greatest importance to detect tender areas, or to fill out parts of the stomach or duodenum under the pressure of the fingers. Thus ulcers and tumors are readily detected. X-ray pictures are made of all abnormal appearances not merely to detect minute changes but to keep a permanent record. This furnishes definite information which is most valuable in the diagnosis.

It is surprising what a large number of people who worry about stomach trouble have no X-ray evidence of anything wrong with the stomach. This is due to the fact that diseased conditions outside of the stomach often give rise to digestive disorders or to symptoms in the digestive tract.

If a certain dye, called sodium tetra-iodo phenolphthalein, is given either by mouth or injected directly into the blood, it finds its way into the gall bladder. This dye has a special affinity for the liver and is passed by the liver cells into the small "canals," and later into the larger "canals," and finally into the gall bladder. Furthermore, this dye casts a shadow on an X-ray film when the person who has taken it is exposed to X-rays. This permits the doctor to make more accurate diagnoses and also makes treatment, both medical and surgical, more definite.

Formerly gallstones were rarely detected by the X-ray, the chance depending on the amount of calcium (or lime salt) which they contained. Now early cancer of the gall bladder may be recognized in some cases by this method. This gall-bladder dye test was based on a test of the function of the liver.

Occasionally, when the doctor wants special information as to normal and abnormal conditions of the duodenum, which is the first portion of the small intestine just beyond the stomach, he allows a small tube with a metal perforated tip to pass through the stomach until it reaches the duodenum, where it can be retained. Thus duodenal juice is collected and may be studied for its constituents, as outlined under the physiological considerations. This is especially important in studying the secretion of the pancreas, which also empties into the duodenum and plays an important part in digestion.

EXAMINATION OF EXCRETED MATERIALS

A routine and systematic examination of the stool (feces or bowel movements) of every patient is of great importance. This enables recognition of diseases of the stomach, liver, pancreas, gall bladder, and intestine. The consistency, shape, size, color, odor of the stools, and gross admixtures of mucus, blood, pus, and worms are all important. Chemical tests are made for blood and bile. The fermentation test determines whether the stool inclines too much to carbohydrates or protein putrefaction. The stools are examined with the microscope for the presence of undigested muscle fiber, fat, pus, or blood, or the eggs of parasites; and then stained with dyes to determine the bacteria present. Bacterial cultures are made of the stool to determine the type of living organisms existing in the stool.

ACUTE INDIGESTION

Acute indigestion usually follows the intake of substances that are obnoxious to the stomach. Consumption of too great quantities of food or of unsuitable articles may irritate the lining of the stomach, or these substances may decompose in the stomach and thus initiate acute dyspepsia. A frequent cause is the taking of food which has begun to decompose, particularly in hot weather. In children the fermentative processes are apt to induce enteritis (inflammation of the intestines) as well. Another common cause is the abuse of alcohol, especially "modern alcohol." The tendency to disturbances of the stomach varies in certain individuals who may have *per se*, or inherently, the so-called "vulnerable stomach." The lining of such a stomach is swollen and reddened, covered with much mucus, and in some cases even minute or large hemorrhages.

In mild cases, the symptoms are those of slight indigestion such as an uncomfortable feeling in the abdomen, headache, depression, nausea, belching, and vomiting, which usually gives relief. The tongue is heavily coated, and the saliva is increased. In children there are also intestinal symptoms, such as diarrhea, colicky pains, and often fever. The duration is rarely more than twenty-four hours. The severer attacks may begin with a chill, followed by fever which may reach 102 or 103 degrees. The tongue becomes furred; the breath is heavy, and vomiting is frequent. The material vomited first contains food particles and later becomes bile-stained. There may be an associated constipation or diarrhea. The abdomen becomes distended and tender. Herpes (cold sores) may appear on the lips, and these severe attacks may last from one to three days.

Many acute infectious diseases may begin the same way, and great care must be taken to be certain of the diagnosis. In addition, one must ascertain at once if poison such as phosphorus, corrosive sublimate (bichloride of mercury), ammonia, arsenic, lysol, iodine, or similar substances, has been swallowed, so that a proper antidote may be promptly administered. Furthermore, one dare not overlook the fact that appendicitis, peritonitis, or other infections in the abdomen may also begin in this manner. Any delay in making a conclusive and accurate diagnosis of these conditions may be fraught with danger. Finally, many of the deaths reported from so-called "acute indigestion" are actually acute heart attacks, in which the symptoms are more related to the abdomen than the heart. It is rare for anybody to succumb suddenly to a so-called attack of "acute indigestion" which has no other basis than disease of the stomach.

TREATMENT OF INDIGESTION

Some people with indigestion get the idea that there is some one food substance that is responsible for the feeling of fullness, the discomfort, the pain, and the eructation of gas that follow eating. Some of them force themselves to eat with the idea that this will make them well; others eliminate one food substance after another in the hope of finding the offending food substance, almost starving themselves to death.

After the doctor has made a complete examination and finds out that there is nothing organically wrong with the patient that can be reached, and after he assures the patient that he does not have cancer, heart disease, or some equally serious disturbance, he next tries to find what troubles are in the family which cause the patient to lose his appetite and ruin his digestion. In most cases of acute indigestion, according to Dr. W. C. Alvarez, it is common to find women who lead cat-and-dog existences with their husbands and who wrangle at mealtimes.

Sometimes rest or vacation will have a favorable effect on the person with acute indigestion or dyspepsia, particularly if he goes away from his household and all the people around him. This does not mean a strenuous holiday but an actual rest.

Many persons who seem to be having trouble with their digestions do better with a certain amount of massage and mild exercise. This is particularly the case in stoutly built men who were once athletic and who, following a business career, become flabby and fat. Most important in these cases, however, is the developing of a diet that the patient can take and the teaching of the patient to eat as he should. The smooth diet is the one most frequently prescribed for such patients. In one of the largest clinics in the United States the following smooth diet is regularly advised for persons with chronic digestive trouble:

If you are to give this diet a fair trial, eat no coarse foods with fiber, skins, seeds or gristle. Avoid particularly salads with celery, tomatoes, cucumbers, and pineapple, many of the green vegetables, raisins, berries, jams full of seeds, nuts, and many of the raw fruits. Beans, cabbage, onions, green or red peppers, melons, cucumbers and peanuts are notoriously gassy. If you are living in a boarding house you can stick to this diet by simply avoiding the forbidden foods and eating more of the digestible ones which are put before you.

Avoid sugar in concentrated form and take no candy or other food between meals. Hot cakes and waffles might not be bad if they are properly fried, that is, totally immersed in fat at the right temperature. Avoid eating when in a rush and when mentally upset. Family rows should be held away from the table. Chewing gum may cause distress, as much air is swallowed with the saliva. Digestion is greatly helped by a good chewing surface. If there are any gaps in your teeth have your dentist fill them with bridges. Purgatives often cause flatulence and distress in the abdomen.

The following are suggestions for breakfast: Orange juice, grapefruit (avoid the fiber in the compartments); cantaloupe and melons are inadvisable. Coffee, if desired, is allowed in moderation; it sometimes causes flatulence. If you are sensitive to caffeine try Kaffee Hag or Instant Postum. Chocolate, cocoa or tea, one or two eggs with ham or bacon (avoid the tougher part of the bacon), white bread, toast or Zwieback with butter, any smooth mush such as farina, germea, cream of wheat, cornmeal, or rolled oats (a fine oatmeal can be obtained by calling for Robinson's Scotch Groats); puffed cereals and cornflakes are also allowed. Shredded wheat biscuits and other coarse breakfast foods are not allowed. Bran is particularly harmful. Graham bread is permitted but not the coarser whole-wheat bread.

Suggestions for lunch and dinner: In fruit cocktails avoid the pieces of orange and pineapple. Broths, bouillon, cream soups and chowder are allowed, also meat, fish or chicken, squab or game, excepting duck (avoid the fibrous parts and gristle). Veal may be tried; it is not digested well by many persons. Eat no smoked fish or pork. Crab and lobster had better be left alone. Oysters and sausage may be tried later.

Bread and butter are allowed, and hot biscuits if they are made small so as to consist mainly of crust. Rice, potatoes, mashed, hashed brown, or French fried, are allowed; and later may be added sweet potatoes, hominy, tomatoes stewed, strained and thickened with cracker or bread crumbs, well-cooked cauliflower tops with cream sauce, asparagus tips, Brussels sprouts, squash, beets, turnips, creamed spinach, Italian pastes, noodles, macaroni and spaghetti cooked soft, purées of peas, beans, lentils, lima beans, or artichoke hearts. All skins or fiber should be removed by passing the food through a ricer. Sweet corn may be used if passed through a colander. There are practically no other vegetables that can be puréed to advantage. String beans (large tender string beans which can be used as a vegetable or salad can now be obtained in cans) are allowed if they are young and tender.

No salad should be taken at first. Later you may try a little tender lettuce with apples or bananas, tomato jelly, or boiled eggs. Mayonnaise and French dressing are allowed. Potato salad without much onion may be tried.

Suggestions for dessert are: Simple puddings, custards, ice cream, jello, plain cake and canned or stewed fruits, particularly pears and peaches. Cottage cheese is permissible; other cheeses often cause trouble. Apple, peach, apricot, custard and lemon cream pie may be tried if only the filling is eaten.

In case of constipation, stewed fruit may be taken once or twice a day. In winter the dried pared fruit may be used for stewing. Prunes are probably the most laxative of fruits and if eaten every other morning they will relieve the average case of constipation. They should be cooked slowly until they almost go to pieces. If the skins are still tough they should be discarded. Apple sauce is much more palatable if made from unpared and uncored apples. The sauce is strained later. It may be mixed with a little tapioca or sago. The apples may be baked. Apples, even when cooked, often cause distress. Blackberries and loganberries can be stewed and strained and the sweetened juice thickened with corn-starch. This makes a delicious dish with the full flavor of the berries. Later you may try fully ripe pears and peaches.

Make no effort to drink water. Be guided by your thirst. Avoid excessive use of salt or other seasoning. If you wish to gain in weight eat as much cream, butter, fat and starch as you can. If you wish to lose or stay thin, live largely on vegetables, fruits and salads, with a moderate amount of lean meat.

DIFFICULTY IN SWALLOWING

Many people have difficulty in swallowing. The scientific term is dysphagia. This may be of no importance or it may signify something serious. Many nervous people suffer from "lump in the throat." In purely functional or nervous trouble of this kind, there is seldom loss of weight and strength, such as occurs in actual changes of the tissues of the esophagus (the food pipe leading to the stomach). Such actual changes may be malignant or non malignant (benign). Simple spas-modic contractions of the esophagus may be due either to disease of the wall or to a so-called reflex (referred) spasm from disease elsewhere. The most common type of spasm is at the end of the esophagus (called cardiospasm), where it enters the stomach. Here the esophagus closes down and does not allow the food to enter the stomach. The esophagus becomes larger above the constriction, food is not taken satisfactorily, and the patients lose weight and strength. Sometimes people with this condition become nauseated and may even vomit. In severe cases food may remain in the esophagus for a few days. As a rule these cases recover when the opening is stretched repeatedly at suitable intervals with proper instruments.

In cases of cancer of the esophagus the early signs and symptoms may go unnoticed. However, there ensues gradually increasing difficulty in swallowing, associated with loss of weight and strength. There are numerous other causes of disturbed swallowing because foreign bodies are swallowed and stick. Sometimes patients swallow too much air (called aërophagia). The stomach becomes dilated and swollen, and then it is difficult to force any food down.

The diagnosis of any of these conditions is based on a careful record of the events and, in addition, accurate X-ray observation. Occasionally a long metal (lighted) tube is put down the esophagus and direct observation can be made of the trouble. Sometimes the condition can be treated directly through this tube. In doubtful cases pieces of growths or tumors can be taken out and examined with the microscope to determine their exact nature.

DYSPEPSIA

"Dyspepsia" means difficult or painful digestion. It is not a definite disease but a particular set of symptoms. Indigestion, strictly speaking, is perhaps somewhat different from dyspepsia; it denotes failure of digestion rather than difficulty or pain in the process. The two terms are commonly used synonymously and may be understood to include every condition which is associated with an abdominal sensation referable to the stomach after the ingestion of food. There is not always an organic disease present. Sometimes the imagination may conjure up what seems like a real disease of the stomach. Unfortunately, it is not always possible to make an accurate diagnosis as to the causes.

The outstanding symptom of dyspepsia is abdominal discomfort or pain. The healthy person is unconscious of the existence of his stomach; the dyspeptic rarely forgets it. The intensity of the sensation may vary in degree from a slight feeling of heaviness to agonizing pain which is almost beyond endurance. This occurs usually immediately after the intake of food. When the discomfort becomes more evident, it may be a dull, aching pain, or it may be boring, cutting, stabbing, burning, or griping. Occasionally it is so severe that the sufferer is "doubled up" and writhing in pain. It may be aggravated by pressure over the stomach. Vomiting may afford relief, especially when associated with belching, which relieves pressure.

Heartburn is a peculiarly appropriate word. It exactly describes a sensation; a characteristic burning pain felt immediately behind the "chest bone," rising upward and occasionally spreading to the throat. Heartburn is a frequent symptom of stomach disturbance. It is supposed to be due to increased acidity of the stomach and a regurgitation of the contents upwards into the esophagus through a relaxed muscle at its lower end. The acid supposedly irritates the lining of the esophagus. However, in some patients with no acidity in the stomach, heartburn may be present. Posture may, at times, seem to favor its development. Occasionally change of position from one side to another, sitting up, rather than lying down, may afford relief. Heartburn tends to occur especially at night and may cause considerable distress by interfering with sleep.

"Water brash," or eructation of sour fluid, may follow a burning sensation in the stomach. It is due to increased flow of saliva, associated with acid eructations and heartburn. Increased salivation is frequently an accompaniment of many forms of dyspepsia. Acid eructations are similar to heartburn, except that the acid is brought up with gas by belching. Many dyspeptics complain of a feeling of distention after meals. This may be associated with flatulence or "gas on the stomach." The latter may be caused by the swallowing of air. A certain amount of air is normally swallowed by everyone with food and saliva, but in some people the quantity is excessive. This is called aërophagia. Flatulence may also be caused by fermentation of the stomach contents. Various gases arise in this manner from starches and sugars and also vegetables with much cellulose. Oxygen and carbon dioxide are normally absorbed in the stomach, but disease of the lining of the stomach may prevent normal absorption and may lead to distention.

Vomiting often accompanies indigestion. It may be associated with pain, which is relieved when the stomach is emptied by vomiting. Closing of the upper end of the stomach and the attempt to vomit without bringing up anything is called retching, which is always accompanied by nausea.

Hiccup is a sudden inspiration of air due to spasm of the diaphragm and sudden closure of the glottis (Adam's apple). It may be a symptom of stomach irritation, or it may be due to many other causes.

In dyspepsia, the appetite is variable. The tongue is often furred, especially when thirst is severe. The breath is offensive, and there is a bad taste in the mouth. However, bad breath may also be due to disease of the nose and throat.

In general, all of the conditions described may be classified as dyspepsia. Modern medicine tends to correlate the symptoms that are related to disease of one or more organs so that the treatment may be more scientific and accurate, as well as to determine the necessity for medical or surgical procedures.

GASTROPTOSIS

Many thin, weak people suffer from time to time with vague stomach complaints which, until the advent of the X-ray, were not well understood. The condition called gastroptosis or falling of the stomach is not uncommon. It occurs more often in women than in men. There are many theories as to its cause. Pregnancy, loss of body tone and vigor, and great loss of weight may be factors. Some people are born with the condition.

The symptoms vary from mild and vague to severe. Most people with gastroptosis are dull and apathetic, have dizziness and headaches and are without appetite. There may be some nausea and even vomiting. The skin may be dry and the cheeks lack their normal color. Pain, feeling of pressure, weight, fullness or distention of the stomach are common. Small amounts of food satiate them, and they have little desire for food after the first mouthfuls. Sometimes there is a splashing sound in the stomach as water enters it. Occasionally the distress simulates the pains of ulcer. If the disease is of long standing, patients begin to lose weight and strength. Many remote changes in the body may be referable to the "fallen stomach." It has always been interesting to know why such a condition causes so many symptoms. It is apparently due to the inability of the food and secretions to get out of the stomach into the small intestine. The duodenum, which is the first part of the small intestine beyond the stomach, may be four to six inches long, or longer. Because of the stagnation and pressure caused by the drag of the stomach the duodenum becomes dilated and larger. When substances are absorbed from the duodenum they are poisonous, and an overwhelming amount, as in the case of this disease, is more than the body can take care of. Therefore, headache, dizziness, nausea, lack of appetite, and consequent loss of weight appear.

The X-ray clearly reveals this difficulty. Furthermore, these patients are more comfortable when they lie down, or even better, if the end of the bed is elevated so that the pressure is relieved from the duodenum. With proper diet and sedatives, these patients begin to gain in weight and vigor. If the treatment is to be accomplished without rest in bed, then a suitable corset and pad to elevate the stomach, to favor more rapid emptying, has been used successfully by some physicians. In obstinate and severe cases, operative procedures have been designed to correct the trouble. All in all, a hopeless, "taken-for-granted" disease now is subject to a ray of hope that relief may be brought about in some cases.

Ulcer of the Stomach and Duodenum

An ulcer is a raw spot in the inner lining of the stomach or duodenum, representing destruction of tissues. The life history of an ulcer is extremely varied. Some heal; others burrow deeper and become chronic; others bleed (hemorrhage); some penetrate through the tissues or perforate. Occasionally this perforation may be sealed by nature. The ulcer may be adjacent to a neighboring organ, such as the pancreas, or it may be sealed by that great protective pad or veil of fat in the abdomen, called the omentum. Sometimes the perforation may remain unsealed and the contents of the stomach or duodenum, or both, get into the free abdominal cavity, called the peritoneal cavity. Then a serious condition of inflammation and infection develops which is called perforation peritonitis. The peritoneum, or membrane covering the organs and lining the abdominal cavity, is involved.

The exact cause of ulcer is unknown. There are, however, many predisposing factors. First there is a definite tendency in some families to formation of ulcers. The condition is more common in the third and fourth decades of life, although it is found even in the first decade. Constant abuse of the stomach, eating too highly seasoned foods, or food too hot or too cold, or not properly masticating the food, may be factors. The rôle of infection is still debatable. Many physicians believe that diseases of the tonsils, teeth, gall bladder, and appendix are definitely associated in some cases with formation of ulcer, and that the elimination of all such infections definitely modifies the course and helps in the healing of an ulcer of the stomach. That this is true in a certain percentage of ulcers cannot be doubted, but it is also true that ulcers exist in the absence of such conditions. It has been thought, and experiments done to prove it, that certain ulcers represent the same phenomena that take place in asthma; namely, a reaction of sensitivity. A deficiency of vitamin in foods eaten has been associated with some cases. However, the outstanding fact is that hydrochloric acid, the acid normally present, plays a predominant rôle in making an ulcer chronic. That it is not the cause of ulcer is rather generally accepted. The arguments pro and con are too technical for extended consideration here. The rôle of pepsin is becoming more definitely understood. Nature tends to protect the stomach itself from being digested by secreting a substance called mucin. If a sufficient amount is present, the digestive action of the stomach juice remains inert against the lining of the stomach.

Patients with ulcer have variable symptoms. Most of them complain of a distress which may be a burning sensation (sometimes called heartburn), or a feeling of pressure and weight, or a dull ache, or even a severe pain, sometimes remaining localized to the region of the stomach, occasionally going into the back, or even traveling upward beneath the sternum (chest bone). This distress may come on soon after eating or may be delayed as long as two or three hours. It usually lasts until the next meal, unless it is relieved by taking some medicine. It may awaken the sufferer in the early hours of the morning. It may be seasonal in type, more prone to occur in the spring and fall of the year. As the ulcer becomes chronic, the distress may last throughout the year. But this periodicity of the distress is quite characteristic. Many patients are afraid to eat because eating seems to bring on the pain. Some have found that by eating frequently they are more comfortable. Occasionally, at the height of the pain, vomiting brings relief. This is especially true in those cases in which there is a spasm or constriction at the outlet of the stomach. Patients soon learn to avoid certain foods, especially seasonings, condiments, fried and greasy foods. Tobacco and coffee, as a rule, increase the distress.

While pain is an outstanding feature, occasionally the observant patients may notice tenderness in the abdomen high up, just beneath the sternum (chest bone).

As the ulcer grows older, so to speak, certain manifestations may take place. The pain may become more persistent and severe and may only be relieved by natural or forced vomiting. If the scar of the healing ulcer is located at the outlet of the stomach, an obstruction may develop, which will not permit the stomach to empty itself, or the ulcer may have two important complications; notably, hemorrhage or perforation.

Hemorrhage is associated with certain definite symptoms. Even if no vomiting of blood takes place, the person who is bleeding soon finds himself overcome by a sudden weakness with slight nausea. He may break out in a cold perspiration, become dizzy, feel faint and giddy. If the hemorrhage is large he may become unconscious. Sooner or later his stool, or bowel movement, appears black; this is called a "tarry stool." The face becomes blanched; the expression is anxious. The feeling of fear has a tendency at first to increase rather than decrease the hemorrhage. Nature counteracts this by causing a fall in blood pressure and thus lessens the tendency for hemorrhage.

If the person with ulcer vomits blood, which is more common if the ulcer is located in the stomach rather than in the duodenum, he immediately knows the cause of his distress. Anyone who has experienced the sensation of a hemorrhage recognizes the early symptoms promptly on the second or third repetition of the bleeding.

In the case of perforation, the course is much stormier. Agonizing, excruciating pains develop in the upper abdomen. Cold, clammy sweat appears, and the sufferer becomes anxious, nauseated, and may even vomit. The abdomen becomes tense and board-like, and as conditions become more severe, the symptoms become intensified. Unless the ulcer becomes immediately sealed, or an operation is performed, the outlook is ominous. The life of the patient is hazarded if prompt measures are not taken.

After the ulcer is diagnosed, the choice of treatment depends on the nature of the condition. Some ulcers will never heal with medical treatment alone and should properly undergo surgical operation; others should have medical treatment from the outset. If the patient has ulcer of the stomach and is in or about the cancer age, thirty-five or above, then great care should be exercised as to the choice of treat-

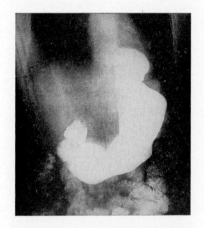

Fig. 50. Normal stomach.

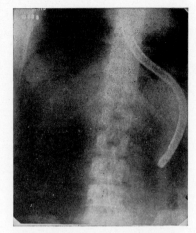

Fig. 51. Tube in stomach.

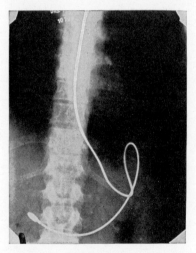

Fig. 52. Duodenal tube at outlet of stomach.

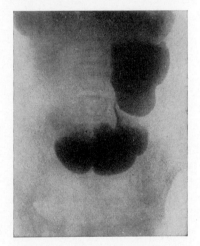

Fig. 53. Hourglass stomach.

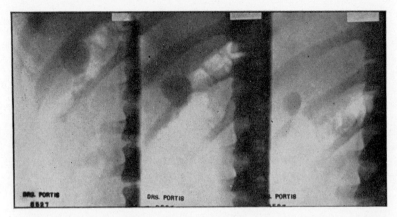

Fig. 54. Normal gall bladder showing injection of dye, indicating normal filling, concentration of bile, and emptying after a meal of fat.

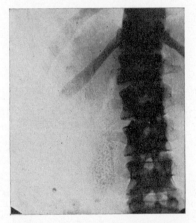

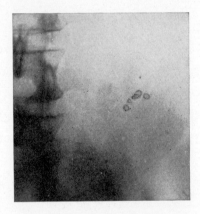

Fig. 55. Gall bladder containing numerous small gallstones.

Fig. 56. Gall bladder containing several large stones.

ment. If the ulcer is in a young person, medical treatment can usually be carried out safely.

If the ulcer is located in the duodenum, medical treatment can usually be carried out unless there is evidence of perforation or obstruction. For these, the surgeon must be called. Repeated menacing hemorrhages may also demand surgical operation. Finally, cases that have not received benefit from thorough medical management should be referred to the surgeon. Ulcers at the outlet of the stomach, which practically close off the exit, make life miserable and unsafe unless surgical measures are instituted. The X-ray is a great aid in deciding whether an operation is advisable in a complicated case.

One outstanding feature of all medical treatment has been the attempt to decrease the acid in the stomach. Efforts should be directed not only to neutralization but to preventing or inhibiting the formation of too much acid. This may be accomplished by change of habits and the use of certain foods and drugs, notably alkalies. Recently gastric mucin (an extract of the wall of the lining of the stomach of animals; e. g., the mucus) has been used. Patients cannot be treated by rule of thumb. Some can stand alkalies (ordinary neutralizing powders); others are made worse by them, and their long continued use in these cases may result in the development of a condition called alkalosis (too much alkali). It is easily recognizable, and treatment when instituted early is prompt and satisfactory. The diet forms the most important part of all medical management of gastric and duodenal ulcers.

An ulcer is best treated by a bland diet and the use of a powder to neutralize the acid secretion. Milk and cream and eggs should form the principal foods; puréed vegetables, and puréed, stewed fruits are all beneficial.

DISEASE OF THE GALL BLADDER

The most common cause of stomach disorders in the adult is disease of the gall bladder. Such diseases as typhoid, pneumonia, influenza, sore throat, and other acute infectious diseases may leave residual disease in the gall bladder. Gall-bladder disease is particularly likely to occur during and after pregnancy, especially in nursing mothers. Fatty or obese people are also likely to develop this disease. Modern methods of dieting, of omitting meals, of allowing the gall bladder to remain filled too long without its physiological emptying are also important factors. The gall bladder empties when food is taken, especially fatty foods. It is best to eat three times a day to keep the gall bladder functioning well. The typical patient with gall-bladder disease is a woman, fair, fat, and forty.

The early signs are usually fullness and distention of the abdomen associated with much belching. The distress comes on, as a rule, immediately after meals. The patient rises from the table with an "overloaded" sensation. Belching affords relief, but occasionally more air is swallowed in the act of belching, and this leads to greater distention. Fatty, greasy, and highly seasoned foods aggravate the distress. Pain may be present. It may be a dull ache, a sensation of weight, or it may be sharp and severe. It may be constant or intermittent. It may be localized beneath the ribs in front on the right side, or it may go to the back and right shoulder. If it is severe enough to "double one up" and is associated with nausea and vomiting, it is significant of gallstones. Occasionally gall-bladder disease causes a spasm of the outlet of the stomach, which is not only painful but may be accompanied by nausea and vomiting. When the outlet relaxes, the vomitus may be yellow or green.

Headache is a common symptom and is associated with disturbed movements of the first portion of the small intestine. Here premature absorption of poisonous products of digestion takes place and causes headaches and dizziness. Such people often are irritable and nervous. Their sleep is disturbed and fitful. Their complexion is often sallow, and they complain of being "bilious." Constipation is a frequent symptom. If the disease progresses, stones may be formed in the gall bladder, which later become dislodged into the larger tubes carrying the bile and obstruct the flow of bile; then "yellow jaundice" supervenes. Jaundice may be present without stones associated with disease of the liver. There are many other causes of jaundice, but it is most commonly associated with gall-bladder disease and its complications.

Jaundice first appears in the whites of the eyes. Later, the skin becomes yellow, and still later the urine grows darker and the excretion from the bowels lighter in color. Itching may be a pronounced and aggravating symptom to the extent that severe scratching and abrasions of the skin take place. The jaundiced person becomes dull, apathetic, and lethargic when cholemia (bile poisoning) takes place. In extreme cases unconsciousness may develop. People with gallstones are frequently miserable because of irritation and pain, and when a positive diagnosis is made they should have an operation, providing contraindications to operation do not exist. The danger of stones in the gall bladder should not be underestimated. Pus may form, which is dangerous, and what is more important, cancer of the gall bladder is associated with stones in approximately 95 per cent of the cases. The early removal of these stones and of the gall bladder before the inception of the cancer is the best method known today in its prevention. The medical treatment in cases of stones affords little or no relief. However, it must be frankly stated that all patients with gallstones are not good surgical risks, and it may be the lesser of two evils to allow patients to go without operation.

Jaundice

Whenever material from the bile, called bilirubin, gets into the blood there follows a yellowish discoloration of the skin. The skin, the mucous membranes, and even the whites of the eyes become jaundiced. There are, however, several different types of conditions that can cause the passage into the blood of this bile. For instance, an obstruction, may occur anywhere in the bile ducts from the smallest channels which develop in the liver to the point at which the bile pours into the intestines. If the obstruction is sufficient, the bile is turned back, and jaundice follows.

The most frequent causes of such jaundice are stones which block the tubes, but occasionally tumors may form and block off the ducts, and in other instances there may be serious infection with inflammation and swelling resulting in obstruction.

Associated with jaundice, itching of the skin is not infrequent. The material is excreted in the urine, and as a result the urine has an intense yellow color. Because the bile is not, as usual, expelled with the excretions from the bowel, these develop a clay color. Frequently the entrance of the bile substance into the blood leads to hemorrhages not only through injury to the walls of the smaller blood vessels, but also because of its effects on the substances in the blood which are involved in clotting.

One form of jaundice, which occurs often in children, lasts from two to twelve weeks. It has been thought that this is infectious, but the proof is not certain. It seems to come on about the same season of the year when colds in general are prevalent. The condition does not actually occur in epidemics. It is often without fever, and definite bacterial organisms have not yet been found in the bile as taken directly from the intestines at the point at which the bile is poured into the intestines.

Various types of poisons which tend to injure the liver as, for example, poison by arsenic, phosphorus, chloroform, and cinchophen, are frequently associated with jaundice. There are also cases in which certain types of infection actually do spread through a community. Much liver damage is frequent. Such cases might well be called infectious or epidemic jaundice.

One of the most common types of bile in the blood is that which, occurs in tiny babies just after birth. This usually tends to clear up in a few days. There are, however, other types of infection at birth associated with jaundice which are more likely to be serious, if not fatal.

APPENDICITIS

Appendicitis, as the name indicates, means an inflammation of the appendix. This small rudimentary organ, located at the beginning of the colon, a portion of the large bowel in the lower right side, occupies an important place in the causation of both acute and chronic abdominal complaints. It is quite large in herbivorous animals, and in action is like the rest of the colon. It is one of the commonest sites for an infection inside the abdomen.

Acute appendicitis now is well recognized as a definite disease. It occurs at all ages, even in infants. The early signs of this condition include mild to severe abdominal pain, which frequently is first felt in the upper portion of the abdomen. After a period of hours the pain tends to localize in the right lower quarter of the abdomen. The pain usually develops suddenly and is cramp-like. It recurs at intervals and at times is most severe. The patient soon has some nausea which may be progressive and associated with vomiting. These early symptoms may increase in severity, and if the inflammation of the appendix progresses there is soon a rise in the temperature of a few degrees. When a blood count is made it shows evidence of infection by an increase in the number of white blood cells. The abdominal muscles on the right side over the region of the appendix are rigid, and to relieve this feeling of tenseness the patient will often bend the right knee. The patient lies on the back and remains quiet, for all motion increases the pain.

The examining physician is able to demonstrate the local tenderness over the appendix and perhaps some increased resistance to touch or muscular rigidity in the same region. This is typical of acute appendicitis, and most physicians usually decide on immediate operation in such cases. If after a few hours the pain suddenly diminishes, there may be gangrene or rupture of the appendix, to be followed within a few hours by peritonitis. Hence, although at times in mild catarrhal appendicitis the pain may subside and the patient begin to improve, in the majority of cases this abrupt change should be considered a danger signal for the beginning of peritonitis.

If the sick person does not have medical attention during the first twelve to twenty-four hours, two possibilities may occur. First, the inflammation may subside and thereafter be followed by mild symptoms of a chronic nature. Second, the acute inflammation of the appendix may progress rapidly, giving rise to the so-called pus appendix, gangrene, or rupture with peritonitis. These complications are, of course, extremely serious and may even terminate fatally. When a member of the family develops a sudden pain in the abdomen, like that described, one should never give a laxative, but should call a doctor at once.

Chronic appendicitis is usually the outcome of one or more mild attacks of previous acute appendicitis. The symptoms may be vague and baffling for a long time. Ordinarily there is some abdominal pain, which has a tendency to be colic-like and may not be associated with any nausea or vomiting. In the chronic cases the doctor must make sure that the symptoms are not due to some other cause, such as gall-bladder disease, or stone in the kidney, or ulcer of the stomach, or disease of the colon; then, when the symptoms are clear and the X-ray gives evidence of disease of the appendix, an operation should be done to remove it.

The diagnosis of chronic appendicitis depends mainly on the past record of the patient, the tenderness over the appendix, and the X-ray demonstration of disease of the appendix.

The treatment is not necessarily an operation in every case, as many individuals with this condition are relieved by proper dieting and medication. However, when the symptoms become severe and persistent, the appendix should be removed.

Dr. John B. Murphy insisted, once the diagnosis of acute appen-

dicitis was made, an operation should be done as soon as possible, and
this is the safest course.

No one can predict just what the subsequent changes may be, and
no one can foretell whether a rupture of an inflamed appendix with
peritonitis may not occur. Operation in the uncomplicated cases is
comparatively simple and safe.

ULCER, GALL-BLADDER DISEASE, AND APPENDICITIS

To distinguish between ulcer, gall-bladder disease and appendicitis
is difficult. At times the three may be similar. It is not safe for anyone
to try to distinguish these for himself. There is severe pain in all of
them. The pain in ulcer comes on one-half hour or longer after eating
and is relieved by taking some milk or bland food or some alkaline
substance. Highly seasoned foods or alcohol make the pain worse.
The pain is felt over the pit of the stomach and remains there. The
pain in appendicitis, although at first felt in the region of the stomach,
later moves to the location of the appendix. The pain has no relation
to the taking of food and is not relieved by food or an alkali. The
pain in gall-bladder disease is first felt in the upper right side of the
abdomen, and it is referred to the right shoulder and back and often
to the right shoulder blade region. The pain may be severe, especially
in cases that have gallstones, and it may be colicky.

In all three diseases, nausea and vomiting may be present. In ulcer
the vomiting brings relief, except in the ulcers that may be in a per-
forating stage. In the gall-bladder disorders or appendicitis vomiting
is persistent, usually without relief.

There is usually fever in acute disease of the gall bladder and
appendix, but seldom in ulcer unless the ulcer has perforated the
wall of the stomach or duodenum. Likewise, the white cells of the
blood increase in number except in the case of ulcer, and they are
usually higher in disease of the gall bladder. The physician determines
this by a blood count.

If the patient is jaundiced or has a history of a previous attack
of jaundice, it is more than likely that the gall bladder contains stones.

At least one half the chronic cases of indigestion are due to disease
of the appendix or gall bladder. It is only by careful laboratory work
and the use of the X-ray that an exact diagnosis can be made. A host
of digestive troubles that are called neuroses are really due to ulcer
of the stomach or duodenum or a diseased gall bladder or appendix.

Cancer of the Stomach

Cancer of the stomach is third in frequency among the parts of the body that cancer attacks. It usually appears after forty years of age, but it has occurred in young persons. The cause is unknown, but the taking of unduly hot or irritating foods or liquids may be a factor. Ulcers in the stomach may change to cancer, but in the duodenum rarely become cancerous. A patient with cancer loses in weight and strength and gets indigestion. If the tumor is at the entrance of the stomach, food cannot enter, and rapid starvation occurs. If the tumor is located at the outlet or pylorus, obstruction occurs, and food will be vomited instead of passing into the bowels. This produces rapid loss in weight. The secretions of the stomach are altered by cancer, and the hydrochloric acid disappears. This interferes with digestion and causes nausea. Sooner or later the tumor ulcerates and bleeding occurs. Due to the fact that the blood remains in the stomach for some time, it becomes dark and altered, and in the vomitus looks much like coffee grounds. Most patients with cancer have pain; the pain may be a dull ache or be boring or severe, depending on the location of the tumor. The pain is usually made worse by food and is not relieved by alkalies, but it may be diminished by vomiting.

Any person in or beyond the middle period of life who develops indigestion, with nausea and pain and loss of weight and strength, should be examined immediately and most thoroughly. Only careful examination of the contents of the stomach and of the excretion from the bowels, and an examination with the X-ray, will enable one to make a positive diagnosis. The X-ray usually shows a defect or deformity in the normal shadow of the stomach and is of greatest aid in the diagnosis.

The only possible treatment in most cases is an operation to remove the growth; if that is not possible, then X-ray or radium treatments may be of benefit. When obstruction occurs, it is necessary to make a new opening between the stomach and bowels, or a gastro-enterostomy. This gives relief from symptoms and may prolong life for several months.

Constipation

In constipation there may be retention of the material that should be excreted, for an abnormal time, or merely difficult evacuation of the bowels. Few other subjects in medicine have received more thought and attention. Volumes have been written on it. From the moment of birth until death the question of the daily bowel movement is paramount. The child is asked daily over and over again whether its bowels have moved; naturally this emphasis makes a strong impression which lasts the rest of its life. No other drugs have had greater sales than those that contain laxatives; fortunes have been made by clever advertising of patent medicines, taking advantage of this all-absorbing question of the human animal.

Actually, it is not necessary for the bowels to move every day. It is normal for some people to have an evacuation every other day; in others several days may elapse between actions of the bowels and still complete health be possible.

Until the food eaten reaches the colon, digestive processes are going on in the long small bowel, with absorption of all digestible portions. The material which reaches the colon is in a semi-solid state, and its passage through the large bowel occurs slowly. During this time a good part of the liquid content is absorbed, leaving a more solid residue which finally is expressed as a stool or bowel movement. Naturally, as more food keeps coming along, the bowel contents are finally forced into the terminal portion of the bowels, called the rectum. Normally the rectum does not contain material; when the excrement is forced into it, reflex contractions occur, and the bowels empty themselves of their contents in the terminal portion. This constitutes the act of defecation. Usually this occurs once or twice in twenty-four hours.

There are many different possible causes of constipation. Failure to pay attention to the desire for a bowel movement or to devote sufficient time to it will lead first to a retarded movement and later to constipation. There must be a sufficient amount of residual material or bulk to form a mass of stool to excite activity; hence the food must contain enough vegetables and fruit and salads, if normal evacuations are to continue. Likewise, for normal digestion, the body demands a necessary supply of fluids. If the material in the colon is dehydrated or dried out, the desiccated stool will be difficult to evacuate. For this reason profuse sweating or the loss of fluids due to fever may induce constipation. All diseases which cause body weakness or wasting may be attended by constipation, due to the fact that the muscles necessary for expelling the bowel contents are too weak to act. Any disease causing a narrowing of the caliber of the bowel may be attended by constipation for mechanical reasons.

Finally, the habitual use of purgatives is a frequent cause of constipation. Owing to the irritation of the drugs the colon becomes contracted and tight, or owing to repeated overstimulation it finally becomes exhausted or atonic.

In some cases there may be no symptoms, whereas in others there may be conditions simulating a wasting disease. Early there is, as a rule, a loss of appetite. The patients complain of a foul breath and often notice a coated tongue. Later, mental depression supervenes, and the individual wonders why he has become dull and listless; why his ordinary activities, which formerly caused him no fatigue, now cause undue fatigue; why he is not as alert as formerly; why ordinary problems befuddle him; why it takes him longer to work out things mentally than formerly. He may have headaches, complain of dizziness, and often of ringing in his ears. His friends tell him that he does not look well, that he has a pallor to his skin, and this may be associated with a resulting beginning anemia. Often, in young people, skin eruptions and skin manifestations may be associated with habitual constipation.

Constipation is usually associated with indigestion, so-called dyspepsia; such patients may feel full after a relatively small meal. They frequently belch and complain of undue distention. Often, cramp-like pains are noted, and little relief is obtained from the small, constipated bowel movement. If this condition persists long enough, actual disease of the large bowel may follow. In many cases ulcers of the bowels seem to have their origin in long-standing constipation.

It is important to correct any tendency to delayed bowel movement, especially when this occurs in childhood. Regularity should be insisted on. The bowels should be trained to move the first thing in the morning. An effort should be made to have them move after breakfast each morning.

Exercise and diet are important. The diet should consist of plenty of vegetables, salads, and fruit, in addition to milk, cereals, eggs, and meats. An outdoor, active life is also beneficial for people with sluggishness of the bowels. An occasional enema or mineral oil may be helpful, but the use of laxatives regularly is distinctly harmful.

Along with diet, exercises intended especially to strengthen the abdominal muscles, massage of the bowels, and the drinking of large amounts of water on arising are of distinct help in stubborn cases.

Cathartics are at times necessary for temporary help. Mineral oil and agar are usually tried first, since their action is that of a lubricant or of stimulation by bulk. An enema consisting of olive oil or mineral oil is frequently necessary when the bowel is in an irritable condition, and plain tap water may be used for an enema without harm.

More recently it has been found that acidophilus milk, taken regularly between meals and at bedtime, is of great value in chronic constipation. It transforms the intestinal bacterial flora to a normal type. This has a wholesome effect not only on the constipation but on the body in general.

Laxative medicines are put up today in tempting forms, such as candy and gum or in chocolate and cookies. Children frequently take these too often and thus lay the foundation for stubborn constipation in later life. When a cathartic is really needed, one of the simpler drugs or measures advised should be used. It is best not to take even laxatives, and certainly not cathartics, without the advice of a physician.

COLITIS AND DIARRHEA

"Colitis" is a misnomer. More accurately it is an inflammation, either acute or chronic, of the large intestine. The inflammation may be limited to the lining or may involve the other layers of the colon. If the outer coats are involved, adhesions to the intestines may form. The essential cause is bacterial, or it may be a parasitic infection. Constipation is doubtless a predisposing factor of importance, especially in the chronic forms. The large bowel symptoms are often due to faulty digestion higher up in the intestinal tract. When the improperly digested material enters the lower bowel it may give rise to disturbed function. Because the symptoms are referable to the large bowel, the condition is diagnosed as colitis, when in reality inflammation is not present.

Inflammation of the colon frequently accompanies diarrheal diseases. Sometimes such inflammation is a secondary manifestation of certain infectious diseases, such as blood poisoning, pneumonia, smallpox, measles, influenza, and typhoid, and also kidney conditions with anemia.

The causes of the acute form of diarrhea include faulty diet or the use of spoiled and contaminated foods. Foods which decompose readily, such as unripe or overripe fruit, ice cream, and sea foods, may cause diarrhea. Sometimes water may carry grave infection. Indeed, infected water is the most common source of such serious diseases as dysentery, cholera, typhoid fever, and paratyphoid fever. In the tropics and even in temperate climates, amebic dysentery is often due to infected water. In the temperate climates bacillary dysentery is the more common.

In certain cases, spoiled meat is the cause. Poisons, such as arsenic, mercury, silver salts, and various cathartic medicines often provoke diarrhea. General toxic conditions, such as blood poisoning, measles, exophthalmic (inward or ingrowing) goiter, pneumonia, cancer, and Bright's disease may cause diarrhea. Certain food deficiencies where lack of vitamins plays a rôle, as in pellagra, cause frequent movements. In some cases, absence of the acid of gastric juice may cause diarrhea.

Simple acute diarrhea, ordinarily due to ingestion of infected drinks or food or unripe fruit, is characterized by frequent evacuation of material, which is at first solid or soft but soon becomes chiefly liquid. Colic with pains is common, and straining at stool with a sense of a desire to purge further is evident. There may be thirst, coated tongue, tenderness in the abdomen, and in some cases even fever, especially in younger people. If the attack becomes severe, mucus— slimy material—is noted in the excrement. In severe cases even blood or blood-tinged material may be noted. Chronic diarrheas usually follow acute attacks, and when they persist, further search for the causative factor must be made by the doctor. If allowed to continue without abatement, loss of weight, anemia, profound weakness, loss of appetite, and susceptibility to infections may develop.

CHRONIC DIARRHEA AND DYSENTERY

The two most common forms of chronic diarrhea of the infectious type are bacillary dysentery and amebic dysentery. Bacillary dysentery is due to a specific infection with the germs of dysentery of which there are many types. It is a communicable disease and due, for the most part, to bad sanitation. After one person in a community has the disease, another may come down with it from two to seven days later. The onset is sudden, with griping pains in the abdomen, followed by diarrhea. The bowel movements show much mucus and later pus and blood. There is practically always fever. Along with this, there may be headache, vomiting, malaise, or drowsiness. The abdomen may be tender over the course of the large bowel. Sometimes the onset may be confused with acute appendicitis. If the disease persists, it frequently goes into a chronic form, which may have definite periods of remission during which time the patient may be comfortably free from symptoms.

Early in the disease, the germs can be isolated from the stool and, in some cases, even from the blood. The most important aid in diagnosis is found in the ability of the serum, or fluid matter of the blood, of the affected patient to "clump" dead dysentery germs together. This scientific test is an almost specific method. On the basis of this fact there is a specific treatment using an anti-serum made from the blood of horses. The disease may for years be unrecognized. Many cases of ulcerative colitis (called non-specific ulcerative colitis) are nothing more than chronic bacillary dysentery with a secondary invading or infective organism. Arthritis is the most common complication of the disease and most often the knee, with or without other joints, is involved.

Amebic dysentery was once considered to be a disease confined to the tropics; now it is known that there are few places in the world where the disease does not occur. About 5 per cent of the population of the United States are infected. The causative organism is called endameba histolytica. It is a parasite called for short ameba, and its favorite habitat is the human intestinal tract, especially the large bowel or colon. It frequently penetrates into the blood stream, and thus can travel to any organ in the body. The liver is at times invaded, and an amebic abscess of the liver sometimes results.

In cases with acute dysentery actively moving ameba may be found, while in the chronic cases, even without diarrhea, the ameba may be found in the form of cysts, or collections of fluid. It is in the form of cysts that the disease is usually carried. Individuals who pass these cysts in their stools are called "carriers," though they may themselves never have had the typical acute symptoms.

The infection in the human body can take place only by swallowing the cysts. Food handlers who are carriers have been found occasionally. Some vegetables that are eaten raw may be contaminated when the soil has been contaminated by a carrier. The house fly may carry the cyst from the stool to the food. Hence, one should be careful that vegetables grown in gardens should not be eaten raw, and proper screening should be used to intercept the fly with its burden of filth.

The symptoms of the disease are similar to those of the dysentery caused by the smaller germs. A person may harbor the amebas and have for prolonged periods few, if any, symptoms. The liver is a common site for the amebas to locate outside of the intestinal tract, due to the fact that the blood of the intestinal tract first enters the liver. In the liver, small or large abscesses may result from the action of the invading amebas. The joints are, at times, invaded, producing arthritis, or inflammation of the joints, and the kidneys may be affected, causing bloody urine. The disease is difficult to eradicate, and relapses are frequent.

CANCER OF THE BOWELS

Cancer rarely occurs in the small bowel but is fairly common in the large intestine. In the small bowel the cancerous growth usually does not make itself known until obstruction or blocking occurs, due to its filling the inside of the bowel. At other times, the first warning may be bleeding. The symptoms of an obstruction are at first cramp-like pains and later nausea and vomiting.

Cancers may arise in any part of the colon or large bowel but are more common in the lower portions, called the sigmoid and rectum. In the early stages there may be no symptoms. When the tumor grows large enough to obstruct the inside, the typical symptoms of intestinal obstruction or blocking arise. At other times, the surface of the tumor becomes abraded or bruised by the onward movement of the intestinal contents, and infection or ulceration of the eroded surface takes place. Thus. the blood vessels may become exposed and broken, and bleeding follows.

Cancers in the rectum are commonly located just above the opening and are within easy reach of the doctor who examines for them. The person affected may think he has piles, with some bleeding from time to time. The simple examination to make certain should always be made.

Cancer of the bowels may set up secondary growths, commonly in the liver, with jaundice or yellowness of the skin, but the secondary growths may also appear in the lungs or bones.

Early symptoms are frequently absent, and the patient may come to the physician too late for a cure by operation. The symptoms, when they do appear, are constipation, distention and cramps and sometimes diarrhea, alternating with the constipation. If the tumor is in the lower part of the bowels, some mucus and blood may be present with the stool and the patient frequently feels that he has not emptied his bowels.

The X-ray is of greatest value in diagnosing cancer of the bowels. When some opaque material, like bismuth or barium, is taken by mouth and its course through the bowels is watched by the X-ray, a defect in the shadow can be seen which represents the tumor mass. An enema containing the opaque material can be given and the tumor of the colon readily recognized by the defect in the normal shadow by means of the X-ray. A long metal tube, electrically lighted, can be passed into the rectum for a considerable distance, and through it even small growths may be seen; also a small piece of tissue may be removed for microscopic examination.

As soon as the diagnosis can be made, an operation should be carried out to remove the tumor, if possible, and, if that is not feasible, at least a new opening may be made by bringing the bowel just above the tumor to the skin surface. This procedure is called a colostomy. Inoperable cases can sometimes be helped by X-ray or radium treatments.

Intestinal Obstruction

Intestinal obstruction indicates some abnormal abdominal condition which gives rise to an interference with the onward flow of intestinal contents. This may be produced by a large variety of causes. Adhesions resulting from previous operations are the most common cause, as the intestinal loops become entangled in these strands of tissue and become kinked. Hernia, or rupture, may be complicated by obstruction when the bowel falls through the outlet of the rupture and its return to the abdomen is prevented by swelling of all of the structures. Sometimes one portion of the intestine ensheaths or slips into itself; this is called technically intussusception, and is an especially common form of intestinal obstruction in children. Tumors, of which cancer forms the largest group, may narrow the inside of the intestine by progressive growth and prevent normal onward movement of the intestinal contents. The circulation of the bowels may be destroyed by small clots which may lodge or form in the blood vessels, with subsequent loss of vitality and paralysis of the intestine. Intestinal obstruction, or ileus, as this condition is called, may also be associated with numerous conditions, such as peritonitis, kidney stones, and gallstones.

The symptoms depend usually on the suddenness of the onset and the degree of obstruction. When due to adhesions or ruptures, there is usually a sudden attack of severe abdominal pain followed by repeated severe vomiting. These symptoms become more severe with the passing of hours and soon are followed by distention of the abdomen and inability to have bowel movements. Obstruction due to tumors is usually slow in its development and may be preceded by periods of constipation alternating with diarrhea and abdominal pain. Cancers of the rectum and lower colon frequently are associated with bloody excretions and mucus, and the tumor may be felt by the finger or seen by the use of special instruments. With an enema opaque to the X-ray, obstructing growths and gas-distended intestinal loops above the site of interference may be seen by the doctor. However, even in cancer of the rectum, a sudden obstruction may be the first evidence of its existence.

The diagnosis of an intestinal obstruction is usually obvious, but some cases may remain uncertain until operation. The causative lesion must be carefully localized, as this gives a definite plan for surgical relief. The location of the pain and tenderness are valuable aids. The physician may think it wise to see what can be accomplished by the use of enemas for the relief of the obstruction. Obstinate constipation and impaction of stool may produce symptoms which resemble true obstruction, but in them enemas will bring complete relief.

When there is delay in taking care of intestinal obstruction, an artificial opening must be made above the obstruction to permit complete drainage of the obstructed intestine. In the cases in which this is the only remedy, later on a more complete operation can be carried out to join the bowel above and below the obstruction and at the same time to close the artificial opening. It is all-important to recognize, in the cases with the symptoms described, that intestinal obstruction is present and to call a surgeon at once as a life-saving measure.

INTESTINAL PARASITES OR "WORMS"

Several types of animal parasites may inhabit the human intestine. The more common types encountered are the beef, pork, and fish tapeworms; roundworms, pinworms, hookworms, and flukes. They vary in size and shape, some being long and flat, others shorter and round. There are species which are microscopic in size, while others are many feet in length. They usually enter the body by way of the mouth through the intake of food which has been contaminated with the eggs or the adult parasite. After an interval in the intestinal canal the eggs hatch into the adult worms and continue to live, grow, and reproduce. With certain species the embryonic forms are absorbed into the blood stream and migrate through the body, at times lodging in the liver, brain, lungs, and muscle, to return later to the intestine. Along with the contents of the bowels the parasites are excreted in the form of either the adult or the embryo, to be taken up later by animal or man for repetition of the cycle.

The common sources of the worm are infected beef, pork, fish, and contaminated food and water supplies. In hookworm disease the parasite enters the body through the skin.

There are no absolutely typical symptoms produced by worms, and many cases are long free of symptoms. In many instances there is abdominal pain, irregular evacuation of the bowels, itching about the rectum, vomiting, headache, mental depression, lassitude, and loss of appetite. There may be a severe anemia and marked physical and mental underdevelopment. The bowel content will at times contain blood and mucus, and in most instances the parasite or its eggs. Examination of the blood shows an increase in the percentage of certain cells called eosinophiles. In cases of hookworm or fish tapeworm infestation, the blood may be very watery, owing to a severe grade of anemia induced by the parasite.

The most important feature of the treatment is prophylaxis or prevention. Thousands upon thousands of lives have been spared or made useful through careful attention to sanitation and hygiene. This has been especially true with hookworm. The proper disposal of sewage, careful inspection of cattle and foodstuffs, and proper washing and cooking of vegetables and meats have been responsible for the marked diminution in the number of worm-infested people. The measures used in the treatment of the sick include starvation for a period of twelve to forty-eight hours, purging, and the administration of certain drugs called anthelmintics, which have almost a specific action against the worms. The more common ones in use are male fern, oil of chenopodium, thymol, santonin, and calomel. In cases of fluke infestation, emetine and antimony and potassium tartrate are effective.

Cathartics, Laxatives, and Enemas

The large bowel is one of the most abused organs in the abdomen. This abuse can be attributed, for the most part, to the drastic cathartics and laxatives which people are in the habit of taking. When one considers that the function of this part of the intestinal tract is purely mechanical and that its labors are mostly concerned with excreting the waste products of digestion and metabolism, it is not at all surprising that many patients develop colon disturbances when they irritate it with drastic cathartics. Nature never intended that severe cathartics be used. It supplied suitable roughage in food to supply mass action in the large bowel. While one may get results from a drastic cathartic or purge, it should also be remembered that there is a concomitant obstipation or "tying up" of the bowels for a few days following this irritation. The patient then often desires another laxative or purge, and there soon develops a so-called cathartic habit. Finally, there is a chronic irritation of the colon due to the persistence of the hard small masses of the stool, and many cases of ulceration of the colon or bowel may thus be due to an apparently innocent cathartic habit.

If laxatives must be taken, one should try to use the natural laxatives, particularly those found in fruits and vegetables. Such foods as meats, bread, eggs, fish, potatoes, and milk give little residue in the large bowel, and these, for the most part, form the bulk of the average American diet. If one finds that fruits and vegetables are not enough to stimulate the bowels, mild laxatives may be used.

Many people resort to various types of enemas to relieve constipation. Just as the colon can be abused from above by drastic cathartics, so can it be abused by irritating enemas injected from below. The prime function of an enema is to produce contractions in the lower section of the large bowel so that this expulsive force may bring about the required movement. This expulsive force is directly proportionate to the overdistention with fluid and not to the kind of irritant used. Such simple enemas as tap water or soapsuds enemas may be used. However, when more drastic enemas are required, they should be used under the direction of a physician.

The colon is an innocent organ bearing the brunt and work of the rest of the digestive tract; its main function is to get rid of the waste products. Do not disturb its function by the habitual use of artificial cathartics, laxatives, or enemas.

CHAPTER XVI

The Kidney: Its Diseases and Disturbances
PHILIP S. HENCH, M.D.

INTRODUCTION

MOST OF THE DISEASES *of the kidney are insidious in their onset. The person who has such a disease in an early stage is usually uncon scious of the fact, and the disease is detected by the simple examination of the urine that is part of every examination of any applicant for life insurance. There are all sorts of disturbances of the kidney, varying from the acute inflammation that is associated with or follows some infectious diseases, like scarlet fever, to the gradually developing inflammation of the kidney that is the result of the breaking down of the tissue due to some irritant action, a long continued mild infection, or some similar cause.*

The diseases of the kidney rank high in modern compilations of the causes of death; no doubt, because men live longer than they used to. Today we die of breaking down of the human body associated with wear and tear rather than from the results of sudden severe infections which were the chief causes of death in an earlier generation.

An examination of students entering one of our great universities indicated that 5 per cent of them had changes in the urine, representing the beginning of disturbances in the kidney. Such observations indicate the desirability of having the urine examined at least once each year for the presence of kidney deficiencies and of following up the study with careful examination when any trace of disturbance is found. The finding of albumin in the urine does not indicate necessarily the presence of disease of the kidney, but it does certainly indicate the need for investigation. Such an investigation may lead to determining the presence of symptoms of importance in relationship to health and to life, and may mean a great deal in giving extra years of healthful life to the person concerned.

M. F.

To THE KITCHEN of a great hotel are brought quantities of food, wholesome, pure, catering to each need and taste. In the preparation and consumption of this food waste accumulates; useless material in which food is packed, unused and unusable parts of food itself. Avenues are provided for their ready elimination; boxes and wrappings disappear in fire and in chimney fumes; liquids flow into cisterns; garbage is carted off in wagons of the "reduction company." So too in the organization of our bodies there are veritable human reduction companies.

In the human economy (we have seen in previous chapters) food is the source of all tissue growth and energy. Yet for all our modern laws there is no such thing as "pure food"—at least, in the sense that for the human body there exists no food wholly valuable, completely utilizable. Even from that "perfect product" mother's milk are formed wastes to be discarded. Men foretell perhaps not too seriously the day when a hearty meal will consist, alas, of six courses—each a scientifically compounded pill. Even were the prophecy to come true, waste products would develop in our bodies from the ordinary wear and tear on our own human tissues. The twitch of the tiniest muscle, the lightning wink of an eyelid, the swift flight of a half-formed thought: each is accompanied by, indeed is the result of, the combustion or reduction of some body substance. In the utilization of food and from the growth and repair of body tissues end-products are formed. Carbon dioxide escapes in the flue of the lungs; food residue is discarded by the bowels; water steams out in the breath, escapes in sweat, and is lost in urine. Daily about two quarts of water are eliminated by the lungs, a pint to a pint and a half in the sweat and about one and a half to two quarts in the urine.

The kidneys, forming urine, are one of the chief organs of elimination. Their function is to keep the body free of an excess of substances derived particularly from protein, albuminous or nitrogenous matter

—found for example in meats, milk, eggs, and body muscle. When such food is consumed by the human engine, the ash or residue consists of certain matters which cannot be excreted readily or in quantity by other means than in urine. Those we know most about are urea, uric acid, and creatinine. They must be got rid of, as they are useless; otherwise they would accumulate in the body and be injurious to health and life.

So vital is the need for their proper elimination that nature has included the kidneys among those organs not one but two of which seem necessary to provide a safe margin of reserve. It has been found that man can live, at least for the time being, even after all of one kidney and about half of the other have been removed or destroyed. Yet nature was not unduly profligate in providing us with this reserve, for our kidneys are unfortunately called on to excrete not only the natural waste of wholesome foods, but from time to time must hastily and efficiently help rid the body of products of bad food, germs and their harmful toxins, diseased and dead tissue cells, and chemical poisons.

Every such experience provides a hazard for the kidneys. Repeated, little by little they lower their reserve. Some insults are borne by them silently, without signs, uncomplainingly, without symptoms. To some injurious experiences they temporarily succumb, soon to regain apparently full capabilities. From others they may acquire permanent damage. When the burden is temporarily or permanently too great for the kidneys, when the "threshold of their reserve" is passed, when their function is appreciably deranged, a train of events occurs, the symptoms and signs of which indicate what is called "nephritis." We can readily imagine, considering the great variations in type and degree of such insults met in the course of a lifetime, that there must result different types and degrees of nephritis. One will appreciate that one form of nephritis may be the expression of an essentially minor and transient difficulty, a condition about which no concern need be felt, readily amenable to treatment, and the afflicted person the happy subject of an early cure. Another form, however, may signify grave disease fraught with great danger, which may destine its victim to an early fatal outcome.

The term "nephritis" simply means inflammation of the kidneys. While modern medicine recognizes many different diseases of the kidney, each essentially a type of nephritis, to many the term represents one condition and is synonymous with "Bright's disease." Because the first modern reports of this disease dealt with one of its most serious forms, to some nephritis and Bright's disease remain designations with an evil portent, omens of death. Happily we are getting away from this unfortunate viewpoint, and modern dictionaries define Bright's disease as "a term of very indefinite limitations, meaning in general acute or chronic nephritis," or as "any one of a group of kidney diseases attended by albuminuria" (albumin in urine). Fortunately modern science has provided ways of differentiating between types of kidney disease and of telling whether a given type is serious or not. This is a matter of great importance.

ANATOMY OF THE KIDNEY

The average man has eaten beef or lamb kidneys occasionally, but that is about all he knows of kidneys. For those who wish to learn more, a little description of their interior workings may be of real interest. The kidneys are so placed that they are amply guarded from injury even during such strenuous exercise as the straining and twisting of an athlete at the hurdles, or high jump. Situated in the lumbar region, or small of the back, about the level of the eleventh rib, they are protected by thick spinal muscles behind them and by the peritoneal cavity in front. They are thus not in the abdomen but behind it. They are further surrounded by a tough fibrous coat or capsule, around which is packed a considerable amount of fat.[1] The right kidney is usually about a half inch lower than the left, probably because the liver is above it, and is a little lower in children and women than in men. It is often easily felt on examination. Such a "palpable kidney," if smooth and not enlarged or tender on pressure, is perfectly normal.

Each adult kidney is about 4½ inches long, from 2 to 2½ inches wide, about 1¼ inches thick, and each weighs on an average 1/3 of a pound (150 grams). In shape it resembles a large kidney bean, being rounded and curved with a concave area in the middle of the inner border, the hilus, where the renal[2] artery, vein, and nerves enter

[1] Placed just above each kidney is the adrenal or suprarenal gland, small organs whose physiologic action is different from that of the kidneys but which sometimes become diseased by extensive inflammations around the kidneys.

[2] "Renal" means "pertaining to the kidney." For its derivation see comment on page 428.

and from which arise the ureters, the tubes that carry urine from the kidneys.

On slicing the kidney and laying it open one can see three main areas. The outer zone, called the cortex, contains the pin-point kidney filters, the glomeruli or "little balls." The middle zone, or medulla, is marked by innumerable stripings consisting of microscopic tubules which converge into a number of pyramid-shaped areas. These are connected by many finger-like projections to a fairly large smooth-lined, sac-like collecting chamber called the kidney pelvis. From the pelvis the ureters arise at the hilus. The ureters are tubes about 1/5 of an inch wide with a channel within only ⅛ of an inch in width. They travel 10 to 12 inches down along the spine to the bladder.

Thus each kidney is a tremendously compact area of collecting tubules and of wonderfully small filters, each placed in its minute filter chamber. Before discussing the filters we will describe the filter chambers and tubules, for these are the fundamental anatomic units of the kidney. Each of these units—or nephrons—begins as a little cup-like chamber, 1/200 of an inch in diameter, comprising the filtration chamber named Bowman's capsule, into which are inserted the filters themselves, which are the masses of capillary loops called glomeruli. The walls of the cup-like Bowman's capsule are double, with a narrow space between, since the structure is like a round ball pushed in from one side. These small filter chambers are confined entirely to the cortex, and from them arise small tubules which begin very meandering courses, to end, many of them together, in large collecting tubules that lead to the kidney pelvis. Just after the tubule leaves the filter chamber it enters a series of convolutions in the cortex ("proximal convoluted tubule") and then dips down into the medulla as a very thin descending loop 1/1,200 of an inch (1/3000 cm.) thick, which turns as Henle's loop to ascend again into the cortex where, somewhat thicker (1/600 of an inch or 1/1500 cm.), it becomes even more convoluted ("distal convoluted tubule") before it finally straightens out to join with myriads of others into the collecting tubes which empty into the kidney pelvis. Despite all this wandering, it has traversed a distance of only about 2 inches. As we shall see, the purpose of this extreme migration is to permit it to come in contact, in a minute space, with an extensive meshwork of very fine blood vessels. It has been estimated by some that there are about 1,000,000 (Kittleson-Vimtrup) (others say 4,500,000: Traut) of these filter chambers in each kidney, each with its 2-inch tubule (Möllendorff). In the adult, therefore, the total length of these tubules in each kidney would be from 2,000,000 to 9,000,000 inches, or the equivalent of a channel from about 32 to 140 miles long; 64 to 280 miles long in both kidneys, compressed into a space of only about 20 cubic inches in volume!

Now let us return to the structure and contents of each filter chamber. From the great blood vessel of the abdomen, the aorta, a short thick renal artery, passes to each kidney, entering at the hilus, carrying a large amount of blood under high pressure. At the hilus this artery divides into several branches which pass to the junction between the cortex and medulla where each again divides, at length forming a small but stout little vessel, the efferent artery, or intake pipe which enters the filtration chamber, Bowman's capsule. As it plunges into the cup-like depression constituting the filter chamber, it breaks up into two, then four, and finally into about fifty curling, twisting loops, each about 1/2500 of an inch (10 microns) in diameter, which coil and twine in interlacing fashion and then reunite to pass out of the chamber as the outlet pipe or "efferent artery." The latter soon breaks up into fine capillaries that surround the meandering tubules mentioned above, finally reuniting to leave the kidney as the great renal vein.

The tortuous loops within the filter chambers constitute the glomeruli or filters, and each glomerulus with its little cup-like room forms a marvelous little filtration plant, the basic unit of the kidneys' excretory system. The reason for such an arrangement of glomerular loops can be understood by visualizing the structure of an ordinary room radiator. The steam enters the room through a single pipe which breaks up in the radiator into a large number of coils before leaving the room again as a single pipe. The many coils increase by so much the radiating surface of the apparatus. Although the glomerular loops are only 1/2500 of an inch (10 microns) wide, their length totals about 1 inch (25 mm.) in each glomerulus. If there are about 1,000,-000 glomeruli in each kidney, the surface area of its glomerular capillaries is about 0.78 of a square meter for one kidney, or for both kidneys about 1.56 square meters (15 square feet), the area of a dining-room table top. If, however, there are in each kidney 4,500,000 glomeruli, as some believe, the filtration surface of glomerular capillaries in both kidneys exceeds 7 square meters (about 67 square feet), equivalent to the floor area of a small room.

FUNCTIONS OF THE KIDNEY

In simple terms the purpose of the kidney is to make urine and get rid of it. Our first clue to an understanding of its function is obtained by analysis of whatever is found to be continuously present in "normal" urine, for such is obviously not wanted by the body. We find therein large amounts of water and urea, smaller amounts of sodium chloride (common table salt), potassium, phosphates and sulphates, creatinine and uric acid, and minimal amounts of several other substances. Some are excreted, as they are always and entirely useless; others are got rid of because, while ordinarily useful, the body already has enough of them. The functions of the normal kidney are further demonstrated by observing what happens when they go wrong, noting what substances accumulate in the blood and tissues and what deficiencies appear in the urine.

As a result of such analyses we can summarize the known functions of the kidney as follows:

1. It excretes 40 to 60 per cent of all water liberated from the body. An excess of this vital substance is always present in healthy bodies, derived from what we eat and drink and from cellular activity.

2. It excretes the waste products of protein destruction: urea, uric acid, creatinine.

3. It helps to preserve the normal acid-alkaline balance of our tissues by excreting excess acids. Our system is never "acid," and by "acidosis" we really mean a reduction in the reserve of alkali. All tissues and fluids of the body except the stomach juices and at times the sweat, are faintly alkaline. Although we eat large amounts of acids in food and are constantly producing more by our normal metabolic processes, the reaction (alkalinity) of our tissues remains practically constant. The maintenance of an alkaline reserve is of supreme importance, and the extreme delicacy of this balance is appreciated by realizing that death would occur were the reaction of our blood to be altered by the minute change equivalent to that caused by adding one drop of even a weak acid to a quart of water. Blood becoming as acid as distilled water or as alkaline as ordinary tap water would be incompatible with life (Marriott).

4. By eliminating just the proper amounts of salt and water the kidneys maintain that normal physiochemical state of body fluids responsible for osmotic pressure. When this is disturbed one of two things results: water-logging of tissues (dropsy, hydrops, edema, ascites,

anasarca)[3] or the opposite, a condition of body dehydration, desiccation, or water famine.

5. It has been recently discovered that the kidneys apparently manufacture small amounts of certain substances found in urine: hippuric acid and perhaps ammonia. All other recognized urinary constituents are brought to the kidney already manufactured, and the kidney merely excretes them unchanged. Since the synthesis of hippuric acid and possibly ammonia are but steps in the excretion of unwanted substances, we can still conclude that the known functions of the kidney are chiefly if not entirely excretory.

PHYSIOLOGY OF THE KIDNEY: HOW IT CARRIES ON ITS FUNCTIONS

The striking anatomic arrangement of glomerulus and tubule led early physicians to regard the kidney units as filters and to believe that urinary components passed through glomeruli into tubules by a sort of suction, or a simple process of filtration (resulting from a higher pressure in the glomerular capillaries). Later others insisted that the cells or microscopic units of which living matter is constructed, played more than a passive rôle in formation of urine, and that they had an important part in its manufacture, actually pouring out or "secreting" substances into the tubules. Thus there arose a great dispute between the "mechanists" and the "vitalists." While the details of this argument do not concern us here, a brief statement of the modern viewpoint on kidney physiology will help us to understand some of the different symptoms and signs of kidney disease and the rationale of treatment.

It has been estimated that more than 600 quarts (about 20,000 ounces) of blood (some say 1,000 to 1,500 quarts) flow through the kidneys every day, passing through glomeruli at the very reduced speed of about 18 inches per hour (0.125 mm. per second) (Vimtrup). About 90 per cent of it continues on into the efferent arteries and finally back into the main blood stream, but about 10 per cent of its fluid is taken out in the glomeruli and starts flowing down the tubules. The fluid taken out amounts to more than 60 quarts (cited by Harvey); others say 170 to 290 quarts (Rehberg, cited by Wilbur; Richards). Were all of it allowed to continue on down the tubules and be

[3]Dropsy means "hydrops" or "water." Edema means "swelling." Ascites ("bag") means "dropsy of the abdominal cavity." Anasarca ("throughout flesh") signifies "general dropsy."

lost in urine there would be an enormous waste, causing almost constant urination and producing a tremendous thirst to replenish body fluids. In addition to water this glomerular filtration includes not only wastes (urea, uric acid, creatinine, and so forth) but also large amounts of useful substances (sugar, salt and amino-acids), foods which the body cannot afford to lose. The tubules, therefore, prevent this waste by reabsorbing through the cells, of which the walls of the tubules are built, all of the sugar and amino-acids, and almost all of the water and chlorides, at the same time refusing to take back any of the unwanted substances. As a result of this vigorous reabsorption of water (97 per cent or more) the total amount of fluid that finally reaches the bladder to be excreted as urine is only about 1½ quarts a day (instead of 60 or more quarts) in which there is a high concentration of waste products. The latter are not equally concentrated; for example, there are 60 to 100 times as much urea in a quart of urine as in a quart of blood, but only about 30 times as much uric acid.

Modern studies indicate, then, that substances pass out of the blood going from glomeruli into tubules in one direction only. Lower down in the tubules some useful materials are restored to the blood by passing through the cells lining the tubules. That the passage of materials through the cells lining the tubules may not be just in one direction, as formerly supposed, is suggested by recent evidence indicating that certain tubular cells may actually take out further waste material from the blood capillaries and pour it into the tubules. Thus this waste passes through the walls of the tubules in the opposite direction from the useful substances which are reclaimed by them. By this means the kidneys are given a second chance of throwing off wastes through a "tubular secretion" supplementing glomerular excretion.

The coördinated activity of the myriad cells in each kidney unit reminds one of a scene in an automobile assembling plant where down along the long runways are placed hundreds of men. Here one is adding a part, there another removing some appliance, until at the end of the runway there rolls off a completed car. As flivvers are thus born at so many an hour, so drops of urine roll out into the bladder at the rate of about four a minute, night and day.

In summary: Both the glomerular and tubular cells seem to exhibit definite discrimination in determining just what and how much shall be taken out of the blood, excreted, and what and how much shall be reabsorbed. By a process of filtration the glomeruli excrete a plasma,

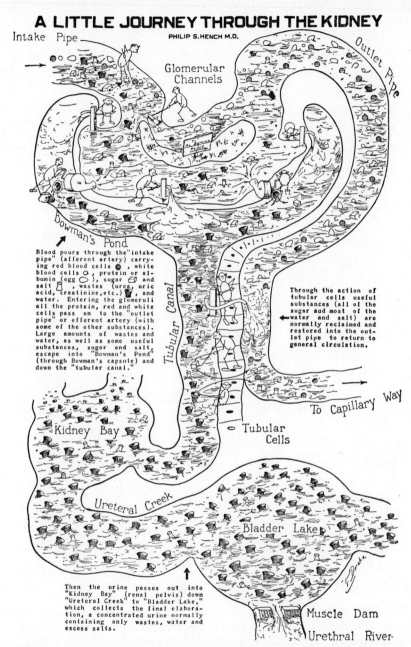

FIG. 57. A little journey through the kidney. The essentials of renal physiology illustrated in the spirit of a modern animated map.

containing substances (except proteins and cellular elements) in about the same concentration as they exist in the blood, and through the selective reabsorption of useful substances and possibly also some secretion by tubular cells, this fluid is further elaborated into the final product, urine.

To demonstrate this graphically, with due apologies for the omission of finer details and at the risk of being taken too literally, I have included a diagram, drawn in the spirit of our modern animated maps, showing the main essentials of renal physiology.

HISTORY OF KIDNEY DISEASE BEFORE THE TIME OF RICHARD BRIGHT

In the light of our present knowledge one may be surprised to learn that almost all we know about the kidney and its diseases we have learned in the last century. The term "Bright's disease" is about one hundred years old, and prior to this little indeed was known of the diseases of the kidney. As a matter of fact, before that it was not even known that albumin in the urine bore any special relation to nephritis. At the time of the American Revolution, doctors recognized in general only two kinds of kidney disease: stones (*nephritis calculosa*) and suppurative or purulent nephritis (so-called ulcerated or pus kidney). This much had been known two thousand years before in the time of Hippocrates, the Father of Medicine, when four diseases of the kidney were described, among them calculus (stone) and abscess.

It may afford an interesting diversion to trace briefly the development of our knowledge of the kidney and its diseases and especially of urine, an analysis of which constitutes modern man's commonest medical experience. Let us recall that time way back when it was not even known where urine came from nor what the kidneys were made for. Philologists tell us the word "kidney" may have been derived from those words meaning womb or egg. Its Latin ancestor *rein* (renal, and so forth) it is thought referred to the midriff, the parts about the heart and liver.[4] Hippocrates (460–370 B.C.) believed the kidneys separated

[4]The Bible contains many references to "reins" and kidneys, using the terms literally and figuratively. In a literal sense it refers only to the kidneys of animals offered in sacrifice. By law the kidneys and their fatty covering were Jehovah's special share of sacrificial victims. Their peculiar sanctity arose from the belief that, next to the blood, the kidneys were the seat of life and should therefore be returned to the Author of Life. A natural extension of

out urine, but Aristotle (384–321 B.C.), who was one of the greatest scientists and philosophers of all times and who carried on extensive anatomic investigations, thought the bladder was the chief site of urine formation. He believed that the kidneys were not essential to life, but "when they are present exist not of actual necessity but as matter of greater finish and perfection." Galen (A.D. 131–201) had no patience with such "nonsense" and considered that the blood serum percolated through the kidneys. A thousand years after Aristotle, errors still persisted in some quarters, and urine was considered by Protospatharius (A.D. 603–641) a filtrate of the portal vein of the liver.

Long before this, although the ancients knew little or nothing about the kidneys or the source and purpose of urine, much was written about urine itself. Records indicate that Babylonian physicians at the dawn of earliest civilization (around 4,000 B.C.) examined it sufficiently to note color changes, "worms of urine" (casts), and "knots of thread" (albumin). In old Sanskrit writings there was described a total of twenty different diseases, each with its characteristic urine, among them "honey urine." Ten of these diseases were said to be due to deranged phlegm, six to deranged bile, and the remaining four to wind. The diagnoses of diseases, as well as prophecies as to their outcome, were made by those ancient worthies from examination of the skin, eyes, and tongue, but "especially the pulse and urine without which all knowledge of physick is obscure, doubtful and uncertain." From observations made on the urine of patients with fever Hippocrates wrote: "One may judge what is to take place, for if the urine be thick and more yellowish so much the better, but if it be thinner and blacker so much the worse. . . . When in fever the urine is turbid, there either is or will be headache." And again: "The most deadly of all kinds of urine are the fetid, watery, black and thick. . . . If the urine is passed in deficient quantity, with a noise, it indicates either that the man stands in need of purging or that the bladder is diseased."

Urine was held by some to have curative properties, an idea re-

this idea led to their being considered the "seats of passion," the organs of feeling, or man's conscience. It is used in this latter sense in Psalms, 26:2— "Examine me, O Lord, try my reins and my heart"—and not as an appeal for a kidney function test as a recent writer implied when he wrote, "Even the Bible mentions as important 'to test a man's heart and kidneys.'"

pulsive to others. "It is said that some who have drunk it in the plague have recovered." It was also drunk as a cure for leprosy, putrid ulcers, sprains of the feet, used as antidote for snake bite and deadly poisons, and as an application for erysipelas! "The urine of mules suits with arthritic remedies, that of goats and camels is laxative of the belly and hence is given in dropsical complaints."

Through the succeeding centuries gradually uroscopy, the art of inspection of urine, became the greater part of medical practice. Many of us will recall the numerous drawings in European art galleries[5] which depict the physician of the thirteenth to the sixteenth centuries practicing this art, a subject particularly fascinating to Dutch painters. We can view them with greater appreciation after reading the interesting descriptions of Garrison, Wellcome, and others. The urine was always contained in a characteristic flask, of transparent "clere glasse," not flat on the bottom, "but the shape of a very bladder (for the urinall should represent the bladder of a man) and so shall every thyng be sene in his dew place and colore." The container being shaped thus "the urine should be in natural position as in the bladder." With the spherical base the container could not stand alone, and it was therefore always carried to the physician in a basket of cylindrical shape. The grave-faced physician, dressed in doctor's robe and cap, is always represented as inspecting the urine in a most judicial way, sometimes holding the flask in his hand, at other times examining it while held in the hand of a patient or servant, as by some a physician was considered too sacred to hold a urine bottle himself. Near by the patient silently awaits the verdict, his attentive expression portraying his pathetic anxiety.

A proper light was most necessary, and the urine was held in such a way that no reflection or refraction from the sun's rays would "make the colour more remisse," and thus interfere with a true observation. As many as twenty different colors were described, each of significance. In addition to the color, the urine was studied as to consistency, transparency, quantity, sediment, odor, froth, scum floating at the top, and substances in the watery part. Grave pronouncements followed such inspection. Cloudy urine at the top of the bottle signified disease of the highest parts of the man's body, alterations in the middle part

[5] I am informed that there are no such originals in the art museums of the United States.

of the urine related to diseases of the spleen, liver, heart, lungs, bowels, and stomach, and the urinary sediment showed the condition of the lowest parts of the body. Bubbles and frothing indicated evil digestion.

"In an epoch when all clinical methods and investigation were unknown," as Wellcome has aptly put it, "it is natural that the urine should be expected to indicate the disease and its nature, and so as time went on it is not surprising to find that inspection of the urine gradually became more popular in medical diagnosis, as doubtless it appealed from the spectacular point of view, as strongly to the patient as to the physician." But as imagination increased, uroscopy became uromancy and quacks flourished everywhere, traveling the land with their urine bottles, preying on the gullibility of the people, diagnosing all kinds of diseases, and prognosticating all manner of events, from the diagnosis of chastity or pregnancy, to the sex of an unborn child.

Naturally a reaction was aroused from time to time against such charlatanism, and frequent tirades were made against the "tricks of the water-doctors" who might go to such limits as did "the physician who saw an oat-grain in a urinal and stated the patient had eaten a horse."

Particularly blameworthy were the attempts of physicians to diagnose the ills of an unseen patient from the analysis of urine sent from a distance. This practice in sixteenth-century England caused the passage of statutes forbidding apothecaries from sending such specimens to physicians, and physicians from pronouncing on any disorder from such an uncertain procedure.

Up to this time the examination of urine was almost entirely by inspection, not analysis. Discoveries in the seventeenth and eighteenth centuries saved it from ill repute and opened the era beginning with Van Helmont's (1577–1644) studies on the variable weight of urine, and ending in the epochal work of Bright (1827) which ushered in the modern period in the study of renal disease. Among these were the demonstration of albumin in urine in the presence of acetic acid (Dekkers, 1694), after boiling (Cotugno, 1764), and in dropsical urine in the presence of nitric acid (Cruickshank, 1798); the determination of its water and solid content (Bellini, 1643–1704), its specific gravity (Booerhaave, 1668–1738), and some of its chemical constituents, such as urea (Booerhaave, 1720; Rouelle, 1771), sugar in diabetic urine (Dobson, 1772), and many others.

THE WORK OF RICHARD BRIGHT

Surpassing all these in importance, as has been said, was the contribution in 1827 of Richard Bright, a distinguished English physician of Guy's Hospital, London, whose name will always be the symbol of kidney disease. To judge the permanency and extent of his reputation even in this day this comment may be made. The rare and great honor paid by physicians to colleagues who have made outstanding contributions in certain diseases is to give that disease an eponymic designation. Of the thousands of known diseases, about 375 are called in modern medical literature after physicians' names. Of all these conditions the layman, happily unacquainted with disease, is familiar, we are sure, with the name of hardly a single one save "Bright's disease." (Saints have fared less well, being honored thus only about twenty-five times.)

In retrospect Bright's contribution seems a simple one, the demonstration that albumin in urine indicated kidney disease. Its importance rested in making with gratifying precision and clarity the differentiation between several diseased states about which there was great confusion.

In Bright's time the significance of dropsy and of albuminuria was unknown. Dropsy, an accumulation of fluid in the tissues (extremities, abdomen, lungs), was thought by some to be a disease in itself; by others it was considered the result of a variety of diseases, among them disease of the liver, ovaries, lungs, heart, or from certain obstructions to circulatory flow. Albumin had recently been found in the urine of dropsical cases (Cotugno, 1764; Cruickshank, 1798; Wells, 1811; Blackall, 1813), but neither dropsy nor albumin was at that time considered significantly related to kidney disease (which was then thought to consist mostly of stones or the inflammation resulting therefrom). This may seem strange when we learn that as early as the sixth century a Roman emperor's physician (Aetius) noted the association of dropsy and hardened kidneys. Four centuries later (Avicenna) the doctor of a Mohammedan caliph commented on the excessive, thin, watery urine in dropsy, and in 1476 Saliceto, an Italian doctor, wrote on the association of scanty urine, hardened kidneys, and dropsy. But this had apparently been long forgotten. It was reserved for Bright first to connect clearly these conditions, albuminuria and dropsy, with kidney disease. He showed indisputably that albuminous urine was present in twenty-four cases of dropsy with kidney disease, but absent in eleven cases of dropsy with liver disease and in four cases of dropsy with heart disease. Thus he demonstrated that there were different kinds of dropsy, that albuminuria was a sign of nephritis, and that the dropsy resulting therefrom could be thus recognized by finding albuminous matter in urine.

Although he mentioned several varieties of nephritis of differing severity, Bright spoke of "this most fatal disease"—fatal enough to bring seventeen of his twenty-four patients to the post-mortem table. While he felt that "where the mischief is less rooted we may undoubtedly do much," he admitted that "some cases defy cure." Thus by the very strength of his clinical and necropsy data, so important to prove the significance of his discoveries, he unwittingly fostered the notion that this new type of nephritis was a hopeless condition. Then began the era when albuminuria doomed many comparatively healthy persons to the fear of an early death. So indiscriminately were dire predictions made on the presence of albumin alone that Bright wrote other papers mainly for the purpose of correcting this misconception. He tried to modify the general pessimistic view by stating that "the disease on which the secretion of albuminous urine depends is in the commencement functional, that as long as it continues in this state it is capable of cure or of relief by various means."

His chemist colleagues, Bostock, Barlow, and Rees, further softened the sting of albuminuria by their careful analyses, demanding that laboratory data necessary for a diagnosis of Bright's disease include other tests on urine (e.g., the nitric acid ring test), besides the heat test. While confirming its general importance as pointed out by Bright, they noted cases where albuminuria was "so trifling in nature as to render it almost a constant occurrence."

MODERN SIGNIFICANCE OF ALBUMINURIA

The development of modern tests of renal function has extended our knowledge of the diseases and disturbances of kidneys so that the finding of albumin in the urine is no longer interpreted as the equivalent of Bright's disease. It is merely a signpost pointing to any one of several different conditions. Its importance lies in the fact that it constitutes the most readily detected aberration of normal renal function. While it is thus usually the earliest sign of renal disturbance, functional or organic, it may occur in persons who in other respects are apparently entirely normal, or it may be initiated by any one of many conditions which can disturb kidney function, disturbances which are frequently not great enough to warrant the term "nephritis." However, when albumin does appear, it generally indicates a kidney of which the function is embarrassed due to some change, slight or great, temporary or permanent, in its cells.

Albumin is a simple protein found in nearly all animal and many vegetable tissues. It is soluble in water and coagulates as egg white (albumin) does on heating. It is formed by the dissolution of dead tissue cells, either of food or from our own bodies, including red and white blood cells. Digested foods form proteins which are absorbed and circulate in blood to be used in human growth. About two thirds of this blood protein is in the form of albumin. As we have seen, healthy kidneys do not allow this useful substance, food albumin, to pass out from the circulation into the kidney tubes and be lost in urine. Hence the liquid which passes through the small filters of the kidney is normally protein or albumin free.

There are two additional sources from which albumin may arise to appear in the urine. When our own tissue cells die, instead of becoming food protein, they are in the blood as waste protein. Other forms of waste or foreign protein may arise from impure foods or injected proteins. These the kidney filters do not try to keep back, but allow to pass into the urine as waste, albumin to be excreted. Albumin in urine must come, therefore, either from food or from waste proteins in the blood passing through the kidneys, or from the breaking down of cells in the kidney itself or along the urinary passages. The loss of food proteins is accidental; that of waste proteins is purposeful.

Because healthy urine is practically albumin free, albuminuria should always be considered an abnormality, even though its significance is exceedingly variable. Found in the course of an examination for life insurance, it serves as the starting point for other than a routine examination.

INCIDENCE

The incidence of albuminuria in a large group of healthy people is approximately 5 per cent. Certain tests demonstrate albumin more readily than others, and in a series of 417 men (Hill, L. C.) in a military training camp almost 30 per cent showed albuminuria on first examination when finer tests were used, as compared to only about 3 per cent when the ordinary nitric acid test was employed. Various workers using this nitric acid method found an incidence of albuminuria on a single test ranging from 3 to 16 per cent, with 5 to 7 per cent most commonly reported. Albuminuria was noted in about 5 per cent of 60,000 healthy soldiers (MacLean) and in a similar proportion of 5,000 healthy students (Lee). In another series of 20,000 male students (Diehl-McKinlay), 5.3 per cent showed albuminuria on the first examination. In 66 per cent of these the albuminuria was transient, discovered only once; it was occasionally present in 13 per cent, and persistent in 12 per cent, without any other evidence indicating kidney damage. In only 6.5 per cent of those with albuminuria were there other signs indicating probable renal disease. About 3 per cent of 100,924 male life insurance policyholders showed definite albumin in the urine, while slight traces were found in about 19 per cent more (Sydenstricker and Britten). Sudden increases in its incidence may be noted as in the case of the "epidemics" of albuminuria seen in healthy West Point cadets (Ashburn).

It is found much more frequently in those who are sick or who consider themselves sick and consult physicians. At a large clinic albumin was detected in the first urine specimen in 39 per cent of 663 patients seen consecutively (Sanford, Conner, Magath, and Heck). Where three different methods were used, albumin was indicated by one or more tests in more than half (59 per cent) of those studied. Further investigations, however, revealed definite kidney disease in less than half (40 per cent) of the 39 per cent in whose urine albumin was found.

Albuminuria bears a definite relationship to age (Calvin, Isaacs and Meyer, Sydenstricker and Britten). There is an increase in its incidence from childhood up to the age of sixteen years. From this peak there is a rapid decline to between thirty and forty years of age, after which a progressive increase again occurs up to seventy years and over.

TYPES OF ALBUMINURIA

The albumin that leaks into urine through or from the kidneys constitutes "renal albuminuria"; that which is added to urine in the lower urinary passages below the kidneys is called "nonrenal albuminuria."

"Renal albuminuria" may be caused by imperfect working of

normal kidneys or by real disease of the kidneys. It occurs (1) when there is disease primarily in the kidneys or when, in a general disease of the body, renal disease constitutes a major part of the disability; (2) from disease primarily arising in other organs but definitely affecting the kidneys; (3) with certain states in which the working of the kidneys is disturbed, thus causing "benign albuminuria" without other signs indicating disease.

The first is the most important, when there is true kidney disease either affecting mainly the kidneys themselves, or mainly some other part of the body, and this, in turn, affecting the kidneys. Here, in general but with certain exceptions, albuminuria is associated with the presence in the urine of casts (plugs of material washed out of the tubules) and sometimes red blood corpuscles but no pus cells, with variations in the amount and composition of urine. There is also a variety of signs and symptoms due to changes in the blood and other organs in addition to the kidneys. The main examples are the various forms of true, acute and chronic Bright's disease (diffuse bilateral nephritis), cysts or tumors of the kidney, disease of kidneys in pregnancy and in chronic gout, plugging of blood vessels (thrombi) to or in kidneys, and disease caused by the presence of renal stones, tuberculosis, or obstruction to urinary flow. Strangely enough, cases of severe kidney disease without albuminuria are occasionally seen, and then the diagnosis rests on other findings.

Secondly, a large variety of diseases in other regions may affect the kidneys to the extent that albumin appears in urine generally without other definite urinary abnormalities. Varying degrees of disturbed kidney function, however, may result. Transient albuminuria may appear in children after a trivial illness, a cold or bronchitis; marked anemia or jaundice may induce it. To enumerate further, this type of renal albuminuria may result from almost any febrile condition, especially scarlet fever, diphtheria, malaria, erysipelas, smallpox, and pneumonia; less frequently from certain drugs, anesthetics (ether, chloroform), poisoning with lead, mercury, arsenic, phosphorus, from alcoholism, burns, toxic goiter, acute gout, from certain diseases of the blood and blood-forming organs, and from parasites. It also occurs with disturbances of circulation ensuing from diseases of the heart with heart failure, and with certain vasomotor neuroses producing spasm of vessels. Many of these conditions produce degeneration of kidney cells, causing a type of kidney disease commonly called nephrosis, which may often clear up.

The third variety of renal albuminuria is that often called physiologic or benign albuminuria, arising from a number of conditions producing alterations in the general circulation and corresponding changes in the normal rate and flow of blood in kidneys. They generally result from certain physical or functional states whose influence on the kidney is reflected by a transient, sometimes a rather persistent, albuminuria without additional evidence of renal impairment. The disability produced may be harmless and insufficient to justify the term "nephritis." Thus, various amounts of albumin may appear in urine after strenuous exercise such as rowing, boxing, running, and so forth, and in emotional states and malnutrition. It is this form which appears in adolescence often without apparent cause. It may occur after a cold shower or exposure to cold, in students cramming for examinations, and in football players after a game. Its relation to malnutrition is shown by the fact that in a series of children of the poor, more than 60 per cent had albuminuria, while in an equal number of children under the best hygienic care only 15 per cent demonstrated it.

Some of these benign forms of albuminuria appear only when the person is in the erect position and hence are called postural orthostatic (cyclic, intermittent) forms of albuminuria. A curious variety, the lordotic type of orthostatic albuminuria, is found occasionally in healthy young persons with an exaggerated spinal curve in the small of the back. Considerable albumin may be present in urine passed in daytime, but that formed at night while in a reclining position or passed on arising in the morning shows none. After being up and about again it reappears. It is thought by some to be due to pressure of abdominal organs on the vein of the left kidney, causing interference with adequate circulation when in the upright position. As body growth is completed, the condition usually disappears, and the patient remains quite healthy. Others believe it is due to mild but persistent kidney damage from an unknown cause.

NONRENAL ALBUMINURIA

We have seen that albumin forms on the dissolution of any tissue cells. In the lower urinary tract cellular débris may give origin to small quantities of albumin which are added to urine after its formation in the kidney and its passage into the tubules. The presence of spermatozoa in the male genital tract or of cast-off cells from the vagina in women may account for a mild albuminuria, contaminating an otherwise normal urine. Catheterized specimens are therefore sometimes necessary when examining women to be certain of the source of albumin. When inflammation occurs, with formation of pus in the urinary tract below the kidneys, such cells may dissolve in varying quantities. A nonrenal albuminuria may thus arise in cystitis (inflammation of the bladder), pyelitis (inflammation of the kidney pelvis), prostatitis, or from stones in the bladder, ureters, or kidneys. In these conditions the kidneys themselves may be playing no part in the production of albuminuria.

CHEMICAL TYPES OF ALBUMINURIA

The term "albuminuria" is not strictly accurate, for the coagulable protein of urine consists generally of a mixture comprising not only albumin but also globulin, mucin, and other proteins. In benign albuminuria proteins besides albumin derived from blood serum are prominently present, such as globulin, nucleo-albumin and mucin. In definite nephritis most of the urinary protein consists of serum albumin and globulin which may be derived from the food proteins in the blood leaking through damaged glomeruli. Occasionally part of the albuminuria comes from proteins other than those normally circulating in blood; one of these is Bence-Jones protein, which will be discussed later. There is some evidence to suggest that in the early stages of diffuse bilateral renal disease at least part of the urinary albumin comes from degenerated liver cells. Later, protein may be liberated from degenerating kidney cells. These, becoming more permeable, then permit the loss of large amounts of serum albumin. Since the methods of easily differentiating these chemical types of albumin are as yet not perfected, these points are in controversy, and such studies are not applicable to routine examinations.

CONCLUSIONS REGARDING ALBUMINURIA

We have discussed the subject of albuminuria in some detail because of the importance popularly attached to it. It is obvious that to determine the type of albuminuria present a doctor is necessary, and not just a microscope or laboratory, as the differentiation between significant and insignificant forms can be made only after a careful history has been taken and physical examination made in addition to chemical studies. It is particularly important to recognize benign, postural, and other forms of functional albuminuria to prevent persons so affected from being limited by unwarranted fears and by needless restrictions in diet and activity, as occurs when confused with true nephritis. In such instances the psychic harm from a dreaded diagnosis may be much greater than the physical harm afforded by the condition itself. Thus are created "albuminuria neurotics." It has been said that "frequently the 'disease' occurs only in the physician's test tube and in the mind of the patient" (Calvin, Isaacs and Meyer).

To the fearful patient the discovery of albuminuria may be a rude awakening arousing concern unduly great. Yet even when significant it sometimes constitutes a positive advantage, a beneficent warning to slow up, thereby preventing serious illness or sudden death. From this viewpoint a great physician once wrote a paper with the paradoxical title, "On the Advantage of a Trace of Albumin and a Few Casts in the Urine of Men over Fifty."

In general, albuminuria in older persons usually represents some organic disease of variable degree, while that of the young is often functional. In many cases either one may be entirely consistent with the prospect of a healthy and active life. Where doubts are entertained, prolonged but not too anxious observation is justified, using such supplementary examinations over a period of several months as seem necessary.

The fallacy of placing much reliance on periodic urinalyses without an accompanying history and physical examination seems evident. Of themselves such analyses are of little value and may do more harm than good. It has been rightfully said that a physical examination with a urinalysis once a year is of far greater value than a urine test alone once a week. Yet a reputable mail-order house of wide activities recently saw fit to offer such service, however, for a short time only. The service was catalogued between a bathtub mat and a bottle of milk of magnesia, and an "analysis covering twenty-nine chemical and microscopical tests" was promised.

We are reminded of the story of a great English physician of the seventeenth century. A woman presented to him a specimen of her husband's urine, requesting a diagnosis and prescription. "Where is he?" asked the doctor, to which she replied, "Sick in bed four miles off." "What is he?" "A boot-maker." Throwing out the urine and substituting a fresh sample the doctor said, "Take this home with you, and if your husband will undertake to fit me with a pair of boots by its inspection, I will diagnose and treat him by a similar examination."

Shakespeare commented similarly when to Falstaff's inquiry, "What says the doctor to my water?" the page replies, "He said, sir, the water itself was a good healthy water, but for the party that owned it he might have more diseases than he knows for." A modern counterpart is the inelegant but pertinent tale of the canny gentleman who on receiving a favorable report from a single, but mixed, specimen sent to a "urine laboratory" happily said, "Good! Mama's well, papa's well, the whole family's well."

MODERN METHODS OF EXAMINING THE KIDNEYS

As Bright found more than one test useful, indeed necessary, so we have benefited by that scientific ingenuity which has provided a number of ways in which to study the condition of the kidneys. A routine urine analysis constitutes the first test to be used and affords the chief point of departure, indicating whether other tests are necessary. While it is true that occasional cases of severe nephritis have been found where the urine was apparently normal, not even containing albumin, generally some abnormality is present. Ordinarily urine is examined for its alkaline or acid reaction, its specific gravity, the presence of albumin, sugar, pus or blood cells, sediment, and casts. The odor and sediment of urine of a normal person can be altered in several ways; by the kind and amount of food eaten, amount of water drunk, length of time the urine has stood, time of day it was passed, and so forth. Odoriferous or cloudy urine, therefore, does not of itself indicate nephritis, nor is clear urine a sure token of healthy kidneys. Casual inspection is valueless, indeed may be misleading.

Casts, as has been said, are small masses of protein material, cylindrical in structure, taking the shape of the kidney tubule. They are of various types. Those most frequently found are the pale, transparent "hyaline" casts. Others with cellular débris attached to them are called granular, fatty, waxy, epithelial, and blood casts. Their origin is not perfectly understood. Normal persons may pass small numbers of hyaline casts which arise from the same conditions that may produce albuminuria. When they are numerous or when other types of casts are present it usually signifies inflammatory or degenerative changes from renal disease.

We have seen that the ability of the kidneys to excrete a large amount of waste in a small amount of fluid, in other words, to elaborate a thick or concentrated urine, is one of their most important functions. By the water-dilution and water-concentration tests we can determine whether their concentrating power is being maintained. On one day a patient is given solid, dry food only; no fluids are permitted. The urine is collected at certain intervals, and it should normally become thick, highly colored, with a specific gravity of about 1.025 or over. On another day 7½ glasses (3 pints, 1,500 c.c.) of water are given on an empty stomach. At least 75 per cent of this should be passed normally within the next four hours; the urine becomes very thin, watery, and with a specific gravity as low as 1.003. When the kidney is seriously impaired this concentrating and diluting ability is lost, and the specific gravity becomes relatively fixed around 1.010. As long as it is partially preserved, maximal renal damage has not yet occurred.

The size, shape, and position of the kidney can be faintly but un-mistakably outlined in an ordinary X-ray picture of the abdomen. The size and shape of the pelvic cavity inside the kidney can be studied also by special means. With the cystoscope and ureteral catheters certain liquids opaque to the X-ray can be forced to flow gently up the ureters to fill the renal pelvis, outlining it sharply like a glove with many projecting fingers (a pyelogram). If disease has destroyed part of the kidney substance or its tubular projections, or if a stone is present, blocking up all or part of the pelvis or ureter, characteristic alterations from the normal shadow are produced which help the trained eye in diagnosis. One of medicine's recent triumphs is the elaboration of a harmless substance which, taken by vein, finds its way to the kidneys and becomes concentrated therein sufficiently to cast such a shadow on X-ray plates, thereby in some cases avoiding the discomfort of the cystoscope.

The excretory ability of the kidneys can be tested by injecting into the muscles or vein certain harmless dyes (phenolsulphonphthalein, indigo carmine, methylene blue) to see how rapidly and completely they are eliminated in the urine. Eight to ten minutes after injection 'phthalein (pronounced thaleen) begins to appear in the urine and 40 to 60 per cent of the amount injected should appear within the following hour. Disease of the kidneys or any block to the free passage of urine below the kidneys in the tubes or bladder (from stone, adjacent tumors, enlarged prostate) will cause a definite reduction in the amount of dye recovered. Since we do not know just which cells, glomeruli or tubules, have most to do with the excretion of dyes, their retention does not imply specifically localizable damage.

By means of dyes and the cystoscope a trained physician can often determine whether one or both kidneys are diseased and how much. Passing small ureteral catheters or collecting tubes into each ureter as they enter the bladder, one can see, in the urine samples collected separately from each kidney, whether blood, pus, or germs (e. g., tubercle bacilli) are coming from one or both sides. The importance of this test can be imagined when it is deemed necessary to remove one kidney. The function of the other must be adequately gauged. Finer details concerning excretory capacity can be determined by giving orally or injecting into veins, not "foreign dyes," but measured amounts of those products which the kidneys naturally handle (urea, uric acid, creatinine), then studying their concentration in blood and urine, and the speed of their elimination. These are called "clearance" or "concentration" tests.

When kidney function is appreciably impaired, waste substances accumulate in the blood so that their concentration therein may rise from ten to fifty times (urea 16 to 700 mg. per 100 c.c.; uric acid 2 to 30 mg.; creatinine 1 to 20 mg. or more, sulphates from 2 to 40 mg. or over). When the kidneys are disturbed sulphates are one of the first substances to increase in blood. Urea and uric acid are excreted fairly readily, and the estimation of urea concentration in blood is the most important and common test of renal function, next to a urine analysis. Since creatinine is excreted very easily it is a very sick kidney that cannot still rid the blood of it, and hence it is the last substance to increase therein. When it rises appreciably and constantly it is generally an omen of impending death, indicating a kidney too disturbed even to carry on this, its simplest function. We can appreciate thus that blood analyses may give information of great value.

As waste substances accumulate in the blood they begin to adulterate all body tissues and appear in abnormal amounts in such fluids as saliva, breast milk, bile, and the fluids that bathe the brain, spinal cord, heart, lungs, and joints. They even accumulate in fluids of the eyeballs and are present excessively in tears. Advantage has been taken of this fact by the author who showed that where blood tests are inconvenient or impossible because people had small veins or swollen, edematous extremities, a simple estimation of the amount of urea in saliva gives a satisfactory index of nitrogen retention in the body. In serious cases these and associated poisons are eliminated excessively in sweat and by bowels and may cause small skin and bowel ulcers. In such cases "uremia" is present, a condition we shall discuss later.

The kidneys are not isolated structures, and their disturbances may affect distant organs and systems, especially the heart-blood vessel (cardiovascular) system. Therefore it is important for the doctor to examine the heart, the blood pressure, and the condition of the blood vessels in the arms, and particularly of the smaller ones in the eye, where at times certain "diagnostic" disturbances may be seen with an ophthalmoscope.

KNOWLEDGE DERIVED FROM KIDNEY TESTS

We have gone far—some say too far—from the simple albumin test in finding ways of diagnosing nephritis. However, no one test tells the whole tale of a kidney's woe. Nor is an elaborate array of expensive tests ordinarily necessary. The intelligent use of four or five of them (urine analysis, dye test or urea estimation, water dilution, and concentration test and blood count), along with the patient's story and a physical examination, will give all necessary information —at least in so-called "medical nephritis." Where pus and blood are present, where stones and other surgical conditions are suspected, advantage of other tests should be taken. In many cases the physician from such studies can with remarkable exactness tell the cause and extent of the disease and the exact parts of the kidney affected. He may venture a prophecy on whether the patient will recover or not, and if not how long he has an average chance of living, and finally what the kidney should look like after death. Sometimes the information gained from such examinations is limited. While they show approximately how badly the kidneys are diseased, one cannot always say "only the tubules are involved" or "the glomeruli are alone concerned." The kidney filters and tubules work together essentially as units, and when one part is diseased the other part is apt to become disturbed also. Often when the kidney is "sick" it is like the boy with the toothache, "sick all over." At other times, when one part of the kidney is too disturbed to carry on its function, that work is apparently take over by another part: a compensatory mechanism. Furthermore, invisible lesions are sometimes present which the microscope and test tube cannot demonstrate. While the doctor cannot see how the kidneys look, he can see how they are working and act accordingly.

GENERAL CAUSES OF KIDNEY DISEASE

Bright's disease, using the term inclusively, is "the response of the kidney to any alteration in its environment, especially to the irritation of toxic substances." As these toxic substances may be very numerous, so the causes of nephritis are many. Nephritis may result from the invasion of the kidneys (1) by germs themselves—bacteria of many kinds; (2) by bacterial poisons either manufactured by germs or formed in infected tissues; (3) by toxins not of bacterial origin, such as from metals; (4) by infectious and intoxications resulting from mechanical interference to the normal passage of urine produced by obstruction (e.g., from stones or an enlarged prostate gland), and (5) by abnormalities of growth, such as cysts and benign or malignant tumors, producing interference in the kidneys' function.

A large variety of germs may be brought to the kidneys and there set up infections which may localize in the kidneys alone or invade surrounding tissues and the lower urinary passages. The commonest germs found in such infections are the colon bacillus, staphylococci and streptococci. The tubercle bacillus is also an important invader. Some of the germs present a curious consistency in the "geography" of their invasion. Thus the colon bacillus usually attacks the interior part of the kidney, its pelvis and urinary tubes, while the cocci fight their battles in the outer part, the cortex and fatty tissues about the kidney. Some germs are especially prone to cause the precipitation of matter which forms stones. These various germs reach the kidney by several routes: they are either brought to it through the blood vessels (i. e., by an infected blood stream), or along infected lymph channels. or come up from infected urine dammed back by any interference with urinary flow, such as are presented by stones, kinks in the ureters, or enlarged prostate gland. Germs which reach the kidneys through the blood arise from foci or infection—small collections of germs in infected teeth, tonsils, ears, or other sites.

Some germs do not themselves invade the kidneys but from a distance liberate toxins or bacterial poisons which injure kidney cells. Or there may arise in distant infected areas toxins from dying infected cells which injure the kidney tissues as they are being excreted from the blood. There are many poisons not of bacterial origin which may produce nephritis. Some of them have been mentioned: certain metals such as mercury, uranium and lead, and poisons arising in burns, goiter, gout, and pregnancy. Some of these disturbing agents arouse rather individualistic reactions and special types of cellular disturbance identified by signs and symptoms fairly peculiar unto themselves. Such, for example, are tuberculous infections or the manifestation of stones. The majority of them, however, initiate changes in function and structure which at least in the beginning arouse in their victims more or less identical complaints.

GENERAL SYMPTOMS AND SIGNS OF KIDNEY DISEASE

In the mildest forms there may be no symptoms, and the patient only accidentally discovers his trouble through an examination for life insurance or examination for some other purpose. The blood pressure may be found a little too high, the heart may be a little inadequate, or the urine test betrays its guilty secret—any of these may introduce the unexpected, brutal revelation of the presence of kidney disease. Some are aware of vague discomfort; they are "out of sorts," or "off color," without knowing why. They may complain of an unaccustomed listlessness, unexplainable fatigue, dull headaches, slight puffiness about the eyes, or a poor appetite. Careful parents will especially be alert to such insidious complaints in their children.

As the kidneys become further diseased, a more or less identical train of events often occurs without regard to cause. Slight disturbances of vision are noted, such as occasional blurring, or spots in front of the eyes. There may be disturbances of sleep because of the desire to void urine at night. Bed-wetting, however, does not necessarily signify nephritis, being caused by a variety of conditions.[6] Dryness of the mouth may appear, with thirst necessitating frequent water

[6]Paulus Ægineta (A.D. 625–690) recommended the following for incontinence of urine (bed-wetting): "Burn the crop of a cock, and give to the patient to drink in tepid water when fasting, or the flowers of the white ox-eye (chrysanthemum) in like manner." (Vol. I, p. 548.)

drinking. There may be weight-loss, or if waterlogging of tissues (edema) occurs, the patient may gain weight, a source of false security, as if he were healthy. When stones, abscesses, or inflammations with pus in the lower urinary passages are present, pain may be present. In the majority of kidney diseases, however, pain is not a feature and may be entirely absent. The well-known advertisement illustrating a man slightly stooped with his hand on a painful flank is very misleading, inferring, as it does, that pain here generally means kidney disease, for which the advertiser has a wonderful medicine for so much a bottle. The great majority of patients with chronic pain in the flanks are not suffering from nephritis at all, but from some other disease, often some form of rheumatism in the muscles or joints of the spine.

As the disease progresses other organs may become disturbed, and a variety of symptoms may arise, such as dizziness, nausea, vomiting, perhaps diarrhea, severe headache, shortness of breath, swelling of feet and arms, enlargement of the abdomen from fluid, and symptoms of congestion in lungs and liver. As the nephritis approaches its most serious phase, unconsciousness may arise from uremic coma, and convulsions may occur.

The general signs of kidney disease may be local or constitutional. The local signs pertain to alterations in quantity, appearance, and quality of the urine. The urine may be pale and thin and voided frequently or in large amounts. In other cases it is dark, cloudy, and diminished in amount. Tests will show alterations in the urine and changes in the amounts of blood wastes present. Signs which reflect constitutional disturbances in association with nephritis may be: an elevated blood pressure, an enlarged heart, fluid in the lungs, small hemorrhages in the skin or in the back of the eyeballs, and especially a pale, pasty complexion and anemia. Verily, a pair of sick kidneys are versatile in the range and scope of their symptomatology.

UREMIA

If both kidneys are removed or both ureters blocked, death results in a few days, due to the retention and formation of poisons. This toxic state is called "uremia," the main characteristic of which is a period of drowsiness interrupted perhaps by convulsions. A similar intoxication may occur in cases of acute or chronic kidney insufficiency. Its first manifestations are often itching of the skin, headache,

,and cramps or twitchings in muscles. Then intense nausea, vomiting, and shortness of breath may occur. If the condition persists it may be distressingly punctuated by convulsive or epileptiform seizures, or the patient may lapse into a drowsy state ending in coma and death.

Uremia is not entirely dependent on the duration or amount of kidney disturbance. It may appear as a tragic surprise early in the course of an acute and seemingly moderate kidney inadequacy, and it may be postponed for long periods in a patient whose kidneys are known to be hardly functioning at all. It may attack with sudden fury a person in active and apparently healthy life, unaware of catastrophe impending. Nor is uremia dependent on the amount of urea dammed back in the blood, for a marked excess may be long present yet the patient escape its symptoms. Furthermore, it may occur in nephrosis, that form of kidney disease with water and salt retention, but where urea is eliminated normally. Here it is thought due to "wet-brain." But to confuse matters, uremia is not apparently dependent on edema alone, for it occurs in its most violent forms in nephritis without dropsy.

The exact substance responsible for uremic poisoning is not known. When his colleague Babington first noted an increase of urea in the blood in nephritis, Bright coined the term "uremia," believing urea toxic. Recent studies seem to indicate that urea is not sufficiently toxic to account for this profound upset. While various minor disturbances can be produced in the body by feeding excess urea, the author, following Hewlett and others, noted only slight muscular fatigue, drowsiness and lassitude after taking sufficiently large amounts of urea to raise the blood concentration for several hours to almost ten times the normal amount. The conclusions of such feeding experiments have only a limited application, however, just as symptoms of acute drunkenness cannot be compared to those in the chronic poisoning of habitual alcoholism.

In some illuminating experiments the physiologists, Bollman and Mann, have recently transplanted animals' ureters into the bowel, thereby causing at least part of the urinary substances to be reabsorbed through the intestines into the blood. The amazing concentration of more than 1,600 mg. of urea for each 100 c.c. of blood was reached (at least fifty times as much as is normally present), yet the animals continued to live with no noticeable effect whatever. This seems to present indisputable evidence that urea is not toxic, and physicians must therefore seek to discover and eliminate some far more potent poison.

When uremia begins to occur, that is, where an appreciable and prolonged rise of blood urea takes place, great caution must be exercised to prevent serious, perhaps fatal, toxicity. A sudden increase of headaches or muscle pains, a rapid elevation of blood pressure or blood urea, should warn of impending danger and prompt the physician to initiate the necessary additions to treatment. Unfortunately, in cases ⌐f progressively failing kidneys the physician's efforts often only postpone an inevitable tragedy but they do make its coming more bearable.

AIMS IN THE TREATMENT OF KIDNEY DISEASE AND KIDNEY FAILURE

Special treatment is required for such forms of kidney trouble as tuberculosis, tumors, pus infections, stones, the kidney poisoning that occasionally occurs in pregnancy, and that caused by obstruction from an enlarged prostate gland producing a backflow of urine. What the doctor tries to do in the treatment of nephritis and of renal insufficiency or kidney failure of other types can be discussed together briefly.

There are two aims in treatment: (1) Where possible, to discover and remove the cause of the kidney trouble, and (2) to lighten the burden on the kidney while it is diseased. The commonest known causes of nephritis are bacterial and chemical poisons. In nephritis of youth and middle age any chronic source of infection should if possible be removed. If this is impossible treatment locally should be provided for disease such as may exist in tonsils, the middle ears and sinuses of children especially, the teeth, prostate gland, and occasionally about the female organs. The time for their removal or treatment must be carefully chosen. The habitual use, by susceptible persons, of certain medicines is occasionally found to be a causal factor. "Cleansing mercury douches," for example, may seriously irritate the kidneys, and when so the use of such medicine should be stopped.

A physician of antiquity (Galen) wrote that "the offices of the kidneys and bladder being incessant, these parts, if diseased, having no rest, can scarcely get well." It has been found, however, that the kidneys as a whole do not work incessantly. Only certain units in a kidney are working at any one time, but when working they do so at full speed (Khanolkar). Richards, a physiologist, recently proved this by watching, through special microscopes, the glomeruli of a frog's kidney actually working. The glomeruli did not all work continuously but in shifts, some taking time off. Through this wise provision of nature the vitality of these delicate but energetic units is conserved.

The units of a sick kidney need even more rest. For them rest is the great restorer of health and life. It is the one measure that may tide them over until such time as they can recuperate fully, or may conserve their energies so they can carry on as long as possible. The kidneys can be rested in several ways: by not adding to their burdens, by shifting part of their work to other organs, and by helping them carry on such work as is unavoidable. During physical activity body tissues are forming wastes which the kidneys must handle. Rest in bed during the acute stage of nephritis is therefore advisable to prevent avoidable and unnecessary formation of body wastes. Some wastes are excreted through sweat and by bowels. A kidney can be spared considerable work by stimulating the skin and intestines to greater activity. This is accomplished by giving in some cases mild laxatives, warm enemas, a daily warm bath, and in severe cases hot packs under careful supervision. Since elimination of wastes through sweat is retarded or prevented by cold, ample clothing is necessary, and at times a sojourn in a warm, dry climate. Catching cold or the "flu" may add a serious burden to the kidney, and protection from prevalent infections should be afforded; avoidance of crowds, keeping away from sick relatives, and so on.

One of the most important measures is a carefully selected diet. A milk diet is by no means universally adequate. In some types of kidney disease such a diet may provide too much fluid; in another type it may contain too much protein. A proper diet for each patient can be planned only by a physician who has carried out the required minimum of laboratory procedures previously mentioned. Those who have found this necessity irksome will sympathize with Bill Nye. "I have just been sent to the hospital. My physician did it. He did it with an analysis. Anybody who amounts to anything nowadays gets analyzed. Sometimes you find casts, sometimes you find maple sugar and sometimes acids, oxides, paints, oils, varnish, white lead, borax, albumin, lime, hair and cement. In these cases the patient should be placed on a strict diet or he will in the course of his life become a corpse. . . . An analysis today shows more casts, fibrin, gelatin and some zinc and copper. The chemist also discovers that in 1853 I fell from an apple tree and tore my pants in two places. He says I will be unhappy with my third wife. She will be unhappy also."

The important features of diet concern the amounts of salt, water, and protein permissible. Where dropsy is present or impending, the amount of salt and fluid allowed must be carefully estimated. When retention of urea (and other wastes) occurs in the blood, it has long seemed best to restrict the proteins ingested. Recently some physicians, as the result of certain experiments, have become more lax, allowing rather generous amounts of protein. Until the effects of such diets are better known, moderate restrictions in meats, eggs, and other proteins seem indicated. A certain amount of fluids and of protein, however, is vitally necessary, and complete abstinence is rarely required. There is no essential difference between so-called red meats and white meats, as far as nephritis is concerned.

The elimination of wastes by kidneys can be increased by the use of a variety of diuretics, substances which cause them to pass through the kidneys in added amounts.[7] Water itself is a diuretic, and some persons after drinking a quart of water will within a short time eliminate perhaps a quart and a half of urine. Concentrated glucose solutions, coffee, tea, certain mineral waters, beer, and a number of drugs will promote an augmented urine flow. Some of these diuretics are indicated when dropsy occurs without the increase of wastes in the tissues. Choice of a proper diuretic is important, as the wrong one may irritate the kidneys and add to their embarrassment, thus causing further damage.

The treatment of kidney disease has been made much more successful by the recent discovery of several new and more efficient diuretics. Contemplating the ease of their administration and their efficacy, one can be thankful to live in modern times. It was only about two centuries ago that the following was advocated by an esteemed physician (Pechey cited by Hewitt) : "Put washed worms into a curcurbit (flask) so well stoppered that nothing can exhale. Place it to digest either in sea water or in the heat of the sun, that the worms may putrefy and ferment. This fermentation is sometimes so very great that it breaks the glass. The fermentation being over, the earthy part sinks to the bottom, and the skins swim on top, the spiritous liquor is in the middle.

[7]"Diuresis" means "to urinate through"; a diuretic is a substance which increases the secretion of urine.

Separate this and distill it, and it will yield a spirit; this spirit is an excellent diuretic."

Dropsy, water-logging of tissues, has been found to occur in some cases where too much common salt (sodium chloride) is eaten. It has been found, however, that when a different salt is used (ammonium chloride, ammonium nitrate, or potassium chloride) dropsy may be relieved, not increased. In Bright's time mercury in certain forms was used but often was found to be harmful. Now a new mercury preparation has been found which is often almost miraculous in its effects, ridding the body of great quantities of dropsical fluid rapidly. When necessary it has been given by injections repeatedly almost weekly for five years without harm. This may prevent ascites, the accumulation of fluid in the abdomen. When the latter occurs and is unrelieved by diuretics, the abdominal cavity may have to be tapped to save the patient's life. An eighteenth-century physician (Mead, cited by Mac-Bride) cited the "remarkable case of Lady Page who in seventy-seven months was tapped seventy-six times and had taken away two hundred and forty gallons of water without ever repining at her case, or ever fearing the operation." Fortunately, modern diets and diuretics have largely done away with this necessity.[8]

When uremia occurs, drastic measures may be necessary to prevent convulsions and unconsciousness, or even death. Then the resources of the physician may be taxed indeed, but often by injections of fluid, transfusions of blood, and other procedures a new lease on life, or at least some comfort, may be provided.

Quack remedies for kidney diseases abound in great numbers. In a recent circular are advertised fifty different "kidney tablets," fifty-one "kidney remedies," and one hundred and twenty-seven "kidney pills," as well as various "kidney-tonics, bitters, cordials, capsules, drops, medicines, treatments and herb teas." Many of them are called "kidney and backache remedies" fostering the classic falsehood of the quacks regarding urinary sediments and pain in the back. The charlatan often recommends a nostrum indiscriminately for nephritis and diabetes, making no distinction between these utterly different types of disease. Scores of them have been analyzed by government

[8]A photograph of the gravestone of Lady Page in Bunhill Fields Cemetery, London, with the quaint inscription readily visible thereon, may be found in the *National Geographic Magazine,* 65:369, March, 1934. The inscription varies slightly from the quotation given above.

and national medical laboratories. Most of them contain drugs that tend to increase the quantity of urine but not the amount of waste excreted. In some cases this is done in a particularly vicious way, by including a powerful irritant to the kidneys which, though it increases the urine, may cause serious damage. Others are harmless but quite useless. One used to "cure Bright's disease, gravel, all urinary troubles and pain in the back or groin from kidney trouble" was found to contain white sugar exclusively! One widely advertised backache and kidney pill which sells for seventy-five cents for a box of forty pills and which has been estimated as costing a cent a box to make, was found to contain one harmless and one equally useless but irritating substance. Another well-known diuretic pill, also quite ineffective, was advertised as worth five dollars a box, sells for twenty-five cents for a box of thirty-five pills, and has been estimated as costing about a quarter of a cent for a full box! Certainly there is no place for alleged cures for the self-treatment of such a potentially dangerous condition as kidney disease.

Classification of Kidney Diseases: Synopsis of Chief Forms

None of the many classifications of kidney diseases is entirely satisfactory. Were the cause of each known it would be simple to designate them accordingly, "tuberculous nephritis," "mercurial nephritis," and so on. In many the cause is obscure, and classifications are based on the part of the kidney chiefly involved, on what the microscope shows after death: "glomerular nephritis," "tubular nephritis." Others are named from the chief symptoms and signs they produce (or from the main functional derangement), "chronic nephritis with edema," "salt and water nephritis." This discussion affords no place for more than a brief mention of the chief forms of kidney disturbance.

They can be divided into four groups. Group I constitutes those diseases which affect primarily the kidneys alone or where the kidney disturbance becomes the chief cause of ill health. Group II includes different types of "nephrosis" or toxic states where the kidneys are disturbed on account of disease elsewhere and become a secondary cause of ill health. In group III we shall discuss certain conditions where there is actually no nephritis (where the kidneys are relatively unaffected) but in which alterations in the quality or quantity of urine afford important signs in diagnosis. Group IV includes disturbances of kidneys dependent on maldevelopment.

GROUP I.   DISEASES WHERE NEPHRITIS BECOMES THE CHIEF CAUSE OF ILL HEALTH

The kidneys do not live to or for themselves alone, and nephritis is rarely if ever strictly a disease solely of the kidneys. They become diseased from poisons and germs brought to them from some distant site; as a result of the subsequent nephritis, other tissues in turn become involved. The blood vessels of the kidneys may participate with those of other organs in a systemic disease affecting vessels throughout the body. One organ may suffer more than others; when the kidney does so, the nephritis becomes the chief cause of ill health. Acute and chronic glomerulonephritis are examples of the latter. The small blood vessels of many organs, heart, brain, muscles, eyes, liver, and so on, are diseased, but the difficulty in the kidney dominates the picture. It is, for example, as if all the pipes in a house become clogged; damage to those in the kitchen where food must be prepared would cause a greater disturbance than to those in the parlor radiator or the bath.

Acute Glomerulonephritis (Acute Bright's Disease)

Acute glomerulonephritis is usually a disease of young people. During the World War it affected many soldiers and acquired the term "war" or "trench" nephritis. Its cause is unknown, but sometimes it disappears after a focus of infection is removed. The urine is cloudy, dark, and scanty and contains albumin, casts, and red blood cells and sometimes even visible blood. Wastes do not often accumulate markedly in the blood. Dropsy occurs, and the blood pressure rises. The death rate is low, perhaps 3 per cent. It often clears entirely in a few months or even weeks. Occasionally it progresses into chronic glomerulonephritis.

Chronic Glomerulonephritis (Chronic Bright's Disease)

Chronic glomerulonephritis is perhaps the most serious of all forms of nephritis. It is that form first described by Bright and from which arose the erroneous idea that all nephritis was very serious. Its onset is usually before the age of forty years, may be insidious, or may follow acute glomerulonephritis. It is often a part of a general disease of blood vessels. The patient may pass thin watery urine at frequent intervals during the day and night, a total of two or three quarts, or more. The urine contains albumin and casts. Dropsy is usually absent or not marked. The blood pressure rises; the complexion becomes pasty from anemia. Wastes accumulate in the blood. The heart enlarges and weakens. Vessels in the brain may be affected. Thus death may result from heart failure, a "stroke," or from uremia. Some patients live several years but as chronic invalids. In others the disease may become latent or quiescent, so that they are able to lead moderately active lives for many years.

Kidney Disease Secondary to High Blood Pressure

While the blood pressure rises with or as a result of certain forms of nephritis, there are types of increased blood pressure (so-called essential hypertension) which come at first without nephritis and indeed may never be associated with significant kidney disturbance. Another form (malignant hypertension) progresses more rapidly to produce disease in the small arteries of the body. When it produces serious prolonged tension in those of the kidney it may cause a condition similar to chronic glomerulonephritis.

Chronic Renal Arteriosclerosis (Arteriosclerotic Kidneys, Nephritis of Old Age)

Chronic renal arteriosclerosis may occur in elderly persons (over the age of forty-five or fifty years) with hardening of large arteries elsewhere, at the "temples," wrists, and so on. The condition is often discovered by chance during a yearly check-up or from urinalysis in the course of an examination for life insurance. It may reveal itself by causing the patient to pass thin, albuminous urine frequently and at night. The larger, not the small, vessels of the kidney are chiefly diseased; hence, a degree of accommodation takes place whereby the patient may not be noticeably incapacitated. The blood pressure rises to force blood through the stiffened vessels. Dropsy is rare. Some anemia may occur, and there may be a lag in ridding the blood of wastes. No special cause for alarm need be felt. Under supervision the patient may lead a comparatively comfortable and useful existence for a number of years. Plenty of fluids are required to rid the body of wastes, but because excretion of water is slowed, fluids should be taken mostly before supper to avoid interruption of sleep.

Pyelonephritis

Pyelonephritis is caused by bacteria invading the kidneys in the course of infection of the blood stream, or by an infection secondary to obstruction of urinary flow by stones or an enlarged prostate blocking the ureters. Chills, fever, vomiting, and sweating occur, and there may be severe pain and tenderness or merely a dull ache in the kidney region. The urine contains pus, red blood cells, albumin, and bacteria. Wastes accumulate in the blood, but dropsy and high blood pressure are uncommon. When the infection is apparently confined chiefly to the pelvis of the kidney it is called pyelitis, a condition not uncommon in infants and in pregnancy. It usually disappears but sometimes causes chronic nephritis, even uremia. Pyelonephritis may be associated with inflammation in the bladder (cystitis) and urethra with burning on urination and the desire to void frequently and urgently.

Perinephritic Abscess

Perinephritic abscess, another form of "pus kidney," is a localized purulent infection in fat pads about the kidney, usually only on one side. The kidney tissues themselves may escape entirely or share in the infection. Severe pain in the flanks, chills, and fever are present. Where the kidneys are not invaded the urine may contain no pus cells. An operation to drain the abscess is necessary.

Renal Lithiasis

A stone in the kidney (renal lithiasis) may give no symptoms, or may produce kidney colic, one of the most agonizing pains known to man. Pain is produced only when a stone tries to pass out of the kidney into the narrow ureter. Large stones, too big to enter the ureters, may therefore be painless. Small stones traversing the ureters may cause great suffering, unless, and until, they pass out into the bladder. Some pass spontaneously or can be removed by instruments. Others must be removed by operation, or they may cause obstruction to the flow of urine with resulting pyelonephritis or even complete destruction of kidneys. No known medicines or mineral waters have any effect whatsoever on dissolving stones, the multitudinous promises of quacks, ancient and modern, to the contrary. Stones are of various types, most of which (though not all) cast shadows in a roentgenogram. They consist of urinary salts and albuminous substances precipitated together. The reasons why these salts, normally kept in solution, become precipitated is not known, but such an event is probably induced by chemical alterations and bacterial infections.

Kidney Disturbances During Pregnancy

Most women are able to complete pregnancy with little or no real kidney trouble. In the last three or four months of pregnancy the womb may so crowd the bladder and ureters that free passage of urine is interfered with. When slowing of urinary flow results, a mild bacterial infection of bladder urine often occurs. Occasionally more serious trouble arises, formerly called "kidney of pregnancy" or "nephritis of pregnancy" and believed to be essentially one form of kidney trouble. Now it is recognized that this term really includes several quite different disturbances: pyelitis, pyelonephritis, acute or chronic glomerulonephritis, acute nephrosis, preëclampsia, or eclampsia. A glomerulonephritis or nephrosis, existing prior to pregnancy but so mild as to go unrecognized, may flare up acutely under the stress of childbearing. More serious are those conditions called eclampsia and preëclamptic toxemia, manifestations of a poisoning caused presumably by toxic products thrown off from the uterus or from the growing baby. The manifestations of such a poisoning are headache, disturbances of vision, nausea, vomiting, dizziness, restlessness, dropsy, albuminuria, and high blood pressure. Without convulsions they indicate preëclampsia. "Eclampsia" means convulsions and represents the most serious phenomenon of this condition. It arises more frequently in first pregnancies (about one in every 250); only about once in every 1,200 later pregnancies. In all it occurs only about once for every 500 or 600 births, generally during the last three months of pregnancy. A degeneration of the liver and the kidney tubules is present and a special form of glomerulonephritis. Under appropriate treatment the pregnancy may occasionally be completed. Sometimes premature completion is necessary to spare the patient's life. Thereafter kidney function may be remarkably restored. Obviously it is most important for an expectant mother to coöperate with her physician in the routine and repeated examination of urine and blood pressure.

Tuberculosis of Kidneys

Tuberculosis of kidneys is always secondary to tuberculosis elsewhere—in lungs, lymph nodes, bones, or joints. Usually bilateral to a degree at least, it invades one kidney especially and may destroy it entirely. The urine contains albumin, blood, pus, and tubercle bacilli. The latter may be difficult to find, and guinea-pig tests may be necessary. Tuberculosis in kidneys practically never heals spontaneously, and if the kidney is not removed the disease may invade other tissues and endanger the other kidney. The operation is generally quite safe and the outcome hopeful. Half of a group of patients recently studied were found to be apparently completely relieved ten years after operation (Wildbolz).

Kidney Disease from Enlarged Prostate Gland

For some unknown reason the prostate gland frequently enlarges in men over the age of fifty years. This may cause difficulty in starting urination, frequent urination, and dribbling due to partial blockage of the urethra. If free flow is not reëstablished, infection (pyelitis, pyelonephritis) and destruction of kidney tissue may ensue. Ureters and pelvis may be ballooned out with urine (hydroureter, hydronephrosis). Wastes accumulate in the blood, and uremia may result. If appreciable urinary retention is present, careful drainage of the bladder and surgical removal of the prostate gland, or of a portion of it, are generally necessary, despite long-winded and long-distance radio advice otherwise.

Gouty Nephritis (Gouty Bright's Disease)

Years ago a German physician (Hahn) found that when a patient with gout took small quantities of turpentine, the odor of violets present in the urine of normal persons after taking turpentine was absent. This was one of the earliest tests of renal function. The exact relationship between gout and nephritis is not known, but in chronic gout there is often a disturbed kidney function. A mild form of chronic nephritis with manifestations somewhat like those of renal arteriosclerosis may be present. Kidney stones of uric acid salts are not infrequent, and occasionally the actual precipitation of crystals of uric acid salts occurs in kidney tissue.

Scarlatinal Nephritis

In the course of scarlet fever there is usually some albuminuria with no other signs of renal disease. In about 10 per cent of cases, however, there develops about the second or third week a definite nephritis. If mild, it is signalized by transient dropsy, with albumin, casts, and a few red blood cells in the urine. Others may develop considerable dropsy, and the signs of nephritis may last a number of weeks or so and then gradually disappear. A few patients develop an acute glomerulonephritis which temporarily, at least, may be severe, even accompanied by uremia. More or less complete recovery usually follows, but chronic nephritis occasionally results. It is said to occur, however, in only twenty of 5,000 cases (McCollum).

GROUP II. NEPHROSIS

There are many conditions which produce in kidneys a toxic state affecting chiefly the renal tubules, nephrosis which affords a secondary cause of ill health. In nephrosis there is usually marked albuminuria but no increase in blood pressure or generally of waste products in the blood. In some forms dropsy is absent, in others much dropsy occurs. Chemical nephrosis may be caused by certain metals, drugs, anesthetics, or food poisons such as from meat, fish, or mushrooms. The commonest causes are mercury and salvarsan. Other responsible substances are arsenic, phosphorus, chromates, lead, bismuth, uranium, zinc, turpentine, tar, cresol, carbolic acid, certain alcohols, chloroform, and ether. Toxic nephrosis may be caused, in the absence of fever, by such conditions as jaundice, intestinal obstruction, burns, pernicious anemia, diabetes mellitus, syphilis, and thyroid disease, or by a variety of infectious diseases with fever. Febrile nephroses (febrile albuminuria) may result from pneumonia, malaria, yellow fever, typhoid fever, diphtheria, empyema, blood poisoning, peritonitis, gangrene, injections of foreign protein. Lipoid nephrosis is a special form of kidney toxemia, the cause of which is unknown. I shall comment on only two types of nephrosis.

Mercurial Nephrosis

Excesses of mercury produce serious kidney trouble. The acute form is encountered when tablets of bichloride of mercury are taken by mistake or with suicidal intent. The urine becomes loaded with albumin, casts, and red blood cells. Complete suspension of kidney function with suppression of urine for several days may follow the extensive tubular damage present. Uremia and death may ensue, or slow recovery may follow prompt and vigorous treatment. While the physician is awaited the patient should be given several raw eggs in milk. Chronic mercurial poisoning is an industrial hazard for the makers of thermometers, barometers, felt hats, and other products necessitating the use of the metal or salts of mercury.

Lipoid Nephrosis (Chronic Tubular Nephritis with Dropsy)

Lipoid nephrosis is characterized by marked albuminuria and dropsy, and the presence of peculiar fatty or lipoid bodies in the urine. Anemia, high blood pressure, involvement of the heart and eyes are not present as they are in chronic glomerular nephritis. Kidney function is adequate except for excretion of salt and water, and diets have to be arranged accordingly. Diuretics are especially useful in this condition. The edema clears, and the danger to life is not great, although the patient's resistance to infections seems lowered. Health returns, but albuminuria may continue more or less persistently. Occasionally a "mixed nephritis" follows, however, and the outlook is less favorable.

GROUP III.   CONDITIONS IN WHICH THE URINE IS ABNORMAL BUT NO NEPHRITIS IS PRESENT

There is a group of diseases in which abnormal substances are present in urine but where no nephritis exists. The kidneys are merely excreting material abnormally present or present in unusual amounts. Alterations in the quality or quantity of urine occur, but renal function is normal.

Diabetes Mellitus

In *diabetes mellitus*,[9] a disease of the pancreas, or human sweetbread, the first symptom generally noted (by the patient) is the passage of large amounts of urine, usually three to six quarts, sometimes ten quarts or more daily. In mild cases the output of urine is normal, but in any event sugar is present therein. We have seen that when the blood contains the usual amounts of sugar, the kidneys are

[9]"Diabetes" means "to go through."

able to hold it back. Its loss in urine is prevented. When the blood sugar is highly concentrated, as in diabetes mellitus, the excess slops over into urine.

Renal Diabetes

In *renal diabetes* there exists an unusual permeability of the kidney to even normal amounts of circulating blood sugar, such that, even without diabetes mellitus being present, sugar (glucose) appears in the urine. The patients are not sick, and no diet or other treatment is necessary except, of course, sufficient observation to make sure that true diabetes mellitus is not present. It is an uncommon condition, and the cause is unknown.

Bence-Jones Proteinuria ("White Urine")

Ordinary albumin is invisible in cold urine but becomes apparent as a white cloud after urine is heated. In multiple myeloma, a disease of bones, a special kind of albumin called "Bence-Jones protein" may appear. A patient may pass "white urine" when voiding outdoors in the cold. The white cloud disappears on heating the urine, and reappears on cooling. The kidneys themselves are normal, merely excreting the abnormal substance.

Diabetes Insipidus

In *diabetes insipidus* there is no sugar in the urine, no disease of the pancreas or kidneys, yet the patient passes large amounts of otherwise normal urine (except for its low specific gravity), as a rule four to ten quarts a day, in severe cases from twenty to thirty or more quarts a day. The author recalls a case of a boy sixteen years old who passed thirty-three quarts of urine every twenty-four hours and in forty hours the weight of urine was equivalent to his own body weight. Ten years later he was still passing these enormous amounts. A record was made by a twenty-four-year-old male patient who passed about forty-three quarts (43,000 c.c.) in twenty-four hours (Trousseau). Diabetes insipidus is a rather rare disease and usually afflicts children or young adults, probably as a result of disease of the pituitary gland following infection or injury to the brain. It causes intense thirst constantly day and night. Injection of pituitary extract may temporarily stop the excess thirst and urination.

"Black Urine"

A curious and rare urinary disturbance is that presented by certain persons with an inherited anomaly of nutrition producing "alkaptonuria." The infant's urine may stain its linen brown or black. The urine turns dark when exposed to air. In itself the condition is a trifling matter, inconvenient rather than harmful (Garrod). In rare instances the cartilage of the ears and joints also turn dark. There are no symptoms and no treatment is necessary.

GROUP IV.   DISTURBANCES OF THE KIDNEY DEPENDENT ON MALFORMATION

This includes such conditions as "single," "horseshoe," "floating," and "polycystic" kidney and certain anomalies of the ureters, such as double ureter, absent ureter, and so on. About one in 1,800 persons is born with only one kidney. Persons with this anomaly are unaware of it and there are no symptoms. The kidney present is usually enlarged to compensate for the absence of one. The chief importance of this condition is that when a man's only kidney is diseased, danger to life is great. A diagnosis of single kidney is of course of vital importance when considering kidney removal for any surgical condition therein.

A bridge of renal tissue may extend across from one kidney to the other, generally at the lower pole, connecting them to form a horseshoe kidney. They are symptomless and are recognized almost exclusively by means of a pyelogram, an X-ray of the inside of the kidney. When disease is present in one side of a "horseshoe" kidney it may spread to the other readily and thus the condition of union is dangerous to health and life. It may complicate or prevent surgery when renal tuberculosis or abscesses are present, and therefore its recognition is important.

The normal kidney can move up and down about an inch, and, as we have noted, the right kidney is a little lower and more readily felt than the left. Such a palpable kidney is entirely normal. Where the kidney moves excessively owing to weakness of its supporting structures, it is then known as a "wandering," "movable," or "floating" kidney and may be felt low in the abdomen or even in the pelvis. It is found low in women six times as often as in men, generally on the right side in thin individuals. It usually gives no symptoms. Sometimes a dull ache in the flank is present, or when it moves enough to cause kinking of the ureter severe pain may result. Surgery to tack up the kidney should be done only when exercises to strengthen abdominal muscles, the use of supporting belts, and sometimes rest in bed with nutritious diets to replace fat about the kidney have proved unsuccessful.

Certain abnormalities occur in ureters also, chief of which is the presence of an extra one on one or both sides. These occur in about 1 per cent of people, and when disease is present therein may cause trouble in diagnosis. Special X-rays will reveal their presence.

Polycystic Kidneys

Polycystic kidneys represent a curious congenital anomaly recognized as present in about one in every 3,500 patients seen at the Mayo Clinic (Braasch). Often unrecognized, it occurs actually much more frequently than this, being found in about one of every 1,000 persons examined after death. The cause is unknown but is thought to be related to inadequate fusion of constituent parts of the kidney units during the time the body is developing in the mother's womb. The kidneys swell to various sizes, forming abdominal tumors which are sometimes enormous. A forty-year-old man was recently found to have such kidneys, each weighing about 17 pounds (about 7,300 grams)! (Normal weight of each is about 1/3 of a pound [150 grams].) Although both kidneys become enlarged one is usually felt earlier than the other. The enlargement is due to the accumulation therein of small and large masses of watery or semigelatinous material in multitudinous pockets or cysts. Symptoms rarely arise before the age of thirty or forty years. Weakness appears, and a dull ache may be present in the flank. Sometimes blood appears in the urine. A slow and unusually benign type of uremia develops, and the patient may live several years in relative comfort, even with two to three times the normal amount of wastes present in blood.

Conclusion

The advice of a fifteenth-century physician (Arderne) on "the governance of nephritics" included the admonition that such patients "should put away anger and all strenuous business and intense occupation and all manner of things that disturb the soul or move it in any way save only joy." Easy words those, but in that day the joyous state of mind must have been indeed difficult of adoption. Today, as a result of the enormous advances of the past century, or even of the past score years, it has become possible to remove from many the soul-disturbing fear of nephritis. It has become possible to send many nephritic patients back to their strenuous business. To others more seriously ill it has become the physician's happy lot to bring a degree of physical comfort undreamed of heretofore.

CHAPTER XVII

The Blood and Its Diseases
RAPHAEL ISAACS, M.D.

INTRODUCTION

FROM TIME IMMEMORIAL *the blood has been recognized as essential to life. At the same time, it has generally been thought that there is something more to it than merely a nutrient fluid. The story of the gradual changes of opinion of mankind concerning the nature of the blood is one of the most fascinating histories in science. It involves all sorts of confused ideas, attempts at magic, and extraordinary theories which were only destroyed by the development of the microscope and our modern knowledge of the blood.*

It is interesting to realize that some of the formed elements in the blood were discovered only within the last hundred years, and that actual knowledge of these formed elements has been available only for the last fifty years. For instance, the man who first described pernicious anemia in 1822 apparently never looked at the blood but concerned himself only with the gross symptoms.

The first record of a microscopic examination of the blood in disease was apparently dated about 1845, when an Englishman named Hughes Bennett and the great German Virchow simultaneously described the appearance of the blood in the condition called leukemia, a disease in which the manufacture of the white blood cells runs wild.

Actually most of our modern knowledge of the blood depends on the fact that the great Erhlich, who first discovered salvarsan, began to develop stains which are applied to specimens of blood withdrawn from a vein and dropped on a slide, these stains having the power to bring out the various elements within the blood cells.

The manufacture of blood goes on constantly in the human body. In some diseases, such as pernicious anemia, the destruction goes on rapidly. By the giving of liver, the manufacturing rate may be speeded up. If the blood becomes too thick with blood cells, more work is required on the part of the heart to push the blood around the body. The blood must be sent to every part of the body in order to maintain its health and nutrition.

The white blood cells are increased in times of infection and greatly lowered in certain diseases. Thus the number may vary from two hundred cells for each cubic millimeter of blood to many thousands of cells for each cubic millimeter. The white cells are concerned with the defense of the body against germs, against the poisons developed by germs or by chemicals, and against any foreign material.

Today the study of the blood has become one of the most technical of medical specialties, and actual knowledge of the state of the blood in many cases may mean the difference between life and death.

M. F.

IN SOME DISEASES the blood is affected just as are all the other parts of the body, but in others the blood changes are so definite that they appear to be the outstanding feature. These are the conditions which are sometimes called "diseases of the blood." They are really not diseases of the blood itself, but changes in the blood accompanying disease elsewhere in the body. This idea is important, as the doctor must find the cause of any disease in order to remove it.

The word "blood" is sometimes used rather loosely, as "it's in his blood," or "blood will tell," when in reality it is not the blood at all that is meant. The words "blood poisoning" are another example of referring a disease affecting the whole body to the blood, which, naturally, shows changes just as do the heart, lungs, liver, kidneys, blood vessels, and other parts of the patient. In the diseases here described, the blood refers to the red liquid which is pumped by the heart through the blood vessels to all parts of the body.

THE MEANING OF A "BLOOD COUNT"

RED BLOOD CELLS

In order to understand the changes which take place in the body when one has anemia (too little blood) it is necessary to know something of what blood is and where it is made. The red fluid which runs or oozes from a cut and later becomes jelly-like and semi-solid is really a pale yellow liquid in which are suspended millions of tiny greenish disks. In health they are round and about three ten-thousandths of an inch in diameter. These are the red corpuscles, so called because in thick layers they appear red. Normally there are between four and six million in each cubic millimeter of blood, men having a slightly greater number than women. These corpuscles grow in the bone marrow, especially in the ribs, backbone, and flat bones. In babies, the marrow of all the bones takes part in building blood. When the corpuscles are ripe, they enter the blood stream and serve to carry oxygen from the lungs to the rest of the body. The red coloring matter, called hemoglobin, is a complex substance containing some iron. If the number of red corpuscles falls below normal, or if the amount of hemoglobin is deficient, anemia is present. The doctor can count the number of corpuscles by taking a drop of blood from the tip of the ear or from a finger-tip. (The ear is not especially sensitive to a needle puncture.) As it is rather hard to count the exact number of cells easily, a variation of a quarter of a million between two blood counts is not considered significant.

RED COLORING MATTER

The doctor can estimate the amount of hemoglobin by comparing its color, or the color of the solution when it is mixed with acid, to a piece of colored paper or glass which he calls the standard. He will then say, "your blood is 80 per cent of the standard," or 60 per cent as the case may be. However, it is important to remember that there are many different standards, so that it is rather difficult to compare the results from one doctor's instrument with those from another. This sometimes causes needless fear, as a patient will often say that last week one doctor found the hemoglobin to be 70 per cent and now it has dropped to 60 per cent. Another point that must be appreciated is that blood changes slightly from hour to hour, so that it may be 70 per cent now and 60 or 80 per cent at some other period in the day or night, without meaning that there is any sickness. It is also rather difficult to read the instruments exactly, so that a few points of difference, as from 70 to 74 per cent, may have no real meaning. From this it is apparent that the numbers alone may be misleading, and the doctor will have to consider all the other details of the illness along with the blood count, in order to judge its significance.

WHITE BLOOD CELLS

With the red blood cells are a much smaller number of white blood cells. These are small living cells which develop in the bone marrow, mostly of the long bones, as well as in many of the places where red corpuscles grow, and in the spleen and lymph glands. In normal blood the number is between 6,000 and 10,000 in each cubic millimeter, so that any variation between these two numbers is perfectly normal. The number changes throughout the day and night, so that it may be 7,000 at one time and 9,000 a little later. If it drops below 5,000 in each cubic millimeter, and after repeated examinations does not exceed this, then the doctor will try to find out the cause of the decrease in number. Similarly, if it reaches 12,000 or above and remains elevated, the doctor will investigate the cause. In most infections the number increases, because the white blood cells take part in the war against disease. In some infections, as in typhoid fever and influenza, the number is low instead of being increased. This is a peculiarity of the response of the body to these particular diseases. In this way the white blood-cell count is of great aid to the doctor, for he can often tell a harmless "stomach ache" from more serious appendicitis by counting the cells in a drop of blood. It also tells him whether the body is fighting the infection, or whether the powers of resistance are low and the bacteria are getting the upper hand. It is also an aid in predicting whether the patient will get well or not.

BLOOD PLATELETS

A third structure present in the blood is the blood platelet. This is a minute particle of protoplasm—the material of the cells—about one quarter to one half million in a cubic millimeter, which plays a part in the clotting of blood. When there are too few of these particles, or when they are below standard in their composition, the blood clot is not strong, or the blood may remain fluid for a long time.

The fluid part of the blood is probably formed by contributions from many parts of the body. Much of the liquid comes from the water which one drinks or that in food. The albuminous part is formed partly in the liver and partly elsewhere. Food in a soluble form is carried from the stomach and intestines to the various organs, and these in turn contribute various secretions and waste products. The carbon dioxide is carried to the lungs and eliminated there, and certain other waste products are washed out through the kidneys. The fluid part of the blood can be replaced quickly when it is lost, sometimes in a few hours, or at most a few days. It takes weeks, however, to replace the red corpuscles, and it requires a longer time for the body to make hemoglobin than it does to make corpuscles. Corpuscles made in a hurry, to replace blood which has been lost, are apt to be smaller and paler than normal. Normally there is a supply of red blood corpuscles stored in the spleen, which takes care of minor losses of blood.

Why the Doctor Makes Certain Laboratory Tests and What They Tell Him

When a person has anemia or other conditions in which there is some abnormality of the blood, the doctor makes certain tests to learn the state of the body and the different organs. From the blood count he learns whether there are too many or too few red or white blood corpuscles or blood platelets, and from this he can tell the presence of certain diseases or the ability of the person to fight the disease. From the hemoglobin test he will learn how much coloring matter there is in the blood. He will make a thin film of blood on a piece of glass, and, after staining it to bring out certain details, will study it under the microscope. From this he will learn whether the red blood cells are round and normal in size, or whether their shapes are distorted, as in certain diseases, or whether they are too small, as after a hemorrhage, or too big, as in pernicious anemia. He can tell if they are well colored or pale. He can tell whether the parasites of malaria are present. Certain changes may cause him to suspect lead poisoning or other poisons. From the white blood cells he can discover the presence of infection, or failure to respond to infection, or whether the cells are immature, as in leukemia. He can tell if the patient is subject to asthma or hay fever or similar diseases. He can also see if there are enough blood platelets.

THE WASSERMANN AND KAHN TESTS

He will also take some blood in a small tube for the Wassermann or Kahn test. This is important in determining the presence of syphilis, and it is done routinely on all people as a part of a complete examination, and should not be considered as casting any suspicion on the patient. While syphilis is often called a "blood disease" or "blood poisoning," it is in reality not primarily a disease of the blood but a disease of the whole body.

From the urine analysis the doctor may note whether kidney disease is present, as this may cause anemia at times. In some diseases blood is lost through the kidneys or bladder.

The examination of the stomach contents (gastric analysis) tells the physician whether acid is secreted or not, or if the amount is too great or too little. Patients with true pernicious anemia do not secrete acid. The doctor will want a specimen of the excretions to see if there is any blood in it, and he will look for parasites and their eggs. Hookworm and tapeworm infestations are accompanied by anemia at times. From the character of the blood in the stool, when it is present, the doctor is sometimes able to tell something of the part of the stomach or intestines from which it came.

The blood pressure is important, because there is a tendency for it to fall after hemorrhage, and this is often a guide in telling how severe the loss of blood has been. When the blood pressure is high, there may be bleeding, which may be minor in extent, as a nose bleed, or it may involve an important region of the brain (so-called "stroke" or apoplexy).

There is a "breathing test" or "basal metabolism" test that is valuable in telling the doctor how much oxygen the patient uses per minute. In certain blood diseases, as leukemia and polycythemia, the amount may be greatly increased above normal, and the doctor will be guided by this in gauging his treatment.

There are many other tests which the doctor may perform under special circumstances, such as determining the "bleeding time" and the time it requires for the blood to clot.

THE CAUSES OF ANEMIA

Real anemia means that the number of red blood cells or the amount of hemoglobin in the blood is reduced below normal. It is frequently referred to as "lack of blood," "too little blood," "weak blood," or the blood is popularly said to have "turned to water." The fact that a person is pale does not mean that he has anemia. Some ruddy people may have too little blood. This is evident when a person turns pale with fright. In this case the number of blood corpuscles in the body does not change, but the color of the face does. The skin color depends on many factors, such as thickness, amount of blood in the blood vessels, pigment, and state of nutrition. Sometimes a rough idea of the presence of anemia may be obtained by studying the color of the lining of the eyelids or the mouth.

One may have too few corpuscles or too little coloring matter in them for many different reasons, and the doctor must find the cause before he starts treatment, as each type requires different medicines. The doctor may use the terms "primary" and "secondary" anemia. By "primary" he means an anemia in which the decrease in amount of red corpuscles or hemoglobin is the main disease, whereas in secondary anemia there is some other disease in which anemia is one of the symptoms or consequences.

When much blood is lost from the body, anemia develops. If the loss is rapid, the patient is liable to become pale, weak, and dizzy, and his heart will beat faster. The average person has between five and six quarts of blood in the body, children having proportionately less. The loss of about one third of this, if rapid, will cause serious symptoms, but if this same amount is lost slowly, over days or months, the body can become accustomed to it, and the symptoms are much less definite. It is often hard to judge the amount of blood which is lost, as a small amount in a bucket of water will give an intensely red fluid which appears to be many times its strength. The seriousness of a hemorrhage also differs in regard to the place from which the blood is coming. As a rule internal bleeding is harder to fight than that from external wounds. As the heart pumps harder when a person exerts himself, rest is prescribed when there has been loss of blood. In addition to finding the source of the bleeding, the doctor will try to find out whether the hemorrhage is due to accident, as the injury or disease of a blood vessel, or whether it is due to a failure of the blood to clot properly. For example, in hemophilia, a hereditary disease in males, the blood takes a long time to clot, and so an open blood vessel continues to lose blood. In purpura, the blood clot which forms is not strong enough to hold back the blood, and bleeding continues. Sometimes a change takes place in the blood-vessel walls, and the blood oozes out.

Sometimes anemia develops because the bone marrow is injured and it produces little blood. This is called aplastic anemia and develops in some people who are poisoned with benzine or similar substances, or who have worked too long with radium or X-ray. The amount of X-ray used by the doctor in taking "pictures" of a patient for diagnosing disease is not harmful. Sometimes aplastic anemia develops, and no cause can be found. When the blood cells fail to grow, all the functions of the blood cells are not performed properly, and in addition to the anemia, the patient may bleed, because of few platelets, or may be subject to infections because of few white blood cells.

Another cause for anemia is the failure of the red blood cells to ripen. This is the condition found in pernicious anemia, in some patients who have sprue, and in a few of the people who have a tapeworm. It is believed that in these patients the substance which makes the red cells get ripe is not made in the stomach, where it is usually manufactured from meat and similar foods. The missing substance may be replaced if stomach or liver substance or properly prepared extracts from them are taken. As the stomach defect is permanent, it is necessary to keep up the treatment throughout life. The patients with pernicious anemia may suffer from stomach and intestinal disturbances, sore tongue, and difficulty in feeling objects. Their hands, which feel numb and tingle, are clumsy, and as they cannot feel the floor with their feet, or tell the proper position of their joints, they have difficulty in walking. The real cause of these symptoms is a disease change in the spinal cord, and not in the hands and feet, where the patient feels his trouble.

Sometimes anemia develops when improper food is taken for a long time. Babies who live on milk alone during their first year, without additional food, may show this type of anemia. Young girls, and older people also, who for some reason are unable to use the iron of their food to the best advantage, become anemic. This was the disease known to our grandmothers as chlorosis. Some people are unable to chew their food because of poor or no teeth, others have diseases which make it difficult for them to swallow or digest their food, and constant diarrhea in others makes them lose the benefit of the meals that they have been able to eat. After the doctor has studied these patients carefully to find out the cause of their inability to use their food, he gives iron in some simple form—the simpler the better, as the complicated, fancy, and often expensive preparations are sometimes of little value and are hard for the body to utilize.

There are other causes for anemia, which are somewhat less common. The blood may be made in the bone marrow in a normal manner, but it may be destroyed too quickly after it reaches the blood vessels. It is not known just how long a red blood corpuscle survives, but various estimates place its life at from less than a week to several months. Red blood cells may be stored temporarily in the spleen and other organs, to be used when there is an increased demand for them. When they have finished their period of usefulness, they are taken out of the blood stream by the spleen, which breaks them up and prepares the decomposition products for further use or for elimination. The colored part of the blood eventually gives rise to some of the yellow pigment in the bile, which is secreted by the liver. If the yellow pigment is made too rapidly, or if the liver is unable to control it, the whole body becomes stained yellowish, and the patient is jaundiced. If the spleen works too rapidly, or if certain poisons affect the body, the red cells are destroyed so fast that jaundice develops. This disease sometimes runs in families, or is present at birth (congenital hemolytic jaundice) but in some it develops later in life.

Occasionally some foreign growth or tumor crowds out the bone marrow cells, and so anemia develops. This sometimes happens in cancer or leukemia or related diseases. The doctor will then try to remove the crowding tissue by means of X-ray or radium.

Sometimes there are several causes for the anemia in the same person, and careful study is required to find the proper treatment. After any severe illness in which nutrition is badly disturbed, or in which the bone marrow has been utilized mainly to make white cells to fight the infection, a mild form of anemia develops. Sometimes anemia develops in the course of pregnancy, and this may be caused by any of the factors just described, as hemorrhage, nutritional deficiency, failure of the blood cells to ripen, or destruction of the red cells at too rapid a rate.

TREATMENT OF ANEMIA

Each type of anemia requires a different treatment. It is not economical or wise to buy a bottle of "blood medicine" in the hopes that it will cure the anemia. If iron is needed, it is a waste of money to buy medicines containing other things in addition. If liver or stomach is needed, it is not economical to pay for a lot of other substances, and there is no use at all in taking iron when liver extract is necessary, nor will liver extract help an anemia where iron is needed. There is an old fallacy that "blood will make blood." Now it is known that blood is practically indigestible, and so little is absorbed when taken by mouth that it is practically useless as a treatment of anemia. Furthermore iron itself, or in any form, is useless as a "tonic," unless the patient

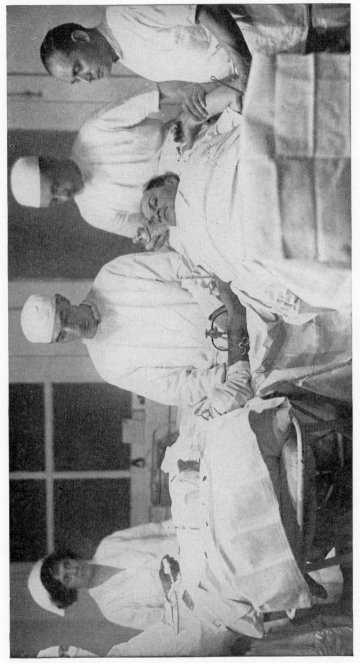

Fig. 58.   Blood transfusion.

needs iron specifically because he has too little in his body. If the body needs more iron than is obtained from the food, it is best to take it as a medicine rather than fill up on spinach and other substances, which, at best, contain but little more than a trace of iron. While good food, fresh air, and sunshine are ideal in the normal life of a patient, they become tedious when taken in abnormal quantities as medicine, so that it is best to find out exactly the treatment that is needed and live an otherwise normal life. There are many so-called patent medicines which claim to cure anemia, but they usually contain but traces of the important material, and the cost to the patient is out of all proportion to the value of the ingredients. When they are taken without direction, they may delay real treatment until it is too late to hope for recovery, or they may cover up a serious underlying disease which should receive urgent attention. Some of these medicines contain nothing of value and are total frauds.

An important feature in the treatment of anemia is the removal of the cause. When this can be corrected, the anemia soon responds to treatment, and the cure is complete. If the cause cannot be removed, as in pernicious anemia where there is a permanent defect in the workings of the stomach, the medicine, which really replaces the missing substances, must be taken during the remainder of the person's life. It is hard to appreciate this, and many patients, feeling perfectly well, discard the medicine, and anemia develops once more in from two weeks to several months. When anemia develops as a result of cancer, it is of course not possible to remove the cause. Fortunately anemia in cancer is rare, despite the general impression that the two are always associated. While much is said about the general importance of vitamins and ultraviolet light, at present there is no real evidence that they make more or better blood.

Blood Transfusion

If the loss of blood has not been serious, the doctor will only give medicines which will supply the body with material to make new blood. If, however, the patient is utterly collapsed, or it is necessary to replace the blood quickly, a blood transfusion will be given. To do this, the doctor must find someone (a donor) whose blood will mix perfectly with that of the patient, without causing it to dissolve or form clumps of corpuscles which would block the tiniest blood vessels. All human beings fall into four main groups as far as their blood is concerned, and only certain groups can be mixed. As long as the blood is compatible and the donor has no disease which the patient can get from his blood, there need be no restrictions as to the person from whom the blood is taken. There is a general feeling that the donor must be a member of the family, but this is not necessary. The loss of a pint or a pint and a half of blood is not harmful to the donor.

Symptoms of Anemia

When one has too little blood, or too little coloring matter (hemoglobin) in the blood, it is more difficult for the body to carry oxygen from the lungs to the different organs. The heart tries to make up for the weakened blood by beating faster, so that the few corpuscles which are present may make more frequent trips to the lungs and tissues and thus accomplish their normal work. As long as the heart succeeds in doing this extra work, the anemic person feels just like a normal one. However, if the heart is not able to compensate for the weakened condition of the blood, the tissues of the body begin to show signs of poor function. The feet and ankles begin to swell, the person becomes short of breath, and pants on the least exertion, and the heart beats fast and thumps. Each organ sends out its own danger signals of defective function. When too little blood goes to the brain, there is dizziness, headache, difficulty in remembering or of concentrating the mind on any kind of "brain work," and if the anemia is severe, or the exertion too great, the blood supply is inadequate to keep the person awake, and he faints or becomes drowsy. The stomach may rebel, and the person loses his appetite, or may become nauseated or vomit. He may lose control over any of the functions of the body. The muscles are not supplied with enough oxygen, and they fatigue easily. The person then tires on slight exertion. There may or may not be pallor of the face, depending on how much blood and how much coloring matter there is in the skin. Paleness may mean anemia, but the real test is the blood count. Some persons are always pale, and sometimes it is hard to tell the difference between the sallow complexion of a person who works indoors and takes but little exercise from the pallor of anemia.

The symptoms which a person with anemia shows are not directly associated with weak blood but are associated with how well or how poorly the heart compensates for the missing corpuscles. One may have one or all of these symptoms when in reality there is no anemia at all but some other condition which has the same effect on the heart. It is futile to guess whether the symptoms are those of anemia or heart disease or kidney trouble without a most thorough examination by one skilled in the diagnosis of these conditions. How dangerous, then, are patent medicines which give a list of "symptoms" of anemia, so that a person may make his own diagnosis without proper study in order that the sales of the medicine may be increased.

In addition to the symptoms of a poorly nourished heart trying to do its best with weak blood, there may be other symptoms and signs associated with the disease which causes or may accompany the anemia. Occasionally too little iron in the blood is associated with iron starvation in the rest of the tissues of the body, as in nutritional anemia. In the disease called pernicious anemia the inability to walk or feel objects, the soreness of the tongue, the troublesome constipation or diarrhoea, the numbness and tingling of the hands and feet are symptoms not directly associated with the anemia itself.

Some types of chronic anemia seem to get better or worse by spells. The doctor calls these remissions and relapses. This sometimes accounts for the mistaken impression that a certain medicine or a peculiar diet has miraculous effects. During the spontaneous remissions many unwary people write testimonials about the treatment which they think brought about the improvement. Many well-intentioned but utterly false testimonials of this character are published to mislead others into anything from buying a given medicine to giving offerings to a patron saint. The good and bad spells are especially marked in pernicious anemia, but appear to a greater or less degree in the hemolytic and nutritional types also.

Another feature which causes the symptoms to vary, besides the strength of the heart, is the rate at which the blood has been lost or destroyed. Whereas utter collapse may follow the sudden loss of blood, many times this amount may be lost slowly, over days or weeks, with comparatively few or much less severe symptoms. There is a popular belief that the blood is weak in the spring, and many people resort to "blood tonics" at this time, frequently urged along by glowing advertisements in the newspapers or magazines of the necessity for the spring rejuvenation. Fortunately the blood is not any weaker in the spring than at any other time, which counteracts the fact that the advertised medicines would not have helped the blood anyway.

Prevention of Anemia

Anemia is not catching and is not inherited. Some families have a greater tendency to anemia than others, and it is in these groups that much misery and loss of efficiency can be avoided if the disease is discovered and treated very early. Occasionally such a patient is discovered during his periodic health examination; at other times because his friends notice that he is pale, or because he seeks relief from some symptom associated with it. The routine pulling of teeth or removal of tonsils should not be looked on as of prime importance in relation to the prevention or cure of anemia. It is extremely rare for diseases in these organs to be the cause of a decrease in the number of red blood cells. Isolated, selected patients, however, are improved when virulent sources of infection in the teeth or tonsils are removed. Removal of the tonsils or teeth will not prevent anemia, because there are many other causes. Removal of all the teeth frequently leads to anemia, unless well fitting plates with artificial teeth are obtained. The question is asked occasionally, "If I eat liver, will that prevent the development of anemia?" The answer is "No, unless you have pernicious anemia, and then only if enough is taken." Odd diets should be avoided, and every effort should be made to obtain, during the course of each week, the essential foods necessary for a healthy body. In health, the appetite is a good guide, and it is only when this becomes perverted, either through mental or physical disease, that outside guidance is necessary. The trace of iron needed daily (about 15 milligrams or about a quarter of a grain) is obtained from the meat, eggs, and vegetables which we eat. A healthy person need not worry about supplementing this. It is only when the body needs more iron, or cannot use the iron in the food, that it is necessary to think of increasing the intake. As chronic nosebleed, or daily loss of blood from bleeding piles or hemorrhoids, or too profuse menstruation may lead to anemia, these conditions should be remedied as soon as possible.

Polycythemia, or Too Many Blood Cells

There is a rare disease in which the red blood corpuscles grow faster than normal, and the red blood-cell count may climb from the normal of 5 million in each cubic millimeter of blood to 8 or 10 million or even higher. The blood becomes quite thick, and the congestion of the blood vessels of the face gives the patient a reddish purple appearance. Quite paradoxically, however, some people with this disease are pale and are mistakenly thought to have anemia. An outstanding symptom is the ease of fatigue and utter weakness. The patients complain that they get no sympathy as they look so ruddy that their friends cannot imagine that they are sick. There may be headaches and body pains and disturbances of digestion with severe constipation. These people are frequently nervous and irritable and try the patience of their nurses or relatives. The well people should sympathize with the patient, as it is not meanness or spite which makes him behave as he does, but the curious changes brought about by the disease. Patients with leukemia or too many white blood cells may also show this same type of nervousness. The spleen, which acts as a storehouse for blood, soon becomes enlarged in trying to hold some of the extra blood. It is enlarged not because it is a cause of disease, but because it is a "safety valve," trying to take some of the extra blood corpuscles out of the circulating blood. This is an example of an organ being greatly enlarged as a protective mechanism, and it is important to differentiate this from other diseases where the same organ may be enlarged because it is the seat of the disease process itself. Because of the sluggish circulation in the smallest blood vessels, bruises are liable to be followed by ulcers. There is also a tendency to bleeding, as the greatly increased numbers of red corpuscles interfere with the formation of a good clot. There is some danger of internal hemorrhage in a vital spot, as in the brain.

The doctor may treat the patient with certain medicines which destroy the extra blood, or he may withdraw a pint or more of blood from the veins. This is one of the few diseases, in modern times, where blood-letting is still practised. In the earlier days of medicine this was the common and accepted practice for the treatment of many diseases, but in the wrong disease the patient must have been harmed more than he was helped. In polycythemia the blood tends to keep on growing, so that the treatment must be repeated frequently.

There may be an increase in the number of red blood cells for other reasons, some of which are beneficial to the patient and do not need treatment. When a person goes up on a high mountain, where the air is rare, he needs more blood to obtain sufficient oxygen. The body responds by increasing the number of corpuscles in the circulating blood. Similarly in patients whose lungs are not perfect and who have some difficulty in absorbing oxygen from the air, the body once more responds with the production of a richer blood, and the normal processes can go on.

LEUKEMIA, OR TOO MANY WHITE BLOOD CELLS

As has been mentioned, the white blood cells are made in the bone marrow and in the lymphatic tissues, such as the spleen, lymph nodes, tonsils, appendix, and similar organs. The white blood cells which are made in the bone marrow are different from those made in the other places, and their function appears to be to fight infection. They accumulate wherever bacteria begin to invade the body, and form the pus or matter which one sees in boils or infected wounds. The white blood cells which form in lymph tissue are probably more concerned with immunity, or the chemical protection of the body. There is still much to be learned about their functions and how they work.

Once in a while the growth of the white blood cells becomes abnormal, and they fail to ripen properly. The immature cells then grow beyond all restraint and cause the lymph glands and spleen to enlarge, and they crowd the red blood cells from the bone marrow. The patient becomes weak and sick, and anemia develops. This disease is called leukemia (meaning "white blood"), because when such blood is allowed to settle, the great numbers of abnormal white cells form a thick whitish layer over the heavier red cells. The white blood cells may increase in number in the blood from the normal of 6,000 or 10,000 in each cubic millimeter to several hundred thousand, sometimes reaching one half to three quarters of a million or more.

One of the symptoms of this disease is nervousness with abnormal perspiration and loss of weight. When anemia develops, all of the symptoms of too few red blood cells appear. Another symptom is ease of bleeding. The white blood cells, being present in too great numbers, interfere with the formation of a good strong clot, and the blood continues to ooze from the injured vessel. The blood platelets, which take part in blood clotting, may also be deficient in number or quality, and this too may lead to abnormal bleeding. As long as this condition is present, operations, even the pulling of a tooth, must be avoided, and the person must be protected from the danger of accidents.

For treatment, the doctor uses X-ray or radium to clear out the abnormal growths and allow the normal cells to develop. There is a tendency for the disease process to reappear again and again, so that the doctor must watch the blood carefully and order treatment when it is needed.

There is an acute type in which the outlook is very bad, but in the chronic form, the patient may live many years, dependent on the mildness of the disease and the resistance of the individual.

Hemophilia, Purpura, and Abnormal Bleeding

Some patients bleed easily because their blood does not clot readily or because the clot is not strong and firm. In hemophilia, the blood will sometimes remain fluid for hours after removal from the body. This disease is curious in that it runs in families. The last Crown Princes of Russia and Spain were said to have this condition. It appears practically entirely in boys and men, and it is exceedingly rare to see the real condition of hemophilia in a woman. There is something in women that appears to counteract the disease, so that when they have it they do not bleed, but their sons may show the trait. Such women are called carriers or conductors, because they appear to carry and transmit the disease, but do not show it themselves. Some of their sons may be perfectly normal, however, and not all of their daughters will be conductors. A daughter will be a "bleeder," as they are sometimes called, only if the father has hemophilia and the mother is a conductor of the disease. A man with hemophilia will have perfectly normal sons, if the wife is not a conductor, but the daughters will all show the tendency to transmit the condition to some of their sons.

These people do not bleed severely from a tiny cut or pin prick, but they may die of hemorrhage if a larger vessel is cut. If an operation is necessary, the patient must be prepared with blood transfusions. Even the pulling of a tooth may be a serious matter, and preparations should be made for a transfusion if the bleeding becomes profuse. Sometimes there is bleeding into the joints, and stiffness may result if the proper treatment is not given. People with hemophilia must lead a protected life, as they cannot run the risks of the accidents which are so common in the everyday routine. A slight accident, which may have little effect on a normal person, may lead to fatal hemorrhage in a hemophiliac.

Purpura is also a condition in which there is abnormal bleeding, but this is due to the fact that the clot, which forms in the proper time, is not strong enough to hold back the flow of blood. In some, it is associated with some abnormality of the smallest blood vessels which causes them to rupture easily. Purpura may be a disease in itself or it may be a symptom of another disease. In some patients the spleen appears to work too fast, destroying the important little blood platelets which are so necessary in the formation of a good, strong blood clot. In others, certain poisons arising from an infection or from drugs which have been taken may lead to the abnormal bleeding. Still others appear to be sensitive to certain foods. In leukemia, the abnormal number of white blood cells, or the abnormal or decreased number of blood platelets may produce the same effect. The bleeding usually shows itself first as reddish spots or areas which remain red even though they are pressed under the finger, later turning "black and blue." A black and blue spot merely means that some blood has escaped under the skin and the body is changing it into a form that can be absorbed and carried away. The spots are familiar to all of us as the ordinary bruise marks which appear whenever an object strikes us.

When the purpura is severe, a blood transfusion may be necessary to stop the bleeding. The disease tends to get better at times of its own accord, to be followed later by reappearance of the symptoms. When the cause of the disease is an abnormal spleen, removal of this organ results in the disappearance of all of the symptoms. When the spleen is removed, other organs in the body take up its normal work, so that the individual is not handicapped in any way.

If a person is subject to nosebleeds, or if black and blue spots appear without the history of striking one's self, or if there is abnormal bleeding from cuts or during menstruation, the doctor must try to find the cause. It may be something simple and of no consequence, or it may be a serious disease which requires active treatment. Some diseases as hemorrhoids, cancer, gastric ulcer, pulmonary tuberculosis, and similar conditions may be accompanied by abnormal bleeding because a blood vessel has been eaten away by the disease and it has ruptured.

Hemorrhage in the newborn is a condition occasionally encountered, in which the baby bleeds, usually from the stomach and intestines, but at times from the cord or elsewhere. The stools are liable to show fresh or changed blood. This condition usually requires a blood transfusion, after which the baby may be perfectly normal.

Enlargement of the Lymph Glands and the Spleen

The lymph glands or lymph nodes are small organs scattered in many parts of the body, especially in the neck, armpits, around the roots of the lungs, around the intestines, and in the groins. They have several functions, one of which is to make lymphocytes, which are one of the types of white blood cells which circulate in the blood stream. The lymph nodes are like stations along the route of the lymph vessels, and they serve as sieves or blocks to the passage of material causing infection. That is the reason why lymph nodes at the elbow or in the armpits become tender when there is an infection in the hands. The tonsils are really lymph nodes, and when they try to stop virulent infections they sometimes become swollen and inflamed. When the infection manages to get past the tonsils, then the lymph nodes in the neck enlarge in an effort to prevent further passage of the infection into the rest of the body.

Sometimes the lymph nodes themselves are the seat of disease. As has been noted, they may enlarge in leukemia, because of the great increase in the number of white blood cells which fail to get ripe. When tuberculosis affects the lymph nodes they have a tendency to become enlarged, inflamed, and at times they break down and form sinuses or draining ulcers, especially in the neck. This is sometimes referred to as scrofula. There is a group of diseases which cause enlargement of the lymph nodes in all parts of the body and which eventually lead to death. They are something of the nature of cancer, inasmuch as certain cells grow beyond the needs of the body. This group is called lymphoblastomas and includes Hodgkin's disease, lymphosarcoma, and other conditions in which the masses grow at the expense of the rest of the body, finally causing weakness, anemia, loss of weight, and symptoms from the pressure of the enlarged glands on other structures. The doctor controls these growths mostly by the use of X-ray or radium. There are many other diseases which cause enlargement of the lymph nodes, some serious, others of a minor significance, so that a very careful diagnosis is necessary before the condition can be treated properly. For example, there is a condition known as infectious mononucleosis, accompanied by enlargement of the lymph glands, fever, and weakness, which makes one think of leukemia. However, these patients soon get well, whereas the ultimate outlook in leukemia is not as hopeful. In some stages of syphilis the lymph glands increase in size. The spleen may be enlarged in all of these diseases, and it is then necessary to find out if there is a possibility that the person has malaria or typhoid fever. The large spleens in leukemia and polycythemia were mentioned before. There are also some diseases in which abnormal growths in the spleen cause the illness. Examples of this are Gaucher's disease, Banti's disease, Niemann-Pick's disease, Von Jaksch's disease—so-called because these men were among the first to call attention to them. In some of these, the disease spreads to other parts of the body, especially the bones.

From this description it is quite evident that the appearance of a lump or swelling in any part of the body warrants a careful examination by a qualified doctor. There is no first-aid treatment for these, as they may be the outward evidences of serious disease, and no time should be lost in seeking expert help. Under no circumstances should anything ever be "rubbed into" the glands, unless the doctor orders it after very careful study. The "lump" may turn out to be something very minor, or it may mean that drastic measures are necessary to cure the underlying disease. It is too dangerous to apply home remedies, as treatments which help one kind of glandular enlargement aggravate other kinds.

CHAPTER XVIII

Deficiency Diseases

RUSSELL M. WILDER, M.D., and DWIGHT L. WILBUR, M.D.

INTRODUCTION

OUR KNOWLEDGE *of the deficiency diseases is largely a development of the last quarter of century. The mechanisms of disease are varied. For years it has been recognized that many of the diseases of mankind were due to poisons taken into the body. Finally, it came to be believed that all disease was due to outside influence. Then came the knowledge of the vitamins as fundamental constituents of food substances, and that knowledge has introduced an entirely new conception into the study of health and growth.*

The so-called deficiency diseases reviewed by Dr. Russell M. Wilder and Dr. Dwight L. Wilbur include scurvy, beriberi, pellagra, night blindness and a number of other disorders. They are due, however, not to substances included in the body, but to the absence of necessary substances from the diet. They can be reproduced in the human body in each instance by the feeding of a diet in which the vitamins are deficient. The absence of vitamin C from the diet results in scurvy; the absence of vitamin G in pellagra; the absence of vitamin D in rickets; the absence of vitamin A in night blindness and other disturbances.

Moreover, there is also good evidence that relative deficiencies of the diet in some of these vitamins may produce a general lowered resistance of the body to disease, may interfere with proper nutrition and with growth, and altogether be an exceedingly unfortunate thing for the human being who happens to neglect the securing of adequate amounts of vitamins in his food.

While the chapter which follows is concerned largely with deficiency of vitamins in the diet, there may also be deficiencies in the taking of and in the assimilation of proteins of various kinds, of carbohydrates and fat, and of the various mineral salts. From this point of view, the

483

subject is discussed further in the chapter on diet by Dr. Solomon Strouse, which is found elsewhere in the book.

It might be thought that the question of dietary deficiencies is not one which should concern the average American. Nevertheless, so many people voluntarily restrict their diet for purpose of weight reduction or voluntarily avoid substances simply because they do not like to eat them that better knowledge of the hygiene of diet is clearly desirable for the majority of people.

Fortunately, the subject of adequate diet is now taught in most schools, and the child is able to get the necessary information along with its reading, writing, and arithmetic, in its formative years.

M. F.

Most diseases are due to the presence in the body of abnormal factors such as result from infection by germs, from intoxication or poisoning of some sort, or from the growth of tumors, or from accidents. More recently, doctors, chemists, and biologists have been studying a group of diseases known as "deficiency diseases." These are abnormal conditions or diseases due to the absence of certain necessary substances usually found in food. Their discovery has depended on finding in food certain factors which are essential for health. It has long been known that proteins, fats, carbohydrates, salts, and water are necessary for life. Only recently, however, another group of substances, known as the vitamins, has been found. These are just as necessary for the maintenance of health as the other food factors just noted. Both from experience with human beings and laboratory research, it has been established that the body not only requires these substances for the preservation of health, but that a normal food supply furnishes them in adequate amounts.

Fats and carbohydrates, which are used chiefly as fuel in the food of man and animals, are found in almost all food substances. The relative ease of interchangeable use of these substances in the body makes the development of diseases due to their deficiency unusual. The protein of a mixed diet is rarely inadequate. Although deficiencies of certain salts such as those of iron, iodine, and lime will produce disease, the term deficiency disease is usually restricted to deficiency of one or more of the vitamins. The vitamins probably act to speed up or to initiate certain chemical reactions in the body. They do not serve directly as fuel or builders of tissue. They are, therefore, necessary in small quantities only. The separation of man from his natural environment, which has occurred with long travel and the development of civilization, has made the procurement of adequate natural foods steadily more difficult. The preparation of food in highly concentrated and purified form, such as flour, prepared oils, sugar and foods "ready to serve," while it has many benefits, has also limited the amount of food taken in the natural or fresh state. Although properly canned vegetables and fruits are equally wholesome, it is in the natural state that foods are richest in vitamin value.

The beginning of knowledge concerning vitamins is more the product of development than of any isolated discovery. Much of this development came before the first use of the word "vitamin." Eijkman, Hopkins, Funk, Osborne and Mendel, and McCollum and Davis are names which stand out prominently in the investigation and development of present conceptions of deficiency diseases: (1) Animals on a diet of purified foods furnishing adequate proteins, fats, carbohydrates, salts and water, fail to secure normal growth until given some natural food such as milk, butter, or fish oil. (2) Certain diseases of man can be cured by adding to the diet certain natural foodstuffs.

Diseases which are today recognized as being due to vitamin deficiency have occurred for hundreds of years. A summary of the vitamins and the deficiency diseases produced by their absence may be found in the table on p. 502.

With the exception of rickets and pellagra, the United States is relatively free of dietary-deficiency diseases. It must be added immediately, however, that we may not be free of vitamin-deficiency states. In this connection, McCollum and Simmonds said:

> We appreciate the existence of many grades of malnutrition. It is becoming constantly more evident that even a slight departure from the optimum in the composition of food may lead to states of nutritional instability which become contributing factors to physical breakdown when hygienic factors are unfavorable or when infectious processes are operative.

In order to produce a deficiency disease recognizable by its symptoms, the deficiency of a vitamin must be considerable. It is probable that deficiency states exist in which the food is not devoid of sufficient vitamin to produce a recognizable deficiency disease and yet is insufficient for normal nutritional needs. Perhaps such a state might more properly be called not a deficient state but one of failure of enrichment of diet by the vitamin. In the words of Sherman, who is an authority on the subject:

It seems to be true of vitamin G, as also of vitamins A and C, that the optimal amount is much higher than the minimal ("actual") requirement: in other words, that the body is able to make good use of a much more liberal intake than can be proved to be absolutely necessary.

That is, there is a zone between the merely adequate and the optimal in nutrition. This is a relatively new and exceedingly important conception. Although we may be getting enough vitamin to give us "passable" health, we may not be getting enough for "buoyant" health. It seems reasonable that in the future in this country we shall be concerned more with this idea than with the occurrence of actual deficiency diseases, except for rickets and pellagra. Indeed, we may go even further and eventually discover, as suggested by Sherman:

Just as a lack of this factor [vitamin G] brings about a condition of malnutrition which may contribute to premature senility, so a liberal intake of vitamin G contributes to a better than average nutritional condition and thus to what McCollum and Simmonds have aptly termed "the preservation of the characteristics of youth."

Possibly other vitamins in optimal amounts may not only lead to buoyant health but also to the preservation of the characteristics of youth. We are certain of one thing, and that is our incomplete knowledge. As Hess said:

We are only at the threshold of an understanding of the nutritional values of the foods and combinations of foods which enter into our dietaries.

Although diseases produced by deficiency of vitamins are distinct among themselves when clear cut, in the earlier stages and in those states between passable and buoyant health it may be impossible to determine clearly which vitamin is deficient. As a rule, all deficiency states at first lead to failure to gain weight, or loss of weight, exhaustion, lassitude, and weakness.

The knowledge of deficiency diseases gained through animal experiments has been indispensable in our understanding of their nature, prevention, and treatment. The dependability with which such disorders develop among certain animals on suitable diets, and the relative ease with which these experiments allow study of the various dietary-deficiency conditions, has advanced our knowledge further in proportion than in the case of many other diseases. If we were able to produce other diseases experimentally as readily as we do dietary deficiencies, the knowledge gained and the suffering saved would be priceless.

The average American dietary is adequate to prevent the development of dietary-deficiency diseases. It may not be adequate in all cases to maintain buoyant health. It is only under unusual circumstances in this country, such as war, famine, floods, and other deprivations, that actual deficiencies are likely to develop, with the exception of rickets (and pellagra in the South). There are other factors which must be thought of in a consideration of the elements which enter into the development of deficiency diseases, such as differences or disturbances in the assimilation of vitamins from the digestive tract, due to disease, or variability in storage of a vitamin in the body.

The most gratifying feature about deficiency diseases, both to the physician and to the patient, is that these conditions are not only curable but preventable. From the individual standpoint, therefore, their control is easy. From the standpoint of the community, the state, and the nation, the problem is one of public health and economics, and one cannot but hope that the day of deficiency diseases throughout the world will eventually be past. That still greater benefit than eradication of deficiency diseases is available may be surmised from the following expression of Sherman:

One of the most impressive features in recent discoveries regarding the relation of food to health and vitality is that the benefit of better feeding usually becomes fully apparent only when it is continued throughout a large part of the life cycle, and often the benefit is greater to the second generation than to the first.

Vitamin A Deficiency and Xerophthalmia

The most readily appreciated symptoms of vitamin A deficiency are changes occurring in the eyes. In previous years vitamin A deficiency has been considered to be manifested chiefly, if not entirely, in this way. The characteristic abnormality is a dryness of the eyes, so the disease has been known as xerophthalmia (dryness of the eyes). Vitamin A has been called the anti-xerophthalmic or anti-ophthalmic vitamin, since it prevented the occurrence of this condition. In the last few years, however, our knowledge of the function of this vitamin has increased tremendously. We now know that it serves an exceedingly useful and essential purpose in maintaining the skin and other coverings of the body in a healthy state. Because the onset of many infections depends on loss of integrity of these body coverings, and since vitamin A maintains these in a healthy state and is therefore indirectly partially responsible for preventing such infection, the vitamin has also become known as the "anti-infective vitamin." Since it is essential to growth, it has also been called the "growth-promoting vitamin."

HISTORY

It has been known for hundreds of years that certain diseases of the eyes developed after long fasts or after the use of improper foods. It was not until 1913 that we began to understand why they occurred. Osborne and Mendel, and McCollum and Davis, in that year reported that experimental animals such as rats, fed on food mixtures alike in all other respects, would continue to grow and thrive, or would soon cease to grow and shortly thereafter sicken and die, according as the fat in these mixtures was butter fat, cod-liver oil, egg yolk, or lard. Animals having lard as fat failed to grow, were unhealthy, and disease of the eyes developed; those with one of the other three fatty foods mentioned were healthy. This demonstrated that egg yolk, cod-liver oil, and butter contained an essential substance lacking in such a fat as lard; this substance we know as vitamin A.

Bloch, in Denmark, during the World War, suspected a relationship between a condition of malnutrition and eye trouble of children with insufficient amounts of fat in the diet and inadvertently made a remarkable experiment. In 1919, in an institution in Copenhagen he divided thirty-two healthy children, aged from one to four years, into two groups. One group received whole milk with their food; the other, fat or vegetable fat. In eight cases in the second group (those on vegetable fats) dryness of the eyes (xerophthalmia) developed subsequently and was relieved by cod-liver oil, whereas, in the group given whole milk, trouble did not develop. This showed conclusively that butter fat contained some substance essential for the maintenance of the eyes in a healthy state. Widmark, also in Denmark, was able to show a direct relationship between the amount of butter used and the occurrence of xerophthalmia among children.

EFFECTS

A great deal of our knowledge concerning the effects of vitamin A deficiency has been obtained from Denmark and the Orient, where xerophthalmia has been prevalent, and from experiments on animals.

Infants and children, just as young animals, are more susceptible to such deficiency than adults. In the first place, vitamin A is essential for adequate growth of the infant and child; also because its deprivation leads to lessening of resistance to infections, children are subject to severe and perhaps fatal infections if deficiency of vitamin A persists for a considerable length of time.

In the second place, vitamin A is essential for the maintenance in a healthy state of the tissues which serve as a covering for the body, such as the skin and the membranes covering the eyes, digestive tract, urinary tract, respiratory tract, and their associated glands. These covering tissues are known as the epithelial tissues. The essential change, in vitamin A deficiency, in these tissues is a drying, hardening, and thickening, so that they become much more susceptible to the occurrence of infection.

The manifestations in the eyes of vitamin A deficiency are xerophthalmia, or dryness, and night blindness. The xerophthalmia is manifested by drying of the tissues which cover the eye, resulting in dimness of vision and eventually infection, with partial or complete blindness if the disorder has been allowed to continue. This condition is a frequent cause of blindness in the Orient. Night blindness, or inability to see clearly in dusky light, is frequently due to vitamin A deficiency and is a result of disturbance in the delicately balanced mechanism of vision. Sometimes it is the first symptom of vitamin A deficiency to develop.

In cases of vitamin A deficiency, bronchopneumonia is the chief manifestation of infections in the organs of respiration. The effects on the digestive system are as yet uncertain. Possibly such deficiency may be significant in the occurrence of some types of stones in the bladder and kidneys, but such a definite relationship in man cannot as yet be absolutely established, although it is likely to occur among certain animals. The skin of people with vitamin A deficiency is frequently dry, scaly, shriveled, and pigmented.

At present the greatest interest in the importance of vitamin A is in connection with its relationship to infections. Does a normal supply of vitamin A give a person greater resistance to infections than an inadequate supply? More important, does an excessive supply increase the resistance to infection of the person concerned over that of the normal? It is as yet impossible to answer definitely these important questions. Evidence has been offered which would indicate that this vitamin is not only important in increasing the resistance of the body to infection, but that it is of importance in combating infections once they have occurred. However, conservatism leads one to say that at present vitamin A is to be considered as a substance protecting against infection by virtue of the fact that it maintains the integrity of the epithelial linings (coverings) of the various tracts, digestive, respiratory, and urinary, and of the skin, but its anti-infective power, that is, its ability to cure infections when the barrier of these coverings has been passed, or to prevent or cure infections in the blood stream, is questionable. Attempts have been made to show that this vitamin is important in the prevention of the common cold and childbed fever, but such evidence is not as yet convincing.

SOURCE, NATURE, AND ACTION OF VITAMIN A

Vitamin A, formerly known as fat-soluble A (and before its distinction from vitamin D known also as the anti-rachitic vitamin), is generally considered to occur in the fatty foods of animal origin, such as milk, butter, cod-liver oil, and egg yolk. It is now known, however, that the chemical predecessor or precursor of vitamin A is the yellow pigment, carotene, which gives the color to carrots, sweet potatoes, yellow corn, and other vegetables. This substance, carotene, which can be extracted in the chemical laboratory, is exceedingly potent and is converted in the animal body into what we know as vitamin A. Consequently, vitamin A may be obtained from either animal or vegetable sources. The way in which vitamin A acts on the tissues after its formation is unknown. The liver stores large quantities of it, a supply sufficient to last several months. This explains why liver oil is such a rich source of the vitamin. The liver of the cod is particularly rich in the vitamin, but more recently it has been found that liver oil from the halibut is many times richer in vitamin A and, in fact, is almost pure vitamin A.

PREVENTION AND TREATMENT

The prevention and treatment of the vitamin A deficiency states are exceedingly simple and depend on an adequate intake of foods containing vitamin A, which include milk, butter, eggs, and fresh vegetables containing the green and yellow pigments. Various concentrated preparations of vitamin A are also available.

THIAMIN OR VITAMIN B_1 DEFICIENCY

[Vitamin B deficiency was once limited to beriberi, derived from a Singhalese word meaning I cannot. In this disease, the patient cannot do anything because his heart is weak, his limbs become full of fluid, and there is paralysis. The paralysis is due to the fact that a deficiency of vitamin B_1 affects the nerves.

Vitamin B_1 has now been identified as a chemical compound called thiamin hydrochloride. It is recognized as a substance which is deficient in certain forms of neuritis, especially that associated with alcoholism and with overaction of the thyroid gland. Apparently in these conditions it is impossible for a person to get enough vitamin B_1.

This vitamin is also of value in developing and preventing loss of appetite in certain cases, and it is important in maintaining a proper physiologic condition of the bowels. It is known also to be highly effective in securing optimal growth of infants and children.

In the neuritis of scurvy and in the neuritis of pellagra there may be a shortage of vitamin B_1. This appears also when there is great stimulation of the chemistry of the body, such as occurs when there is fever or too much muscular exercise.

Although it was first thought that there was no deficiency of vitamin B_1 in American diets, it is now recognized that there may be widespread deficiency due to the fact that we have been eating too highly refined grains. Nowadays breads are available which have been enriched with vitamin B_1. This vitamin is found largely in meat or grain cereals, dried beans and peas. White cornmeal, egg yolk, milk, butter, green peas, and yeast are also rich in vitamin B_1.

In addition to thiamin, vitamin B complex includes what is scientifically known as riboflavin. This has been studied chiefly in animals, and has been found necessary for the growth of chicks and rats, and for the prevention of cataracts in rats. It seems to be associated in the human body in controlling in a definite way the process of oxidation and reduction which goes on in the individual cells.

Also included is nicotinic acid, a factor which has been found especially effective in the treatment of pellagra in human beings, and in a condition in dogs known as black tongue.

In human beings with pellagra the giving of nicotinic acid will lead to a disappearance of the disturbances of digestion and of the skin which are characteristic of the disease. Moreover, some of the mental symptoms which do not represent complete degeneration in the tissues of the nervous system will also improve. Nicotinic acid does not, however, seem to influence neuritis, frequently seen in pellagra. In such cases it is necessary to give also vitamin B_1 or thiamin.

OTHER VITAMIN B FACTORS

There is a factor which is important for the prevention of a form of skin disease which occurs in chickens, known as B_3. Factors B_3, $_4$ and $_5$, are important in the health of birds. Another factor, known as B_6, is related to certain disturbances of the skin, particularly, as has recently been reported, a cracking which occurs in the corners of the mouth in persons who do not get sufficient amounts of this vitamin. The vitamin B_6 factor is also believed to be quite definitely related to the early graying of the hair and it is believed that an adequate amount of this vitamin will, to some extent, postpone the appearance of this condition.—Ed.]

SCURVY, OR VITAMIN C DEFICIENCY

Scurvy is a disease produced as a result of deficiency of vitamin C in the diet. It is characterized chiefly by marked weakness, bleeding into the tissues, and softening of the bones. The occurrence of scurvy in times of deprivation of food, and particularly among sailors, is a matter of common knowledge. At present the occurrence of well-developed scurvy among adult persons is rare.

HISTORY

The first account of scurvy among sailors is to be found in the descriptions of the voyage of Vasco da Gama to the East Indies, by the Cape of Good Hope, in 1497, during which 100 of his 160 men died of scurvy. The seriousness of this disease in past centuries is difficult to appreciate today in our relative freedom from it and in its ease of control. The anti-scorbutic value of citrous fruits has long been known. In 1795 the British admiralty introduced one ounce of lemon juice daily as a regular item of the navy ration; this eradicated scurvy from the British navy and was unquestionably one of the great public health improvements of all time.

SYMPTOMS

Scurvy does not develop immediately on the deprivation of foods containing vitamin C. As a rule, from four to seven months are required before such deprivation leads to the development of symptoms of scurvy. This period is known as the depletion period and corresponds roughly to the incubation period of infectious diseases.

The number, situation, and amount of the hemorrhages into the tissues decide, in large part, the symptoms of which the patient will complain. The bleeding probably is not due to changes in the blood but to alterations in the substances which help to hold together the cells which compose the walls of the blood vessels. Areas in which hemorrhages occur are the gums, skin, muscles, bones, and nose. The gums swell and become red and spongy or fungus-like.

COURSE

It is amazing to consider the rapidity with which individuals with scurvy recover as soon as the diet becomes adequate. Just a few days may be required, unless permanent injury has been done.

Interest among physicians considering scurvy at the present time is chiefly concerned with scurvy of infants. Infantile scurvy is not seen, as a rule, before the child is aged six months. It is usually manifested by some of the following symptoms: swelling and bleeding of the gums, tenderness of the legs due to bleeding into the muscles or beneath the periosteum (tissue covering the bones), anemia, dental decay, susceptibility to infection, and cessation of growth. It has recently been claimed that dental caries (decay of teeth) is the result of vitamin C deficiency. This may be of the greatest significance, for if consumption of adequate amounts of vitamin C will in part prevent the development of such dental decay, its importance can hardly be overestimated.

X-ray studies of the bones help to establish the diagnosis of scurvy if hemorrhages in the bone are present.

TREATMENT

The treatment of scurvy is simple and consists in giving a diet high in value of foods containing vitamin C. Oranges, lemons, limes, germinating seeds and fresh fruits, especially tomatoes, and vegetables are the most abundant sources of this element.

Heating is detrimental if not destructive to vitamin C. This apparently explained the insufficiency of pasteurized or boiled milk, canned and cooked foods, as substances useful against scurvy until Hess pointed out that it was not the actual heat which destroyed the vitamin, but oxidation. Consequently, the preparation of canned foods has been fitted to this fact. Many canned foods, and especially canned tomato juice, contain almost as much if not as much vitamin C as the fresh substance.

RICKETS: A VITAMIN D DEFICIENCY

Rickets is a chronic nutritional disorder of infants and children, producing alterations chiefly in the bones, and considered by many to be a deficiency disease due to a lack of vitamin D. Rickets affects infants and children. The deficiency is most apparent during rapid growth, but a similar disease of adults, called osteomalacia (destructive disease of bones) is thought to be closely related. The origin of the word "rickets" is not known for certain, but it probably is derived from the Anglo-Saxon word, "wrickken" (to twist), and was applied because of the deformities it produced. Almost everyone is familiar with the term rickety chair or table, which has a somewhat similar significance.

HISTORY

In previous centuries rickets was a disabling disease, leading to severe crippling of children. Today, as with such a deficiency disease as scurvy, it is rarely seen in its worst form and generally is quite mild in this country, except among the Negro and Italian populations in our larger cities.

INCIDENCE

Rickets is the most common nutritional disease occurring among children of the temperate zone, and it is primarily a disease of this geographic area. It occurs chiefly in the large cities and industrial districts. It has been estimated, for example, that at least 50 per cent of all infants in New York and London have rickets. It must be remembered, however, that this does not mean severe rickets, as was known in previous centuries and still exists, in the minds of many laymen. The disorder is frequently so mild in the present day as to be unrecognized except by experts.

The intensity and incidence of rickets throughout the world corresponds fairly closely to the amount of sunshine present. It is the sun's ultraviolet rays, invisible to the human eye, which are significant anti-rachitic factors.

There is a distinct seasonal incidence in the occurrence of rickets. The incidence of the disorder begins to increase, for example, in the autumn of the year, reaches its peak of the greatest number of cases in March, and then disappears rapidly.

Premature infants and those who grow rapidly seem to be predisposed to rickets, probably because of the rapid rate of growth. Infants aged from six to eighteen months are most often affected by rickets, since the infant is much less exposed to sunlight than is the older child who runs about.

CAUSE

Many factors which have a direct bearing on the development of rickets are now known, and there are several specific measures for the successful prevention and treatment of the disease.

The diet and condition of the mother before birth of her child probably have some effect on the subsequent development of rickets. Bottle-fed babies are much more likely to develop rickets than are breast-fed babies, but the latter do sometimes have rickets.

The distinguishing characteristic of rickets is that the bone which is formed is not of normal composition, since it is improperly and inadequately calcified (hardened). The result is that the bone is abnormally soft, and deformity, bending, and twisting occur. Naturally, the more abundant the growth of bone, the more likely is the hardening to be insufficient, which explains the increasing frequency of rickets in the more rapidly growing and well-nourished child.

The greatest recent advance in the study of rickets has been in the understanding of the precise nature of the effect of sunlight on the disease. It has been established that the ultraviolet rays of the sunlight are the significant factors. It is remarkable that these rays of invisible light are of such great importance in the hardening of bone. It is still more remarkable, and certainly beyond our present comprehension, that only those ultraviolet waves of a certain length (290 to 313 millimicrons) are effective, and that a difference of as little as from ten to twenty millionths of a millimeter (25 mm. to an inch) is sufficient to render ultraviolet light effective or ineffective in curing or preventing rickets. During the winter months the absorption of these ultraviolet waves by moisture, dust, smoke, and other foreign substances in the air makes their quantity reaching the skin of the well-covered infant extremely small, even though the child is out of doors. Direct sunlight is not essential, since it has been shown that the so-called skyshine, light reflected from the sky, clouds, and so forth, possesses approximately from half to two thirds the anti-rachitic effect of sunshine. This is an extremely important observation. An infant obtains considerable ultraviolet irradiation without being in the direct sunlight. Ordinary window glass removes the ultraviolet rays, so that sunshine which passes through a windowpane is ineffective against rickets. Special kinds of glass are made which do not remove these rays.

The exact mechanism of action of the ultraviolet waves in hardening bone is unknown. Probably the ultraviolet light acts by producing chemical changes in the traces of ergosterol (one of the fatty materials) of the skin, with the production of a substance known as vitamin D. Ultraviolet waves from artificial sources, for example, mercury vapor lamps, are quite as effective, if not more so, against rickets when properly given than is direct sunlight.

The factor leading to the hardening (calcification) of the bones, may be obtained not only by the action of sunlight on the skin but by the ingestion of certain foods (anti-rachitic) such as cod-liver oil, egg yolk, foods which have been treated with ultraviolet light (irradiated foods), to some extent breast milk, and irradiated ergosterol (viosterol). These substances all contain vitamin D.

SYMPTOMS

The earliest signs of rickets are restlessness, irritability, and sweating of the head. These signs are, however, only suggestive and not conclusive; they also occur under other circumstances. In the bones will be found definite evidence of rickets, which shows itself by enlargement of the ends of the bones (epiphysial areas) and by softening. The most reliable early sign is thickening or beading of the ends of the ribs about the nipple line, at the points where the bony and cartilaginous ribs join. This swelling or beading is known as the "rachitic rosary." There is also enlargement of the bones, particularly about the wrist and the knee, squaring of the head, failure of the soft areas (fontanels) in the head to close at the proper time, and softness of the bones of the head. These symptoms are not all necessarily present in one case. Subsequently, enlargement of the abdomen, grooving in of the lower ribs (Harrison's groove), squaring of the head, and bowlegs or knock knees may develop. The muscles become soft and flabby; the physical development is poor, so that rachitic children usually are slow in sitting and walking; the eruption of the teeth is tardy, and occasionally curvature of the spine occurs. The importance of rickets as a factor in causing delay in the development and eruption of the teeth and in the subsequent development of dental decay is as yet unknown, but the relationship seems significant.

The diagnosis of rickets is easily made in a classical, well-developed case. In the early stages, it may be necessary to resort to laboratory measures, such as X-ray examinations of the bones, and studies of the phosphorus content of the blood, which is generally below normal.

The outlook for recovery of the rachitic infant is excellent, especially if treatment is given. As a rule, the mild condition recovers spontaneously during the summer. Occasionally deformities persist if the condition remains too long untreated; rickets is readily cured by adequate treatment.

PREVENTION AND TREATMENT

Rickets can be prevented. People are so rapidly becoming educated in the matter of prevention and cure of rickets that the disease becomes less serious and perhaps less common as time goes on.

The prevention and treatment of rickets is unique; it is the only disease for which there are several specific methods of cure. These are the use of cod-liver oil, ultraviolet light, irradiated foods (foods treated with ultraviolet light), and irradiated ergosterol. The efficacy of cod-liver oil has been definitely established within the last few years, and its effectiveness definitely shown on experimental animals with rickets.

The amount of cod-liver oil to be used in preventing or treating rickets is variable and depends on the age of the patient, the severity of the disease, the vitamin D and anti-rachitic value of the cod-liver oil, as well as the associated treatment applied. It is difficult to make a general statement concerning the matter, and this should be left to the discretion of the physician in a given case. The Council on Pharmacy and Chemistry of the American Medical Association has decided that a dosage of 3 teaspoonfuls (12 c.c., 3 fluid drachms) daily may tentatively be set as the standard optimal dosage of standard cod-liver oil for the average infant aged three months.

Sunlight or ultraviolet light artificially produced, as for instance by the mercury vapor lamp, is perhaps as effective as any other measure in the prevention and treatment of rickets. Sunlight and sky-shine, as mentioned, should be more generally used, especially in cities, than they are at present.

Irradiated ergosterol (viosterol), which is highly specific for rickets, should be used only under the direct supervision of a physician. The tremendous anti-rachitic power of irradiated ergosterol can be seen from the fact that 5 mg. $\frac{5}{1000}$ of a gram) of this substance is estimated to be equivalent to one quart of cod-liver oil. Excessive doses of this potent substance are known to have produced undesirable effects.

It should be remembered, also, that breast milk, although not a specific for rickets itself, is one of the most valuable measures for combating the disease.

Pellagra

The name "pellagra" is probably derived from the Italian words *pelle*, for skin and *agra*, for rough, since roughened skin is one of the most frequently observed symptoms in this disease.

Probably pellagra occurred occasionally in the United States during the nineteenth century, but scientific reports of its occurrence in this country were almost lacking until 1907, when an investigator named Searcy made the first report. Perhaps previous failure of recognition in the United States was due to the fact that pellagra was considered a disease of the tropics or of Europe only, and therefore it received practically no recognition in medical textbooks published in this country before that time. However, knowledge of the disease spread rapidly throughout the southern part of the United States, and numerous reports of cases and of epidemics were recorded; thus a great deal of knowledge has been acquired concerning pellagra since 1907.

CAUSE

Dr. J. Goldberger and his associates of the United States Public Health Service have shown that most, if not all, cases of pellagra are closely associated with a deficiency in the intake of food. Goldberger said:

> Indeed it may be stated that our knowledge of the nature of the dietary deficiency has now been sufficiently clarified to warrant placing pellagra in a category closely related to, if not identical with, that of beriberi and scurvy.

The substance which is lacking in the dietary of the individual suffering from pellagra is vitamin G, known also as the P-P factor of Goldberger and, in England, as vitamin B_2. Recently a substance called nicotinic acid has been isolated as a part of vitamin G or B_2 necessary to control pellagra.

INCIDENCE

Pellagra is endemic in the South; that is, it is constantly occurring, chiefly in the spring and summer months. There also seems to be a close relationship between the number of cases and economic depression. Individuals who are victims of pellagra usually fall into three groups: (1) those with simple deficiencies of diet; (2) those with deficiencies of food due to prolonged use of large amounts of alcohol, and (3) those with deficiencies because of organic disease of the digestive system.

SYMPTOMS

For many years medical students have been taught that the great triad of symptoms in pellagra was "the three D's," dermatitis, dementia, and diarrhea; that is, inflammation of the skin, abnormal mental symptoms, and looseness of the bowels. but there are few existing diseases which are more variable in nature than is pellagra. The occurrence of these three symptoms together, or in the same patient, is found only in the severest cases and usually means that the outlook is bad. The skin, the digestive tract, and the nervous system are, how-ever, the three parts of the body which are particularly affected when pellagra occurs. Goldberger said:

> The eruption is the most characteristic telltale of the disease and the main reliance in its recognition. When the eruption first shows itself it may look much like, and frequently is mistaken for, a sunburn. The sun-burned appearance soon changes and in many cases the reddened skin turns to a somewhat dirty brown and frequently acquires a parchment-like appearance, then quickly becomes rough and scaly, or cracks and peels. . . . Among the most distinctive peculiarities of the eruption is its preference for certain parts of the body surface. The backs of the hands, forearms, and the backs of the feet are its favorite sites. [It also occurs on the face, neck, trunk, and legs.] Another marked peculiarity of the eruption is its tendency to appear at about the same time and to cover similar areas, both as to extent and peculiarities of outline, on both sides of the body.

The skin may peel and become dark. Eventually, as the disease is overcome, the eruption on the skin may entirely disappear or the area affected may remain dark. The symptoms related to the skin in them-selves are rarely serious, but as a result of them the patient may look old and scrawny.

The digestive symptoms in the early cases are excessive amounts of gas on the stomach and in the bowels, loss of appetite, vague distress in the abdomen, and constipation or diarrhea. Loss of appetite is less common. Diarrhea is common late in the disease and is usually diffi-cult to control. The patient may believe that he has colitis. There is usually a lack of hydrochloric acid in the content of the stomach.

The effects on the nervous system which are first noted are ex-haustion, lassitude, insomnia, and subsequently, in the severe cases, hallucinations, and finally insanity. Only a small proportion of cases go on to this condition, from which recovery is infrequent.

COURSE

The course of pellagra is variable. At times it may begin without any notice save for a little burning of the hands or feet, a sense of heat in the pit of the stomach, and a little nervousness and restlessness at night. In other cases the skin changes only will be present and, because of frequent resemblance to sunburn, may not be particularly noted by the patient. In the absence of skin symptoms, the diagnosis of the disease can be correctly made by an expert only.

Although the disease is frequently completely overcome by patients, it may remain chronic, with flare-ups suggesting repeated acute attacks each spring and summer.

Underhill stated: "In general, pellagra seems no more dangerous than measles." Death occurs in about 3 per cent of the cases of pellagra, although in certain types of cases this incidence may be considerably higher.

TREATMENT

The keystone in considering the treatment of pellagra should be prevention. Goldberger said: "The suspicion of pellagra may with confidence be dismissed in one who is known to be, and to have been, a habitual milk drinker and meat eater." Although a patient may have placed before him an adequate amount of food containing vitamin G, it is to be remembered that individual eccentricity of taste may make the actual vitamin content of food consumed inadequate for his needs. This at times explains the occurrence of pellagra in the well-to-do person with apparently sufficient food.

[The treatment of pellagra is based on an adequate intake of foods containing particularly nicotinic acid, which is specific in the treatment of acute pellagra. If this product is administered in appropriate doses, it leads to the disappearance of practically all of the symptoms. People suffering from pellagra usually have diets insufficient in other important factors. They should be provided with sufficient amounts of thiamin, which is vitamin B_1, and also vitamin B_6.—Ed.]

VITAMIN E

Vitamin E, which has been discovered more recently than the other vitamins, has been shown to be necessary for normal reproduction in certain animals. Its relationship to reproduction in man has not been determined. It has been recommended for habitual abortion.

It is quite possible that other vitamins will be discovered in the course of time, and that certain of the vitamins now considered to be single substances will in fact be found to be a group of substances, all of which are essential for the attainment and maintenance of good health.

RÉSUMÉ OF THE KNOWN VITAMINS, THEIR NAMES, SOURCES, PURPOSES, AND DEFICIENCIES

Vitamin	Other Names	Sources			Excellent Purposes	Deficiency Leads to
		Fair	Good	Excellent		
A	Anti-ophthalmic Anti-infective Growth promoting Fat soluble A Carotin or pro-vitamin A	Green vegetables Fruits	Tomatoes Whole yellow corn Hens' eggs Ordinary green vegetables	Butter Cod liver oil Other liver oils Spinach Kale Turnip greens	Maintains integrity of epithelial (covering) tissues thereby helping in part to prevent infections Promotes growth and vigor Essential for reproduction	Lowered resistance to infection of many organs, especially of the eyes (xerophthalmia) Failure of growth of children Loss of vigor Night blindness
B	B_1 Anti-neuritic Anti-beriberi Thiamin chloride	Lean muscle meat	Heart, liver, kidney, eggs, milk Whole cereals Green vegetables	Wheat germ Asparagus Yeast	Promotes appetite and digestion Stimulates body activity Overcomes some forms of neuritis Prevents beriberi	Beriberi Loss of tone of digestive tract Sterility Forms of neuritis Loss of appetite
C	Anti-scorbutic Ascorbic acid Cevitamic acid	Fresh apples and onions	Bananas Pineapple Collards Green peas	Green peppers Tomatoes Grapefruit Lemons Oranges Tomato juice Cabbage	Protects body from scurvy Required for proper formation of bones and teeth	Scurvy Softening of bones Decay of teeth Loss of muscle strength Hemorrhage

					Function	Deficiency
D	Anti-rachitic Irradiated ergosterol Viosterol	Milk or butter	Eggs	Cod liver oil Sunlight Artificial ultra-violet lights Irradiated ergosterol (viosterol)	Proper calcification (hardening) of bones Prevents rickets	Rickets Bone deformities Defects and caries of teeth General muscular weakness
E	Anti-sterility	Whole cereals	Whole wheat Lettuce Watercress	Wheat germ	Necessary for reproduction in animals and man?	Sterility (noted in animals only) Failure of reproduction (noted in animals only)
G	B₂ Riboflavin Lactoflavin	Whole wheat Dried beans Soya beans	Wheat germ Meat Green vegetables	Dried yeast Milk Eggs Heart Kidney	Extrinsic factor in pernicious anemia (Castle)? Necessary for normal growth Development of cells	Disorders of growth Digestive disturbances Nervous weakness Infection
P.P. Factor	Nicotinic acid Pellagra preventive factor	Milk Wheat germ Lean meats	Green vegetables Beans	Yeast	Prevention of complications in pellagra	Pellagra, including nerve, skin and intestinal disturbances Black tongue in dogs
K	Anti-hemorrhagic vitamin	Grass	Alfalfa	Concentrates	Prevention of hemorrhage by maintaining concentration of prothrombin in blood	Tendency to bleed, particularly in new-born
Vitamin B Complex	Vitamin B complex includes also filtrate factor; vitamin B₃ " ₅ and ₆				These factors are known particularly for effects in absence in animals but have been related to complications of pellagra and similar disturbances in human beings. Pantothenic acid (filtrate factor) is related to graying of hair in human beings. Vitamin B₆ (pyridoxine) is related to some chronic nervous disturbances.	

CHAPTER XIX

Allergy and Hypersensitivity

INCLUDING HAY FEVER, ASTHMA, HIVES, ECZEMA, HEADACHE, STOMACH AND INTESTINAL DISORDERS, AND OTHER FUNCTIONAL AND ORGANIC DISEASES

WILLIAM W. DUKE, M.D.

INTRODUCTION

ONE OF THE MOST REMARKABLE *advances in modern medical science has been discovery of the fact that human beings may be specifically sensitive to certain substances in their diet, in the air, or in their environment which causes them to react by development of severe symptoms, including skin eruptions, hay fever, or asthmatic attacks, and not infrequently complete prostration. By means of skin tests with extracts of the suspected substances it is possible to show the nature of the things to which the person may be sensitive. Among the leading causes of such sensitization, specialists have found some people are sensitive to glue, others to feathers, or to various types of dust, to pollens, to strawberries, or indeed to almost every type of plant or animal product.*

About one hundred years ago several medical writers mentioned as curiosities patients who began to sneeze and wheeze at the time of the blooming of the roses. In 1819, an English physician named Bostock described his own symptoms, which included a sense of heat and swelling of the eyes, with itching and smarting and with much running of tears when he looked at the light. This was followed by a fullness in the head and irritation in the nose, with fits of severe sneezing, sometimes so violent as to cause pain in the chest.

Naturally a person afflicted with these symptoms would feel generally ill and be tired most of the time, because of inability to rest at night. Usually the symptoms appeared about the beginning or middle of June and disappeared toward the end of July. After more and

more cases of the disease were studied, it was found that there were also cases which appeared in the early summer and some which came on in the late summer and in the fall, and that persons in different sections of the country were likely to succumb at different times to the disease.

The very earliest investigator, Bostock, gave to the disease the name of summer catarrh and also suggested the term "hay fever." Later investigators differed with that suggestion and experimented with extracts of the pollens of all sorts of flowers and grasses. The earliest observations disclosed that the appearance of the disease was definitely associated with the pollination of plants. Another English physician, named Blackley, experimented on himself between 1856 and 1877 with the pollens of more than one hundred grasses and flowers, inhaling pollen and applying it to the membranes of his nose and eyes.

Later Dunbar proved that it is the protein portion of the pollen which brings on the symptoms in the more intense form, and that neither the whole pollen nor the protein extract would have any effect on normal persons, although they did produce the most severe symptoms in persons who were subject to the disease.

The average person may not be particularly interested in the details of the investigations that have been made, but these have established beyond the shadow of a doubt that hay fever is the result of a definite sensitivity of the person to the protein portions of the pollens of various flowers and grasses. It is not contagious, but a history of the disease in the ancestry is found in from 58 to 68 per cent of persons affected. This may indicate a possible hereditary relationship.

It is surprising how many thousands of sufferers from hay fever and asthma accept their condition with despair or equanimity and do not realize how much they may be helped by proper scientific medical attention. This is, no doubt, due to the fact that dissemination of the information as to what can be accomplished has not been sufficient to get these persons into the hands of those able to be of service.

In the article which follows, Dr. Duke explains some of the methods by which the modern physician determines the nature of hay fever or asthma in the individual case, and then the methods used for prevention and relief.

It should be clear that the best and most important of the methods of treatment are those which make certain of strict avoidance of any contact with the actual excitant. The determination of these excitants is one of the finest examples of the methods of detection used by the modern physician in his study and control of disease.

M. F.

Persons with allergy are hyperresponsive, hyperactive, and hypersensitive to certain things, often things with which they are intimately associated; often to things which they dislike, and sometimes to things which they may need or crave. Examples include certain pollens, dust, foods, animals, fowl, insects, drugs, smoke, light, heat and cold. Success in treatment depends primarily on finding the substances to which the person is sensitive and thereafter avoiding these substances or getting accustomed to them.

Unfortunately, the agents which sensitize such people are usually infinitesimal in size and are encountered in excessively minute amounts, so that their discovery may tax the ingenuity of both patient and physician to the limit.

Defining Allergy

The person with allergy is an individual who inherits some peculiar constitutional make-up which causes him to become sensitive to certain things. Thereafter these particular things become violently poisonous to him, even when encountered in minute amounts. Allergy patients may become sensitive not only to material things but also to physical agents such as light, heat, or cold. Sensitiveness may develop to such an extreme in certain people that they may be badly affected by a millionth of a milligram of a substance which may be devoured as a food by a nonsensitive person.

The allergic trait is not altogether bad if it does not develop to such a degree as to cause an illness or get the patient into trouble. Some famous historical characters have been allergic, and probably on account of the acuteness caused by this abnormality enjoyed unusual success in the vocation in which they happened to fall. A person may become so sensitive to pollen that the trace of pollen in the air at certain seasons gives him hay fever and asthma followed by frequent colds during the winter season. A baby may become so sensitive to egg or milk that even while on an egg- or milk-free diet, the quantity obtained from the lips and bands of the mother suffices to cause unsightly eczema and asthma. A patient may be so sensitive to fish that the trace of fish glue absorbed from licking a postage stamp, or from the handling of books, or from the putting on of shoes which have been repaired with glue, or the picking up of a beer bottle with a wet label suffices to cause illness which proves all but fatal. All these instances are true illustrations.

Sensitiveness of this grade handicaps the individual and incapacitates him for many types of mental or physical work. An individual was so sensitive to hog fat that the eating of bread containing a trace of lard caused migraine and what was presumed to be a bad cold. Another was so sensitive to bedbugs that one or two bites caused nausea, vomiting, and diarrhea and a general illness which reduced him to a state of coma within a period of hours. A young gallant was so sensitive to a perfume used by his fiancée that he tried to break his engagement the day before the wedding. A social leader became so sensitive to the heat generated by effort that a vivacious conversation with interesting company caused her to have an immediate evacuation of the bowels and forced her finally to lead a life of seclusion. Such sensitivities are intolerable afflictions.

Allergy is a real condition. Its manifestations are grave. Whenever a person of allergic strain comes in intimate contact with an agent to which he is sensitive, he is certain to have a definite illness which may be mild, severe, or grave, depending on the degree of contact.

The agents responsible for allergy are usually infinitesimal in size and inconspicuous. For this reason, a patient sensitive to a certain agent may be inclined falsely to blame his illness on something to which he is exposed simultaneously which he can see. For example, a person sensitive to the inconspicuous ragweed usually places the blame for his illness on some flowering plant blooming at the same time: for example, goldenrod, sunflower, or daisy. The fact is that goldenrod, sunflower, or daisy are practically never a cause of hay fever or asthma. A person sensitive to some fungus in house dust may blame some odor in the house for his trouble or actually lay the blame for his illness to his wife.

HISTORY

Illnesses which were eventually called hay fever, asthma, and eczema were recognized by Hippocrates. The cause of such troubles however, was not referred to in any detail until 1565, when Botallus said that certain patients had headache, itching of the nose, and sneezing from the odor of roses. Bostock, in 1819, was one of the first to give a description of the disease hay fever, and in describing his own troubles said that they were caused by heat and the sun's rays. He mentioned patients, however, who had summer catarrh or hay fever if they walked out into the fields at certain seasons.

Blackley, in 1880, made the first comprehensive study of the cause, diagnosis, and treatment of hay fever, and his work, remarkable for detail and accuracy, stands in line with present-day knowledge. In 1910, Meltzer, a worker in the Rockefeller Institute, stated that he believed that bronchial asthma is a phenomenon of anaphylaxis or allergy. Probably 15 per cent of people are afflicted by allergy in greater or lesser degree.

HEREDITY

Allergy is one of the most consistently hereditary of all diseases. If heredity comes from both sides of a family, the illness is likely to appear in the child at an early age. Since it appears that persons of allergic strain tend to intermarry, this is an important factor so far as the age of onset of the trouble is concerned. Whereas the allergic constitution is hereditary, different members of the same family may become sensitized to widely differing substances.

AGE OF ONSET

Allergy can make its appearance in earliest infancy; in fact, some infants are born with it, caused, apparently, by sensitiveness to some constituent of the mother's diet. In infancy, the chief cause of trouble is food, often some food eaten by the mother and transferred to the infant by the lips and hands. Sometimes the offending substance is obtained through secretion in the milk of traces of some food eaten by the mother. Many of the cases of skin eruptions, food disagreements, nausea, vomiting, diarrhea, and asthma in infancy are traceable to foods eaten by the mother or infant.

Whereas sensitiveness to foods can appear in infancy, sensitiveness to pollen, dust, and other materials obtained from the outside air rarely becomes manifest until early childhood. Sensitiveness of this type can appear at any time between childhood and maturity and rarely appears for the first time after mature age is reached. Allergy which appears for the first time during adult years is due, as a rule, to sensitiveness to heat and effort or to cold or to some organic disease.

Natural and Acquired Sensitiveness

We are at a loss to know why one individual becomes sensitive to one foreign agent and others to another. It seems in many cases that an illness has something to do with it. For example, rather frequently a patient will date the onset of pollen disease from an attack of measles, scarlet fever, pneumonia, or influenza. As a general rule people are most likely to become sensitive to something with which they are in intimate contact at frequent intervals and which they meet with in traces rather than in quantity, such, for example, as the common pollens of the environment in which they live, or dust material which they meet with in their homes or places of business. Contact must have something to do with the development of sensitiveness, for Europeans were never found sensitive to American ragweed. Ragweed does not thrive in European countries.

Some persons are sensitized in mild degree to serum and horses by injections of antitoxin. This type of sensitiveness is rarely grave. Sensitiveness to horse serum which is so severe as to cause desperate illness after the use of antitoxin is practically always spontaneously acquired by persons who have never before had antitoxin.

Effect of Environment and Climate

Environment bears an interesting relationship to the symptomatology which a sensitive patient displays. This is almost always due to the fact that he either does or does not come in contact with the agent to which he reacts. Many patients obtain relief by a relatively small change in environment. Sometimes they need only move from one house to another to avoid a certain type of mold, animal, or fowl which makes them sick, or from one state to another to avoid certain pollens or animals which make them sick, or from one climate to another to avoid certain degrees of heat or cold or air moisture which makes them sick. However, an allergic person who blindly tries one locality after another in an effort to find relief is likely to waste time and money unless he knows the source of his illness. Likely as not, he will meet with the elements which make him ill in many different places.

For example, a person sensitive to egg, milk, or wheat will meet with these substances everywhere and is not likely to be benefited by a change in environment. One sensitive to pollen, however, may obtain relief by removal to an area where the particular pollen to which he reacts does not exist. Sea air is always free of pollen and is good for people sensitive to pollen but may be bad for those sensitive to heat, effort, and air moisture. Consequently, if a person with hay fever, asthma, or eczema wishes relief by change in environment, all causes for his trouble must be discovered in advance of the change. Otherwise, he may accomplish nothing by a change which may entail sacrifice in social, business, or financial status. A careless change is likely to do much more harm than good.

Permanence of Sensitiveness

The constitutional make-up of allergic persons is permanent. The types of sensitiveness developed, however, may or may not be permanent. Sensitiveness to foods, for example, varies sometimes with general health and normalcy of digestion. Sensitiveness to both foods and heat is made worse by fatigue and depression but frequently relieved temporarily by fever. Sensitiveness to pollen, dust, insects, perfumes, and other inhalants, however, is almost always permanent unless changed by specific treatment. Any relief which is apparent is almost always due to some change in the habits of the patient which exposes him to smaller amounts of the agent to which he reacts. Persons sensitive to ragweed can move to a seashore and enjoy years of freedom from hay fever but suffer relapse immediately on their return to the original environment.

Multiple Sensitiveness

Persons with allergy, throughout their lives, may become sensitive to one thing after another through no apparent cause unless possibly through repeated exposure to some substance or during an illness. An infant, as a rule, is sensitive to only one or several agents, whereas an adult in middle life is almost always sensitive to several different things. Some sensitive people think they react to everything, but this is rarely the case. They are usually sensitive to one of several materials which are encountered frequently, and falsely blame their illness on things which they can see.

SPECIFICITY OF SENSITIVENESS

Some patients are sensitive to one specific thing; in fact, so specific a thing that they can eat cantaloupe grown in one district and are made ill by cantaloupe of another district, or can eat strawberries of one district and cannot tolerate strawberries of another. However, what is known as group specificity is the more common, that is, a person sensitive to egg may not be sensitive to one particular variety of egg from certain hens but to eggs in general.

DEGREE OF SENSITIVENESS

Sensitiveness varies in degree in different individuals. Some, for example, who are sensitive to egg cannot tolerate infinitesimal amounts of egg and are made ill even by the quantity of egg they encounter on the hands and lips of other individuals. Others, who are less sensitive, can tolerate small amounts of egg contained in cooked foods, such as cake, but may be made ill by eating eggs as such. There are still others who can tolerate eggs at odd intervals but cannot take them several days in succession without experiencing a definite and severe illness. The high degree to which sensitiveness develops in certain people is almost beyond belief. Some, for example, sensitive to bees, cannot tolerate the bee matter contained in one drop of honey. Some, sensitive to egg, cannot tolerate the quantity of egg contained in hen meat but can eat rooster meat with impunity. Some, sensitive to hog fat, cannot tolerate the quantity of lard contained in one bit of bread, and others, sensitive to cotton seed, cannot tolerate the infinitesimal amounts of Crisco used in the cooking of certain foods. Linseed or cottonseed cases can be made ill by contact with small amounts of fertilizer or fodder. Their contact with the material may be almost infinitesimal. Several people sensitive to chicken feathers could not remain in districts where chickens were raised even though they were not raised in the exact locality in which they resided. These statements sound fantastic, but similar examples have been observed repeatedly by every specialist who has had any experience in this work.

PERIODICITY OF ALLERGY

The manifestations of allergy are usually periodic. Frequently attacks are seasonal. Occasionally, they occur at weekly or monthly intervals. In the majority of cases, the height of attack is reached at certain times of the day or night. This frequently depends on contact with certain substances at certain times or seasons. The majority of cases of asthma, however, are worse at night, or rather, during the early morning hours. This may be due to the fact that vitality at that time is at a low ebb and that body temperature at that time is most highly subnormal. Also, the change from a state of sleep to a state of wakefulness marks the greatest change between rest and activity that occurs at any time during the twenty-four hours and is inclined to cause symptoms in patients sensitive to heat and effort. Night asthma is often, though not as a general rule, caused by sensitiveness to feathers or something contained in pillows or mattresses or dust in the room.

The Nature of the Cause of Allergy

At present nothing is infallibly proven in explanation of this remarkable condition except the hereditary factor. Cohen has suggested that the allergy reaction is an effort of nature to keep out of the blood certain substances which cause the patient to react—that is, substances to which the patient is sensitive. For example, during the pollen season, Cohen can detect pollen substances in the blood of normal individuals but cannot detect it in the blood of individuals sensitive to pollen. This is important in relationship to treatment. After treatment, this tendency to exclude pollen through symptoms such as hay fever and asthma disappears. The patient gains in health. Apparently this effort of nature to exclude noxious substances from the body even in traces, is not altogether desirable. The patients would probably be much better off if their tissues, as in normal people, allowed traces of foreign matter to enter the blood stream.

Relationship of Allergy to General Health

So far as general health is concerned, there are two types of allergic persons: those sensitive to agents with which they come in contact in the outside air, and those sensitive to foods, heat, or cold. The former type enjoy immunity from certain illnesses and as a rule are strong and well except for their sensitiveness to certain agents. They enjoy relative immunity from both tuberculosis and syphilis, and in case they acquire either disease, have a tendency to recover which is definitely greater than that observed in normal people. This is fortunate. However, some of the acute infections run a violent course in people with hay fever and asthma. Such illnesses, for example, as measles, tonsillitis, or pneumonia may be intense, but recovery is likely to be rapid. Those sensitive to foods, heat, or cold are subject to winter colds, pneumonia, and other illnesses which may cause them to run down badly. People sensitive to heat are inclined to emaciate and become excessively thin. Their muscles are small, soft, and lack tone. Some are fat, but even though fat, their muscles are small and flabby.

People with hay fever and asthma usually ask whether or not symptoms of hay fever and asthma will tend to subside if general health improves. Hopes of this sort are almost always ill founded, and efforts to cure asthma is this way almost always disappoint. Regardless of the state of health, a patient sensitive to pollen will react to pollen invariably if he comes in contact with a sufficient amount. The exception is the patient sensitive to heat and effort. Patients sensitive to heat and effort can gain tolerance for heat and effort through building up muscular structures by systematic exercise.

PERSONALITY OF THE ALLERGY PATIENT

A majority of patients who have allergy have a personality and manner which can be recognized by physicians of experience. Whether or not they are having hay fever or asthma at a given time, their manner is usually one of quickness, brightness, acuteness, over-responsiveness, and over-reactiveness to things which interest them, such as their children or parents, their home, and financial status. Conversing with parents concerning a child with asthma, the doctor can usually surmise from which side of the family the heredity comes or whether it comes from one or both sides of the family. The parent from whom allergy is inherited is over-responsive to questions which concern the child and is on edge while the history is being taken. This over-reactability may or may not be unfortunate for the child. It certainly keeps the parent too deeply concerned about its welfare and about remedial suggestions which are made, whether right or wrong. This peculiarity of the allergic individual is not bad if it is not so extreme as to cause him to jump into things or out of things without due consideration of true merit.

In addition, there is an actual change in the disposition of many allergy patients with the onset of allergic symptoms, even though the allergic symptoms may be too mild at the time to cause actual discomfort. One child who had asthma had a vile behavior. He would stick his fingers in the inkwell and thought it a good joke to smear the ink over everything and everybody in the room. He was nicknamed Sunny because of his customary sunny disposition. His mother said that he was a joy to everyone who knew him except during attacks of hay fever or asthma. Many sufferers appear neurotic, high strung, emotional, and hard to get along with during hay fever, hives, or asthma attacks. At other times they may be angelic. This fact should always be given due consideration by the relatives of allergic people, because their actions during attacks may be beyond their own control. This also handicaps the doctor in treatment because, during periods of this kind, these patients are inclined to disregard a physician's instructions, may be pessimistic about continuance of important treatment, and may jump into things which may not be so easy to get out of. Some become delirious and are so nervous as to be unable to take simple remedies for their relief. Some actually become suicidal in their tendencies.

The Ill Effects of Careless Advice

Careless advice given by neighbors, members of the family, or even by friendly physicians handicaps every physician who treats allergy. Tales are told about serum treatments which would terrify anyone. The fact is that serum is never used in the treatment of allergy; in fact, is contra-indicated.

The person with allergy should remember that careless advice is one of the most worthless things in existence; in fact, it is often dangerous. It costs nothing and is worth less. If a friend, neighbor, member of the family has nothing to give except advice, he is as useless to the allergy patient as his advice.

Agents Which Tend to Sensitize

POLLEN

Pollen is apparently the commonest of all causes of allergy. Symptoms caused by it are usually hay fever and asthma. Occasionally, it causes eczema of the hands and face and neck. In this case the oil of the plant can have the same effect, so that this type of eczema can occur during summer months.

Pollen cases usually have seasonal symptoms in temperate climates occurring in the spring, summer, or fall. Cases which occur in the spring are caused, as a rule, by tree pollen which is set free in temperate climates between March and May. In the southern climates, however, mountain cedar may pollinate during the winter months. Summer is the great grass season. In temperate climates, one or another of the grasses pollenate between the middle of May and the middle or latter part of July. In southern climates, however, Bermuda grass may pollenate throughout a much longer season or even during the winter months. The weed season starts during the fall months in temperate climates between the first to the twenty-fifth of August and terminates, as a rule, with frost. Patients who have symptoms following the fall season which last throughout the winter months are sensitive, as a rule, in addition, to heat, effort, or cold, or to some other object which they encounter during the winter months.

The important pollens of a given district are the pollens of some tree, grass, or weed which grows in abundance and blooms inconspicuously. A flowering tree or grass or weed rarely causes trouble because of the fact that little pollen is produced by a flower and little escapes from the plant. Even the pollen of corn is rarely carried far enough from the cornfield to affect people who do not live in the immediate vicinity of the growing corn.

FOODS

Patients may become sensitive apparently to almost any type of food and sometimes to a certain group of foods. The commonest offenders in children are milk, eggs, and wheat. The same is true, though to a less extent, in adults. Adults are, however, frequently sensitive to pork fat, sea foods, nuts, and less frequently to some of the fruits or vegetables. Meats, except pork, appear to be the least offensive of the foods. If patients are highly sensitive to egg, milk, hog fat, wheat, linseed, or cottonseed they are unfortunate because of the wide use of these materials in cookery. Also, patients sensitive to orris are unfortunate because of the use of orris not only in perfumes and toilet articles but also in flavoring extracts.

ANIMAL HAIR AND FEATHERS

Sensitiveness to animal hair and feathers is an important cause of hay fever and asthma but is rarely to be compared with sensitiveness to pollen or foods. Patients may be sensitive to one or several animals,

They may be sensitive to the animal itself, its cured products, or both. The latter, however, is rare as compared with the former. Horse sensitiveness is the commonest type of animal sensitiveness. Less often there is sensitiveness to cattle, sheep, hogs, dogs, cats, rabbits, or guinea pigs. Of the fowl, sensitiveness to chickens, ducks, geese, or pigeons is more common. Less common are sensitivities to the cured products used in pillows and mattresses.

COTTONSEED, LINSEED, ORRIS, GLUE, AND CORN PRODUCTS

These agents are possibly worthy of special mention because of their wide sphere of use. One need only recall various uses to which these products are put to wonder how a person sensitive to any of them could ever escape one of them.

MOLDS AND FUNGI

During the summer months, spores of fungi known as wheat rust or corn smoot fill the air; in fact, in quantity, frequently exceed grass pollen. Also, molds that grow on the leaves of trees and bushes are important. One man was sensitive to a mold which grows on the bark of trees and was subject to unsightly eczema of the face and hands during the winter months owing to the escape of spores from the bark of firewood. Certain molds grow in houses in dry places, in rugs, curtains, and upholstery, and are responsible apparently for hay fever and asthma in people who have trouble in certain houses but who are free from disturbance in other houses.

INSECTS

Two types of allergy are caused by insects, one by the bite of insects, the other by scales and hairs which are thrown off from insects of the moth and butterfly group. The former can cause violent general reactions, even death, as a result of one or several bites or stings of some particular variety of insect. The latter type (moth and butterfly group) can cause hay fever, asthma, and eczema in certain districts in which insects of this variety abound. This discovery is a recent important advance. The insects commonly responsible for this type of allergy are inconspicuous in color and size. They can be observed above lawns at night during the summer months if lights from an automobile are cast across the lawn. They are found on the screens and

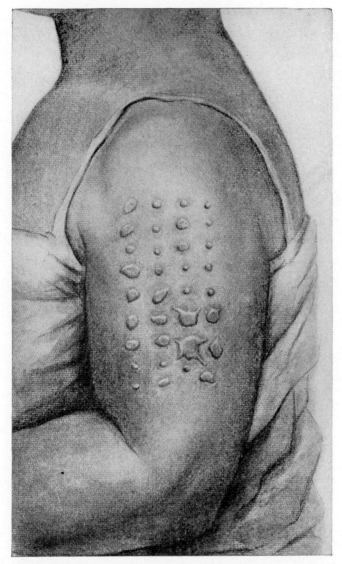

Fig. 59. The large wheals indicate hyper-sensitivity
to ragweed pollen.

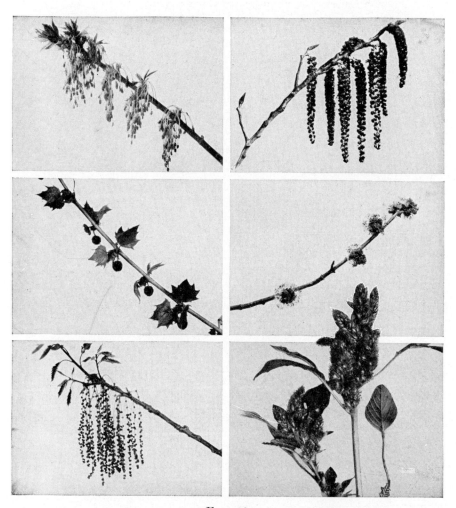

FIG. 60.

Top left: Box elder. Middle left: Sycamore. Bottom left: Oak.

Top right: Cottonwood. Middle
right: Maple. Bottom right: Pigweed.

around lights. Insects of the beetle and cockroach group are apparently unimportant in relationship to allergy,

DUST

Patients can become sensitive to certain specific types of dust accumulating in certain places, especially in the dark corners of certain rooms, in curtains, upholstery, under the beds, and in carpets. This fact has proved most useful in the diagnosis and treatment of asthma, especially of the type called house asthma. The element in dust which is primarily responsible for this sort of illness probably varies. In one case it was proved definitely to be a fungus. One patient who suffered from asthma constantly for eight years was proved sensitive to something which could be extracted from one rug. Her illness dated from the purchase of the rug, and she was cured completely by removal of the rug from the house.

SMOKE

Certain people become sensitive to certain varieties of smoke: wood smoke, coal smoke, tobacco smoke, cigarette smoke or the smoke from burning leaves. This type of sensitiveness can be so specific that a person sensitive to cigarette smoke may tolerate cigar smoke. One patient was so sensitive to cigar smoke that the quantity carried home on the clothes of her husband at odd times would cause her to have asthma. Another patient highly sensitive to wood smoke could not live in houses with open fireplaces even though the fire was not burning. Apparently, enough of the fumes of wood smoke could be retained in the carpets and curtains and upholstery to cause her to have asthma.

DRUG IDIOSYNCRASIES

Individuals of allergic strain frequently become sensitive to one of the drugs such as quinine, aspirin, the iodides, drugs of cocaine series or morphine series. This type of sensitiveness frequently develops to such a degree that one aspirin tablet can cause a desperate illness of several days' to several weeks' duration; in fact, a small quantity of aspirin or cocaine can prove fatal or all but fatal to a highly sensitive case. It is extremely important for people to be acquainted with sensitiveness of this type, since the drugs which are commonly used in the symptomatic treatment of asthma are the ones which tend to sensitize.

ANIMAL PARASITES

Patients occasionally become sensitive to intestinal worms or skin parasites, such as scabies, or to fungi such as trychophyton. Illnesses of this sort may be severe.

BACTERIA

Apparently people can become sensitive to bacterial products and can have allergic symptoms due to absorption of bacterial products.

THERAPEUTIC SERUMS

Some people are naturally sensitive to the serum of one animal or another, especially horse serum. This is important in relationship to administration of antitoxin in treatment of diphtheria or tetanus because if a patient naturally sensitive to serum receives a serum injection he is likely to react with terrific symptoms of asthma, hives, eczema, swelling of the skin, and shock which may terminate fatally within a short period. For this reason, it is important before administering horse serum to inquire for a history of hay fever, asthma, or hives, and in case of a positive history either in patient or family, to avoid the use of serum unless the emergency justifies.

SENSITIVENESS OF ONE INDIVIDUAL TO ANOTHER

This apparently fantastic concept is actually established. One patient may be sensitive to the blood of another patient. In case of blood transfusion, a recipient may be shocked on receiving as little as 20 c.c. of blood from one particular donor. It is rare but well known that babies may be sensitive to the mother's menstrual secretion and can have asthma of severe grade whenever the mother menstruates. One man was sure he was sensitive to his wife, and several Southerners thought they were sensitive to Negroes.

SENSITIVENESS TO HEAT AND EFFORT, COLD, LIGHT, AND SCRATCHES

People may be sensitive to the effect of heat and effort, or to the effect of cold, or to the effect of light, and manifest the same types of illness under the effect of exposure as those which appear in patients sensitive to pollen, foods, or animals. This type of sensitiveness is not identical to allergy, but it is closely related to it.

A patient who is sensitive to heat is almost always sensitive to mental or physical effort; in fact, those sensitive to heat may be made ill with such symptoms as hay fever, asthma, hives, nausea, vomiting, prostration, nervousness, or collapse by the drinking of a hot cup of coffee or by getting up out of a chair quickly, and can be relieved as quickly by the application of ice-cold water to the hands and fore-arms.

Those sensitive to heat instinctively shun activities and situations which expose them to heat or which subject them to the effect of effort which is beyond their tolerance. They seldom realize, however, that they are sensitive to heat. They lead a quiet life and usually give an appearance of laziness. They frequently restrict their activities to small districts or even to a yard, house, or to a room in which they can obtain the condition of quiet and coolness necessary to their feelings of well being. The fact is, however, that they are not lazy. Their physical capacity is incapable of keeping pace with normal desires. Those sensitive to cold seek activity in both their business careers and their games. Possibly many historical characters whose lives have been typified by constant activity and tireless energy owe their motivation to this condition. Such people are happy and comfortable so long as they are active, or hot, and are likely to be ill and incompetent under the influence of cold and enforced quiet. Napoleon may have been cold sensitive. Such an assumption would account for the frequent hot baths and constant activity which typified his life, and also for his gross failures under the effect of cold and quiet.

It is unfortunate if necessity forces a patient who is heat and effort sensitive or cold sensitive to change an environment or occupation which he has instinctively chosen. This occurred in many instances during the war. Many who were thoroughly successful in a chosen vocation proved hopeless failures in the army. Heat sensitive cases, under the effect of drilling in the hot sun, would fall out of line and were frequently falsely accused of willfully shirking duty.

Patients who are sensitive to light frequently have stoppage of the nose and occasionally asthma and also eczema of the exposed parts such as the face, neck, and hands on exposure to sunlight. Exposure of the face to light may cause pain in the eyes, blinding of the eyes, associated with redness and excessive secretion of tears. This condition is often diagnosed "vernal catarrh."

Patients sensitive to mechanical irritation frequently have itching and hives caused by the rubbing of the skin by rough garments or by scratching the skin. The condition may be so extreme as to render a patient miserable for years.

DEFORMITIES CAUSED BY ALLERGY

Allergy has never been looked on as a deforming disease; in fact, has never been looked on as a disease which causes real changes in the tissues. This is true in seasonal cases, because the tissues regain normalcy during the well periods. It is grossly wrong, however, in the case of perennial allergy—that is, allergy which persists throughout the year. Perennial nasal allergy, even though extremely mild in grade, almost always causes nasal polyps which handicap an individual for years, predispose him to colds and sinus infection, and furnish an excuse for one or even ten or fifteen nasal operations which are usually damaging to the patient and do not remove the cause of the illness. The polyps, therefore, even if successfully removed, return and cause more trouble than before. Allergy of the skin can cause organic changes in the skin. Also, allergy of the orbit and bladder can cause organic changes in the tissues and chronic perennial bronchial allergy. Asthma is associated with muscle hypertrophy, swelling, and infiltration of the bronchial tissues with cells which grossly handicap the physician in his efforts to cure the illness.

Chronic allergy in children can cause gross deformity of the face, chest, and spine and stunting of growth. A stooped posture caused by spinal twisting, also pigeon breast and the so-called barrel chest are typical results of neglected asthma in children. If the condition starts during the period of growth, it may be fixed on the patient for life. If asthma is relieved during the period of growth, even for part of the time, at least half of each year, the deformities tend to disappear.

Chronic nasal allergy in children, even though so inconspicuous as not to be noticed by parents or physician, can cause maldevelopment of the nasal sinuses that results in a characteristic facial appearance. A doctor acquainted with the illness can tell at a glance whether or not certain patients have or have not had nasal allergy during their period of growth. The characteristic appearance is a pushed-in appearance on each side of the nose—in other words, a flattening of the face between the cheekbones and nose caused by the fact that the nasal sinuses are too small. This smallness of the sinuses is due to the fact that their openings into the nose have been obstructed during the period of growth by swollen membranes so that their development has been impaired.

Stunting of growth caused by allergy in childhood is common in patients who are afflicted with it perennially in severe grade. It may actually cause them to come in the class of dwarfism. Children of this sort, if relieved of allergy, grow like mushrooms. If the condition persists until the age of growth is completed, the deformity becomes permanent. For this reason, treatment of children with allergy is far more important than treatment of adults with the same illness.

Symptoms of Allergy

GENERAL SYMPTOMS

General symptoms of allergy occur whenever a sensitive patient encounters and absorbs an amount of some substance to which he is sensitive in quantity which is in excess of his tolerance. With the onset of a reaction of this type, a person usually feels a sense of itching followed frequently by redness of the skin, or hives, and frequently by pain in the head and back. This is often associated with attacks of sneezing, coughing, or asthma; also frequently nausea, vomiting, diarrhea, and prostration. The blood pressure usually falls, and the patient's pulse gets rapid or weak. The patient may lose consciousness, get blue and have a convulsion. This condition can be quickly relieved by the prompt use of adrenalin.

EYE SYMPTOMS

Puffiness and itching of the eyelids, slight redness of the lid margins, a tendency to tears and discomfort on exposure of eyes to light are frequent symptoms.

NASAL SYMPTOMS

Hay fever, sneezing, swelling of the membranes of the nose, nasal voice tones, excessive watery or clear mucous secretion, and, in chronic cases, polyps affect the nose.

MOUTH AND THROAT SYMPTOMS

Swelling of the lips and tongue, itching of the roof of the mouth, swelling of the soft palate, hoarseness, and a tendency to choke, are manifestations in the mouth and throat.

LUNG SYMPTOMS

Asthma, chronic cough, spasmodic cough, shortness of breath on exertion, a tendency to wheeze on breathing, and expectoration of clear mucous sputum, are signs of difficulty in the lungs. The difficulty in breathing may reach extreme grades and make it almost impossible for a person to get enough air to sustain life. In this case, the color of the skin is blue.

STOMACH AND INTESTINAL SYMPTOMS

Nausea, vomiting, abdominal pain and diarrhea, sometimes severe, indicate that the condition concerns the stomach and intestinal tract.

SKIN SYMPTOMS

Hives, swelling either general or local, itching of the skin, redness, eczema, increased secretion of moisture and grease, or dryness and scaling are reactions of the skin to sensitivity.

HEADACHE

Headache is a common symptom of allergy. It may be extreme, in fact, may torture a person almost into a state of unconsciousness. Allergic migraine is relatively common. Vaughan and Rowe believe food allergy is a common cause of migraine.

NERVE MANIFESTATIONS

Weakness, prostration, nervousness, trembling, convulsions, transitory paralysis, numbness of the hands or feet, or dizziness, are various grades of reaction of the nervous system.

BLADDER SYMPTOMS

Frequent painful urination, with tenderness and soreness over the bladder, is the response of that organ to allergy.

MISCELLANEOUS SYMPTOMS

There are many other less common or less conspicuous symptoms such as renal colic, disturbance in menstruation, certain types of rheumatism, lowered blood pressure, and changes in the blood.

DIAGNOSIS OF ALLERGY

The story told by the patient with allergy is usually typical. Furthermore, a past and family record usually discloses the fact that the patient or relatives have had typical manifestations of the illness, such as hay fever, asthma, recurring headache, hives, or eczema.

If illnesses of this sort are common in a family, and if an obscure illness in a member of the family does not fit well with known disease patterns, allergy should always be suspected as its cause. In addition, symptoms caused definitely by allergy, if uncomplicated, can almost always be relieved quickly by injection of adrenalin. This serves as a simple and important diagnostic aid.

The discovery of the specific cause of allergy is often difficult. There is nothing in the practice of medicine which taxes the ingenuity, knowledge and experience of a physician as much as studying out an obscure case of allergy. Certain tests of the skin, eye, nose, and diet are useful in unraveling the allergy problem. Skin tests are truly valuable in the diagnosis of reactions caused by pollen, dander, flies, feathers, and molds, but are often hopelessly inadequate and misleading in the working out of food cases. Specific tests with heat, cold, light, and scratches are likely to give accurate information if carried out according to indications given by the history of a case.

Seasonal cases of hay fever, asthma, or eczema of the exposed parts are usually caused by pollen, fungi, or flies, occasionally by animals or fowl, or occasionally, in the case of eczema, by certain oils of pollen or plants, and rather frequently by heat, effort, cold, or light, and sometimes by a combination of two or more of these factors. When symptoms occur the year around, dust, foods, heat, effort, or cold, or some material encountered throughout the year in homes or place of business, must be suspected.

Careful diagnosis of the cause of allergy is essential to success in treatment. The patient, however, should not expect a complete diagnosis on his first or second visit to a physician. After one cause is found, others must be sought in case of recurrence.

Recurrence of an allergic illness after weeks or months of freedom from symptoms has a serious effect on the patient—often one of disappointment, discouragement, or despair. The period of health unfits him for his illness. Forewarned is forearmed. This chance of recurrence is practically sure sooner or later. It is certain to be discouraging unless expected and understood. A person with allergy who considers himself well is almost certain to have recurrence of his illness sooner or later owing to invisible contact with some substance which he thinks he is avoiding, or to contact with an overwhelming dose of some substance with which he has been treated, or owing to contact with some new substance which has not been discovered by the physician.

A man who was sensitive to orris rid himself of a serious chronic illness through complete avoidance of orris, such as he had encountered in toilet articles, tooth pastes, perfumes, soap, and the like. After months of relief, he had a serious recurrence, caused by flavoring materials used in butterscotch pie. Because of freedom from the illness he was unprepared for the recurrence; in fact, had lost his tolerance for illness and was actually despondent to a point of suicide because of the fear that his former troubles had returned.

TREATMENT

There seem to be at least nine different types of allergy each of which needs to be treated according to its special indication. Most important in the treatment of allergy is a physician who understands the illness and who understands the patient.

ALLERGIC SHOCK AND GENERAL ILLNESSES

General illnesses and dangerous illnesses called allergic shock are caused by exposure of a sensitive patient to quantities of an agent which exceed his tolerance. This, and also serum sickness, must be treated quickly and effectively by any physician who is handy. Adrenalin is injected in quantity sufficient to cause slight or marked tremor of the hands but not to the point of causing pounding of the heart, or excessive pallor of the face. If these symptoms appear as a result of overdosage, they can be stopped almost immediately through the use of a tourniquet applied above the site at which the adrenalin was injected. This so reduces the rate of absorption that symptoms of excess usually begin to disappear within thirty seconds. The absorption can be controlled perfectly by the physician since administration can be repeated as often as desired and the drug given in doses of from one to five drops subcutaneously. Then overdose is controlled by the application, release, and reapplication of tourniquets.

In many patients who react to a material substance such as food or antitoxin and who are also sensitive to heat, the effect of adrenalin

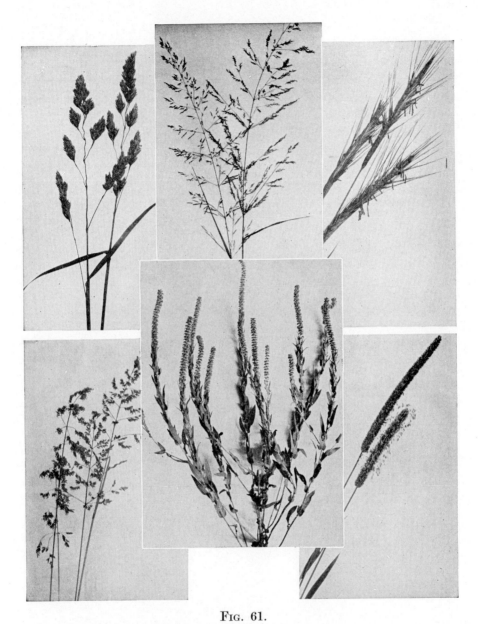

Fig. 61.

Top: Orchard grass.   Redtop.   Rye.
Bottom: Bluegrass.   Southern ragweed.   Timothy.

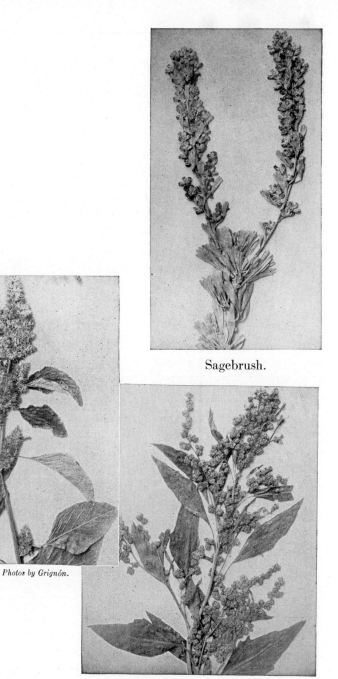

Sagebrush.

Pigweed.

Photos by Grignón.

Lambs'-quarters.

Fig. 62.

can be grossly fortified by rubbing the skin of the chest, arms, and legs with ice, or by the application of cold cloths soaked with ice water to the chest, arms, legs and back, or by a cold bath or cold shower. Cold applications should not be pushed, however, to the point of causing shivering.

In severe general illness caused by food, serum, drugs, or heat and effort, this line of treatment may have to be continued for several days. The mistake usually made is in not using adrenalin adequately or in giving it in gross overdosage after tremor has appeared.

Hay fever, asthma, eczema, headache, or stomach trouble due to sensitivity can be treated along five lines, depending on the causes of the illness.

1. Avoidance or removal of specific cause of illness.
2. Avoidance or removal of contributory causes of illness.
3. Specific treatment with the agents responsible for the illness.
4. So-called nonspecific protein treatment.
5. Symptomatic treatment.

Success in treatment depends primarily on a correct and complete diagnosis. Failure is almost always due to a wrong or incomplete diagnosis.

REMOVAL OF CAUSE

Removal of cause is the simplest of all methods if the cause can be removed. This is easy if the afflicted person is sensitive to a pet, or some uncommon article of food, or a pollen which does not grow in great abundance in his district; or a perfume, plant, insect, fungus, dust, or animal which is found in restricted vicinities. However, removal of cause is difficult or absolutely impossible in the case of high-grade sensitiveness to certain pollens which abound in the air over wide areas and over prolonged periods of time; or to certain articles which are used commonly in toilet articles and cosmetics, as orris; or in the case of sensitiveness to articles used commonly in cookery, as milk, eggs, wheat, cottonseed, flaxseed; or in the case of sensitiveness to ever present heat and effort, cold, scratches, or light. If a person is badly affected by any of these, his only recourse may lie in gaining immunity from the things which make him ill so that he can tolerate them in quantity which he cannot easily avoid. There is no point in giving a person immunity from an agent such as egg, for example, to such an extent that he can eat eggs, nor to pollen to such an extent that he can take railroad trips, auto trips, or go into weed patches during the height of the pollen season. It is better to be satisfied with giving him a lesser grade of tolerance but of such grade that he can enjoy perfect health by partly avoiding the noxious agent and without grossly handicapping him in his normal activities. This is all important to a majority of patients, especially in the case of children who frequently are in constant contact with invisible quantities of the agent responsible for their illness.

POLLEN AVOIDANCE AND POLLEN DISEASE

Pollen symptoms such as hay fever, asthma, and eczema depend largely on the intensity of exposure of the patient to pollen. Symptoms of this sort can be lightened by a knowledge of dates and places where pollen abounds and by knowledge of dates and places where it is scarce during the pollen season.

Weeds, such as ragweed, pollinate during and through a season from about August 1st to frost. They pollinate most profusely from the twenty-fifth of August on, and more profusely still on sunny days. Wind dislodges pollen and carries it for miles, even across a state. Ragweed-sensitive cases have their severest trials on sunny windy days after August 25th, especially, whether or not they are in the immediate vicinity of ragweed patches. Possibly the most intense exposures occur during railroad trips or automobile trips in the country on sunny days. A rain will frequently rid the air of pollen for a few hours or a day or so.

Pollen is heavier than air and sinks rather rapidly if it is not held up by wind. Consequently, still air is inclined to be relatively free of pollen. A person can practically escape from pollen by going into a cave or into a closed cellar or into a house if the windows have been kept closed for a number of hours. Pollen sufferers do better during the pollen season if they keep the windows shut day and night. It is better to keep cool by frequent cold baths or by rubbing the hands and arms with ice, or even by an electric fan. Outside breezes may be laden with pollen and pour it on the afflicted individual through an open window. Patients under treatment with pollen should be especially cautious about exposure to pollen-laden air on days they receive a therapeutic pollen treatment. In this case, they may get a double dose and may hold the innocent physician responsible for an unpleasant result.

SPECIFIC TREATMENT

Specific treatment with the use of infinitesimal, gradually increasing doses of the agents which make the patient ill is the most useful, lasting, and practical means of treatment.

Specific treatment depends primarily on finding the various agents responsible for the illness and then administering them hypodermically or otherwise in doses which do not affect the patient. Then the dose is increased gradually and systematically, preferably also without affecting the person, up to doses which may eventually reach one thousand or ten thousand or more times the original dose. Surprising to relate, this can be done in the case of pollen, animal dander, scales of insects, oils and extracts from certain plants, and extracts from certain foods, without the production of an illness which is noticed in the least by the patient at any time. This, however, depends on knowledge and care for detail on the part of both physician and patient.

In the early part of this line of work certain reactions were experienced by the patient consisting usually of recurrence of the symptoms of which they complained associated often in addition with itching of the skin, hives, asthma, and symptoms resembling hay fever. There was also a feeling of fear. This was due to a too rapid rate of absorption of the material injected. This method of treatment is now perfected through mixing the materials to be used with certain substances which constrict the blood vessels locally and prevent too rapid absorption. The injections can now be given safely and without discomfort or reactions by applying a tourniquet around the arm and injecting the material with vessel-constricting substances on the side of the tourniquet away from the heart. The tourniquet is not released until the vessels have been constricted so that from then on the injected material itself prevents absorption. This gives rise always to a slow rate of absorption of the injected material; in fact, so slow that reactions never occur if the treatment is given correctly and if the patient heeds advice. Following an injection of this sort, the patient should avoid severe exercise in hot weather for the remainder of the day—in other words, should avoid getting hot. He should also carry a tourniquet in his pocket so that in the case of the feeling of something resembling reaction, he can reapply the tourniquet and stop absorption within thirty seconds. The tourniquet need be applied, as a rule, for little more than two or three minutes. This almost always suffices to retard absorption within the limits of tolerance of the patient. It makes treatment safe and free from reaction if both physician and patient understand the requirements for absolute safety of this method.

NONSPECIFIC TREATMENT

Nonspecific protein treatment obtains benefit by raising body temperature from gross subnormalcy toward normal, or actually sometimes to fever. It seems to be of doubtful merit in the treatment of cases sensitive to pollen, dander, feathers, flies, dust, or orris. It may prove useful in the case of sensitiveness to heat and effort. It is most frequently tried in cases of incomplete diagnosis or when it is impossible for the patient to take the specific treatment which he actually needs.

Such remedies as adrenalin, ephedrine, pituitrin, the iodides, and salicylates are used to give relief when the specific cause of illness cannot be found, or during the time when a study and diagnosis of the case is being made.

Unfortunately, people of the sensitive type are inclined to become sensitive to the drugs used. About 10 per cent of asthmatics are highly sensitive to aspirin, so that many may be made desperately ill by as little as one tablet.

Hypnotics such as barbital, luminol, amytal, and ipral, combined with ephedrine, are gaining widespread use at present. This form of treatment is not justifiable except under a physician's guidance. The barbital preparations are potent hypnotics which cannot be used continuously over prolonged periods without ill effect. The barbitals given in adequate dose cause complete anesthesia.

TREATMENT WITH HEAT, COLD, EXERCISE, LIGHT, AND SCRATCHES

In the treatment of any person who is sensitive, among other things, to heat and effort or cold or scratches or sunlight, the condition can be relieved for the moment by an agent the opposite of the one which made the patient ill. Constructive treatment, however, which is necessary for permanent relief, depends on careful graduating doses of the agent which makes the patient sick; in fact, in the case of heat and effort sensitiveness, it is necessary not only to increase the patient's tolerance for heat and effort but actually to build up the wasted muscular tissue through graduated exercise to such an extent that muscle tone constantly generates heat enough to keep him immune from the effect of heat. By persistence in this rather tedious nonin-spirational line of treatment a wasted asthmatic invalid can be built into a healthy strong person who finally craves the things that formerly made him ill.

Results of Therapy

There is nothing in the field of medicine which exceeds in its excellence good treatment in a completely diagnosed case of allergy. The results amount to the transformation of an invalid into a normal human being, or to the transformation of a hideous, eczematous dwarf into a beautiful, normally developed child, or in the transformation of a despicable character into a popular person; in fact, in the minds of some successfully treated patients, the change amounts to a transference from Hades into heaven.

Treatment is especially indicated and especially beneficial in children whose normal development and growth depend on freedom from allergic symptoms. An asthmatic child cannot behave normally, study normally, nor develop normally. His future depends on freedom from allergic symptoms—at least for a larger portion of each year. Here the future of a child frequently depends on the capabilities of his physician in this line, and on the patience, sanity, and coöperation of his parents.

CHAPTER XX

The Internal Glandular System
I. The Glands
WALTER TIMME, M.D.

INTRODUCTION

MEDICAL SCIENCE *is beginning to accumulate more and more information about the glands and the manner in which they and their secretions affect the general condition of the body. When it first began to be realized how important were the functions of such tissues as the thyroid, the hypophysis, the parathyroid, the pancreas, the adrenals and other glandular organs, philosopher physicians began to develop all sorts of queer notions regarding the importance of these tissues to the human body.*

After the first flight of fancy passed, however, research workers in laboratories began to study simple problems and to accumulate real facts of importance in understanding these mysterious glands. For instance, the glands known as the adrenals, which lie just above the kidneys, are sometimes destroyed by serious disease. When this occurs, the person is likely to develop a condition known as Addison's disease, in which there is usually great weakness, dizziness, shortness of breath, loss of weight, soreness of the joints, and gradual breaking down of the human body. Usually the skin becomes pigmented and turns to a sort of bronze color. In the absence of the secretion of the adrenal glands, the person is likely to die.

The hypophysis is a small gland lying near the brain. Its overgrowth may be associated with peculiar changes in the structure of the body. Giantism and dwarfism are not infrequent in relation to changes in this gland. The pancreas secretes the substance that is important in the handling of sugar by the body. Destruction of portions of the cells of the pancreas results in diabetes. The thyroid gland is associated with goiter. Changes in the sex glands result in anomalies being developed which are of great interest. The extracts of these glands seem to have important effects on the body in some cases. Unfortunately, the American market is flooded with preparations of glands and extracts that are worthless.

One of the most remarkable outgrowths of interest in the glands has been the attempt to apply that knowledge to control of the human personality, thus giving both men and women longer life and eternal youth. As will be seen in the article by Dr. Timme, which follows, enough has already been learned to permit an evaluation of the fact, and perhaps to cause the credulous to believe that almost anything is possible. Books have been written to prove that the glands regulate our personality. Charlatans have capitalized public interest by offering youthfulness and longevity.

It is too soon, however, to fly in the face of biologic laws. The human tissues are built for a cycle of seventy years, including twenty years of growth, thirty years of maturity, and twenty years of degeneration and decay. It has not yet been established by any scientific investigation that the administration of glandular extracts seriously modifies this process, and it is safe to say that rejuvenation is not yet even in sight.

Man's search for the elixir of youth is eternal. Since the first announcement by Voronoff and by Steinach that their methods would rejuvenate the elderly, hundreds of experiments have been made to control their claims, but none of these experiments has confirmed their notions. Recently a delegation from the British Ministry of Agriculture visited Algiers to study the Voronoff technic of gland grafting as done on animals. Their report did not endorse his method. Furthermore, the commission did not consider the evidence sufficient to warrant the claims.

It is interesting to have the views of the pathologist Warthin on this subject. An investigation of human bodies postmortem indicates that few men over fifty-five years of age have the power of reproduction, and that certainly the stories of reproductive ability much later in life are to be viewed with skepticism. It is interesting to have the view of the distinguished pathologist as to the possibilities of rejuvenation. He says:

"What philosophy then may we draw from this? Is old age inevitable? Yes, escape from it is possible only for those who meet a premature pathologic death.

"For those who live to their biologic limit, age cannot be escaped Nor can it be deferred. Nor is rejuvenescence possible. The deferring of old age, the rejuvenating of the senescent individual is but idle and foolish talk, and we have had much of this in the last decade.

"What modern medicine has accomplished along the lines of hygiene and the prevention of disease has been only to increase the number of human individuals, both the fit and unfit—unfortunately too many of the latter kind—who come to maturity and to the period of senescence.

"More individuals will achieve their biologic life limit; and this means what?—ultimately a much greater increase in the number of senile, more or less useless, human beings in the age decades of the eighties and the nineties.

"There will be some increase in the number who will reach the age of one hundred years or even pass it, due to their own family inheritance, but this number will not be greatly increased in the present period of evolution."

M. F.

THE INTERNAL GLANDULAR SYSTEM or glands of internal secretion include a number of organs specially adapted for the production of complex substances which have controlling influences on all the other tissues and organs of the body. These influences modify the speed, the intensity, the regularity, and the efficiency of the activities of the organs and in some instances seem even to initiate vital processes such as menstruation and childbirth. The number of glands in the body and their relative size apparently vary in different genera and species. The term "internal glandular system" was first "glands of internal secretion," indicating those glands that gave their product or "secretion" directly to the blood as contrasted with those of "external secretion," which delivered their product through a duct or tube to the tissue where it was needed. The glands of external secretion originally included the liver, the pancreas, the salivary glands, and the sex organs in part. Recently, however, it has been found that some of these glands, besides the material furnished through their ducts, also manufacture

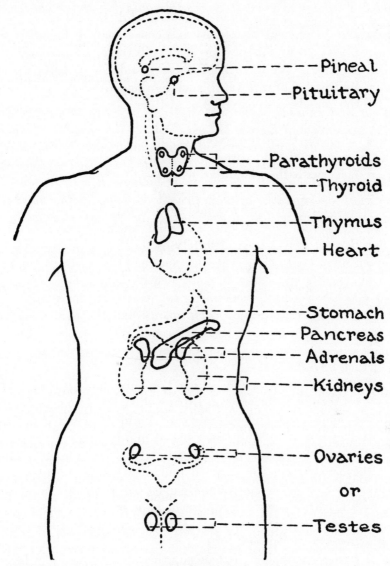

Pineal
Pituitary

Parathyroids
Thyroid
Thymus
Heart

Stomach
Pancreas
Adrenals
Kidneys

Ovaries
or
Testes

Fig. 63. Location of various important glands in the human body.

other chemical substances delivered directly to the circulating blood or lymph. These substances have all the properties of internal glandular biochemical products; thus these organs are of dual nature.

The glands at present of interest and considered in this series are: thymus, pineal, thyroid, parathyroid, pituitary, suprarenal, and gonads (genitals). While each of these glandular structures seems superficially to be a unit, several, such as the pituitary, the suprarenals, and the gonads, are composed of distinct parts, each of which has properties entirely different from those of other parts of the same gland. This makes the investigation of the glandular properties most difficult and intricate. Moreover, practically all laboratory investigations are made with the glandular secretion of animals—frogs, mice, rats, rabbits, cats, dogs, and all types of cattle. Seldom indeed are human glandular secretions available for study. While the absolute chemical identity of the various better known secretions of animals and man has not as yet been definitely established, the analogies and correspondences are so close that they may be assumed to be identical.

The human life span may be conveniently divided into three well-defined epochs: the first from birth to maturity; the second from maturity through the acme of performance and the prime; and the third from the end of our greatest performances through senescence to death. As each of these epochs has a different goal, so must the equipment of each be different.

The first is the time during which the individual grows and develops—it is the time of accretion. During this period he must acquire the stature and power and mentality that will fit him for his life's work in this world of difficulty and enable him to procreate his kind. During the second epoch he must use all his abilities to maintain himself in the competition for survival and, if possible, to advance in every way the cause of civilization. He must also procreate his species. Then, with his life's work accomplished, he is of little further use in Nature's scheme, and gradually goes through his third and last epoch through senescence to his end.

The internal glandular mechanism, therefore, governing largely growth and development, must vary in its activity during those epochs, for in each one it has different ends to subserve. In the first epoch, the two glandular elements, the thymus gland and the pineal gland, are evidently of great importance, for both rise and fall during the first period. By the end of this interval, both have gone through their period of activity and are entirely, or almost, quiescent. With this inactivity they normally undergo involution and practically disappear. The other glands gradually acquire more and more importance and are at the acme of their usefulness during the second period.

THYMUS GLAND

The thymus gland lies in the upper part of the chest between the lungs and above the heart, and in front of the trachea. In this situation it comes in contact with some of the large blood vessels and some important nerves. Should it enlarge greatly, it might exert pressure on these structures, causing difficulty in breathing and circulation. Indeed, it has been thought that some sudden deaths in children are produced by this pressure. Frequently, in deep breathing, all of these structures are caught in the funnel of the neck and chest, then spasms of coughing with gasping and blueness of the face follow. When such symptoms occur an immediate examination by a physician is advised.

There is no agreement as to the effects of the thymus upon the body. Some German investigators found that dogs from which the thymus gland was removed developed a bony skeleton that was deformed, small, and distorted. Their view that the thymus gland produced normal skeletal growth and helped to prevent rickets was held for some time. When thymus gland was fed to tadpoles they increased to an enormous size but did not develop into frogs. They grew but *did not develop* into frogs, i.e., did not become differentiated. Recent experiments on dogs in this country produced contrary evidence. Following removal of the thymus the bony structure was not affected. Perhaps other glands, such as the suprarenal glands, were modified in their activity by the removal so that the thymus gland was not necessary to life. The American workers suggested that the reason for the deformed dogs in the earlier experiments was the fact that they were kept in cages too small for them! However, it has been suggested that particles of thymus gland might have remained attached to other tissue in the chest after seemingly complete removal of the gland. Such remains may grow rapidly, so that enough tissue may be produced to carry on. A different series of trials with birds gave most interesting results. When the thymus glands of fowls were removed, the eggs that were laid were not protected by a shell, but after feeding these same birds with thymus gland the shell again was produced. Even this seemingly conclusive work is now criticized. This discussion may serve to indicate the difficulties and complexities which beset the workers in this field. At present the function of the thymus gland seems to be that it influences the growth of the skeleton; that it partially controls calcium metabolism, and that it holds in abeyance differentiation of development, so that the gonads—the sex glands—remain immature during its activity. In the actual examination of children who have large thymus glands, or in whom the activity of the gland persists after the age of puberty should have been reached, interesting conditions are often seen. These individuals grow large, but disproportionately, usually. The torso is too small for the legs, the arms too long for the body. Furthermore, all the joints are so loosely bound together that there is undue freedom of motion. The arms and legs are like flails. The various joints are easily dislocated, so that the jaw snaps out of place on opening the mouth too wide, or the shoulder or hip joints are similarly "thrown out," and fingers likewise "double-jointed." There is undue freedom of motion in the so-called fixed joints, so that the spinal column and the pelvic bones move against each other, giving rise at times to great pain and distress in the lower back—producing long-standing backache. The bones of the arch of the foot also are so lightly bound together that the arch cannot maintain itself and becomes flat. All other structures of the body seemingly also are victims of the irregular development in these cases, and so definite are the disturbances that a technical medical term has been used to designate them. This term was *status-thymico-lymphaticus*, indicating that the thymus gland and other lymphatic glands such as the tonsils, or the spleen, were enlarged. Recently, because it was found that many more important structures than these were too small to carry out their functions properly, a new name was applied to the condition, namely, "status hypoplasticus," meaning that the condition was one of underdevelopment generally. This name much more properly carries out the significance of the situation. The structures that are found to be too small and inadequate are particularly the heart and blood vessels, the pituitary gland, the gonads or sex glands, the suprarenal glands, and often the thyroid gland also. The blood characteristics are also different from the normally developed type. While there is not necessarily any anemia, yet the white blood cells are usually increased in number and the proportions of the various types of white cell different. The clotting time of the blood is prolonged. The amount of sugar in the blood is lessened, the blood pressure usually low, and the tendency to acidosis is marked. The features also are noticeable. Because of the slow development, youthful characteristics are maintained too long. The skin is smooth and soft and of velvety texture—"peaches and cream." The hair is soft and silky, and in the male no mustache or beard hair appears until quite late. The teeth are of a bluish white color and quite regular except for the central incisors of the upper jaw, which are unduly large and prominent. The canines, which normally are somewhat pigmented and have a sharp tearing fang, are not so in these cases and instead of a fang have a cutting edge such as the incisors. One other curious anomaly is frequently seen: at the central line of the roof of the mouth, instead of a smooth junction of the two lateral halves, there is seen a protuberance, sometimes as large as an olive. This is called the *torus palatinus* because of its similarity to a bulging muscle mass; it is produced by a fibrous cartilaginous junction of the bones rather than by a real bony union.

It seems surprising that all these conditions should be dependent on the improper functioning of one gland. As a result of this seeming imbalance of cause and effect, it has been suggested that the enlarged and overactive thymus gland is only a part of the whole picture of status hypoplasticus, and not the cause of all of its manifestations.

What happens to these poorly equipped individuals? Can they carry on? Throughout our lives there is a natural force or tendency towards "self-repair." Injuries, diseases, disabilities almost invariably call forth this reparative force. In these cases, nature helps by causing an enlargement and overactivity of those structures that would help in the emergency. Thus, because of the low blood sugar and the low blood pressure, overactivity of the suprarenal glands and the pituitary help out, because these glands increase both of these factors. Smallness of the genitals is also overcome by certain parts of the pituitary gland, as will be discussed later on. Practically all of the disabilities can be eventually overcome by the requisite compensatory adjustments. These adjustments take time. Therefore the hypoplasic individual who compensates for his deficiencies completely, arrives at a normal level to begin his second period of life quite a few years later than normally. Nevertheless, even though it takes longer, he is quite as good in all respects when he does arrive. In fact, some brilliant men and women belong to this group.

There are many individuals of this group, however, that do not thoroughly compensate. For them life is a continuous struggle against undue fatigue, lack of initiative and concentration, and lack of courage. They are easily led by stronger minds and bodies, and often take to artificial means for help. Many become addicts to alcohol and drugs and generally go the paths of least resistance.

PINEAL GLAND

The activity of the pineal gland apparently ceases at maturity. For long its character as a gland was disputed, for no evident change took place in animals treated with it. However, recently it has been found microscopically to consist of actual glandular secreting cells. Certain experiments and observations seem to indicate that it does have an influence on the body. It is extremely small—perhaps the size of a pea flattened out. It is located in the central part of the brain at the entrance of an important canal for the circulation of the spinal fluid— hence, when it is enlarged from any cause, it tends to close up this canal, leading to high pressure in the skull with severe and dangerous symptoms. Right next to it is found a structure which was originally the stem of the amphibian third eye. For this reason the gland was formerly supposed to represent this archaic eye. It is difficult to remove the pineal gland without causing death; therefore experimental work is meager. Feeding experiments have been interesting. When small particles of the gland are fed to tadpoles these lose their dark olive color and become almost translucent. Feeding guinea pigs, mice and rats with glandular substance produces rather contradictory results. Generally, the animals thus fed grow larger and stronger muscularly, with some lack of growth and development of the genitals. When guinea pigs had the pineal destroyed experimentally, the genitals of the animals thus operated on grew more rapidly and became larger than those of animals which had not had the pineal gland destroyed. It has also been found that when the pineal gland begins to deteriorate it becomes the repository of calcium salts. An X-ray picture of the skull then shows a shadow at the site of the gland. This shadow usually appears normally in the third decade of life. When it appears early, before the age of twenty years, there are usually symptoms associated with such deterioration. An unusually large genital system but a weak musculature frequently is then encountered. Indeed, many cases of great and undue muscular fatigue in adolescence have such a pineal shadow. A certain proportion of cases of that devastating disease—progressive muscular atrophy—show such a pineal shadow. The pineal gland is apparently a gland of internal secretion, and possibly is concerned with proper muscular development. It evidently plays a rôle in keeping the genital system from becoming developed too soon in life before the other factors of development are ready for it. It has been experimentally fed to mentally deficient children but without any success.

THYROID GLAND[1]

This exceedingly important organ is normally situated in the neck on either side of the windpipe and larynx. An isthmus of glandular tissue connects the sides or lobes. Occasionally the gland extends downwards into the upper chest in direct contact with the thymus, and at times is found entirely in this region. Then it is said to be a thoracic or sub-sternal thyroid because it lies under the breastbone. The importance of this gland to the normal activity of the entire organism can hardly be exaggerated. When it is absent or almost so, congenitally, then the entire development of the individual suffers. Every organ and tissue becomes underactive from the brain to the skin. The beings thus afflicted are occasionally met with in various parts of the world especially in southeastern Europe and occasionally sporadically in other parts of the world. They are the curious old-young type of dwarf known as "cretins." Some remain as small as three feet in height. They have a sallow leathery-colored skin, little or no body hair, high-pitched voice, and small genitalia. If in the course of life of normal individuals, the thyroid gland, through disease or accident, becomes destroyed, then similar disturbances occur, though not so profound. The individual becomes sluggish, he loses hair, grows obese, and cannot cope with his problems. This condition is known as myxoedema. In the first years of thyroid operation for goiter—especially in Switzerland—the removal of the entire gland gave rise to these symptoms. It was some time before this was recognized. Soon thereafter, however, surgeons would leave intact part of the thyroid in their operation, and then this condition of myxoedema did not occur, for even small, active portions of the gland were sufficient to overcome it. In the meanwhile an English physician who had one of these cases of myxoedema under his care conceived the idea of feeding thyroid gland to her to overcome the difficulty. He succeeded brilliantly. She lived

[1]See also article by Dr. O. P. Kimball.

for many years in comparative health and comfort under this treatment, and died only recently at an old age. This was actually the beginning of modern internal glandular therapy. What actually is the basis of these disturbances? Now it is known that the thyroid gland produces a substance or substances that are necessary for the proper activity of every cell of every organ and tissue of the body. Under this influence the cell can utilize the oxygen that is brought to it by the blood to burn up its foodstuffs and get rid of the products of this combustion. If therefore the thyroid substance is deficient, then the oxidation in the cell is diminished, and the partially burnt up material is largely retained. It is much like a furnace to which insufficient air is supplied—there is less consumption of coal, and the partially converted fuel clogs up the little draught there is. Opening the damper increases the draft of air with its oxygen, and the coal burns rapidly with production of much heat and almost complete combustion. Similarly, the thyroid acts to increase the combustion in each cell to a state at which the ash is made easy for removal by the emunctories: the bowels, the kidneys, and the lungs; and so releases the cell for further activity. When the thyroid is deficient, then this chain is weakened—everything slows down; the body temperature is diminished, pulse and heart are slowed, mind and body become sluggish, and as the products of partial combustion cannot be removed, weight is increased.

On the contrary, an overactive thyroid produces increase in body temperature, increased pulse and heart action, increased body and mental activity, and a decrease in weight. It might be thought in this age of speed and action that this latter state is highly desirable, but remember that it is procured at a tremendous cost! The continuous overactivity of the heart alone gradually produces a weakened heart muscle from which, after due lapse of time, there is no escape, and the individual succumbs. An active principle of the thyroid gland known as thyroxin, possibly containing the entire active ingredients of the gland, was discovered a decade or so ago and since then has been produced synthetically—a real and brilliant triumph for the biochemical laboratory in its attack upon the problems of the internal glandular system.

In the various studies upon thyroid activity, it has invariably been found that one ingredient is absolutely indispensable to its normal function, and that is iodine. When this is lacking, or too minute in amount, thyroid activity lags. This is extremely interesting and has exceedingly great economic and practical import, for there are many regions on this earth that lack this element. Not only certain parts of Switzerland and southeastern Europe are thus afflicted, but in our own country there is a zone with ramifications extending from the Berkshires in the East, through Central New York, the Ohio Valley, the Great Lakes, thence through Wisconsin, Minnesota, and the Western states clear through to the Pacific, in which iodine is quite deficient. In these regions, because of this deficiency, many thyroid disturbances and their concomitant and after effects are found. These vary enormously in their symptoms. Because of the lack of iodine the otherwise normal thyroid secretion is bound up in the thyroid gland combined in various chemical ways. This is seen as an enlargement of the thyroid known generally as goiter. The individuals thus affected show many signs of thyroid underactivity, notably gain in weight, sluggishness in all life's activities, and frequently in mental disturbances. When it was found that lack of iodine underlay this condition, its administration was promptly advised and in some regions even compulsorily ordered. The change was almost immediately noticed. The so-called simple goiters became fewer and fewer, and all the other symptoms showed amelioration. A personal survey of these goiters in an affected city over ten years ago and again two years ago indicated the astonishing result that they had diminished almost 80 per cent—all due to the iodine administration. However, a warning ought to be issued in the matter of wholesale iodine treatment. A few individuals have a form of goiter—not of the simple variety—that does not adequately respond to iodine, but curiously enough increases activity under its use to toxic levels; at times these goiters are latent and not recognized. Iodine constantly administered in these cases produces such overactivity as to be harmful to the point at which surgical intervention is the only remedy. People living in the goiter zone should always have a professional opinion as to whether constant iodine usage, either through iodized salt or through water from a reservoir to which iodine is added, is advisable.

Goiter means simply a swelling of the thyroid gland. This swelling may mean any one of a number of things. It may signify an overactive gland, or an underactive gland, or a gland in which one or more tumors exist with a toxic glandular secretion, or a combination of these. Each type needs careful expert examination before a diagnosis can be made, and no treatment ought to be inaugurated until such a diagnosis has been established. Recently there has been devised a method for the determination of an individual's thyroid activity on the basis of his oxygen consumption in relation to height, weight, age, and other factors entering the computation. Any rate between minus 10 per cent and plus 10 per cent of an established base is regarded as within normal variation. This test is the now well-known basal metabolism determination, and is fairly reliable.

Thyroid activity varies in the same person during each day, and seasonally also. At menstrual periods there are wide variations, and at the menopause likewise. These variations account for many of the changes of temperament seen at these critical times. During the last epoch of life, the thyroid gland undergoes changes which gradually diminish its activity.

Just as all other tissues and organs of the body are dependent on thyroid action, so do the other glands of internal secretion depend on it largely for their own normal activity. Some of the interrelationships between the various glands might be indicated here by saying that when the thyroid gland becomes underactive, parts of the pituitary gland enlarge, the suprarenal cortex enlarges, the thymus gland also enlarges. The converse is also true to an extent. Many compensations are possible—as is true in all living structures—for the defections of part of the mechanism, by overactivity of other parts.

PARATHYROID GLANDS

These are small nodules situated within the lobes of the thyroid gland in two pairs of two nodules each. At first they were neglected in operations for removal of the thyroid gland, and were also removed with the whole glandular mass. Later it was found that when these small masses were taken away, the aftermath of the operation included violent spasmodic attacks of the muscles of the body, known as tetany. These attacks did not occur when the parathyroids were allowed to remain, or if the parathyroids were removed and a calcium solution introduced into the circulating blood. Investigation further has shown that deprivation of calcium from the food of animals caused in them similar attacks of tetany. Gradually it became known that the parathyroid glands and calcium utilization by the body were closely linked. This discovery stimulated intensive research into the effects of calcium on the organism. Now it is known that a diminution of the amount of calcium circulating in the blood gives rise to symptoms dependent on increased irritability of the muscular and nervous apparatus of the individual. If this diminution reaches certain low levels, then tetany results. Even before such low levels are reached, an increased muscle and nerve irritability make themselves felt. The individual becomes tense, has no repose, cannot relax, sleeps poorly, and is overirritable at the slightest pretext. In his sudden accessions of anger he does and says things for which he is hardly accountable. Actually they emanate from him too fast for judgment to enter and control his responses. Many cases of incorrigibility in children and assaultive acts in adults may belong in this group. Parathyroid gland, because it increases the mobilization and utilization of calcium, modifies these conditions rapidly. In recent years the active principle of the parathyroids has been isolated and is now available for prescription by physicians under various trade names. An important consideration in its use is the fact that parathyroid administration gets its calcium for use from the nearest available source, if not sufficient calcium is available in the food of the individual. The calcium of the bones of the skeleton is pulled into the blood—a possible danger.

At times the parathyroids will be so overactive, or treatment with parathyroid gland so intensive, that too much calcium will be found in the blood. This then becomes a source of much disturbance to many organs such as the kidneys—and becomes a further danger. Any artificial attempt on our part to correct body ills must always be attended by admonitions not to cause disturbance to organs that previously were normal.

PITUITARY GLAND

In recent years the pituitary gland has awakened probably the most interest. The biochemical laboratories throughout the world are at present engaged in separating the many principles produced by this glandular element from one another and in clarifying the situation from the chaos heretofore prevalent.

The pituitary gland occupies a unique situation and is probably the best protected tissue in the body. It is enclosed almost completely in a bony capsule within the skull, at its base, and so actually is in a skull within a skull. The bony cavity enclosing the pituitary gland is known as the *sella turcica* from its resemblance to a Turkish saddle. It has the most remarkable blood circulatory arrangement about it that is found in the body. Short of death, nothing can deprive it of its blood supply. It is about the size of a hazel nut and consists of two sections, or lobes, the anterior and the posterior, between which are found a few layers of cells called the intermediate portions of the gland. These three parts have entirely distinct functions and possibly give their secretions to the body through different channels. The posterior lobe communicates with one of the large cavities of the brain directly through a tubular canal, and this is one of the channels for the dissemination of some of the secretions. Other methods, particularly for the anterior lobe, are by means of the blood vessels directly and the lymph channels, to say nothing of direct diffusion through brain tissue at the base. What particularly interests us here is the effect on the body of the secretions of these various parts. The following scheme, which is by no means complete and about which opinion is divided, represents these various effects.

Anterior lobe:
1. Controls growth of the skeleton and of particular organs and tissues.
2. Controls the development of the sex glands and is responsible for maturity.
3. Controls periodicity of menstruation, and initiates the bleeding.
4. Has compensatory effect on the thyroid gland.
5. Controls the specific energy in the body produced by foods.
6. Assists in the proper utilization of nitrogenous compounds.
7. Assists in the utilization of fats and carbohydrates.

Intermediate part:
Controls the water exchange of the body: i.e., the relation of intake to output.

Posterior lobe:
1. Controls contractions of uterus.
2. Assists in blood-pressure control.
3. Controls contraction of smooth muscle fibers.
4. Assists in control of carbohydrate metabolism.
5. Partly controls water exchange.

There is no doubt that a specific growth factor is produced by the anterior lobe of the pituitary. In early life, that is, before the long bones have reached their fullest possibility of length, this factor is busy. If now it is increased artificially by injecting into the body a solution containing the growth factor derived from the anterior lobe of the pituitary of animals, the growth of the animal or human being thus injected with material is excessively increased. If the injections are long continued, giantism may be produced. This means excessive height, though proportionate, and includes all tissues and organs as well as the skeleton—all are increased in size. When, however, these injections of the anterior lobe are given *after* the long bones have reached their full extent of growth, then, instead of further length, breadth and grotesqueness of form are produced in the skeleton. The face grows broad, the nose broad and flat, the chin broad and pronouncedly forward, the lower jaw protrudes, the spinal column curves on itself to produce a hunchback appearance, the hands and feet grow broad and clumsy and spatulate. The appearance is known as *acromegaly*. Even without these artificial injections, there occur at times enlargement and overactivity of these cells of the anterior lobe that produce the growth hormone, and acromegaly is the result. Because such growth is usually, though not always, of the tumor variety, the signs of a tumor in the skull accompany the acromegaly. With this increase in the size of the anterior lobe, the sella turcica enlarges materially—a fact which may be substantiated by X-ray examination of the skull.

Another important principle of the anterior lobe is the sex hormone. This stimulates the growth of the genitals and brings on maturity and menstruation. When, because of pregnancy, menstruation ceases, the hormone is not apparently utilized and hence finds its way into the urine. This fact forms the basis for the most recent and certain test for early pregnancy. A few weeks after the onset of pregnancy, the urine of the patient is injected into immature mice or rabbits; and within two to three days these animals develop maturity of their ovaries with the bleeding attendant upon such maturity. Nonpregnant urine does not cause this result. The test is accurate in about 98 to 99 per cent of cases. This is a brilliant example of the application of endocrine (internal glandular) knowledge to vital function.

The intermediate portion of the pituitary gland produces a substance which causes normal relationship between the fluids taken into the body and those excreted. Its disturbance may bring on the disease known as *diabetes insipidus*, in which huge quantities of water are daily excreted. This symptom may be at once ameliorated by injections of one of the posterior lobe secretions known as pituitrin.

The posterior lobe of the pituitary gland produces various active principles. There is some discussion as to whether these substances are actually produced in this lobe or are merely stored there, having been formed previously in the other parts of the gland. At any rate, the substance known as pituitrin has been derived from the posterior lobe and seems to represent some, if not all, of the active principles. It produces increase in smooth muscle fiber contraction and hence increase in blood pressure; contraction of the uterus; diminution of urine output at first, followed by increase; stimulation of motion of the bowels, and increase of blood sugar. Many of these conditions are profoundly wanting in shock of all kinds; hence pituitrin is an excellent remedy in such states. Recently it was found that pituitrin consists of two quite different substances, which can be separated from it. One, known as pitocin or oxytocin, is the part that produces uterine contractions and no rise in blood pressure; whereas the other, known as pitressin or vasopressin, has the blood-raising principle without the uterine one.

Some general statements may be made regarding the gland as a whole in its effects on the body. When it is underactive, the patient becomes slow and sluggish, both mentally and physically; fat deposits in various parts of the body; he falls asleep readily—even during the daytime. If this occurs during developmental life, then mental development is retarded, concentration becomes difficult, the sex glands remain small, and maturity is delayed; there is lack of initiative and inability to stick to a task or problem, and a lack of courage in meeting difficulties. When this condition is quite severe, including especially the fat deposits and the small genitals, the condition is known as the *adiposo-genital dystrophy* of Froehlich. On the contrary, when the gland is overactive, all mental and physical powers seem to be enhanced, although at a cost of a rise of blood pressure and early fatigue.

In cases of status hypoplasticus (see under Thymus Gland, p. 535) an overactive pituitary gland may bring about restoration towards normality by increasing the blood sugar, the blood pressure, and resistance generally. This means that the gland gets larger to perform this extra work. But, as the gland is encased in a bony capsule, the enlargement is sometimes accompanied by pressure against this, producing pain—headache—*within the skull*. Such a headache really represents a curative process, for if the gland continues to exert this pressure, the bony capsule gradually enlarges until it is big enough to include the gland at all times without undue pressure—when the headaches spontaneously cease—although this may take many years. These attacks of headache come on from any cause producing fatigue: worry, chagrin, too great mental effort and concentration, menstruation, fasting, or going even a few hours too long without food; all of these states call out the best efforts of the pituitary gland, with resulting enlargement and pressure. The headaches have many of the symptoms of the so-called migraine. Oftentimes the eyesight is involved as well, because the pituitary gland comes into contact with the nerves controlling motion of the eyeball and of vision itself. There are many conditions that have balked medical science in the past that now are becoming known to be caused by disturbances in the pituitary gland.

THE SUPRARENAL GLANDS

These are two in number. Situated on either side of the back of the abdominal cavity above the kidneys, each gland consists of two parts, the medulla or interior portion, and the cortex or the capsular outer part. These are apparently entirely different in their function. Indeed, in some of the fishes, the cortical portion is entirely distinct from the medulla, and the cortical parts of both glands are united by an isthmus across the spinal column—this distinct unity being called the inter-renal gland. The medulla of each gland forms the smaller part by far, being only about one eighth of the bulk of the entire gland. This medulla is composed of cells that are much like the nerve cells of the sympathetic nervous system and produces a substance which is known as adrenalin, which has a special effect upon the sympathetic nervous system. This adrenalin was the first of the active products of the internal glandular system to be isolated. It causes stimulation and contraction of the smooth muscle fibers of the various organs and by this means diminishes or even closes temporarily the caliber of the blood vessels. This produces diminution or even cessation of hemorrhage from wounds, especially from those of the mucous membranes of the mouth and nose—if adrenalin is applied directly to the spot. Indeed almost bloodless operations can be performed if adrenalin is applied before the operation takes place, for the blood vessels close, and the tissue is seen to blanch under its use. In asthma, with the swelling and congestion of the mucous membranes of the bronchial tubes, the application of adrenalin through spraying directly, or even if given hypodermically, brings almost immediate relief, because of its blanching effect upon the mucous membranes due to contraction of the blood vessels. Here again it must be remembered that it has effects also which may be dangerous. Because it causes contraction of the walls of the blood vessels, it produces an increase in blood pressure. And this increase in blood pressure in some cases can work much harm—either in overloading a diseased heart or in causing actual rupture of an artery. Sometimes in cases of extreme cardiac weakness after the heart has actually stopped beating, an injection of adrenalin directly into the cardiac muscle has resuscitated the heart and prevented death—due to stimulation of the heart muscle fibers and nerve centers. Adrenalin produces by its stimulation of the sympathetic nerve fibers to the liver a release of the sugar contained therein for circulation in the blood and thus produces increase in muscular energy. This makes it of great importance in the treatment of shock. The amount of adrenalin in normal blood is only one part in several millions; an estimate of its potency may be thus realized.

The cortex of the suprarenal glands has thus far eluded all attempts to determine its importance in the life of the individual. Its destruction causes death, but why is unknown. Recently several independent investigators have isolated from the cortex an active principle which prevents death when the cortex is either destroyed experimentally or so diseased that it cannot carry on. The condition which is produced by a diseased cortex is called Addison's disease. In Addison's disease the vital functions are gradually so lowered that death finally results. In the course of this disease there is progressive bronzing of the skin and mucous membranes, among other symptoms. This discoloration is probably due to the release of the pigment from a certain zone of the suprarenal glands which contains it. Until the recent isolation of the cortical hormone, death was the certain outcome of Addison's disease. Now, however, it is possible to maintain these patients in moderate health by the use of this hormone, given, however, continuously. There is one objection to its use: it is exceedingly expensive and can be furnished only in small amounts. In the future, however, it may become possible to produce it synthetically, as has been done in the case of both adrenalin and thyroxin.

Addison's Disease

Addison's disease is a condition affecting the adrenal glands, two small bodies which lie just above the kidneys. As a result of the breaking down or degeneration of these glands, the secretion of the glandular structures is not provided to the body. One of the most prominent symptoms of the disease is a gradual bronzing of the skin, but there are cases in which the characteristic signs and symptoms are not easily apparent and which represent lessened function of the gland rather than complete loss of action.

The most common cause is tuberculous infection of the glands, usually secondary to tuberculosis elsewhere in the body. However, there are other cases, in which cancer may destroy the tissue, and still others, in which the glands are not found grossly affected, yet the function apparently is absent. There seem to be cases in which the loss of function of the gland results from interference with its nerve supply.

The great weakness of the person affected is the most serious symptom. People who have this disease are always tired; the muscles become quickly exhausted. Indeed, the patients become so weak they are even too tired to eat. Naturally, disturbances of the intestinal tract are pronounced because the bowel muscles do not act well; patients lose their appetites and have both constipation and diarrhea. Because they cannot take food and digest it properly, they become greatly emaciated.

Another prominent feature is the weakness of the circulation of the blood. The blood pressure falls to less than half of what it usually is, and people tend to faint or become unconscious because of lack of blood supply to the brain. When anybody is so extremely exhausted, as is apparently the case in this disease, there are associated disturbances of vision and of all of the special senses.

Previous to the last ten years, cases of Addison's disease were invariably fatal; indeed, recovery from a fully developed case was unheard of. However, the advance of modern science and recognition of cases in their early stages have brought about a change, so that modern medicine permits prolongation of life, even if not a cure.

More than seventy-five years ago, the English physician Addison described the disease which bears his name as a clinical entity. Shortly thereafter the French investigator Brown-Sequard proved that re-

moval of suprarenal glands, situated near the kidneys, was incompatible with life. Some thirty-five years ago, British physiologists found within those glands a substance which was associated with marked blood-pressure raising effects. This substance was later isolated and is now commonly known as epenephrine or adrenalin. Promptly it was shown, however, that this was not the indispensable substance in the suprarenal glands. Large doses failed to prevent the development of Addison's disease.

[Within recent years evidence accumulated in various laboratories led to the development of what is known now to be the active substance of the cortex of the suprarenal gland, a substance, therefore, called cortin. The use of this substance in cases of Addison's disease has, it is reported, prevented the development of the disease and maintained life. Since the cost of this substance was considerable, efforts were continued in the laboratories toward developing a chemically pure substance which would be identical. In 1938 such a chemical substance was isolated and applied in the treatment of insufficiency of the adrenal glands. The substance is called desoxicortico sterone and has already been widely used in the treatment of Addison's disease.

When this substance is injected into the human body, the blood pressure values are elevated, which symptom has given some concern to those who have used the remedy. Most of the patients who had weakness, nausea, vomiting, loss of appetite and loss of weight showed much improvement following the use of this new chemical substance. The chief value of the product when injected into the body is its ability to conserve sodium and water in the body and to cause the excretion from the body of the element called potassium.

The extensive studies that have been made seem to indicate also that while it can largely replace certain functions of the adrenal gland, this substance is not a complete substitute for the action of the normal cortex of the adrenal gland. It is not, therefore, the true hormone or glandular principle of the adrenal cortex but only one of the active substances produced by that gland.

The giving of a remedy of such powers is difficult because the physician who is using the remedy must watch constantly the amounts of sodium and potassium in the diet. Unless he does relate the giving of the glandular product to the sodium and potassium, the patient may develop accumulation of fluid in the body and high blood pressure.

The use of the newer preparations will keep most patients in at

least a subnormal state of health for a long period of time and will
postpone death in practically all patients. Actually the temporary use
of this substance permits a recovery of the function of the adrenal
gland and thus what might be called a cure of the patient.

—M. F.]

The suprarenal cortex has some interesting interglandular relationships. Together with the posterior lobe of the pituitary and high fat ingestion, considerable blood-pressure rise takes place. Underactivity of the cortex is conducive to overactivity of the thyroid. It has even been shown experimentally that a marked disturbance of the cortex can produce goiter with exophthalmos. Another interesting relationship is with the gonads—the sex glands. The same character of cell forms the suprarenal cortex as forms part of the ovary. It seems also that the secondary sex characteristics are governed at least in part by the cortex. When it is disturbed, the feminine hair distribution becomes masculine, so that mustache and beard are evident, and the abdominal hair takes on the male character.

The Gonads or Sex Glands

In both the male and the female there are at least two distinct types of cell with separate secretions and different effects. The one group produces, in the male, spermatozoa, and in the female, the ova. The other group, known as the interstitial cells, produces secretions which are just at the present time awakening widespread discussion, although their actual effects are still not known. They probably have to do with secondary sex characteristics, with sex appetite, the libido, so called. Together with the hormones of the anterior pituitary gland, they may control the important and much involved menstrual cycle with the attendant uterine changes. In the male, the fact that the spermatozoa are delivered through a duct to the seminal vesicles, there to remain until discharged in the sexual act, while the interstitial secretions are given to the blood stream directly, forms the basis for the operation to "preserve" youth—if by that is meant the maintenance of the "libido." The operation consists of tying off on one side the vas deferens (the duct for the spermatozoa). This produces with a damming back of the spermatozoa a congestion of the testicle on that side with an increase in the blood stream. While it produces an atrophy of the cells producing the spermatozoa, it increases the growth and activity of the interstitial cells, producing thereby an increase in all the secondary sex characteristics with an increase in sexual life. If both sides are operated on, the result is even more apparent, but of course the ability then to reproduce is nil. The striking and sensational results claimed for these procedures are only occasionally seen. An increase in sexual virility during the third period of life—when the blood vessels are sclerotic and the blood pressure tends to high levels —is of doubtful advantage. The possibility of apoplexy is always present. In the female similar effects are produced by radium and X-ray attempts to stimulate the interstitial tissue. One need hardly point out the difficulty of correctly estimating the dosage of these dangerous expedients to prevent after effects.

The numerous experiments on the gonads are of extreme interest. Thus it has been shown in some animals that the sex can be practically altered by extracting their natural sex glands and substituting therefor the sex glands of the opposite gender.

Mechanism of Menstruation

Menstruation is one of the most interesting of all vital functions. Here, in a most marvelous way, is a regular procession of symptoms and events, repeated month after month, with the utmost regularity, as though controlled by clockwork. After the ovum is released from the ovary, a clot of blood remains at its old site. Cellular material develops in the clot. This is known as the *corpus luteum*, which gives off a secretion known as lutein, that controls many of the events of the cycle. Particularly it inhibits menstruation. If pregnancy occurs, this corpus luteum maintains its activity with its secretion during almost the entire period of carrying the child. If no pregnancy intervenes, then the corpus luteum gradually degenerates, and its secretion ceases. Thereupon menstruation with its bleeding recurs, the ovum is again formed and released, and a new corpus luteum produced. It seems as though the luteal secretion keeps menstruation in abeyance. In this entire procedure the anterior lobe of the pituitary gland takes on the part of a controlling agent and motor of the ovary. Indeed, on this function depends the most interesting of all internal glandular tests: the reaction for pregnancy. As soon as impregnation takes place, the menstrual cycle ceases.

The ovaries and the suprarenal cortex have some mutual interworkings, and the thyroid gland as well seems to play an important part in their proper functioning. Therefore during a menstrual cycle of four weeks there is a constant change and interchange between these various internal glandular units, the pituitary, the suprarenals, the thyroid, and the ovaries, and the reactions on the individual are many times evident of these perturbations. The excitement, the depression, the headaches, the hypersensitiveness to environmental changes followed by calmness and mental clearness, all mark the monthly mercurial levels of many women. They actually represent many individuals in one body. Even lordly man does not entirely escape, for many of his unaccountable changes of temperament can be credited to a more or less periodic readjustment of like character. At the menopause, because of a lack of synchronous involutionary changes in these internal glandular structures, the result is an imbalance. Then changes are seen such as waves of heat or "flushings" over the entire body, followed by chilliness or perspiration, tingling and numbness in different members, and mental disturbances chiefly depressive in character. Strange ideas develop such as the belief that the nearest and dearest of one's family and friends seem to be untrue and persecutory. These symptoms last over a course of years, coming and going constantly. If their true basis is understood and their victim is reassured that the fear engendered by them of "paralysis" or "insanity" is groundless, much mental perturbation and anguish may be spared. Brilliant results are often secured in these cases by the use of glandular medication prescribed by physicians.

There are also changes that occur in the body when the genitals are diseased so that they no longer function or are removed. If this occurs early in life, as is the case with the eunuchs of the orient, it seems that the growth hormone of the anterior pituitary gland, no longer balanced by the sex hormone, overacts. Then comes the tremendous overgrowth of the entire body, with the giant and powerful frame characteristic of eunuchism. Mental changes also occur: the victims become sullen, morose, stubborn, and are not easily amenable. The voice remains high-pitched, and the entire being is as one from another order of life. If the disturbance occurs later in life, then much modification of the symptoms ensues. The inordinate growth does not occur, though many of the mental changes do. Occasionally, after an attack of mumps involving both sides, the genitals also are affected, and if this also is bilateral, then this modification is seen. Later in life, if the ovaries are removed surgically the patient goes through an earlier menopause than usual, often with predominant mental symptoms.

II. Goiter: the Cause and Prevention

OLIVER P. KIMBALL, M.D.

Goiter is one of the oldest diseases known. There are references to goiter, or big neck, in every ancient language, in some instances dating back three or four thousand years b.c. The term "goiter" comes from the old word guttural, meaning throat. Not until the last century was it definitely known that goiter was an enlargement of the thyroid gland. Enlargements of the lymph glands of the neck or tumors of the neck are not called goiter. The term endemic, or simple, goiter comes from the word "endemic," meaning pertaining to that locality; for instance, the Alps mountain region is an endemic goiter district; also the Great Lakes basin in this country. Some condition in the locality is responsible for the goiter, hence it is called endemic, or in some way related to the district. Simple goiter is another term for the same condition, meaning just thyroid enlargement and not related to any other condition. This is in contrast to the so-called nervous goiter, exophthalmic goiter, Graves' disease, or Basedow's disease, all of which mean the same. In these conditions the thyroid enlargement, or goiter, is only a part of a complex disease. The term goiter in this discussion always means simple or endemic goiter.

A few centuries ago goiter, or big neck, was considered a mark of beauty; indeed, the girls with the largest necks were first to marry. It was thought that in some way the goiter was related to the sexual development, and the woman with a large goiter could bear more children. About the middle of the seventeenth century Paracelsus, the famous Swiss physician, pointed out that goiter was in some way related to cretinism, deaf-mutism, and feeble-mindedness. This same impression was again emphasized by the French physician Morel in the middle of the eighteenth century. From the scientific researches of the last fifty years it is now definitely known that instead of goiter being a mark of beauty it is the remains of a deficiency disease. The girl with a large goiter will not be as well developed as if her thyroid had remained normal. Unless preventive measures are taken, her children may be defective mentally or physically, or both, as in cretinism.

ENDEMIC GOITER DISTRICTS

The best known endemic goiter district in the world is the Alps mountain region, especially Switzerland. This is best known, not because of the greater prevalence of goiter, but because of its location in Europe where travel has been more extensive. Their physicians have been studying the problem and writing about it in medical literature for three hundred years. It was in Berne, Switzerland, that the operation for the treatment of goiter originated. Endemic goiter with cretinism and feeble-mindedness are common in some sections of the Himalaya Mountains. A medical missionary told of a section on the western border of China in the Himalaya Mountains where he found a community of Mongolian people where every man, woman, and child had a large goiter. These people felt that they were of a superior race and called the rest of humanity Little Necks. He also counted two hundred cretins in this comparatively small district, yet this superior race had never thought of this condition being the result of their big neck, or endemic goiter. In North America the Rocky Mountain region from northern Canada down through Mexico is an endemic goiter district, some localities being worse than others. The whole Great Lakes basin is also an endemic goiter district, but the region around Lake Superior is decidedly worse than the remaining section. In South America the Andes mountain region is an endemic goiter district. The Peruvian plateau is undoubtedly one of the worst endemic goiter districts in the world. In this region the early explorers found tribes of dwarfs which they described as being not only small and physically immature, but mentally like children. In fact, the missionaries thought them so low in the scale of intelligence that they could not be converted. Now it is known that they were only cretins and cretin imbeciles, the end result of endemic goiter through many generations. Comparatively, the Great Lakes basin is a mildly endemic district. Before the prevention of goiter was started, approximately 40 to 50 per cent of girls and women and 10 to 15 per cent of boys and men had small goiters. In cities the size of Detroit and Cleveland approximately one hundred cretins were found in the school population. The city of Berne, Switzerland, with a population of two hundred thousand, has a cretin farm where approximately two thousand cretins of all ages are cared for.

THE THYROID GLAND

The thyroid is a small gland in the front of the neck, between the larynx or voice-box and the upper end of the sternum or breastbone. It is divided into three small lobes or masses which lie close to the trachea or windpipe. The lobes on either side are the size of a lima bean, while the medium lobe, in front of the windpipe, is smaller. The normal thyroid is small; if the thyroid can be seen going up and down on swallowing, it is enlarged and would technically be called a small goiter. Goiters vary in size from barely visible to those in which each lobe of the gland may be six inches in diameter.

PERIODS WHEN GOITER IS MOST LIKELY TO OCCUR

As stated, goiter is an enlargement of the thyroid gland. In order to appreciate why the thyroid enlarges and why the condition occurs more frequently at certain ages, one must think of its normal activity. The thyroid secretion, which goes directly into the blood and is therefore called an internal secretion, plays a most important part in growth and development from early childhood to maturity; for instance, if for some reason the thyroid stopped functioning soon after birth, the child would not grow beyond the size of a five- or six-year-old. It would not go through the normal changes at puberty, and would remain infantile sexually and mentally. Its personality and characteristics would remain childish. Also, the entire development before birth depends to a great extent on the normal thyroid function of the mother. If the mother's thyroid should stop functioning soon after pregnancy started, the child would most likely die before birth. This was frequently seen among domestic animals in the Rocky Mountain section before the prevention of goiter in animals was instituted in 1918. If there was only a marked deficiency of the mother's thyroid due to an old goiter or exhaustion from any cause, the child would be born with a large goiter or might even be a cretin; or this temporary deficiency might occur just at the right time (fourteen to sixteen weeks of congenital life) to interfere with proper mental development, but might not interfere with physical development (cretinoid feeble-mindedness). The mother is likely to develop a goiter during every pregnancy because of the unusual demand for thyroid secretion; therefore, normal thyroid function is important through the congenital period, through the entire period of growth and

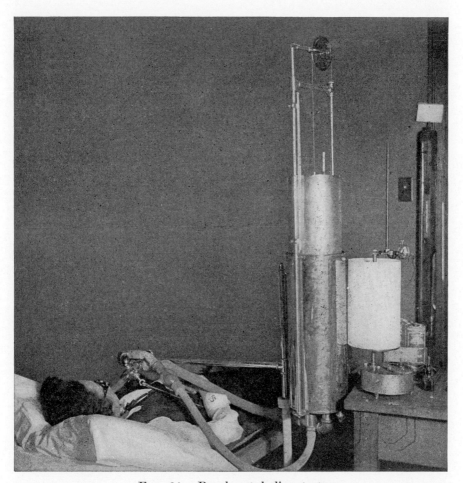

FIG. 64.   Basal metabolism test.

development, exceedingly important through the years of puberty, and in women through the entire period of pregnancy and menopause.

In babies and children goiter is as frequent in boys as it is in girls. In goiter surveys in Ohio and Michigan it was found that up to the ages ten or eleven the incidence of goiter was about the same in boys as in girls; approximately 30 per cent in this district. By the time they reached the age of fifteen the incidence of goiter in girls was twice as high, or 60 per cent, while in boys it was half as high, or 15 per cent. In this mildly endemic goiter district there were from 4 to 6 times as many goiters among girls and women as there were among boys and men. This difference is because of the important relation of thyroid hormone to the sexual development, recurrent menstruation, and pregnancies.

CHEMISTRY OF THE THYROID SECRETION

The normal secretion from the thyroid gland is a compound containing iodine. Iodine in this secretion is as important as iron is to the red blood cells or calcium to the bones. This thyroid secretion is 65 per cent iodine, and no other element can take its place. From his researches, Dr. David Marine found that so long as the iodine content was $\frac{1}{10}$ of 1 per cent, or more, of the thyroid gland, no changes towards the development of the goiter would occur, but as soon as the iodine dropped below $\frac{1}{10}$ of 1 per cent changes such as multiplication of cells (hyperplasia) and enlargement of each cell with consequent enlargement of the gland (hypertrophy) began immediately. From these studies Dr. Marine deduced the simple principle that goiter is due to a deficiency of iodine and all that is necessary to prevent thyroid enlargement is to feed the thyroid the necessary food element. This is the basis of all the work in the prevention of goiter.

PREVENTION OF GOITER

The prevention of goiter among children was first started on a large scale through the schools of Akron, O., from 1916 to 1920. Only girls from the fifth to twelfth grade inclusive were studied, because goiter is so much more prevalent among girls of this age. In this first observation the simplest salt of iodine was used in the drinking water twice a year, spring and fall. Only those girls who were desirous of carrying out this preventive measure and whose parents gave a written request for this treatment received the prophylactic iodine regularly throughout this period. Approximately one half of the girls took the iodine, but the same careful observations were made on all girls, regardless of whether or not they took the iodine. The results were most striking. Not a single healthy girl whose thyroid was normal in the beginning and who took the prophylactic treatment developed goiter. Among those who were free from goiter but did not take the iodine, 27 per cent developed goiter within the period of observation. Among girls who had small goiters to begin with and who took iodine twice a year, 65 per cent had gone back to normal size at the end of this period. Less than 10 per cent of those who had small goiters and did not choose to take iodine decreased in size during this same period. As stated, not a single healthy girl developed a goiter, but 5 developed a small goiter in spite of this amount of food iodine because they had chronic infection, such as tuberculosis, badly infected tonsils, or other diseases of malnutrition. Those who develop a small goiter while taking iodine in amounts sufficient to prevent goiter are few, however, and represent the exceptional case, where the need for thyroid hormone is great, such as chronic infection, severe acute illness, or unusual growth. In such cases it is only necessary to increase the amount of iodine to meet the unusual need.

The use of iodized salt spread rapidly after the demonstration in Akron, and by 1924 the prevention of goiter was being carried out through schools in many cities in the Great Lakes basin, West Virginia, Utah, Oregon, and Washington; also in Switzerland, Italy, New Zealand, Venezuela, South America. In the spring of 1924 the State Health Department of Michigan, after considerable study, attempted to meet this deficiency of food iodine by putting a small amount of iodine in the salt. This was a most natural suggestion. Formerly most food iodine was obtained from salt, but by the process of refining which was worked out in 1898 all of the iodine which was in the salt naturally was driven off. Thus an important source of food iodine was lost. This point was demonstrated convincingly in a study made in West Virginia in the spring of 1922. Several of the older physicians in Charleston pointed out that before 1900 endemic goiter was an exceedingly rare condition in this valley, but soon after this date the doctors noticed a definite increase in simple goiter. A survey of the schools of Charleston and Huntington showed that 60 per cent of the schoolgirls had enlarged thyroids. This was indeed a challenging problem. By the assistance of the State Health Department it was found after considerable study that the condition stated was true of the section, and that the only change in the food supply was in the salt. Until about 1900 all the table salt used in this valley came from wells in this region. Salt wells were common all through the Kanawha River valley, and in 1922 old shacks could be seen that had marked a salt well twenty-five years previously. It was within the memory of every citizen fifty years of age that the table salt mined and used in this vicinity was a crude salt, described by everyone as being coarse and containing dirty brown particles. In 1898 the salt companies of Ohio and Michigan worked out and put into actual practice the new process of refining crude salt, and within a few years this whole section was flooded with refined white salt. Naturally the local salt companies with their crude, dirty brown salt could not compete. This change in salt was the only change in food or water in this district, yet within a quarter of a century the incidence of endemic goiter increased from practically nothing to a point where endemic goiter was as prevalent in this valley as around the Great Lakes.

As a result of using iodized salt almost exclusively throughout Michigan since 1924 goiter has been practically prevented among the school children. In 1928 the school children in several sections of Michigan were reëxamined, and where the incidence of goiter had been as high as 60 per cent among the girls around Lake Superior in 1924, only 8 or 9 per cent was found. The yearly reports of the school physicians in Detroit show that the incidence of goiter in that city has decreased gradually from 36 per cent in 1924 to 2.1 per cent in 1931. During this period approximately 94 per cent of the homes had used iodized salt continuously.

OTHER SOURCES OF FOOD IODINE

All sea foods are rich in iodine. Water obtained from deep artesian wells in Kansas contains the highest iodine content yet found in drinking water. By actual analysis this water contains eighteen hundred times as much as drinking water of cities in the Great Lakes district, as Chicago, Detroit, or Cleveland. Other sections of the country have small amounts of iodine in the soil so that the vegetables are fairly rich with this important food element. This is true of some Southern states, especially South Carolina.

The amount of iodine needed for the average healthy child when the thyroid is normal is comparatively small. In the majority of cases one grain distributed throughout the year would be sufficient. One who uses the average amount of iodized salt would get approximately five grains of iodine during the year. This should be sufficient to meet such emergencies as puberty, pregnancy, and unusual growth or illnesses. As far as can be determined it has met the needs efficiently and is entirely safe.

The use of iodized salt is not original with this generation. It was used for several years in the treatment of goiter by Dr. M. Grange of Geneva, Switzerland, as early as 1840. A paper was read before the Academy of Medicine at Paris, in 1858, on this treatment, in which the writers emphasized the possibility of harm because four cases so treated had developed what is now called toxic goiter. Also, two cases were described who left the mountains and went to the seashore for a short period and developed the same symptoms of toxic goiter. This was most probably the origin of the statement which may still be heard, that it is dangerous to use iodine for goiter. Now it is known that iodine in amounts sufficient to prevent goiter is perfectly safe; and it should be considered food for the thyroid gland just as the iron from spinach is food for the red blood cells.

The Results of Goiter

In endemic goiter districts, where everyone is fairly well acquainted with goiter, the question is asked frequently, "What ill effects might come from goiter?" To the majority of persons the most serious effect is the disfigurement of a so-called big neck. Most of the results of goiter have been pointed out indirectly by telling what the thyroid secretion does normally. Here briefly are the possible ill effects of goiter: The first important period when goiter is likely to affect an individual is the congenital period, i.e., before birth. The mother's thyroid maintains the normal rate of growth and development from conception to a normally developed baby within the short period of nine months. If the mother's thyroid should cease functioning for any reason early in pregnancy (6th week), the development of the child, especially his nervous system, would be retarded to such an extent that he would probably die. If the child should survive it would be abnormal mentally and physically. This is the lowest type of feeble-mindedness called Mongolian idiocy. If this same condition occurs just a little later in the period before the child is born (14th to 15th week), the mental and physical development are again retarded, and the child would most likely be a cretin. If a deficiency occurs a little later in congenital life, or is less severe than that which causes cretinism, the retardation seems to effect the mentality more than the physical, and the child would be apparently normal physically but subnormal mentally. These children show a peculiar type of mental growth; i.e., they reach their maximum mental development early, as do cretins. Recently the condition has been called the cretinoid type of feeble-mindedness.

During the study of retarded children in the public schools of Detroit many such children were discovered, and as near as could be estimated 10 per cent of the feeble-mindedness in the state of Michigan was of this type and indirectly due to endemic goiter. In one family the mother had a moderate-sized, hard, fibrous goiter. The expression of her face and the swelling of the legs were typical of lack of thyroid in adult life, called myxedema. Her older children were normal physically and mentally. Her little girl, age seven and a half, was almost normal physically, but had the mentality of a three-year-old (cretinoid feeble-mindedness). Her son, a year younger than the girl, or six and a half years old, was unable to walk or talk. His tongue and abdomen were large, and his skin was dry and thick. He was a typical cretin imbecile, resembling in some respects the Mongolian type of idiocy already described. His condition was the result of the lack of thyroid function in the mother during pregnancy. Another daughter might have been mistaken for a small, shy girl of five. She was fifteen and a half years of age, but her mental age was only six years. She showed infantile characteristics, or lack of development for one her age. Her condition was recognized soon after birth, and she had had some thyroid treatment since she was a baby; otherwise she would have been similar to her brother. This only emphasizes the important point that the physical appearance can be changed by substitution of thyroid after birth, but the mental development cannot be changed to any great extent, because the brain did not develop properly during the congenital period.

From his experiments on animals Dr. David Marine taught as early as 1912 that endemic goiter was the easiest known disease to prevent. The prevention of goiter in every locality, where carried out scientifically, has proved this statement. Considering the ease with which goiter can be prevented and the suffering and unhappiness that this disease may cause, goiter will stand out in the future not only as a deficiency disease, but as a mark of ignorance or carelessness on the part of someone.

CHAPTER XXI

Diabetes
ELLIOTT P. JOSLIN, M.D.

INTRODUCTION

DEATHS FROM DIABETES *in the United States have risen as much as fifteen times the rate of a little more than half a century ago. In New York, for example, the rate per 100,000 population in 1866 was 2.1. In 1933, it was 29.2. Perhaps even more serious is the fact that more women have been dying of diabetes than men. The death rates for men and women were about the same until about 1905. Then the rate among women began to rise more rapidly, so that by 1932 about' twice as many women as men died of diabetes. Sound conclusions regarding diabetes, however, cannot be drawn, because insulin was introduced around 1923, and diagnosis has become more frequent.*

A part of the reason for the greater number of cases found among women in recent years has been the improvement in diagnosis and the fact that women are being examined more frequently and regularly than they were in an earlier day. Not all the people who have diabetes get an early diagnosis. The condition appears insidiously, and the symptoms are relatively mild in the early stages. Moreover, a laboratory examination is required to make a positive diagnosis. This, and the fact that women are appearing more frequently in industry and similar occupations requiring physical examinations, likely explains some of the increase in diabetes as found in women.

An interesting change brought about by the use of insulin in relationship to diabetes is the manner in which death occurs. In an earlier day, people who died of diabetes used to die in coma—a form of unconsciousness which resulted from chemical changes in the body. Today the number of deaths from this cause has decreased greatly. For instance, from 1900 to 1930 the number of diabetic deaths due to coma dropped 50 per cent. At the same time there was a rise of about

35 per cent in the deaths from diabetes associated with changes in the heart, the circulation, the kidneys, and with gangrene.

Persons who have diabetes live much longer nowadays than those in former years. As a diabetic lives longer, he dies of other conditions. It must be realized that the person who develops diabetes has a life-long problem. He must watch his condition carefully if he is to gain the maximum benefit from methods of treatment. It is known that in some cases the changes that have taken place in the body resulting from diabetes are hereditary. By use of insulin, children with diabetes —which used to be especially fatal to youngsters—now live and are likely to have children. Hence the question of heredity in diabetes will, in the future, be an increasingly important problem.

Diabetes was described by a Greek physician, Aretæus, who lived in the reign of the Emperor Hadrian about A.D. *300. His description of it can be improved according to our knowledge today, only in some terms of chemistry and physiology.*

"The nature of the disease," he said, "is chronic and it takes a long period to form; but the patient is short lived if the constitution of the disease becomes completely established; for the melting is rapid; the death speedy. Moreover, life is disgusting and painful; thirst unquenchable, excessive drinking, which, however, is disproportionate to the larger quantity of fluid excreted; for more fluid is excreted; and one cannot stop them either from drinking or excreting fluid. Or, if for a time they abstain from drinking, their mouth becomes parched and their body dry; the organs seem as if scorched up; they are affected with nausea, restlessness and a burning thirst; and at no distant time they expire."

The term "diabetes" came either from the Greek word meaning fountain, or from another term meaning to "pass through," because the essential feature of the disease is the rapid passing of sugar and fluid through the body. In 1674 an English physician named Willis found that the fluid excreted in diabetes is sweeter in character than normally, and a hundred years later another physician showed that the sweetness was due to sugar. Afterward it was found by German investigators that removal or inactivity of a gland called the pancreas is followed by the development of this disturbance of the body, and later that it was the cells in the pancreas, known as the islands of Langerhans, that are associated with the way in which sugar is handled by the body.

The Canadian investigators, Banting and Macleod, received the Nobel Prize for their investigations of this disease and for their discovery of insulin. They prepared an extract of the pancreas which is apparently largely composed of the tissues of the islands of Langerhans. The use of this extract has greatly modified the method of control of diabetes today. By its use the patient may eat the food necessary to keep him in normal weight and strength without further injury to his pancreas. It is not a cure for the disease, but a method of control.

In the attack on diabetes in the United States, one of the most important contributors has been Dr. E. P. Joslin, whose article follows. He is author of a popular handbook on the subject, as well as of a scientific text widely used by physicians throughout the world. In the article which follows, he classifies the subject for the average reader and indicates at the same time the manner in which the afflicted may coöperate with the physician to the best advantage of their health. While recognizing that the average person may be competent to regulate his own diet under the advice of the doctor and also to administer remedies to himself, Dr. Joslin does not suggest either self-diagnosis or self-treatment as safe for anyone suffering from this disorder.

M. F.

DEATH RATE FROM DIABETES

IT IS HARD WORK to keep up with the modern story of diabetes, and no wonder: first, because the number of cases increases so fast, and second, because the treatment improves so much from year to year. In the closing twenty years of the last century the death rate from diabetes in the registration area of the United States trebled, rising from 2.8 per 100,000 in 1880 to 9.3 in 1900, and in the first thirty years of this century it has doubled, being 19.0 per 100,000 in 1930, and 22.0 in 1932. During 1931 in New York City the mortality was 27.1 per 100,000, 29.3 in 1932, and 29.2 in 1933. But this is only part of the story.

Fifty years ago diabetic patients lived on the average a scant three years. Today diabetic patients expect to live indefinitely, and, in fact, some live longer with the disease than, from insurance tables, one would expect them to live without it. I believe they are living on the average three to five times as long, and if it were not that so many people over fifty years old developed the disease, the average duration would be still greater. In Massachusetts the Board of Health has made a survey and has found that there are approximately fifteen living diabetics for each diabetic fatality during the year. It is a conservative estimate to state that the young doctor of today will have thirty times as much diabetes, i.e., thirty times as many years of diabetes, to treat as the old doctor who began practice in 1880.

THE NINE LEADING CAUSES OF DEATH, AND RANK IN THE UNITED STATES, FOR TWO FIVE-YEAR PERIODS ENDING 1904 AND 1929

Cause of Death (per 100,000)	Annual Average 1904	Cause of Death (per 100,000)	Annual Average 1929
1. Tuberculosis	185	1. Organic heart disease	220
2. Pneumonia	162	2. Cancer	114
3. Heart disease	128	3. Pneumonia	103
4. Nephritis	94	4. Nephritis	97
5. Diarrhea and enteritis (under 2 years)	91	5. Apoplexy	88
6. Apoplexy	76	6. Tuberculosis	77
7. Cancer	68	7. Premature birth	33
8. Ill-defined causes	48	8. Influenza	25
9. Old age	45	9. Diabetes mellitus	23

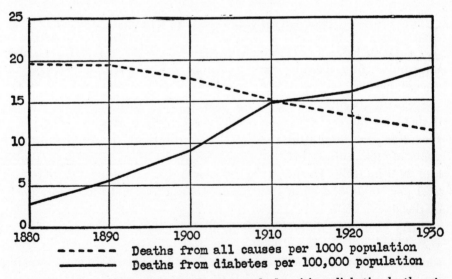

- - - - - - Deaths from all causes per 1000 population
———— Deaths from diabetes per 100,000 population

FIG. 65. The falling total death rate and the rising diabetic death rate United States Registration Area, 1880–1930.

The chart (Fig. 65) shows in more accurate form the death rate per 100,000 for diabetes in the United States in the decades between 1880 and 1930. It is obvious that if diabetes continued to increase as it did between 1880 and 1900 it would transcend all other diseases in importance before half of the twentieth century had expired. Fortunately such a rapid increase has been stayed, but, on the other hand, when compared with other diseases, it has forged ahead so much that now it is of serious concern to insurance companies and health authorities, to say nothing of those who are liable to acquire it. Even twenty years ago, diabetes did not figure in the twenty principal causes of death in the United States, but in 1930 it was ninth in importance, and if one drops out accidents and premature births it would be seventh in importance. Furthermore, if one grouped all those diseases under one heading which relate to hardening of the arteries, such as chronic heart disease, apoplexy, and Bright's disease, it would be fifth in importance. The table on p. 566 shows the nine principal causes of death in the United States in 1904 and 1929, and the table on p. 567 shows for a large insurance company, whose policyholders number some twenty-one or more millions in the United States and Canada, the relative importance of diabetes in their group.

WHAT IS DIABETES?

Diabetes is a chronic disease, and doctors seldom claim to cure it. It is a disease in which the patient fails to get the benefit of the food which he eats, particularly the sugar and starch (carbohydrate foods), but to a lesser degree of the meat, fish, eggs, and cheese (protein

DEATH RATES PER 100,000 FOR PRINCIPAL CAUSES, JANUARY TO APRIL, 1932

METROPOLITAN LIFE INSURANCE CO.

Causes of Death	Cumulative January to April, 1932
1. Organic diseases of heart	170
2. Pneumonia	97
3. Cancer	90
4. Tuberculosis	74
5. Bright's disease	74
6. Cerebral hemorrhage	68
7. Other external causes (excluding suicides and homicides)	50
8. Influenza	31
9. Diabetes mellitus	25

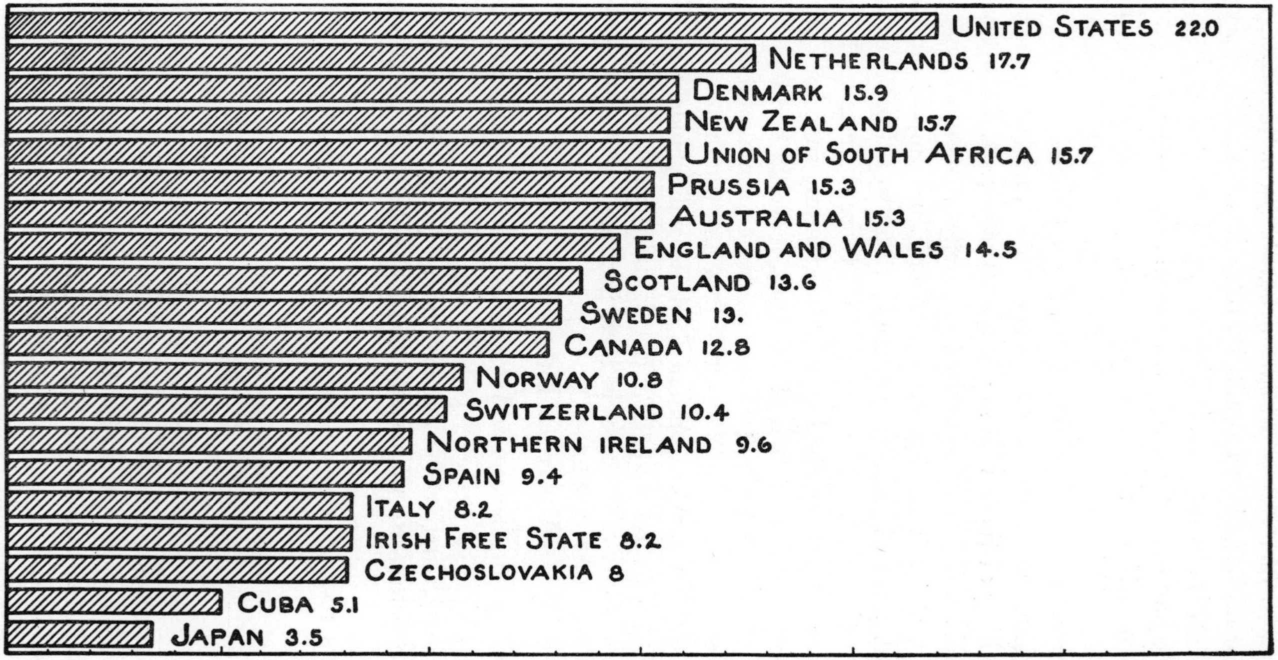

United States 22.0
Netherlands 17.7
Denmark 15.9
New Zealand 15.7
Union of South Africa 15.7
Prussia 15.3
Australia 15.3
England and Wales 14.5
Scotland 13.6
Sweden 13.
Canada 12.8
Norway 10.8
Switzerland 10.4
Northern Ireland 9.6
Spain 9.4
Italy 8.2
Irish Free State 8.2
Czechoslovakia 8
Cuba 5.1
Japan 3.5

FIG. 66. The mortality rates for diabetes throughout the world (per 100,000 of population).

Today, even the patient with severe diabetes can live for years in good health if only he will diet intelligently, and, when necessary, use insulin. In spite of the fact that the disease is controllable, the mortality rate is mounting rapidly, particularly in the United States.

568

foods), and even of the fatty foods such as the fat on meat, cream, butter, oil, and the fat in nuts. The diabetic fails to get the value of these foods because the pancreas, commonly known as the sweetbread and situated behind the stomach, produces an insufficient quantity of a substance named insulin. As a result of this lack of insulin, much of the

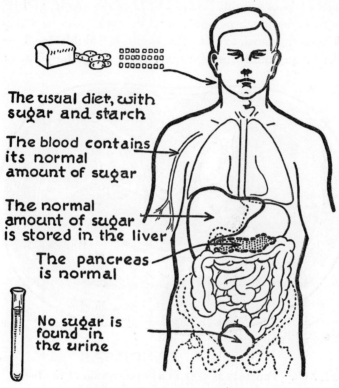

The usual diet, with sugar and starch

The blood contains its normal amount of sugar

The normal amount of sugar is stored in the liver

The pancreas is normal

No sugar is found in the urine

FIG. 67. A normal person.

The pancreas of a normal person makes enough insulin to take care of all the sugar derived from food. No excess is left to injure the body.

food, including most of the carbohydrate, a notable quantity of the protein, but only a small portion of the fat, changes to sugar, and this sugar accumulates to excess in the blood and tissues. Usually this sugar is quickly removed from the blood and stored in the liver, muscles, and skin, or burned up to keep the body warm or furnish energy. But in diabetes this normal routine is broken, and the sugar spills over and passes out of the body through the kidneys, escaping with the urine.

Years ago it was noticed that the urine was sweet, as sweet as honey, and so the disease was called diabetes mellitus in contrast to a much rarer disease, diabetes insipidus, in which the urine is simply watery. The sugar is thus lost to the body, and from this fact anyone can imagine what most of the symptoms of diabetes must be. The untreated patient loses weight, because he loses the sugar, and this sugar may amount to as much as one pound or even more in a day. He is thirsty because he must excrete the sugar in soluble form and to do this drinks large quantities of water. As a result he gives out large

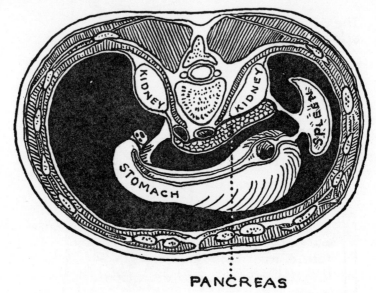

PANCREAS

Fig. 68.   Pancreas as seen in a cross-section of the body.

quantities of urine. Of course he is thirsty, of course he loses weight, of course he becomes weak and debilitated, and years ago, when treatment was unsatisfactory, he became a prey to almost any disease. But now all this is changed, and thanks to a better knowledge of diet and the discovery and use of insulin the diabetic patient can live indefinitely. There may be thirty times as much diabetes to treat as fifty years ago, but it is largely because the treatment has correspondingly improved.

Diabetes is not a very bad disease, because it is clean and not contagious, and the patient who learns the rules of treatment and follows them can keep it largely under control. Many of the most celebrated people in the world have had diabetes. There is some ground for the belief that the diabetic, through the training of mind to control his condition, is more capable than the usual person. Therefore the diabetic should not be discouraged. There may be compensations. With courage and persistence he can prove himself to be the master of his fate.

Why Is Diabetes Increasing?

This is a simple question to answer. Diabetes is increasing because people refuse to die as young as did the brothers and sisters of their grandfathers. Sixty years ago our mothers and fathers, when they were born, could count on living only some thirty-eight years on the average, but today we expect the new-born baby to live at least sixty years. In other words, diabetes is a disease which comes on in adult life rather than in young people. Two thirds of the cases begin after the age of forty years; in women the most common year for it to develop is fifty years, and in men, one or two years later. Today the average youngster will live long enough to reach the diabetic danger zone between forty-five and fifty-five years and therefore through age alone will be exposed to diabetes.

Prevention of Diabetes

My friend Richard Wagner in Vienna, who has had many diabetic children to treat and has just written an excellent book with Richard Priesel on the disease,[1] divides diabetics into two classes according to the origin of the disease: the blameless diabetics and the blamable diabetics. Let us consider the blamable diabetics first.

If a man gets smallpox today we say he is to be blamed for it; he is blamable. If he gets drunk and has an accident we blame him; if he is an adult and gets typhoid fever we say he could have avoided it, he is blamable. No man needs to get smallpox, needs to get drunk, needs to get typhoid fever, because he can be vaccinated against smallpox, leave alcohol alone, and be immunized from typhoid. So it is with a large group of diabetics. Most of those who have diabetes in middle life were fat before they got it. Take any group of diabetics of the age of fifty years or more, and most any ten of them put together weighed a ton before they developed the disease. Over and over again I have demonstrated this to my classes of patients, and this is what we can

[1] *Die Zuckerkrankheit und ihre Behandlung im Kindesalter,* George Thieme, Leipzig.

call blamable diabetes, because one cannot help the conclusion that in the vast majority of instances, if obesity had been avoided, diabetes might have been prevented. This type of diabetes contrasts sharply with blameless diabetes.

Blameless diabetes is the diabetes preëminently of children and those under forty years of age. The rule of obesity, as provocative of diabetes, does not hold in the first three decades of life, and there is evidently another reason for the breaking out of diabetes in the young. Blameless diabetes is the diabetes, then, of the child, and why is his diabetes blameless and that of the poor old man or woman blamable? The diabetic child could not follow Oliver Wendell Holmes's rule and pick out his parents. Although Naunyn suspected and recognized heredity as the cause of diabetes, it is only recently that the proof of its influence has arrived. At first heredity did not seem to be of great importance, because in only 20 per cent of our cases in children could we trace a relative who had the disease. We did not realize years ago that this was simply because the children only lived a year or two and so we lost track of them. Their families were so sad at the death of their children that one did not feel justified in seeking information in after years about the later appearance of the disease in the parents or other members of the family. But today we have a sufficiently large group of diabetic children for statistical purposes who have already lived ten years. And now we find that, instead of one child in five, or 20 per cent, having a relative with the disease, today, according to Dr. Priscilla White, every other child (actually 53 per cent) has a diabetic relative and in fact one in sixteen a diabetic parent. As the parents of our diabetic children are still young, they have hardly entered the diabetic zone of fifty years, the year in which diabetes is most common, and it is probable that still more may show it before they die. Dr. White has studied this most carefully, and with the help of Dr. Pincus of the Biological Department of Harvard University has recorded all her results in her book.[2] The diabetic child, therefore, was born with a tendency to diabetes. The facts correspond with the theory. Consequently, if you do not want diabetes, first of all pick out non-diabetic parents!

The tendency to diabetes appears to be transmitted as a so-called recessive characteristic. If the tendency is strong, the disease comes on soon after birth; if the tendency is slight, it takes some secondary

[2]*Diabetes in Childhood and Adolescence*, Lea and Febiger, Philadelphia.

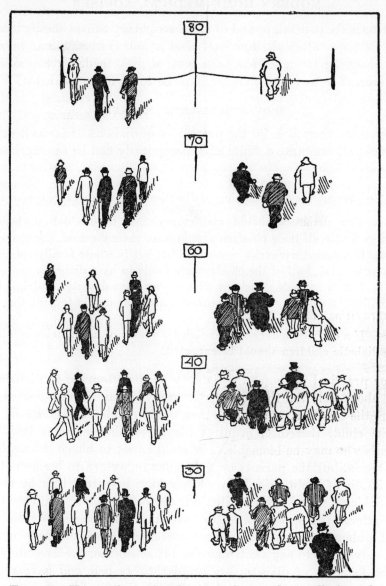

FIG. 69. How 10 fat and 10 lean men fare as they walk through life.

Diabetes is most likely to attack those who overeat and grow fat. It appears most commonly after the age of forty years. To avoid diabetes, eat moderately, and stay thin! The fat person is in danger of diabetes. The person who stays thin often avoids diabetes.

cause to make it develop, and of these secondary causes obesity stands first. Perhaps, after all, our fat friend is not so blamable as we may have thought; he may have been born with a tendency to diabetes. However, if he had kept thin, perhaps he could have avoided it.

SHOULD A DIABETIC MARRY?

The rules, therefore, for the prevention of diabetes as far as heredity is concerned are quite definite and theoretically can be summarized as follows:

To prevent the transmission of the disease to the offspring:

1. Two diabetics should not marry and have children, because theoretically all their children should have their disease.
2. If a diabetic marries a nondiabetic, but in whose family there is a diabetic taint, half of the children are liable to have diabetes.
3. If two individuals marry who do not have diabetes, but in whose families the disease exists, the chances are that one in four of the children will develop the disease.
4. If a diabetic marries a nondiabetic who is of a nondiabetic family, no diabetic children should be expected.

For practical purposes the liability of the offspring to diabetes is only about half the theoretical, because they die from other causes before the time arrives at which they would develop diabetes.

The child, therefore, acquires blameless diabetes, and it is the parents who may be blamable. The child is not to blame if he dies of diphtheria, but the parents or guardians today are to blame if they let him die of diphtheria, because they have been told that by means of a Schick test and toxin antitoxin it can be prevented, and they have been offered the opportunities to have such tests made. The diabetic child is blameless, but, as for the parents of a diabetic child, at present it is only right to say that they are blameless too, because the facts of the heredity of diabetes are comparatively new and have seldom been stated as plainly and as strongly as here written.

THE WISE CONTROL THEIR WEIGHT

Wise people, and particularly the wise relatives of a diabetic, remembering the frequency of diabetes among the fat and the possibility of heredity, will strive to keep their weight under control. If they are under the age of thirty-five they should not try to lose weight, because the young man or young woman who is underweight has a lower expectancy of life than the one of normal weight or above and furthermore overweight as a cause of diabetes is not so important in the young. But being wise people, when they reach forty years of age they will keep their weight under control. To do this, exercise helps. Avoidance of overeating of any kind of food helps. And particularly and most easily can one control body weight by limiting sugar and starch, and especially and most safely by lowering the fat in the diet, such as the butter, cream, oil, and the fat on meat.

When do people get fat and then get diabetes? They get fat when exercise ceases and a sedentary life develops. An officer in the field is given an assignment at headquarters, and diabetes breaks out. A boy breaks his leg, his activity ceases, and friends place a box of candy at his elbow, and diabetes appears. A woman has gallstones, is successfully operated on, and her friends send food instead of flowers; she rapidly becomes fat, and diabetes breaks forth. It develops particularly with patients who have gallstones, because the gall tract is so near the pancreas that inflammation can extend from the one to the other. Fortunately, in the head of the pancreas, which is near the gall bladder, there are only a few of the cells which make insulin, and so only a few are destroyed, and the diabetes which results is fairly mild. Most doctors recommend that patients with gallstones should be operated on so as to lessen the possibility of a later development of cancer as a result of the irritation of the gallstones, but also for another reason, namely, to lessen the possibility of injury to the pancreas, which in time might lead to diabetes.

If you want to dodge diabetes, therefore, pick out your ancestors, don't get fat, and keep active, and if you have diabetes, or if it is in your family and you do not want to hand it down, fall in love with someone who does not have the disease or whose family is free from it. Of course, this may be a hardship, because you may not find anyone to marry who is as nice and bright as a diabetic, but still there are compensations, because your grandchildren may rise up and call you blessed.

AND IF YOU DISCOVER DIABETES IN A RELATIVE

Every once in a while a diabetic discovers diabetes in a relative, and contrary to his expectations he is rewarded by finding that his relative does better with treatment than he himself. The reason is that he has discovered the relative's disease at an earlier stage than that at which his own was recognized, and so treatment was started early, which is always a help. Furthermore, any diabetic who picks up the disease in a relative can be encouraged, because the treatment of diabetes is improving so rapidly that his relative, who develops it a few years after his own disease began, will be able to begin the treatment under improved conditions and so will do particularly well. I have seen this occur in various families where a second child has come down with the disease, and recently it was a great comfort to me to note the attitude of the parents when they found out that their second child had diabetes. They were sorry but not overwhelmed, because from their experience with their older boy they were confident they could keep the disease under control. This is about the best confirmatory evidence of improvement in the treatment of diabetes that I have.

The relative of a diabetic, if he is fond of his family, will not only point out to them the dangers of being fat but will go a step farther and along with the tests which he makes of his own urine he will make similar tests for his relatives. The following episode taught me this:

LOUISA DRUMM AND WHAT SHE DID

March 30, 1920, there came to my office a woman with diabetes. She was given the usual examination with suggestions for treatment, and as it was impracticable for her to enter the hospital, she was taught on the spot to examine her urine. She went home and shortly after contracted pneumonia and died. But in the intervening days, amid her household cares, she found time and took enough interest to examine the urine of ten others in her boarding house, and in so doing discovered the presence of diabetes in a boy. She gave him sound advice and sent him to his own physician, who also subsequently died, and a few days later the boy came to me, telling this story. On the day she learned the Benedict test and made these ten urinary examinations for her friends, Louisa Drumm was seventy-nine years and four months old! Can one not appropriately say to younger diabetic patients, "Go thou and do likewise"?

"A Little Child Shall Lead Them"

Today the diabetic children are the pathfinders for the diabetic adults. Every honest diabetic day which a child lives teaches a lesson which helps a feeble old diabetic man or woman to live more com-

fortably. Children are exploring unknown diabetic regions. When I
began practice I used to keep a record of the days a diabetic child
lived, so as to see if the next diabetic child would live a day or two
longer. Gradually little improvements in treatment occurred, and I
could measure the life of a child by months, but up until the discovery of insulin the span of life of the diabetic child was less than
two years. Today, the younger the child the longer can be the length
of his life, and instead of saying, as we used to do, the older you are
the milder the diabetes, now all agree the younger you are the greater
the diabetic life expectancy.

DIABETES IS BEST STUDIED IN CHILDREN

Children have done so much for the diabetic adult. Diabetic children
are active and happy and prove that restrictions in diet need not make
one sad, morose, and down-hearted. Children were the first to show that
they were better in the summer time and worse in the winter time, because in the summer they have more exercise, sunshine, fresh air, and
freedom from infections, whereas in the winter, when they are less
active and are exposed to infections in school, their diabetes is worse,
as is evident from their difficulty in keeping the urine sugar free.
Diabetic children demonstrate that diabetics nowadays can do almost
everything. They go to school, to college; they surprise and cheer
their elders by having high marks and winning prizes. Dr. Priscilla
White found out that at the time when their diabetes begins they are
a little taller than the ordinary child. Along with their mental precocity and early development in height, there is also an early development of their bones. In fact, from the child we learn that in some
respects the diabetic is an extraordinary person and that likely there
is a connection between his brain and his pancreas. Thus the children
have made us pay more and more attention to the diabetic adults, and
we recognize that many of them have been noted men such as Clemenceau, Joffre, Eastman, and Edison.

Another outstanding contribution of the diabetic children is the
opportunity they present for the study of diabetic heredity. Certainly
all will agree that if diabetes is hereditary we should seek to prevent
its transmission. Most people do not know why their great-great-
great-great-great-grandfathers died, unless they were hanged as
witches on Gallows Hill in Salem Town or had some similar honor
conferred upon them, and so they cannot say whether diabetes runs in

their family. But with a child we can generally find out why his grand-mother and his grandfather and his uncles and aunts died, and so in this way from children we have found out the importance of heredity as a cause of diabetes.

THE DIABETIC CHILD'S SPLENDID TEETH

To the amazement of all it has developed that the teeth of diabetic children are better than the teeth of normal children. Not only may a diabetic child have the best teeth of anyone in his class and in his school, but his may be the best in his whole school district. These incidents occur too frequently to be chance happenings. There must be a cause, and it may be it is due to the preponderance of green vegetables and fruit in the diet and the invariable inclusion of an egg and milk and meat, with the exclusion of soft breads, pastry, and candy.

THE DIABETIC CHILD AND EARLY OLD AGE

From the diabetic children also we have learned how not to grow old too fast, and I am inclined to predict that this is their greatest gift to humanity—an idea which seems impossible, another claim for a fountain of youth; but keep an open mind, for there may be more than a grain of truth in it. The facts are these: Some of our children, who developed diabetes just before modern treatment began, escaped the then usual diabetic coma long enough to allow us to watch the development of the disease. Among these exceptional children we observed that several had the blood vessels of old men, and in certain children cataracts were discovered in the eyes. In contrast to these discomforting findings our present diabetic children, who have now lived quite as long, do not show either of these conditions, provided their diabetes was discovered reasonably promptly after its onset and treated well. In short, there is something in the modern treatment of diabetes which has prevented the appearance of two of the signs of old age which were manifest in the diabetic child of a few years ago. If one therefore can stop the early onset of old age in the child, the inference is plain that if an old diabetic is treated carefully the chances are overwhelming that he will age less rapidly. Finally, is it not reasonable to conclude that if we apply to the general population those same dietetic or other measures which have led diabetics to live longer it may grow old less rapidly too?

Dogs and Diabetics

The diabetic child does well because he leads a routine life, having regular hours for meals, exercise, and sleep. Note this, you older diabetics. You will do well to follow the example of a child, just as he in turn follows that of his dog and cleaves to him. In fact, I like every diabetic to own a dog, because a dog is a diabetic's thoughtful friend. A dog never says to a diabetic, "You are thin," never speaks about his diet, never tempts him to break it and to eat a little more, never refers to the delicacies he himself has eaten or the good bones he expects to eat; in fact, never implies by any sign or action in public or in private that he knows his master has diabetes. A diabetic is never embarrassed by his dog. How often he wishes his friends were as considerate!

A dog is a diabetic's teacher. His dog shows the diabetic how to rest and sleep at odd moments, shows him how to exercise and play, indicates the value of sunshine, and sets him a good example by cleaning his paws every night. A dog is cheerful. The friends of a diabetic sometimes wish that he would take lessons from his dog.

From experiments on a dog Minkowski found out that diabetes originated in the pancreas. From experiments on a dog Allen learned that undereating helped and overeating harmed diabetes. From experiments on a dog Banting and Best discovered insulin.

When I see this little boy, George, and his dog, Bob, and their devotion to each other, I am reminded of the million diabetics and future diabetics in the United States who may not be holding dogs in their arms, yet are alive today or will be alive, enjoying better health and happiness, all because a few dogs, through the instrumentality of multitudes of scientific workers, have revolutionized the treatment of diabetes.

Would you want to be a member of a society if it had for its object the prevention of a dog's saving the life of a child? Do you think this dog, Bob, would want to join such a society?

Treatment of Diabetes

The treatment of diabetes is both simple and complex. It is simple in that a child can learn it; it is complex in that it is based on a combination of diet, exercise, and insulin. To bring out the point of the necessity for coöperation and harmony of action between all these three factors, it is a good plan for the diabetic to think of himself as a charioteer and that his three steeds are Diet, Exercise, and Insulin. If he is fortunate enough to have a country background he will know that to drive three horses successfully one must have training and practice. So it is with the charioteer of diabetes: he too must have training and practice, and there is no doubt that the diabetic who knows the most lives the longest.

Where shall the diabetic acquire his education? Shall he teach himself by listening to the radio and reading in books, by having a tutor in his home, by visiting the doctor's office or going to a hospital? It takes a bright individual to learn medicine over the wire or from the printed page, and even medical students can't do it; it is expensive to have a tutor. On the other hand, a few visits to a doctor's office, supplemented by the help of books and the radio, can start a patient on a right course. In the end, however, I recommend the hospital as the best and cheapest method for a diabetic to begin the treatment of his disease. In a hospital he learns from those about him and automatically learns from observation of other patients what treatment of his disease can accomplish or, because of ignorance or lack of coöperation on the part of the patient, has failed to accomplish. He can attend classes in diabetes. He can see the dangerous complications of the disease—coma, gangrene, and carbuncles—which careful attention on his part will enable him to avoid. His worries about diet and insulin largely disappear when he finds that children follow a diet without complaint and take their insulin as a matter of course. When one child watches another having his daily dose he gets ready for his own, realizing that after insulin comes food.

WEEK-END HOSPITAL TREATMENT

A day in a hospital is worth many visits to a doctor's office, and so strongly has experience forced this home upon me that in these days of financial depression I urge the week-end treatment of diabetes. In this way a patient spends on one or two occasions from Friday night to Monday morning at the hospital, and in this short time, if he is observant, he learns most of what he would acquire if he remained in the hospital a week, which is about the average stay of the uncomplicated diabetic today. During his week-end the teaching diabetic nurse will most likely hold a diabetic Sunday-school class and thus supplement her individual instruction. Week-end treatment protects

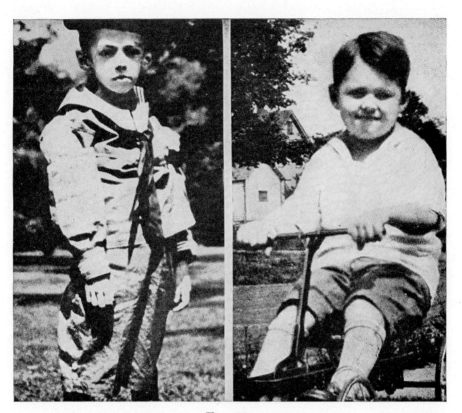

FIG. 70.

Left: A poor, starved diabetic boy, as he looked before insulin was available.
Right: The same boy as he looked afterwards.

the courage and the pocketbook of the patient, because he holds his job. Week-end treatment makes the hospital happy, because it raises the hospital Sunday census; and finally, the doctor does not complain, because it is a part of his life, and if he saves his patient a dollar, there is more chance that he will secure one for his own services. Indeed, it is a rather good plan to have the idea circulate through the community that a doctor expects to work at odd moments, that he will get up at night to bring your next baby into the world and that technicians, nurses and assistants are also willing to work for your health even though it is inconvenient.

HOME TREATMENT

Home treatment can be carried out, but it is most time-consuming for the physician. It is rendered easier if the neighboring hospital has a wandering diabetic nurse at the disposal of the physicians in its radius. Such a nurse can spend an hour or two a day in the home and gradually instruct the patient and his family. Such a nurse, well trained in diabetes, is of great advantage, because she knows from contact with many other patients the points in diet, exercise, and insulin which should be emphasized. Diabetics are not yet quite numerous enough to furnish practice for all nurses to learn about the disease in their courses of training, but I suspect that soon on the staff of every hospital and the staff of every community health organization, one or more nurses will be educated especially along diabetic lines and so be available for expert advice. Home treatment is all right if the doctors have the time for it and the patients the desire to learn.

PLAN YOUR VISIT TO YOUR DOCTOR

If you go to a doctor's office, save your time and his by handing him a list of what you ate at the last three meals. Have your questions ready, preferably in writing in a notebook with spaces reserved for the answers. Having learned how to make the simple Benedict test for sugar in the urine, show him your neat records of the results, so that he can decide what change, if any, shall be made in your treatment. It is a great thing to learn how to utilize a visit to a doctor. Plan for it, so that you can get the most out of it.

DIABETIC DIETS

A diabetic must live on a diet, but there is no one diet which will do for all diabetic patients. Furthermore, the same type of patient can be treated successfully by different sorts of diets providing one adheres to the principle *that the diabetic should never overeat* of any kind of food. Overeating helps to bring on diabetes; overeating makes the diabetes worse; overeating brings on the dread complication diabetic coma and therefore should always be avoided. This is the fundamental principle of diet to which all doctors adhere.

COMPOSITION OF DIET

The composition of the diabetic diet varies not only with the needs of each patient but also with the ideas of each doctor. Some physicians feel that the diabetic mechanism of the pancreas and liver should be protected, and as long as the body does not take care of the sugar and starch in the food we should give very little of these substances—the carbohydrates. Others believe excess of fat in the diet is harmful, that it interferes with the utilization of carbohydrate, and that if we keep the fat extremely low in the diet a patient's diabetic pancreas will be, so to speak, renovated and trained to use more carbohydrate. Of course, whether one gives a low carbohydrate or a high carbohydrate diet, the rest of the diet must be adjusted. It is just like a seesaw with one child Carbohydrate sitting on one end of the board and with the other child Fat on the other, and a third child, the third and essential component of the diet, Protein, in the center, helping the other two. When Carbohydrate goes up Fat must go down, and vice versa, or the patient will get too little or too much food. The whole question of the relative advantages of carbohydrate and fat is not settled. My advice is: do not go to extremes either way, and in the general directions which are listed below it is my purpose to state a mean which will represent the advice most doctors in the United States now give.

Carbohydrates

Diabetics like to eat. Therefore, give them bulky foods in which the percentage of sugar and starch, the so-called carbohydrate foods, is low. Such foods are the vegetables (the green vegetables, the vegetables which generally grow above ground), often termed 5 and 10 per cent vegetables. A saucerful of these vegetables contains about the same quantity of carbohydrate as is in a lump of sugar, and our trained diabetic children know that the weights of a lump of sugar and a five-cent piece are alike. In fact the nickel, with the buffalo on one side of it, is exactly five grams, or approximately one sixth of an ounce. Most patients today can eat four liberal portions of these vegetables each day, and as most of us are happy when eating, and these bulky vegetables require a long time to be eaten, their use permits many minutes of happiness. Consequently, four portions of these 5 per cent vegetables contain the equivalent of four lumps of sugar, the weight of four buffalo nickels, or 20 grams of carbohydrate. The

FOODS ARRANGED APPROXIMATELY ACCORDING TO CONTENT OF CARBOHYDRATE

5 per cent		10 per cent	15 per cent	20 per cent
1 per cent to 3 per cent	3 per cent to 5 per cent	10 per cent*	15 per cent	20 per cent
Lettuce	Tomatoes	String beans	Green peas	Potatoes
Cucumbers	Brussels	Pumpkin	Jerusalem	Shell beans
Spinach	sprouts	Turnip	artichokes	Baked beans
Asparagus	Watercress	Kohl-rabi	Parsnips	Green corn
Rhubarb	Sea kale	Squash	Lima beans,	Boiled rice
Endive	Okra	Beets	very young	Boiled
Marrow	Cauliflower	Carrots		macaroni
Sorrel	Eggplant	Onions		
Sauerkraut	Cabbages	Green peas,		
Beet greens	Leeks	very young		
Dandelions	String beans,			
Swiss chard	very young	Strawberries	Raspberries	Plums
Celery	Broccoli	Lemons	Currants	Bananas
Mushrooms	French	Cranberries	Apricots	Prunes
	artichokes	Peaches	Pears	Ice cream
		Pineapple	Apples	
Grapefruit		Blackberries	Blueberries	
		Oranges	Cherries	

*Reckon average carbohydrate in 5 per cent vegetables as 3 per cent; of 10 per cent vegetables as 6 per cent.

pleasure of eating one lump of sugar is over in a moment, but the satisfaction of eating an attractive portion of nice fresh vegetables lasts a good many minutes, and your stomach does not feel so hollow after it, either. Grapefruit is the safest fruit for a diabetic in that it contains only about 5 per cent carbohydrate. Half a medium-sized grapefruit is the equivalent in sugar of two buffalo nickels or 10 grams. Oranges contain 10 per cent carbohydrate, and a small orange weighs 100 grams and is equal to 10 grams of sugar, which is the same as the half medium-sized grapefruit represents. A banana contains 20 per cent carbohydrate, and as the ordinary banana weighs about 100 grams, half a banana would be equivalent in turn to the carbohydrate in a small orange or half a medium grapefruit. Often a cracker or biscuit can be found which contains 5 grams carbohydrate, because dry biscuits and toast are about 80 per cent starch. Such a one is a Uneeda biscuit. Potatoes and bananas, weight for weight, are alike in the percentage of carbohydrate, and it makes no difference whether they are cooked or not so far as the carbohydrate is concerned. Bread is three times as rich in carbohydrate as potatoes, and so, if a doctor allowed 90 grams or 3 ounces of potato, the patient could replace it with one third the amount of bread or 30 grams, 1 ounce, and this would be an ordinary slice of bread.

Diabetic vegetables, however, have other advantages in addition to the pleasure one derives while eating them. The sugar and starch in these low-carbohydrate vegetables take so long to get from the stomach into the blood that when the patient takes them his blood is not suddenly swamped with sugar, which would be the case if he took pure carbohydrate such as sugar or cornstarch. I often tell my patients that the carbohydrate in vegetables *creeps* into the blood, the carbohydrate in potatoes and in cooked rice or macaroni *walks* right into the blood, whereas actual sugar in the diet *runs* into the blood, and if the blood is overloaded with sugar, it spills over and leaks out through the kidneys. Still another great advantage which comes to the diabetic who eats freely of green vegetables and fruits is due to the vitamins which they contain. As I have said, perhaps it is because of all these vitamins in vegetables and fruits that diabetic children have such good teeth.

Protein

Tiny cells make up our bodies, and the essential component of these is protein. A horse likes his oats because there is more protein in the oats than in the straw. Protein we must have to replace old cells and to add new ones. Diabetics need protein just like the rest of us. Protein is found in concentrated form in meat, in fish, in eggs, and in its purest state in the white of an egg. The baby gets his protein in the curd or cheese of milk. The younger you are, the more protein you require, because not only have children worn-out cells to repair, but they need new cells to grow. Instinct teaches the baby to take three or four times as much protein for his weight as the old man. (Milk is an ideal food partly because it contains so much protein.)

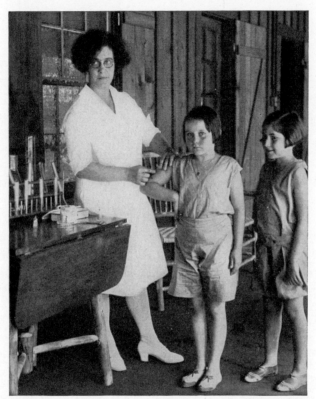

Courtesy of Wide World Photos, Cleveland.

FIG. 71.   Administration of insulin to children.

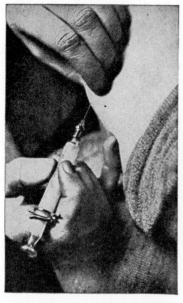

FIG. 73. Pinching up a fold of skin.

A fold of skin is pinched up; the syringe is held by the barrel, *not* by the plunger. Some spots feel the prick more than others; feel around with the needle.

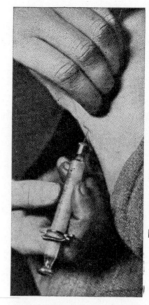

FIG. 75. Inserting the needle.

Then the plunger is pushed in; some prefer slowly, some fast. After pulling the needle out, it is conventional to hold the alcoholic cotton on the spot for a few seconds, rubbing it in!

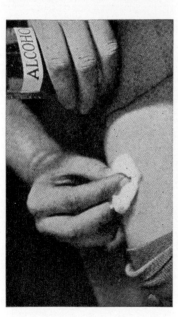

FIG. 72. Cleaning the skin.

The chosen spot on the skin is smartly rubbed with alcohol, a *different spot* each time: any convenient place on the body where a fold of skin can be picked up, but avoiding the *inner* surfaces of limbs.

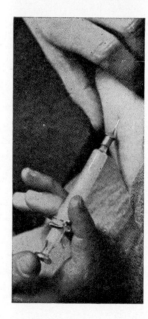

FIG. 74. Injecting the insulin.

The needle is *suddenly* jabbed home, its point landing about midway between the tips of thumb and finger, well beneath the skin, yet not into the solid muscle; either hurts more. The needle goes *straight ahead*, so as not to bend or break it.

Fortunately diabetics can have as much protein as the ordinary individual and only seldom should have more.

Fat

Fat is the third component of the diet. This is to be found in a pure state in oil. Butter is 85 per cent fat, and cream is a transition from this percentage to the 3 per cent in milk as established by law. There is fat in meat and fish, and one should never forget that in nuts and cheese the percentages of fat are high. A generation ago we doctors reduced the carbohydrate (sugar and starch) in the diet of our dia-

CARBOHYDRATE, PROTEIN, FAT, AND CALORIES IN VARIOUS FOODS*

30 Grams 1 oz. Contain approximately	Carbohydrate Grams	Protein Grams	Fat Grams	Calories
Vegetables 5 per cent	1	0.5	0	6
Vegetables 10 per cent	2	0.5	0	10
Shredded wheat	23	3	0	104
Uneedas, two	10	1	1	53
Potato	6	1	0	28
Bread	18	3	0	84
Oatmeal, dry wgt.	20	5	2	118
Milk	1.5	1	1	19
Meat (cooked, lean)	0	8	5	77
Fish	0	6	0	24
Egg (one)	0	6	6	78
Cheese	0	8	11	131
Bacon	0	5	15	155
Cream, 20 per cent	1	1	6	62
Cream, 40 per cent	1	1	12	116
Brazil nuts........................	2	5	20	208
Butter	0	0	25	225
Oil	0	0	30	270

*Convenient values for a diabetic to know:
1 gram protein   = 4 calories.   1 kilogram = 2.2 pounds.
1 gram carbohydrate = 4 calories.   30 grams (g.) or cubic centimeters (c.c.) = 1 ounce.
1 gram fat   = 9 calories.   A patient "at rest" requires 25 calories per kg.

betic patients so low that we were compelled to raise the fat to furnish them enough nourishment to keep alive, and we overdid it. What happened? We satisfied their hunger, but we poisoned them with fat, because in the fat lurked danger. Soon we found out through the painstaking work of many laboratories that if the proportion of fat to carbohydrate in any diet was unduly high, the fat failed to be of use and indeed broke up into fatty acids which in turn caused acid poisoning and death from coma. For this reason today the fat in the diet of diabetics is watched quite as closely as the carbohydrate, and for this same reason we are testing the fat in the blood as well as the sugar to be sure it is not in excess.

As a rule the diabetic is given as much sugar and starch (carbohydrate) as he can take without sugar appearing in the urine, and if he cannot tolerate a considerable quantity, he is given insulin to help him get the benefit of it. He takes as much protein as the ordinary individual. As for the quantity of fat, he regulates that by what he needs to hold his weight, which seldom if ever should long remain above normal standards.

In the tables on p. 583 are recorded foods with varying percentages of carbohydrate, and, for certain commonly used foods, the quantities of carbohydrate, protein, and fat per 30 grams or one ounce. The values are approximate and not absolute.

A Diabetic's Menu

The average diet prescribed for a diabetic in the United States today, I suspect, is about as follows, and if it is not tolerated, the patient's doctor will probably give him insulin.

Breakfast:
Half a grapefruit, a medium portion of oatmeal or a little less of any other cereal, two eggs or one egg and bacon, a pat of butter, coffee and cream.

Dinner (noon):
A moderate portion of meat or fish, two liberal portions of 5 per cent vegetables or somewhat less of 10 per cent vegetables, a slice of bread or a medium-sized potato, a pat of butter, an orange or its equivalent.

Night:
A similar meal to that at noon.

During the day:
Half a pint of medium cream.

With such a diet as a working basis, it is easy to add to it or detract from it according to the needs of the individual patient and to make definite the quantity of carbohydrate, protein, and fat. Such a diet probably contains carbohydrate 100 to 120 grams, protein 65 to 75 grams, and fat 80 to 120 grams.

Calories

If one wishes, such a diet can be reckoned in calories.

Food	Calories per Gram	Carbohydrate in Diet	Total Calories
Carbohydrate	4	100	400
Protein	4	75	300
Fat	9	100	900
			1600

An individual needs from 100 to 25 calories per kilogram (2.2 pounds) body weight, according to whether he is a baby or an old man. The above diet would be about right for a young adult who weighs 110 pounds or 50 kilograms, because it would furnish a little over 30 calories per kilogram body weight.

EXERCISE

The second steed in the diabetic's three-horse chariot is exercise. Years ago I learned his value from a diabetic patient who did unusually well. His favorable progress puzzled me, but after studying his case, it finally came over me that besides being a reliable patient and adhering to his diet, he did well because he exercised. He worked on a railroad, and railroad workmen are reliable, but apart from this I found out that his particular job was to drive an old-fashioned handcar and inspect the tracks over a stretch of many miles. Back and forth he bent his back to turn the crank of his handcar morning and afternoon in those days when one's motor was made of muscles, not steel, and in this way he could assimilate the carbohydrate which he ate. This man showed me the value of exercise in diabetes. About the same time I had a diabetic doctor, and he told me there was less sugar in his urine when he was camping and tramping and carrying his canoe in the depths of the woods in Maine than at home, where his diet was more strict and his exercise far less. Then I began to have all my patients exercise. Exercise does everything for a diabetic, but there are limitations. To drive this horse, Exercise, along with Diet and Insulin, requires judgment, and one must often lower the load for Exercise and increase it for Insulin. Exercise is good for the diabetic of mild or moderate severity, but for the severest diabetics before we had insulin, exercise did harm, and only recently a few patients told me they got along better if they stayed abed. They found out they must not work their machine too hard. In general, however, any patient who cannot exercise is handicapped. Such was the fate of the rare diabetic prior to the use of insulin who was crippled with rheumatism. One reliable patient tells me a game of golf is worth five units of insulin. Today doctors are careful to provide exercise in one form or another for their diabetics who must stay abed as a result of operations or for other reasons. Exercise should be utilized in the treatment of nearly every case of diabetes, but this steed must not be overdriven.

INSULIN

The announcement of the discovery of insulin in Toronto in 1921 brought hope to the diabetic, and its general introduction in 1922 brought him life. It is one of the three major medical discoveries thus far of the twentieth century. Even today none of us wholly realizes the good which insulin has done. *First of all, insulin enables a diabetic child to live, but, best of all, to grow and be happy.* Insulin protects the diabetic mother. Insulin allows the diabetic doctor, lawyer, teacher, laborer to resume his occupation and again to play an active part in the community. Years ago, before we had insulin or knew as much as we do now about diet, nearly one fifth of all diabetics died the very first year of their disease, and most of them were invalids. Today only one twenty-fifth die the first year, and this number is made up almost exclusively of old men and old women and of diabetics who have sustained medical or other accidents. Even if we do not grant to insulin the whole responsibility for the prolongation and protection of the lives of diabetics, it surely is responsible for 99 per cent of their joy, because it affords them the opportunity to satisfy their longing for food and their desire to act as live men and live women and, if children, to rejoice in their play.

Insulin comes from a gland, the pancreas or the sweetbread, which lies behind the stomach in the upper abdomen. No one can live without insulin. Insulin regulates the percentage of sugar in the blood. If this percentage is too high, insulin removes the excess sugar and stores it as starch in the liver and muscles and skin. Starch is an insoluble form of carbohydrate and thus is suitable for storage just as sugar is soluble and, if not used, is lost in the urine. For most of us our own pancreases suffice. The cells of the pancreas are so closely in touch with the demand and supply of insulin in the body that if there is ever a surplus or deficit of insulin in a normal person we consider

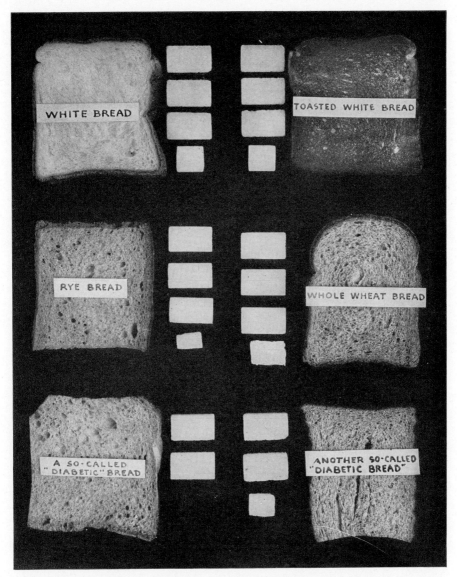

FIG. 76. Portions of different breads, all with dimensions the same as those of the slice of white bread in the upper left-hand corner.

The sugar-forming power of each bread is illustrated by lumps of table sugar. Thus, the slice of white bread yields three lumps and a fraction. The diabetic breads yield less sugar but not enough less to make them useful for rigidly restricted diets.

it an anomaly. If we eat much carbohydrate, the pancreas makes enough insulin to care for it, and the insulin factory is so delicately adjusted to the amount of sugar which should be in the blood that it does not allow this to vary as much as a teaspoonful. Sometimes normal individuals who burn up during violent exercise most of their

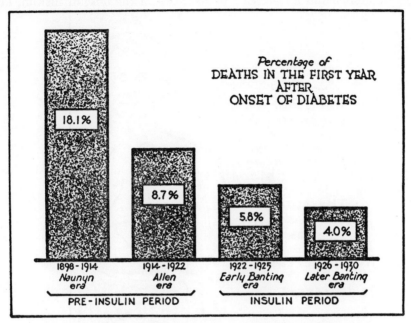

FIG. 77. Decline in mortality among diabetics. Comparison between pre-insulin and insulin period.

The value of insulin in the treatment of diabetics is clearly shown by the rapidly decreasing proportion of deaths in the first year of the disease.

reserve starch (glycogen) and sugar in the body as a result of a Marathon run, a football game, or a four-mile boat race, suffer because exercise has done the work of insulin. Today trainers give to such athletes carbohydrate, tea with sugar, orange juice, etc., to offset the deficiency. Even a healthy child may go without a meal, and his pancreas may not stop manufacturing insulin soon enough, and as a result the blood sugar is reduced so low that he becomes unconscious. Recently four such cases were reported. The diabetic differs chiefly from the normal person in that his pancreas produces too little insulin, and to make up for the lack of insulin he must buy it. Few persons' intelligence is equal to their instinct, and so it is not strange that the diabetic occasionally buys too much and gives himself an overdose of insulin. He is the one above all others who must learn what he needs, and no doctor can decide as well as the patient himself what the dose of insulin should be. Few patients at first recognize the symptoms which demand an increase or decrease in the dose of insulin, but

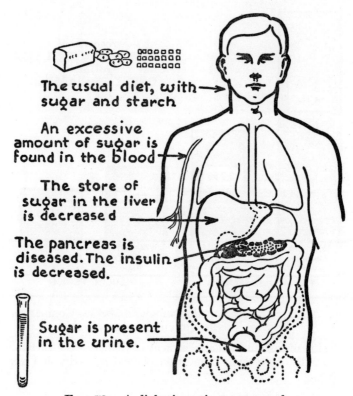

The usual diet, with sugar and starch →

An excessive amount of sugar is found in the blood

The store of sugar in the liver is decreased

The pancreas is diseased. The insulin is decreased.

Sugar is present in the urine.

FIG. 78.   A diabetic patient untreated.

The pancreas of a person with diabetes makes so little insulin that an excess of sugar is left in the body.

the diabetic of several years' duration does know these, and with the help of his physician he finally arrives at the proper amount which his system requires from day to day.

At one time it was the belief that a diabetic got worse the longer he lived, but today we know that this is not necessarily true. Diabetics can improve, and now it is a fact that the doctor must be as alert to

detect his patient's getting better as he was formerly to note a downward course. Fortunately, every diabetic manufactures some insulin, even though the quantity is small, but we cannot tell yet how much a pancreas can be repaired, renewed, or how much it can grow when conditions are favorable. It is my impression that the belief is becoming general among doctors that the diabetic's pancreas is not so bad

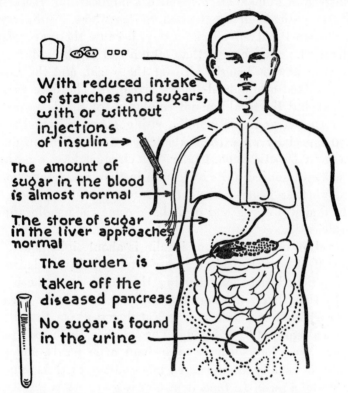

With reduced intake of starches and sugars, with or without injections of insulin →

The amount of sugar in the blood is almost normal

The store of sugar in the liver approaches normal

The burden is taken off the diseased pancreas

No sugar is found in the urine

FIG. 79. A diabetic patient adequately treated.

Before each meal, the patient with severe diabetes must supplement his small supply of insulin with an extra amount obtained from an animal.

a pancreas after all, and that the reason a diabetic acquires his disease is not because his pancreas is destroyed, but rather because it is not acting as it should. The possibility is still open that someone will discover a means by which the lazy cells in the diabetic's pancreas can be waked up and made to go to work, and I am hoping that in diabetes that discovery will be the next one. My idea is that there is greater hope for the diabetic along this line than for a form of insulin which can be given by mouth instead of under the skin.

For patients who complain about taking insulin under the skin I have no sympathy. When I see a child who is six years old or even two and a half years old who gives himself or herself insulin and does not complain about it, it disgusts me to have an adult find fault. To buy insulin instead of to make it one's self is a bugbear, but there are very few diabetic patients in the United States whose insulin need cost them more than twenty-five cents a day, because there are very, very few patients who require more than 50 units of insulin a day.

Insulin can now be bought all over the world, and the League of Nations has fixed a standard for its strength. The dose varies with each patient, but the total amount employed for the day ranges, as a rule, between ten and thirty units, rising above this in the severer cases, and especially when the diabetic has a complication due to an infection or to diabetic coma. Under such circumstances a patient may require several hundred units of insulin in the twenty-four hours. An infection, whether general like influenza or local like a boil, always makes the diabetes worse, and in diabetic coma the insulin appears to act less efficiently.

The duration of the action of insulin is about eight hours, and its maximum effect occurs within an hour after it is injected. Insulin, as already mentioned, acts by removing the sugar from the blood and storing it in the liver, the muscles, and the skin in the form of an insoluble carbohydrate, animal starch (glycogen) so that it can be utilized when required by the body. The sugar in the blood rises to its highest level from half an hour to an hour after meals, and to offset this, insulin is usually administered one quarter to three quarters of an hour before a meal. In fact, if insulin is given when the stomach is empty, it may lower the sugar in the blood so quickly that the symptoms of an overdose, the so-called insulin reaction, appear. Many patients require insulin before only one meal a day, but most patients require it twice, a few three times, and rarely it is necessary to give it four times. During infections the patient may require it every three or four hours, and in the treatment of a patient unconscious with diabetic coma it is often administered every thirty minutes until improvement begins to take place.

Insulin is given by injection just under the skin. The patient should be systematic about this and not use the same spot of the skin for an

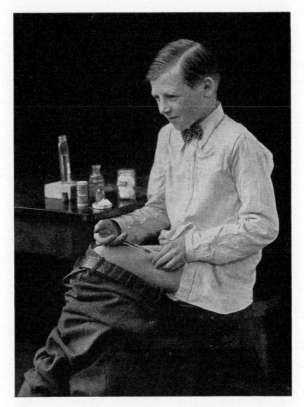

FIG. 80.   Self subcutaneous administration of
insulin by child.

It doesn't hurt. Insulin cannot be taken by
mouth. It must be injected hypodermically because it is destroyed in the stomach by the
digestive juices. Beware of the quack who
claims that his medicine, to be taken by mouth,
is as good as insulin. Along his road lies death.

injection oftener than once a month. A little planning will provide for this. If insulin is always injected in one place, lumps may appear, because the tissues are injured. As a result the insulin is incompletely absorbed, and the patient does not get his money's worth. And this is not the whole story, because in the injured tissue an infection may start. Abscesses from the injection of insulin, however, are exceptionally rare and usually are due only to gross neglect. This is partly accounted for by the antiseptic which is added to the insulin during its preparation.

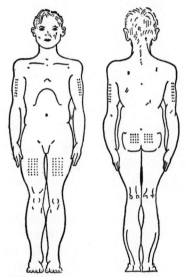

Fig. 81. These insulin maps shows the regions of the body where insulin may best be injected.

The proper dose of insulin is not always easily determined because of the uncertainty as to when or how much the patient will eat or the amount of exercise that he has had or is to take. Obviously the trained patient who injects his own insulin can decide all this better than the doctor. Furthermore, sometimes people eat a meal—and this especially occurs with children—but fail to digest it, or, if seasick, lose it, and so the insulin which may have been given with the expectation that the patient would eat has no food to work upon. If food remains in the stomach and so does not reach the blood, it is the same as if no food had been taken at all. For all these reasons it is not uncommon to see a patient who has had an overdose of insulin with a resulting "insulin reaction." Insulin is a drug, and from an overdose of any drug symptoms will result.

The symptoms which result from an overdose of insulin are much the same as those which occur in several other well known states. Thus if one has been without food for many hours and even fasted, the percentage of sugar in the blood is lowered and may fall as low as after too much insulin. Above I referred to the report of normal children who were taken to the hospital unconscious because of delayed meals. I suspect that the old monks and anchorites, who wandered about the deserts and undertook long periods of fasting, often had experiences akin to those who have an insulin reaction: The sugar in their blood dropped; they became faint and feeble; their hands trembled; their minds were clouded and hallucinations appeared; they fell into trance-like states and could not be aroused. The common symptoms of an insulin reaction are weakness, faintness and hunger; because trembling occurs patients often call these reactions the "shakes." Sweating, numbness, tingling of the lips, even unconsciousness, can come on quite rapidly and if the dose of insulin has been extreme the patient may have a convulsion. Indeed there are on record occasional instances where the diabetic has been supposed to have epilepsy when in reality he had nothing of the sort. An examination of the sugar in the blood will quickly show the true nature of the condition. All diabetics are warned about these reactions, and all diabetics taking insulin are in the habit of carrying one or two lumps of sugar or an orange in their pockets. By eating the sugar or the orange when they recognize the approach of a reaction, they can quickly raise the sugar in the blood and ward off untoward symptoms. If the sugar is taken, it acts rapidly. I have seen a child lying unconscious on the floor in an insulin reaction and three minutes after he was given a teaspoonful of syrup get up and chase his little railroad cars around the room. Obviously it is too dangerous for a locomotive engineer to take insulin unless it is given before his evening meal, so that twelve or more hours will intervene before he gets into his cab. An insulin reaction might come on quickly. Automobilists who take insulin invariably should eat 10 grams of carbohydrate (an orange, two lumps of sugar, or the equivalent of half a slice of bread or half a banana) if they drive a car more than two hours after a meal. A patient using insulin should carry his name, address and directions for treatment of an insulin reaction, so that he can be protected if such a reaction comes on unawares and in strange surroundings. Nondiabetics can also advantageously bear in mind the dangers of being too hungry.

Various attempts have been made to give insulin in other ways than under the skin, but none are practicable. One must allow that there are annoyances in giving insulin, but it is surprising to see how few patients are disturbed by the injections. These are the least of their troubles, and this holds particularly for children who become accustomed to the treatment. However, it is always wise to teach a child early how to take his insulin for himself. He soon will find out that when he gives the injection himself it causes far less discomfort than when it is given by anyone else, and he soon adopts this plan as a matter of course because of its comfort and convenience and the independence which it allows. Furthermore, unless a child is taught at the beginning to accept the injections of insulin, he may get the habit of resisting them, and needless trouble to the family ensues. "Train up a child in the way he should go and when he is old he will not depart therefrom."

The Usefulness of Diabetes

It seems hardly conceivable that a disease should be useful, but really diabetes is a disease which has much to recommend it. We need our diabetics. The diabetic sets an example in cleanliness to his family, his friends, and, in fact, to all his neighbors. He is taught to be the cleanest citizen in the community, because if he keeps his skin in good condition, the chances for complications are slight, and in this way he avoids the carbuncles and boils and inflammations of the skin which years ago were a most annoying accompaniment of the disease. The diabetic is useful because he sets an example for temperance in eating, for control of weight. He is an instructor in dietetics, and he diffuses through his family a practical knowledge of the properties and values of foods. He understands the meaning of a balanced diet. He knows that his 5 per cent vegetables, his fruit, his cream, his egg, and his cod-liver oil contain priceless vitamins. Diabetes is particularly useful because it is so evidently associated with overweight that it directs attention to the dangers of overweight in general, for these are by no means limited to diabetes. For years the insurance companies have pointed out that the expectation of life of the fat person is far less than that of the one of standard weight, because the fat person is more liable to diseases of the heart and the arteries.

Diabetes is useful because it brings before the public the advantage of coöperation between the physician and patient in the treatment of a chronic disease. The diabetic patient who does the best is the one who knows the most about the disease, and this soon becomes apparent to all onlookers. He thus demonstrates that it is desirable for the ordinary individual to know something about diseases, and particularly his own disease, so that he and his doctor can work in partnership. The diabetic is useful because today we know that diabetes is to a certain extent hereditary, and, having the disease, the patient must stop and think before he gets married. Not only must he consider whether he can take care of himself or herself, but he also must consider the health of his future partner before he gets engaged, because one diabetic should not marry another diabetic. In other words, the diabetic will spread the knowledge of eugenics, and when we remember the one million diabetics, or diabetics to be, now living in the United States, the necessity of thoughtfulness on their part before they have children will be taught them and through them pass to the community as a whole. One can see how this idea of more care in contracting marriages will be spread. Almost any thoughtful father today demands a report of the physical examination and Wassermann reaction of the suitor of his daughter before he consents to her marriage.

I feel that the diabetic who lives long lives usefully and that he deserves recognition. Unless he had used judgment in diet and treatment and care of his body his duration of life would have been short. Therefore, I believe a diabetic who has lived longer with his disease than he was expected to live without it at the time it began should be given a medal in recognition of it. Such a practice has been followed, and for the encouragement of patients I can say that I know of more than two hundred diabetics who have received such medals. And Amelia Peabody, the designer, placed on the reverse side of the medal a child in a boat sailing toward the rising sun with this inscription, *"Explorers of Diabetes,"* because it is the child who is leading the way.

A diabetic in the home after all may be an asset. To sum up, he knows about cleanliness, diet, the dangers of overweight, the use of a drug, the importance of heredity, and hence it is no wonder that often he lives long. He and his confrères constitute a great experimental laboratory for the benefit of the human race. I tell my diabetic children that each honest diabetic day they live is a great help to some diabetic old man or old woman, because from their young lives we learn how to treat those whose vitality and recuperative powers are less.

DIABETICS AND OLD AGE

As I have already said, diabetes is predominantly a disease of older people. Two thirds of the cases begin above the age of forty years, the most common years for its onset are fifty for women and fifty-three years for men. The patients live long, and the average age at death, which half a generation ago was forty-four years, is now well above sixty years. Finally, medals have been given in one clinic alone to more than 200 patients who have lived longer with the disease than they were expected to live without it when it was first acquired. But despite all this it is regrettably true that up to the present time it has been the rule for diabetics to grow old too fast. This had long been suspected for the middle-aged diabetic, but it is in the children that the proof appeared. When the children lived only two or three years, of course this was rarely evident, but as improvements in diet came and children lived longer, the very same changes were noted in them which one sees in aging adults. Their arteries began to harden, the condition known as arteriosclerosis, and one could not only feel the hardening, but see the deposits of lime by X-ray examinations of the blood vessels of the legs. More important than the changes in the blood vessels of the legs were those in the arteries of the heart, and in comparatively young people it was found that clots in these vessels (coronary thrombosis) caused death just as in mature individuals. Sadder by far was another change of old age, which came on in the eyes, and as many as fourteen diabetic children in one clinic showed cataracts. I should hesitate even to record all this if it were not possible to add that in the last few years we know that in children this early aging has stopped or at least has been deferred. Today we do not see it in the children who have been treated with the more liberal diets which insulin allows.

Old age has been deferred because insulin permits the diabetic today to eat nearly as freely as the normal individual. How can we help advancing the argument that if modern treatment has stopped arteriosclerosis in diabetic children and is deferring it in the middle-aged diabetics there must have been something harmful in his disease or perhaps in our treatment of it years ago which was responsible for it? And is it not fascinating to seek for the greatest common divisor in the multitude of factors which caused this rapid growing old?

First of all, the evidence points to overeating, and particularly to the diabetic's having overeaten, because we doctors urged it, I must allow, of fat. For a long while the insurance companies have insisted that the man or woman above fifty was not a good risk if he or she was fat, and although this has appeared to be due to the overweight itself, it is possible the additional fat tissue itself in the body has been the reason. At any rate, since our diabetic children have eaten less fat and have assimilated it better, and replaced it with more carhohydrate food which insulin has permitted, we have noticed less hardening of the arteries.

In our deductions we come from overweight to fat, fat tissue, and fat food and diet. One would like to find out what special kind of fatty food it is which makes people grow old. As yet we are not certain, but research in chemistry is helping us make progress. This special fat, cholesterol, in eggs is the same sort which is present in the arteries of diabetics, but up to now we are unable to say that eggs are really bad for diabetics or are productive of old age in anyone. However, eggs seem more appropriate for chickens and children than for old roosters and hens or men and women, and after fifty years of age it is a pretty good bet that one egg a day is enough for anybody. We are, however, absolutely sure of this: that diabetics especially should not be fat, and that if they cannot get a reasonably balanced diet without insulin it is safer for them to take it so as to be able to have more carbohydrate and less fat than in the old days.

It is not easy to tell a diabetic how to avoid the accidents which occur from hardening of the arteries in the heart, such as coronary thrombosis and angina pectoris, in the brain, such as a stroke, a shock, or in the kidneys, Bright's disease, except that he must live the simple life and one free from mental, physical, and emotional excitements. On the other hand, there are very specific directions which the diabetic should follow to prevent the serious effects which go with hardening of the arteries of the legs: namely, gangrene.

DIABETIC GANGRENE

Diabetic gangrene, next to heart disease, is responsible for more deaths among diabetics than any other cause. The hardened arteries m the legs make the circulation poor. An injury to the skin, which would be of little or no account in a young or healthy person, in a diabetic heals slowly or not at all. Unless the skin is kept scrupulously clean, poisonous germs may get into superficial wounds, grow and spread, and very often a leg must be sacrificed to save a life. Old diabetics suffer especially from gangrene. This is not strange, because old people hear less well, see less clearly, and feel less acutely, too, than the young, and thus they often cut themselves when they are caring for their feet, and then either don't see what they have done or don't feel it. In this way trifling injuries progress, and the poor old man or woman may not realize for days or even weeks that a serious condition has developed. It all goes on so gradually that when at last the patients go to a surgeon and he says a toe, a foot, a leg, must be amputated, it comes as a great shock. Every diabetic should care for his feet, or if he can't see well, get someone to do this for him. Chiropodists are a great help to diabetics. They know the dangers of neglected conditions in the feet of a diabetic and can recognize when the patient should see a surgeon.

Care of the Feet

Injuries to the feet in the old must be avoided. New shoes should first be put on at night and worn for an hour or two. Shoe linings should not be broken; one should carefully avoid protruding nails in the shoe. The shoes should be large enough and long enough and flexible enough. The stockings should be whole, and if the feet are deformed with bunions, calluses, or corns, the shoes should be adjusted to overcome these difficulties. As the sensation is poor in the feet the diabetic should avoid exposure to their being burned or frozen. A woman from cold Canada came to the hospital having burned her toes before an open fire; a woman from Cape Cod with its relatively mild climate entered, having frostbitten toes. A great many burn their feet with hot-water bottles and electric pads or even with hot water. We don't dare to trust the patients to use hot applications, because their skins are so lacking in sensation that they often do not feel pain.

The circulation in the legs of old people and of diabetics particularly should not be obstructed with round garters or by crossing the knees. It is a good plan to teach them to change the position of the legs often. Therefore we encourage patients to move about, and then to place their feet on a chair or stool or chaise longue, and sometimes go so far as to have them raise their legs for two minutes on an inclined board placed in the bed at an angle of forty-five degrees, then hang them down out of the bed for three minutes, then rest them in a horizontal position for five minutes, repeating this cycle six times an hour for even three hours a day. Repeatedly I have known this to stop pains and help to heal an indolent ulcer on a toe. But it is far better to prevent the ulcer.

Diabetics cannot be too careful of their feet.

Nearly half of the diabetics who die in hospitals die of gangrene, and fully one fifth of all diabetics reach their end because of troubles with their legs.

Every diabetic should keep his feet as clean as his face.

Every old diabetic should show his feet to his doctor at each visit.

So serious have we found these complications in the feet that each year we increase preventive measures. Kind friends have been so impressed with the necessity of the prevention of all this nearly useless sadness and pain that they have provided in the hospital a beauty parlor for diabetic feet, and each diabetic is there instructed. Similarly I believe each hospital which treats diabetics should have a chiropodist on its staff.

INFECTIONS

Infections make a diabetic worse. Before the discovery and use of insulin the occurrence of an infection in a diabetic was a very serious matter, and a great number of patients succumbed to them. I remember one well-known physician who in the pre-insulin days predicted that pneumonia in a diabetic would invariably be fatal, but in these days of insulin we can combat infections successfully, although we recognize their gravity. During an infection it may be necessary to double, triple, or even quadruple the dose of insulin to hold the disease in control. Therefore, whenever possible, infections should be avoided and sources of infections should be removed. Abscessed teeth should be extracted; really infected tonsils should be taken out; an infected gall bladder or appendix should be eliminated, and any pimple, boil, or run-a-round about a nail or callus on a foot should receive prompt attention. Particularly is it desirable in children to remove an appendix if there is history of an attack of appendicitis, because the early symptoms and signs of diabetic coma can be easily confused with appendicitis.

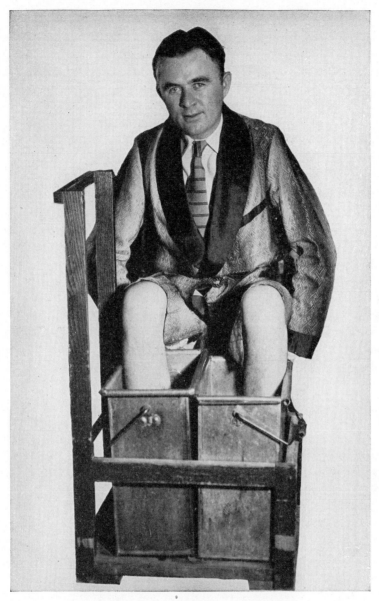

FIG. 82.   Contrast baths.

The diabetic with poor circulation in the feet can be helped by "contrast baths." To exercise the nerves to the blood vessels, the feet are placed alternately in warm and in cool water. They are left in each bath for one minute, and the exercise is continued for fifteen minutes.

When an infection is in progress in a diabetic it may be necessary to give the insulin every three or four hours; it is administered according to the results of the tests of the urine for sugar. Thus some doctors prescribe fifteen units for a red test with Benedict's solution, ten for a yellow test, five for a green test, and no insulin if the test is blue, showing no sugar. Mothers soon learn to vary the dosage of insulin which even so mild an infection as a common cold in a child may demand. Fortunately, when the infection subsides, the dose of insulin can be reduced to its former level. This makes us conclude that infections do not injure the pancreas or indeed cause diabetes, but in some other way interfere with the diabetic state. By having all his lurking infections promptly treated, the diabetic may score a few points of health over the nondiabetic who is neglectful or careless about the same.

Remember an infection makes the diabetics worse.

Get rid of all infections.

DIABETIC COMA

Only a generation ago sixty diabetics in each one hundred died of diabetic coma, yet today a death from diabetic coma is as needless as a death from diphtheria. All patients must learn how to escape it. Once we thought diabetic coma was the culmination of the disease, its final stage, and that it came on only in the severe diabetic, but now we know that it may occur in many of the milder cases and frequently in the very earliest stages, so that the diagnosis of the disease is first made when the patient is unconscious.

If you are a diabetic and want to dodge diabetic coma, or if you are a relative or a friend of a diabetic and wish to prevent it in your relative or friend, the rules are plain.

RULES TO AVOID AND PREVENT DIABETIC COMA

If you feel sick, take no chances, but call it coma and

1. Go to bed.
2. Call the doctor.
3. Take a cupful of a hot drink—water, coffee, tea, broth, strained oatmeal gruel—every hour.
4. Get someone to care for you.
5. Move the bowels with an enema.
6. Keep warm.

The symptoms of the onset of diabetic coma are notoriously obscure, and long ago I gave up trying to teach them. The patient usually feels "sick" and has nausea or vomiting; often he has broken his diet; he may have developed an infection and not realized that he required more insulin; he may have drawn too heavily on his own body fat because of extreme exercise or lack of food. (Too much fat is bad for

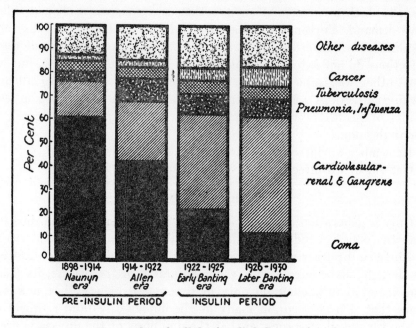

FIG. 83. From what do diabetics die? Comparison between pre-insulin and insulin period.

Thanks to insulin, diabetics now live longer. Deaths among them today are usually due to conditions typical of old age and much less often from coma.

a diabetic, no matter whether it is his own body fat or some other kind of fat.) Perhaps he has been seasick, perhaps he has goiter and thus, not getting enough food, he is living on his own body fat for nourishment to the exclusion of carbohydrate, which either he has not taken or has been unable to utilize because of want of insulin, either his own or that which he buys. He is weak, irritable, tired, nervous, and begins to have difficulty in breathing. All this comes on slowly and slyly: that is the reason for telling him if he feels sick to go to bed, get the doctor, and to call it the onset of diabetic coma until the doctor proves it otherwise. Even before the doctor arrives, the cupful of hot liquid every hour will help to wash out of the body the fatty acids which cause the coma.

The onset of coma is slow, but its course is fast, and its outcome in death or recovery usually takes place in twenty-four hours, so that treatment must be prompt and active. Hence the patient needs a nurse or someone to care for him at once. As one patient put it, even get your mother-in-law, because it is touch and go. What is done for you the first two hours is worth more than what can be done for you the next twelve hours. The children know this. So do the well-trained hospital patients. When they get sick they telephone their doctors and start treatment immediately, and thus the coma is stopped before it gets a headway. If the patient becomes advanced so far in coma that he is nearly unconscious, then it means a day-and-night job for the doctor and the nurse to bring him out of it and maybe a week or two to convalesce. An hour of prevention or early treatment saves a week of hospital stay.

DIABETIC COMA NEEDLESS

Diabetic patients will never go into diabetic coma if they live on their diets, keep their urines sugar free, and are careful about their insulin. They must remember, however, that infections make a diabetic worse and so make necessary changes in the doses of insulin. Patients must not omit a regular dose of insulin without testing the urine within six hours to note its effect. A little experience will protect them.

DANGERS OF DIABETIC COMA

If a diabetic patient can get into a hospital with a laboratory in which tests can be performed by night as well as by day, his chances for recovery from coma are good, and the younger he is the better they are. Of seventy children with diabetic coma only one died, but I have heard of only one person as old as seventy-three who had an attack and lived. That patient is now seventy-five years old and is bright and happy.

The patient may be unconscious and yet not have diabetic coma, but be unconscious from other causes, and the danger is then imminent that he be treated for the wrong condition. Accidentally he may have taken too much of a drug to produce sleep or relieve pain. He may have had too much insulin. He may have had a stroke of apoplexy or some temporary nervous trouble which has made him unconscious. Children not uncommonly are unconscious at the beginning of various diseases, or even in health if long without food. The picture is very confusing if an appendicitis is beginning, and that is why it is so desirable to remove the appendix in a diabetic if there is a history of its being diseased.

The consequences of a wrong diagnosis between the unconsciousness of diabetic coma and an overdose of insulin (insulin shock) are tragic and, I regret to say, in a few instances fatal. Therefore every diabetic should carry an identification card in his pocket, so that if by accident he should become unconscious from any cause, the strange doctor who first sees him will be given a hint of his condition.

An example of such a confusing situation is shown by the following incident. An old colored preacher whose kidneys were bad and his blood pressure high in pipe-stem arteries became unconscious, and his wife thought he was having a stroke. At first, on reaching the hospital, this appeared to be the diagnosis, but a bright young house officer examined his blood and found the blood sugar to be below normal. He injected a little sugar into the vein and—a miracle—the colored clergyman was brought back to life. If that young doctor had made a mistake and treated him for diabetic coma and injected insulin instead of sugar, in the place of a miracle there would have been a funeral. What happened was this: The pious old darkey took his insulin as usual before breakfast, and then went into his garden. He worked hard, so hard, in fact, that his steed Exercise did all the work of his steed Insulin. Insulin ran away with his blood sugar and sent it 'way below normal. The patient should have realized that the diabetic who takes unwonted exercise is entitled to an orange or a little additional carbohydrate in some other form. The extra carbohydrate would have protected him.

DIABETIC CAMPS

Although the lot of diabetic children is steadily improving and they now enter into all the activities of a normal child, they carry heavy responsibilities. At each meal they are reminded of their disease; two or three times a day they must have an insulin injection;

constantly their every act is watched, and they cannot help seeing the apprehension which their parents feel for them. Diabetic children need a respite, and for them the late Dr. Wendt of Detroit some six years ago planned a diabetic camp. In the following year Mrs. Devine at Ogunquit opened her camp for diabetic children, and little by little these camps have sprung up in various parts of the country. Under the supervision of Dr. Priscilla White at the New England Deaconess Hospital, eighty-seven diabetic girls and boys are attending such camps this summer. We have found these camps to be most advantageous and strongly recommend their enlargement.

The change of food and surroundings, which a trip away from home involves, and the contact with many others, who have the same disease, along with the pleasures of camp life, are splendid for the children. The revision of diets and dosage of insulin while under supervision which is as close as that in a hospital and yet not so obvious gives an excellent opportunity to improve treatment. But these camps soon disclosed another useful feature of almost equal value, and that was the vacation they provided for the parents and the entire household. It is no joke to have the responsibility of a diabetic child day and night for years, and we soon learned that the mothers were quite as thankful for the freedom from care and the vacation they received as were the children themselves.

The diabetic camp is an educational institution. To the Clara Barton Camp at North Oxford, Worcester County, Mass., we invited several hundred doctors. For them were given demonstrations by the doctors, nurses, dietitian, and technician associated with the camp, and by the children themselves. These camps will not make permanent islands of safety within a radius of twenty miles of every diabetic, but at least they will serve as floating islands from which the knowledge of diabetes can diffuse in widening circles.

When I see these happy diabetic children in their camp I realize more than ever that a diabetic should go to a school instead of to a hospital, because he needs to be classed with students rather than with the sick, and that hospitalization should be reserved chiefly for diabetic emergencies and as a preliminary introduction to treatment.

Half a million diabetics are now in our midst, and another half million and more are on the way. Let us recognize the importance of this immigrant host which is springing up in every city and town in our country. Let us treat them rationally, appreciate all the good they do from their example in cleanliness and their temperance in diet and their useful disease, not forgetting their precocity and their wonderful leaders like Edison and Eastman, and strive to help them in their diabetic studies knowing full well that in the end they are the experimental laboratory and already the teachers of us all.

PROTAMINE ZINC INSULIN

One of the greatest discoveries of recent years in relationship to the control of diabetes has been the modification of insulin which is known as protamine zinc insulin. This product is more slowly absorbed and used up by the body than is the ordinary insulin. Now in many instances the diabetic who formerly took two doses daily may get along with one of the new insulin and those who took three doses daily may be kept in good condition with two doses of the protamine zinc insulin. Every diabetic patient is, however, an individual in relationship to his requirement of insulin and of carbohydrates so that the dosage of both the protamine zinc insulin and of food must be figured out for the patient by his own physician.

CHAPTER XXII

Blood Pressure
WINGATE M. JOHNSON, M.D.

INTRODUCTION

O NE OUT OF FIVE PEOPLE *who die in the United States lose their lives as a result of one of the complications of high blood pressure. Yet high blood pressure is in itself not a disease, but the symptom of a variety of conditions.*

The rapidity with which hardening of the arteries occurs in different people varies greatly. Some are old at forty; others not until after seventy. There is an old saying that a man is as old as his arteries. Much depends on what Osler calls the vital rubber in the vessels that carry the blood. The exact cause of hardening of the arteries, with which high blood pressure is usually associated, is not known. It may be the result of a hard life involving overstrain; it might be in response to repeated infection, to intoxication with alcohol, tobacco, and other poisons, to overeating and abuse of the body generally. In his article on blood pressure Dr. Wingate M. Johnson considers it not as a disease but as a condition.

Everybody has some blood pressure, exactly as everyone has some temperature, but not everyone has a fever; neither does everyone have either a high or low blood pressure. It is only when the blood pressure is abnormally high in relationship to the general condition of the person concerned, or abnormally low, that it requires any attention. Simply because so much attention has been paid to blood pressure during the last quarter century, and simply because insurance companies focus a great deal of their attention on this condition in relationship to granting life insurance to any individual, it has been given a special chapter in this book.

M. F.

Blood pressure has been well defined as "the pressure exerted by the blood on the walls of the vessels in which it is flowing." The heart beats on an average seventy-two times a minute. With every beat, as is described in the chapter on heart disease, blood is forced from the left side of the heart into the great artery known as the aorta, and from it into smaller and smaller branches throughout the body until it reaches the meshwork of capillary vessels which connect the arteries and veins. From these it passes back through the veins into the right side of the heart, whence it is pumped through the lungs to be charged with oxygen and sent back to the left side of the heart.

A number of factors influence blood pressure: for example, the force of the heartbeat, the elasticity or rigidity of the vessel walls, and the secretions of certain ductless glands which, in turn, are controlled somewhat by the emotions. Exercise raises the pressure. Some drugs raise, others lower it.

Measuring the Blood Pressure

The blood pressure is measured by an instrument known technically as the sphygmomanometer, or, more generally, blood pressure apparatus. This consists of a rectangular rubber bag 5 inches wide by 9½ inches long, encased in one end of a long cloth sleeve. Two pieces of rubber tubing are attached to the bag and pass through an opening in the sleeve. To one of these tubes is attached a bulb for inflating the bag. The bulb is provided with a valve to regulate the inflow and outflow of air. The other tube is connected with a column of mercury in a glass tube graduated in millimeters (mercury instrument) or with a dial the hand of which registers a corresponding pressure against a spring (aneroid instrument).

In taking the blood pressure, the sleeve containing the rubber bag is wrapped around either upper arm, usually the left. In the method usually practised—by listening or auscultation—a stethoscope is placed over the artery in the bend of the elbow and the bag in the arm band inflated until the impulse of the heartbeat—the pulse—is cut off. Then the pressure is slowly released until the sound of this impulse is heard, when the height of the mercury column or the figure on the dial is noted. This is the systolic pressure and represents the maximum pressure of the heart as it contracts—the systole. The pres-

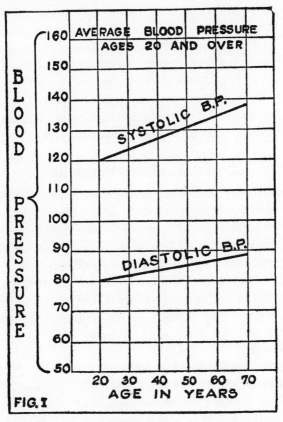

FIG. 84.

This illustrates the average blood pressure, both systolic and diastolic, from ages 20 to 70. It will be noted that the average blood pressure is lower than many people realize. The old idea that the systolic blood pressure should be 100 plus the age is erroneous. The average systolic blood pressure is more accurately expressed by the formula $113 + \frac{\text{age}}{3}$ for ages 20 and over. The average diastolic pressure may be estimated from the formula $75 + \frac{\text{age}}{5}$ for ages 20 and over.

The average systolic blood pressure is as follows:

At age 20....................120
"   "   30....................122
"   "   40....................125
"   "   50....................129
"   "   60....................134
"   "   70....................138

And the average diastolic pressure at the fifth phase is:

At age 20....................79
"   "   30....................81
"   "   40....................83
"   "   50....................85
"   "   60....................87
"   "   70....................89

Continued study seems to indicate that the average diastolic pressure is probably somewhat lower.

sure is released still slowly until the sound of the pulse disappears, when the reading is recorded as the diastolic or minimum pressure, corresponding to the resting period or diastole of the heart. The difference between them is called the pulse pressure. The diastolic pressure is normally about two thirds the systolic.

In the palpation method only the systolic pressure can be taken. With the finger on the pulse at the wrist, the operator notes the reading of the instrument when the impulse is first felt.

Normal Blood Pressure

It is difficult to say just what constitutes normal or average blood pressure. By fairly common consent, as a starting point a systolic pressure of 120 millimeters of mercury is considered a normal average for a male twenty years old. The pressure increases slowly with age. The rule commonly known, "the age plus 100," increases it too rapidly. Nicholson's rule, "Start at twenty with a systolic pressure of 120 and add half a point a year," is more accurate, but even this gives a higher reading than the averages reached by the combined statistics of insurance companies. Women have slightly lower blood pressures, on the average, than men.

If 110 or less be considered as hypotension or low blood pressure, and 140 or more as hypertension or high blood pressure, for average adults, it will be found that there are about twice as many people outside these limits as within them. Some time ago two of my medical friends and I pooled the blood-pressure readings of several hundred office patients. A little less than a third of them were between 110 and 140, virtually the same number above 140, and decidedly more than a third were below 110. This illustrates the well-known characteristic of Americans to go to extremes, even in their physical make-up.

Either high or low blood pressure has its advantages and disadvantages, as will be shown in the discussion of each condition.

High Blood Pressure, or Hypertension

It is not more than twenty years since it became the medical fashion to take blood pressure; and it is a debatable question whether mankind has been the worse or the better for the discovery. According to the manufacturers of an expensive instrument for taking blood pressure, "The eminent physiologist Ludwig has said that the discovery of blood pressure was more important than that of circulation." On the other hand, Sir James Mackenzie, who has added more to our knowledge of the heart than any other man since Harvey discovered the circulation, attached little importance to it. And I think it was Dr. Christian, of Boston, who said in a medical meeting that he was prepared to debate with anybody, anywhere, the affirmative of the query that the invention of the blood pressure apparatus had done mankind more harm than good.

Like most other debatable and debated questions, the truth lies somewhere between the two extremes. If hypertension is taken as a symptom instead of a disease in itself, if its importance and its danger do not become exaggerated in the mind of the patient, and if its treatment does not overshadow the treatment of the patient, it may be a valuable aid. If, on the other hand, a person who is inclined to be hypochondriacal meets a doctor who exaggerates the condition into a disease, who insists on taking the victim's pressure at frequent intervals and telling him just how high it is, and who punishes him with a too strict regimen of living, it were better for him that a millstone were hanged about his neck, and his misery quickly ended.

Many reasons have been suggested for high blood pressure, but the last word has not yet been said. While no one cause can be given, there are a few factors most often associated with it which probably play some part. These are heredity, emotional strain, overeating, overwork, certain diseases, and focal infections.

Heredity is almost unanimously given first place among the causes of hypertension. In the present stage of our civilization, however, Mark Twain's remark about the weather applies here: "Everybody talks about it, but nobody ever does anything about it." Dr. Logan Clendening says that if one could be given the privilege of mating human beings as animals are mated, he could produce a race whose average lifetime would be a hundred years, or one whose members would die of arteriosclerosis at twenty. But such a dictatorship is out of the question, and the well-known law of nature whereby opposites attract militates against such a plan. As to the other factors, however, it is possible to be less Calvinistic.

Emotional strain is perhaps the next most important factor. It includes such causes as unhappy family life, fear, anger, excitement, jealousy, and, perhaps chief of all, anxiety over finances.

An uncongenial atmosphere in the home is doubly harmful, in that the unpleasant emotions engendered are themselves harmful and that they interfere with digestion. The wisest man in the world said, "Better is a dinner of herbs where love is, than a stalled ox and hatred therewith"; and again, "It is better to dwell in a corner of the housetop than with a brawling woman in a wide house."

Fits of temper always cause a temporary rise of pressure and, often repeated, tend to make it stay up. The celebrated John Hunter, one of the greatest surgeons of all time, suffered from anginal attacks for twenty years before he died. He is often quoted as saying, "My life is in the hands of any rascal who chooses to tease or annoy me," meaning that the rise of blood pressure thus caused might bring on a fatal attack. Great excitement serves the same purpose. More than one football and baseball fan has paid with his life for seeing a crucial game.

Fear is in a class by itself as a cause of high blood pressure. It is one of the most subtle of all evils. Often morbid fears are instilled in childhood that are never outgrown. One of the most wholesome trends in modern child training is the stress laid on the harmful effects of fear and the means by which it may be prevented or overcome. Some of the fears most often met are the fear of financial reverse, of losing a position, of failing to make good in some undertaking, of committing the unpardonable sin, of disease, and of dying. Even the fear of high blood pressure may be one of the most potent reasons for its existence. One of the great objections to periodic health examinations is the danger of centering the patient's attention too much upon himself. This is especially true if the custom of the so-called life extension institutes is followed, and the patient given a detailed report, with elaborate pamphlets on the dangers of constipation, smoking, improper diet, the neglect of the teeth, and others.

Overeating refers more to the quantity than to the kind of diet. A reasonable amount of fat is needed for padding and protection of certain organs, but excessive fat acts as a parasite on the body. It adds enormously to the burden on the heart, and also contributes much more waste matter to be eliminated by the kidneys. Any life insurance man will testify that the expectation of life of an over-weight or obese person is far less than that of a normal or under-weight man. Verily, a man's belt line is his life line. Moderation in weight is to be obtained more by temperance in eating than anything else, though exercise helps. Nor should this doctrine go so far as the utterly ridiculous and dangerous starvation that many women have suffered in order to get and to keep a boyish figure.

Overwork may be either mental or physical. Prolonged and intense use of either brain or muscles raises the blood pressure, and sufficient rest should be taken to allow the circulation to relax. If kept tightened up for long intervals, it has a tendency to stay at a higher level. This is particularly true if the work is accompanied by emotional strain. Such is the life led by the average doctor, and its results are shown by the fact that of 173 physicians whose obituaries were published in one month in the *Journal of the American Medical Association*, 100 died of diseases of the circulation, which is far more than the general average.

Certain diseases, notably syphilis, tend to cause arterial degeneration and hypertension. The improvements made within this century in the diagnosis and treatment of this disease should eventually greatly lessen its importance as a factor.

Focal infections, such as abscessed teeth, diseased tonsils, infected sinuses and gall bladders, were once thought to play an important rôle in producing hypertension, but their importance is now being questioned. This is not meant to encourage anybody to harbor pockets of pus anywhere in his system, for occasionally a high blood pressure is lowered markedly after the removal of such a focus; besides, the body should be rid of such cesspools on general principles.

One condition which was long considered a chief cause but which is now practically abandoned is constipation and its consort, auto-intoxication. On the contrary, it seems that the opposite condition of low blood pressure is more likely to be associated with persistent constipation.

Caffeine, in the form of coffee, tea, or certain soft drinks, undoubtedly raises the blood pressure for a while, and further predisposes to a permanently high level by stimulating both brain and muscle, especially the brain, to unduly prolonged exertion. As Dr. H. A. Hare used to say, "Caffeine is a key to one's reserve energy, which should be saved for emergencies." The great popularity of certain soda-fountain beverages undoubtedly adds to the high-tension life of today. Although I voted for prohibition, it is my firm conviction that the unlimited sale of beer over the soda-fountain counter would be less harmful to the American nation than the unlimited sale of caffeinated beverages.

As to alcohol and tobacco, one is impressed with the free use of dogmatic statements of opinion and the lack of accurate observation. One cannot but regard as appropriate the words of old Omar:

> *Myself when young did eagerly frequent*
> *Doctor and Saint, and heard great argument*
> *About it and about: but evermore*
> *Came out by the same door wherein I went.*

The immediate effect of a single dose of alcohol is to lower the blood pressure; and only after its long abuse has wrought changes in the kidneys or arteries will it be raised. Even this is a doubtful point. In passing, it may be observed that one who habitually uses the high-explosive type of liquor dispensed by most bootleggers is not likely to live long enough to develop hypertension.

As to tobacco, opinions have long varied. According to some observations I made a few years ago, its effect on blood pressure is almost negligible. It is interesting that Sir Armand Marc Ruffer, in his dissection of Egyptian mummies, found arteriosclerosis as common among them as among Europeans. He remarks that whatever it was due to, it was not due to tobacco.

TREATMENT OF HIGH BLOOD PRESSURE

The treatment of high blood pressure has largely been anticipated in the foregoing discussion of its causes. It is evident that the chief cause, heredity, must be accepted as philosophically as possible, for it has been fixed before the patient's arrival in the world. Much can be done, however, to lessen the influence of some of the other factors.

Emotional strain can be controlled to some extent. One of the first things a person should do when told that he has high blood pressure is to make up his mind that he will not let it ruin the rest of his life. He must adopt a philosophic attitude toward it, amend his habits so far as necessary and possible, and then forget it.

It is not a good idea to have the blood pressure taken too often, nor to press the doctor for the exact reading in figures. Anybody's pressure may fluctuate widely within a day, and even a well-balanced layman who does not realize this can hardly help worrying if told that his reading is a few points higher than it was last week. Let the doctor worry over it, anyhow; that is what he is paid for.

The advice perhaps most often given and the least often taken is "Don't worry." When one has learned how not to worry, he has learned the philosophy of life. Would that I were genius enough to formulate a universal rule for casting out the demon of worry, but every man must work out his own salvation. One can only offer a few bits of general advice.

Of prime importance is not to work against the pressure of time. Plan the day's work so it will not be overcrowded, even if something has to be left until tomorrow or delegated to someone else. Allow plenty of time for every task. For example, if it is necessary to catch a train and it takes ten minutes to drive to the station, allow fifteen minutes, so there will not be a feeling of uncertainty in case of an unexpected traffic jam.

Far be it from a humble practitioner of medicine to offer any advice about finance, except that my professional observation has taught me most men pay dearly, from a physical standpoint, for profits made by marginal trading and for highly speculative dealing of any kind. I have long had a conviction that Freud was wrong in teaching that sex maladjustment was responsible for all the mental and most of the physical ills the flesh is heir to. Where sex has destroyed its thousands of happy homes, financial worry has destroyed its ten thousands. One of the greatest trials in the practice of medicine is the inability to relieve a condition when a diagnosis is made. A doctor would need the resources of a Rockefeller to treat successfully a large proportion of his patients, the prescriptions needed for them being checks for amounts varying from $5 to $50,000 or more.

Fear and worry are closely akin. Undoubtedly fear is one of the most potent causes of unhappiness and of high blood pressure. One of the best prescriptions for any victim of hypertension or of morbid anxieties is that remarkable book called *Fear*, by Dr. John Rathbone Oliver of Baltimore. In fascinating novel form, Dr. Oliver gives a clear, sensible discussion of fears: how they come into one's life and how they may be eliminated.

Overeating, as has been said, refers more to the quantity than the kind of food, though rich, highly seasoned food and an excess of meats, especially pork, are to be shunned. One should learn from one of the numerous reference tables what his weight should be and try to keep it within bounds. A word of caution here, however, is necessary. These tables are merely averages, and a man with a large frame and big bones should weigh more than another man of the same height but with a slender framework. It is not sufficiently emphasized in our Sunday schools that it is possible to be just as intemperate in eating as in drinking. Indeed, one objection to alcohol for the average man is its appetizing effect. Of a preacher who was famous as a valiant trencherman the remark was made that it was blasphemous for him to preach a sermon on temperance; yet it was his favorite topic. He died in middle age of apoplexy.

Work is not nearly as dangerous as worry. In fact, within reasonable limits it is one of the best antidotes for worry. My experience has convinced me that the worst thing that can happen to the average man is to be deprived of his work. It is often wise for an overworked man to cut down his activity by delegating more authority to others and by taking more or less frequent rest periods; but to require the average man with hypertension to stop all work is usually to kick the last prop from under him. The medical director of a great life insurance company once told me that policyholders who quit all work on finding they had high blood pressure did not live nearly so long, as a class, as those who carried on.

To be guarded against, however, are prolonged periods of intense application to work without sufficient rest to compensate. A rest period in the middle of the day, of one half to two hours, helps to keep the pressure at a lower level. Frequent holidays, not too strenuously used, are beneficial. Longer vacations once or several times a year help to prolong life for a victim of hypertension.

To quote my friend Dr. Clendening again: "The treatment of hypertension should be made as nearly painless as possible." Every physician of experience knows that finding high blood pressure does not mean signing a patient's death warrant, for there are numerous persons with hypertension who have been enjoying reasonably good health and leading active, useful lives for long periods of time—many of them as long as we have been taking blood pressures.

There is no better summary of the treatment of high blood pressure than the advice given by Chauncey Depew toward the end of his long and useful life: "Do anything you want to, but do it in moderation." And this was based on scriptural authority: "Let your moderation be known of all men."

Low Blood Pressure, or Hypotension

While one hears a great deal more about high blood pressure than about the opposite condition, more people have low blood pressure. And since the great influenza epidemic of 1918 the proportion of individuals with abnormally low pressure has been increasing. Probably other factors than influenza are responsible, such as the decreased popularity of walking and the semi-starvation women will undergo to attain a boyish figure.

Fortunately hypotension is not nearly so serious as hypertension. Indeed, the experience of life insurance companies indicates that a moderately low blood pressure adds materially to one's expectation of life after the age of twenty-five; but it may take so much of the joy out of living that its victim would gladly exchange his chances of a hypothetical extra year or so of life for the dynamic energy of his neighbor with a higher reading. Having been a victim myself, I speak feelingly.

As a typical example of acute or temporary hypotension I may use my own case. Following an attack of influenza so mild that I spent little time in bed but was kept from practice because laryngitis deprived me of my voice for several days, I felt weaker than ever before. By noon I would feel as tired as if a full day's work were behind me, and the rest of the day was a fight against exhaustion. It was hard to make a decision, and paths of least resistance were followed when possible. A reasonably good memory became exceedingly treacherous. An unwonted tendency to look on the dark side of life became apparent. After two or three months of this, a colleague and I were one day testing our blood-pressure instruments against a mercury gauge. I was astounded to find my systolic pressure only 104, when shortly before my illness it had been 124. Then it dawned upon me that here was an explanation for my chronic weariness, and it was gradually forgotten in looking for the same condition in other influenza victims. Invariably these patients would show a marked reduction in pressure that lasted from a few days to several months. Two of my patients fainted when they first got out of bed, and in each the systolic pressure was below 80. Only a prolonged rest in bed and tonic treatment restored it to normal.

Another interesting observation was that patients with hypertension would after influenza also show a great drop in pressure: in one case from 240 to 170; in another, from 180 to 120. They would seem to feel just as "let down" as do the normal cases, until their usual high level was regained.

Other diseases than influenza cause a similar drop in pressure; but since 1918 influenza has so tremendously overshadowed all other infections that it has been most intensively studied.

Most of the cases following acute infectious diseases might be called acute or temporary hypotension, since they recover far too quickly and completely to have been caused by actual damage to the heart muscle. The most plausible explanation is that during an acute illness there is an increased demand upon the little glands attached to the top of the kidneys and hence called the adrenal or suprarenal glands. They furnish an internal secretion that helps keep up the blood pressure. During an emergency that demands an extra effort on the part of the body—such as the necessity for a fight or a flight—they furnish an increased amount of their secretion. This extra effort is followed by a decrease in this secretion, when the individual feels fatigued or even exhausted. The same idea holds good during an illness, except that the demand is more prolonged and the period of exhaustion following it, longer. The circulation is thus deprived of its natural tonic, and the lack of it is felt by the entire body. The muscles do not get their normal amount of nutrition; hence they tire more easily. The brain suffers likewise, and so rebels at a prolonged or difficult task. The victim of this temporary low blood pressure is apt to feel dizzy on sudden changes of position, to sweat freely on slight exertion, to be more irritable than is his wont, and to feel utterly depressed, physically, mentally, and spiritually.

Its duration depends upon several factors, including the patient's natural vigor and power of recuperation, the care taken of him during and after his illness, and possibly the clearing up of any lurking foci of infection. I have seen a systolic pressure rise twenty points within three days, and have had my own, among others, take three or four months to climb up ten or fifteen points. And of all the factors in recovery, the most important, because the one most easily controlled, is sufficient rest during illness and convalescence. One of the keenest general practitioners I know, despite his seventy-five years, recently said that if he had his professional career to live over again the greatest change he would make in treating his patients would be to keep them in bed longer after acute illnesses, even colds.

Another important part of the treatment is a nutritious diet that is easily digested. And unless there is trouble in sleeping, a temporary low blood pressure furnishes an excellent excuse for an extra cup of coffee or tea.

In considering chronic or persistent low blood pressure, it is necessary first to decide at what level it begins. While it is hard to set an arbitrary limit, I know of no better rule than the one laid down by Dr. Oliver T. Osborne: "A systolic pressure of 110 or lower in an adult should be considered hypotension, anything below 105 calls for treatment, and a systolic pressure of 100 or lower in an adult calls for rest from all active duties." Like all man-made rules, however, this one has numerous exceptions. Every physician of experience can cite individuals who with blood pressures even below 100 go placidly and even cheerfully about their daily duties with apparently no inconvenience, and who could not be persuaded by any means short of physical violence to "rest from all active duties."

Certain chronic diseases, notably tuberculosis, are characterized by low blood pressure. It usually accompanies anemia. It may also be due to a weakened heart muscle (myocarditis). A most sudden and dramatic drop in blood pressure follows the condition known as coronary thrombosis or coronary occlusion, in which the artery that supplies the heart muscle itself is blocked by a blood clot. Here the pressure may fall from above 200 to below 100 in a few hours.

The habitual use of the coal-tar products may cause a very low pressure. Most of the widely advertised remedies for headache, neuralgia, and "colds" contain the coal-tar products and are more or less depressing. By their persistent use the blood pressure may be permanently lowered because the heart muscle is weakened and the quality of the blood impaired. The same is true of "hypnotics"— drugs which produce sleep. Most of these may be identified by their ending in "al"; for example, veronal, trional, chloral, allonal, luminal, amytal, and a host of others. Virtually every physician with whom I have talked of late agrees that the number of people who take such preparations to excess is increasing. The average American does not seem content to be his natural self. In the morning, he wants one or more cups of strong coffee to wake him up, usually followed during the day by one or many glasses of caffeinated beverages from the soda fountain, and more coffee for dinner. At bedtime he wants to shut off the mental activity induced by so much caffeine, and is apt to take a sedative. Even a slight headache is not to be endured for a moment if aspirin or other means of relief can be obtained. The habit of taking such drugs is acquired more easily than most people realize, as the average doctor can testify.

Perhaps the chief cause of persistent hypotension is physique. This, in turn, is determined largely by heredity. It is most apt to occur in the slender, narrow-chested, long-waisted individual. The explanation is one of physics. The heart is on a lower level, and the blood has to be pumped around a sharper bend than in a wide-chested individual. The idiotic fad of dieting to become excessively thin has undoubtedly contributed to the number of hypotension victims.

The point has already been made that hypotension patients, as a class, live longer than those with moderately high or even average pressure; but this advantage is somewhat offset by the fact that they do not feel as alert and vigorous as those with higher pressure. Their condition seems analogous to an automobile with a low-powered motor which has not the speed nor the power of a car with a larger motor, and so wears more slowly. That they do live so long is perhaps due to the fact that their low blood pressure tends to inactivity. This type of individual is more apt to "enjoy poor health" than is the more robust one. The medical director of a great insurance company once told me that his company would gladly accept individuals with low pressure for life insurance, but did not want them for disability insurance.

TREATMENT OF LOW BLOOD PRESSURE

The treatment of chronic or persistent hypotension is, of course, that of the underlying condition. Most people with it need no special treatment beyond the assurance that the condition is not dangerous. Unless it causes its victim to tire too easily, it is quite compatible with an unusually long life of usefulness. Individuals with it need to keep their weight up to normal; to get at least the orthodox eight hours' sleep every night; and to avoid the reckless use of headache remedies and hypnotics. The army "setting-up exercises," Walter Camp's "daily dozen," or similar exercises to strengthen the muscles of the abdomen, will help by overcoming the sagging down of the abdominal contents. Incidentally they will help to combat that condition so horribly portrayed by patent medicine advertisements: constipation. One of the simplest and best of these exercises is while in bed to lock the hands back of the neck and sit up without pushing with the elbows, making the abdominal muscles do the work. This sounds easy—but just try it! This may be done fifteen or twenty times night and morning—with distinct benefit to the waistline as well as to the blood pressure.

As a final encouraging pat on the back for the one with low blood pressure, there is little danger that any doctor will seek to deprive him of coffee, tea, red meats, or any of the most comforting of table comforts.

CHAPTER XXIII

Cancer
FRANCIS CARTER WOOD, M.D.

INTRODUCTION

FOR MANY YEARS *all sorts of agencies have been investigating cancer. From time to time startling discoveries are recorded, but unfortunately most of those dealing with the treatment of cancer, except so far as concerns its early complete removal, have failed to be of permanent value. The present intensified research should probably yield even greater advances within the next few decades.*

Everyone should realize that cancerous growths are not all the same. They vary according to the tissues involved and according to the nature of their growth. It is important to decrease the amount of cancer by educating people as to the value of early diagnosis, early treatment, and particularly the avoidance of causes of needless repeated irritations to the tissues.

The final and probably the greatest problem of all is to determine the exact cause of cancer. It is interesting to know that in the attempt to find the cause practically every method of attack has already been tried. It has been studied as a possible infectious disease; it has been studied from the point of view of inheritance; and from the point of view of chemistry and physics and by every other method.

Cancer statistics have been of the greatest value in attempting to understand the disease, although unfortunately the wrong interpretation of statistics by persons has frequently served to divert attention to unfavorable channels. One of the most important steps to be taken in the study of cancer is the establishment of suitable facilities for diagnosis and for treatment by all of the well established methods in great centers, so that human material may be studied in an attempt to learn more about the cause and control of this disorder.

One of the ideas most promoted by food faddists of one type or another is the notion that the eating of any special food substances may be the cause of cancer and that abstinence from some single article of diet will prevent cancer. In Great Britain research has been undertaken during the past year to find out whether there was any connection between cancer and deficiencies in the diet. Dr. J. A. Murray, director of the Imperial Cancer Research Fund, concludes that there exists no trustworthy evidence, experimental, clinical, or statistical, of a causal relationship between cancer and the absence or presence or excess of any particular constituent of the human diet. Enough is known to say that no definite relationship has been established between vitamin intake and cancer. This announcement will not, however, affect in any way the claims of the food fanatics or food cultists. They are not interested in facts: they are salesmen of propaganda.

Under present conditions the one real hope in cancer is early diagnosis and early operation. Statistical evidence accumulated under the auspices of the Medical Research Council of Great Britain proves the truth of this warning. One group of investigators, studying the lives of women with cancer, found that a woman with cancer of the breast who is not treated at all can expect to live 17.2 per cent of the normal duration of her life. A woman operated on under ordinary conditions may expect to live 30.4 per cent of her normal duration, whereas one operated on under the most favorable conditions may expect to live 68.5 per cent of the normal duration.

In a study of women operated on for cancer of the breast in the medical institutions of Leeds it was found that of those operated on while the growth was still confined to the breast, 90.1 per cent were alive ten years after the operation; of those operated on after the glands under the arm had become involved, 91.3 per cent were dead within ten years after operation. Of the advanced cases, 94.4 per cent were dead within ten years after operation. These figures indicate the extreme importance of undertaking a satisfactory operation while the growth is still confined to the breast.

A woman in England fifty-five years of age may normally expect to live 18.87 years longer. It is estimated that 5,000 cases of cancer of the breast develop among women in England and Wales each year. If all of these were operated on under the most favorable conditions, more than 30,000 years of life would be gained for the entire group. The expectancy of life of women whose cancer is not treated is only

3.25 years, whereas the one operated on under the best conditions has an expectancy of 12.93 years.

A prime topic of consideration is the question as to whether or not the incidence of cancer is increasing. The present consensus seems to be that there may be more cancer now than there used to be because there are more people living to an older age—and cancer is essentially a disease of older age. The children that used to die in infancy and the people who used to succumb to typhoid fever, dysentery, tuberculosis, and similar complaints, now live to an age when they form better soil for the cancerous growth.

According to figures made available by the Metropolitan Life Insurance Company there has been no significant increase of deaths from cancer among white women at any age below sixty-five years. Indeed, they report a significant decrease between the ages of thirty-five and fifty-five. The great majority of people seek aid for cancer at a period of the disease when it is frequently too late to effect any extensive prolongation of life. They come at a time when the cancer has spread so far that it is not possible to eradicate it completely by operation. All must be educated to seek medical treatment on the slightest suspicion of cancer, so that it may be applied while there is still opportunity to save life.

M. F.

THE WORD "CANCER" applies to a number of diseased conditions characterized by the uncontrolled growth of some of the tissues of the body. If not checked, such growth inevitably leads to death.

THE CAUSES OF CANCER

The chemical or other changes which give the cells, the little units of which the tissues of the body are composed, the power to grow in uncontrollable fashion are not known. The exact chemical changes in the cells of the body which are the final causes of the disease known as tuberculosis are not definitely known. We do, however, know the immediate cause of tuberculosis, the germ called the tubercle bacillus. In cancer, the immediate cause of some varieties is known. This cause is loosely termed chronic or repeated irritation. Examples of cancer following chronic irritation are those growths of the skin produced by tar, soot, lubricating oils, and certain synthetic chemicals.

Other types of "irritation cancers" are seen in the mouth, where a sharp tooth or an ill-fitting dental apparatus may irritate the cheek or tongue, and cancer follow. They are seen in the lip where a hot pipe stem irritates the tender skin of the lip, or where a cigarette is repeatedly stuck to the lip and roughly pulled off, bringing some skin with it. The heat and the tarry materials from the tobacco, coupled with the damage to the skin, may, after some months or years, give rise to a cancer of the lip. It is probable also that cancer of the lung and cancer of the throat are produced by inhaling irritating substances. Certain parasites, such as *Bilharzia*, occurring in Egypt and South America, may cause an irritation of the bladder or rectum, and cancer result therefrom. In China, a parasite, *Paragonimus*, occurs which gives rise to cancer of the liver by irritation of that organ. The chewing of betel nut, which is a highly irritating substance, causes cancer of the mouth. The native women of Ceylon have this cancer twenty-five times more frequently than white women, who do not chew. These are the best examples of irritation cancer. It is also probable that irritation anywhere along the intestinal canal may ultimately set up chronic inflammation which may turn into cancer. There are, however, many types of cancer of which even the inciting cause is absolutely unknown.

No relation has been established between diet and cancer; the meat-eating Eskimo and the rice-eating Japanese have the same amount of cancer. Aluminum dishes or canned food do not cause cancer.

DISTRIBUTION OF CANCER

Cancer is apparently a universal disease and has been recognized since ancient times. It has been held that it is due to conditions under which civilized races live, and that the uncivilized tribes were free from the disease. But the more the matter has been investigated, the more certain it is that the Eskimo, the American Indian, the South American savage, the African Negro, all suffer from cancer, and possibly just as frequently as the so-called civilized races. The matter is simply a question of diagnosis and age. For the more skilled the physicians in diagnosis, the more post-mortem examinations are made, the more surgical operations are performed, the larger the number of cases of cancer are recognized and recorded. Hence the highest recorded rates of cancer occur in some of the smaller European states, such as Switzerland, Holland, and Denmark. These high rates are due to a highly educated medical profession, the highly equipped, efficient, and easily accessible hospitals, and the greater number of post-mortem examinations performed. In Switzerland, for example, over 90 per cent of those dying from any disease have post-mortem examinations, which frequently reveal unsuspected cancer. In America, with a much lower cancer rate than in the countries mentioned, only 2 per cent of those dying have post-mortem examinations. In large cities the recorded death rate is higher than in rural districts. This is due to the presence, in such cities, of large hospitals which attract cancer patients from the outlying suburbs to get treatment, and also to the fact that in hospitals post-mortem examinations are more frequently performed than in the private practice of rural physicians.

Striking differences in cancer death rates have been found to be due also to the fact that there are more old people in certain states than in others. For example, the New England states, Maine, New Hampshire, Vermont, and Massachusetts, have high death rates from cancer, the average rate being much higher in these states than in some of those of the West (for instance, Montana, Idaho, and Nevada) where the country has been more recently settled and the population is of average younger age. It has been found by the study of census statistics and of deaths occurring in insured lives that cancer increases steadily from youth to old age, being much greater above the age of forty than it is below. When cancer mortality figures are arranged in age groups, it is found that between the ages of forty and forty-five, or forty-five and fifty, the rate is the same all over the country, so that excessive cancer is evidently due to an older average population. For this reason cancer is less frequently seen in countries where the death rate is high. For instance, in the United States the average life is about fifty-six years. In India it is about twenty-five years; hence, it would be expected that the cancer rate in the United States would be much higher than that in India, a fact which census records show.

In the United States the cancer death rate of the whole population has risen steadily for many years and now amounts to nearly 100 deaths per 100,000. In Switzerland the rate is about 130 per 100,000, and in Denmark about 140 per 100,000. These differences, as explained, are due to improved diagnosis, and unquestionably the recorded death rate in the United States will rise ultimately, when good diagnosis is available everywhere, to the same rates as these

European countries. There is therefore no definite evidence that cancer is actually increasing. The results of educational propaganda in the United States have unquestionably led to the more frequent diagnosis of cancer, both people generally and the medical profession being more interested in the subject, and death certificates are more frequently signed cancer than they used to be. For a long time there has existed a strong feeling that cancer was a disease which carried some hereditary taint and was therefore disgraceful. This is not at all true. With the increase in knowledge, greater frankness concerning the disease has become widespread, so that relatives are willing to have death certificates signed correctly and do not demand that the physician conceal the real cause of death under the title heart failure, pneumonia, or some other term.

CLASSIFICATION OF CANCER

The word "cancer" is an old term derived from the Greek physicians. It is used, as has been said, in a popular way to indicate any malignant tumor, malignant meaning that the growth ultimately destroys life. The word "tumor" is used to designate any lump or new growth in the body, which may or may not be malignant, so that a tumor may be a cancer, or may be a harmless growth. There are a great variety of malignant tumors or cancers which are classified under two main heads, carcinoma, those types of malignant growths which arise from the skin, the lining membrane of the intestine, or anywhere that there may be epithelial or covering cells; and sarcoma, which is about one tenth as frequent as carcinoma and is a malignant growth arising in the supporting tissues of the body as distinct from the covering tissues. Therefore, sarcoma appears in the bones, in the muscles, in the lymph glands, and in similar situations.

THE NATURE OF CANCER

Malignant tumors vary greatly in their appearance and rate of growth. Cancer of the skin of a certain type may exist for many years without causing death of the one affected. Other types of cancer of the skin are much more rapid in their progress and may kill within a year or two. Cancer never disappears of itself. There are occasional examples in which a temporary shrinkage of the growth, or even complete disappearance, has been noted, but if the patients are watched, it will be found that the cancer appears elsewhere and goes on its relentless course. The cells which make up any malignant tumor resemble closely the cells of the normal structures from which the tumor has arisen. A cancer of the thyroid, when examined under the microscope, looks like the tissue of the thyroid; a cancer of the stomach resembles the glands of the stomach. In this way it is sometimes possible to detect an internal cancer from a small external particle which has appeared under the skin and which is removed and examined by the microscope. Death from cancer is "not caused by a poison arising from the cancer"; instead, it is due to some interference with the normal performance of bodily function. If a cancer involves the brain, for example, it destroys a certain amount of brain tissue, and the patient dies for that reason. A cancer of the stomach often interferes with the free passage of food from the stomach; the patient vomits, and therefore gets no nourishment from his food, and ultimately dies of starvation. Cancer of the bowels may close the bowels entirely and cause intestional obstruction. If a cancer decays, as it often does, because it is not well supplied with blood vessels, it may ulcerate, then bacteria get into the ulcer and set up a local or general infection. Pneumonia, for this reason, is not an infrequent cause of death in the late stages of cancer.

HEREDITY

Cancer itself is not inherited. The liability or susceptibility to cancer is, however, inherited under certain conditions. It is well known that certain malformations, such as harelip, extra fingers, color blindness, and certain blood diseases, like hemophilia, are inheritable. If such malformations or diseased conditions are transmissible from parents to children, it is obvious that there may be transmitted certain weaknesses of an organ which would make it susceptible to cancer, provided the necessary irritation or stimulation required to produce cancer occurs. There are families reported, many of whom have died of cancer of the breast; others in which cancer of the stomach is extremely frequent; others with cancer of the rectum. Identical twins are known both of whom have died of the same kind of cancer at about the same time. But these occurrences are rare, and they occur apparently from some unfortunate ancestral combination. For instance, two persons may marry, both of whom have susceptibility to cancer of the stomach. This concentrates such susceptibility in the offspring.

Not that such concentration necessarily means that all the children will die of cancer of the stomach. There are families in which both parents have had the same kind of cancer and yet none of the children died of cancer. It only means that if the proper stimulus is given, such children are more liable to a cancer of the stomach than the average person. If the mother has cancer of the breast and the father has cancer of the rectum, the records do not show that any proportion of the children necessarily die of either of these types of new growth. In those families in which cancer is frequent the strain quickly dies out. The insurance companies have studied this question of inheritance of cancer susceptibility and as yet have not found it of sufficient importance to warrant the refusal of insurance, or even increase in the premiums to persons with a cancerous ancestry. At present the conclusion is warranted that there is no definite basis for the belief that the factor of heredity plays a large part in cancer among human beings.

RACE

There are certain little understood differences in distribution of cancer in different races. The Negro race has but little cancer of the skin as compared to the white race, whereas Negro women have much more cancer of the womb than white women have; the Dutch woman has more cancer of the womb, and the English woman, of the breast.

SEX

Sex plays a part in the distribution of cancer, in that women have certain organs which are extremely susceptible to cancer, notably the breast and the womb, the corresponding tissues in men not being susceptible. Cancer of the breast in men occurs only in about one one-hundredth the frequency in women. Cancer of the stomach in men is a little more frequent than in women. Cancer of the gall bladder is four times as frequent in women as in men. On the other hand, cancer of the lip, tongue, and mouth is much more frequent in men than it is in women. These differences are probably due to habits and social customs. Men smoke more than women and are less apt to keep their mouths clean and their teeth in good order. On the other hand, in the East, cancer of the mouth, in Ceylon, for example, as has been said, is twenty-five times as frequent in the native races as it is in the whites living under the same conditions. Cancer of the penis is practically unknown in the circumcised Jews, whereas it is fairly common in the uncircumcised Christian races.

CONTAGION

It used to be thought that cancer was contagious, but of late years it has been definitely shown that contagion is impossible. There is no record of a surgeon getting a cancer of the hand from operating on a patient, nor of a nurse catching the disease from a patient whom she attends. The reason for this is that cancer is not a germ disease, but a cell disease. These cells are easily damaged, and to transfer a cancer from one person to another would be, from what is known about animal cancer, a difficult thing. Thus it is often necessary to inoculate at least one hundred other animals to obtain three or four growths from a primary tumor. Also it has never been possible to transfer a cancer from a human being to an animal, or from an animal to a human being. Such transference is strictly limited to animals of the same species, and often of the same strain. For instance, cancer of the white mouse can rarely be transferred to the wild black mouse.

If cancer is not contagious, there can be nothing in the stories which appear occasionally concerning cancer villages or cancer houses or cancer districts. So-called cancer villages have been investigated, and they have been found to be small towns from which all the young people have gone to the cities to obtain a better living. The old folks remain, and as the frequency of cancer increases with age, obviously such a village will have a high cancer death rate, but it has nothing to do with the soil, the house, or any other local condition.

VARIETIES OF CANCER AND THEIR SYMPTOMS

The different tissues of the body each have their characteristic cancers. This is due to the fact that these tissues and organs all have different structures with highly specialized cells. A cancer which appears in such a tissue or organ, being derived from these cells, bears strong resemblance to its ancestral source. Cancer of the skin, for example, may occur either from the surface coating cells of the skin, from the hair follicles, from the sweat glands, or from the sebaceous glands, which give off the oily material which keeps our skin soft. Each one of these types of cancer can be recognized by the expert. The treatment of each is different. It is folly, therefore, to assume that just anybody can diagnose a cancer of the skin with any accuracy. It often takes a microscopic study of the tissue to find out to just which group the growth belongs. The most common types are those which arise from the surface layer, known as the squamous or flat-celled epithelioma, and from the deeper layers, known as basal cell epithelioma. The squamous or flat-celled type is dangerous; it grows rapidly, and is difficult to cure; it gives off particles which get into the vessels and may spread to distant parts of the body. The basal cell type, on the other hand, grows more slowly, remains quiescent for long periods, does not give off particles into the circulation, and is quite susceptible to X-ray or radium treatment. However, no one but an expert doctor can tell which treatment should be applied. The other varieties are so rare that they need not be discussed here. A skin cancer begins as a rule as a small, elevated, rounded, or flat-topped area, which is a little sensitive to the touch, and is yellowish or brownish in color. As a rule, a scab forms early which can be pulled off, leaving a bleeding underlying tissue. New scab forms and may be again pulled off, and will re-form, but it will be noticed each time that the scab is thicker, the growth covers a larger area, and gets harder; it takes longer for the scab to form, and there is no tendency to heal. Ultimately a hollow area with raised edges will be produced, which is called an ulcer. These skin tumors may occur anywhere but most often they are on the face. They may appear on the lip, and similar tumors occur in the mouth, inside of the cheeks, on the gums, and elsewhere. Here they are almost always the more dangerous type of squamous cell tumor. Such a growth on the tongue may kill a person in six months unless promptly treated. Occasionally cancer of the dangerous type is seen on the hands, especially in mechanics, where it is probably due to oil or metallic substances with which the skin becomes soiled. They are very rare in those who keep their hands clean.

The treatment of all these skin tumors implies first a diagnosis, and second, proper treatment adjusted to the kind of growth. For instance, with a basal cell tumor, radium and X-ray may be used, if competent persons to handle these methods are available. The safest way, however, is to cut out the growth or burn it out with a cautery. Pastes and caustics are dangerous, as they frequently result in only partial cures. The tumor returns later, and a fresh treatment must be undertaken. The squamous cell cancers should be cut out by a surgeon. They require high doses of X-ray to cure, and the resulting scar is often worse than the surgical one. Cancer of the membranes of the nose, throat, tonsil, and larynx are fortunately rare. They are difficult to treat. Few people survive even with the best treatment, because it is difficult to make a diagnosis when the growth is early and can be completely removed. Cancer of the larynx can be cured if the growth is confined to the larynx, but the operation necessary is obviously mutilating, and it may take a person a long time to learn to talk without the larynx. This operation requires the most skillful and well trained specialist that can be obtained. X-rays and radium are of little value in laryngeal carcinoma, unless applied with great skill and under special conditions.

Cancer of the Breast

Some ten thousand deaths occur in the United States annually from cancer of the breast. Many of these deaths are in persons, who, if they were sufficiently intelligent, could easily have been saved. When cancer of the breast is small, early, and has not spread to the glands in the armpit, a surgical operation will cure three fourths of the patients. When the growth is the size of a lemon and the glands in the armpit have been involved by the disease, or the tumor is stuck to the chest, few people live five years, despite the best type of operation. X-ray and radium are of little value in the main treatment of most cases of cancer of the breast. In men, cancer of the breast is particularly dangerous, because the breast is small, the growth quickly penetrates the chest wall, and the results of surgery are not nearly as good as they are in women.

Cancer of the Womb

Cancer of the womb or birth organs is somewhat more frequent than that of the breast. It is of two types, one involving the cavity of the womb, which occurs usually in old women, after the change of life. Its chief symptom is continuous bleeding after the periods have stopped. This form of cancer is best treated by surgical removal of the whole womb. The other kind grows at the mouth of the womb, spreads early to the surrounding parts, and is best treated by radium combined with X-ray, provided facilities are available. Cures of the first variety may reach as high as 80 per cent in early cases, 20 or 30 per cent in late ones. With cancer of the mouth of the womb, or cervix, as it is called, the best radium treatment gives about 35 per cent of cures. Cancer of the cervix occurs in younger women; the symptoms are bleeding or an offensive discharge which should lead to an immediate examination by a competent physician. Pain unfortunately indicates that the disease is probably hopeless, as it comes from pressure on the nerves where the tumor has extended.

Cancer of the Stomach

About half the cases of cancer occur in the stomach. In the United States some 40,000 people die annually of this disease. Unfortunately, it is extremely difficult to diagnose and equally difficult to treat. The only symptoms may be loss of weight and appetite in a person over fifty. Pain is rare. Dyspepsia may not occur. Vomiting of blood is a late symptom. The disease is so insidious that every person over forty who has any digestive symptoms, or a slight anemia, or a distaste for food, and loss of weight should consult a physician and have an X-ray examination. This may indicate that the stomach is healthy, or it may indicate that a small cancer is present. If the growth is small and favorably situated, it is possible to remove it surgically. If it is large, the only thing which can be done is a short-circuiting operation, which may give the patient comfort for a while. Not more than one person in twenty of all those operated on lives five years. This is the most serious form of cancer, and one in which the medical profession as yet can do but little.

Cancer of the Intestine and Rectum

In this type of cancer, if diagnosed early, good results are obtained by surgical treatment. The diagnosis depends largely on careful examination together with X-ray studies in patients who have noticed that their bowels are a little irregular; that they suffer a little from gas, and that occasionally there is a little blood in their movements. The responsibility for the diagnosis, therefore, rests largely on the patients. Unless they go to a physician and tell their symptoms, they may quickly reach a state in which only relief can be obtained, and not cure. The frequency of cancer of the intestine and rectum is fairly high. Over 6,000 people die of it every year in the United States.

Cancer of the Kidney, Bladder, and Prostate

This type of cancer causes about 5,000 deaths per year in the United States. A reddish urine is the most important sign. Pain is not infrequent. Prostatic cancers are almost inevitably fatal, as it is impossible to cut out all the growth, except in the earliest stages. Cancer of the bladder, on the other hand, if small, can be effectively treated by surgery or by electric cautery methods. Radium and X-ray may bring palliation but seldom cure. Cancer of the kidney is rarely cured.

Sarcoma of the Bone

This type causes some 5,000 deaths per year in the United States. Unfortunately, it can only be diagnosed in the early stages by means of X-ray pictures, but everyone, child or adult, who has rheumatism, growing pains, or sciatica should immediately have an X-ray picture taken of the bones. Sometimes it is possible to diagnose the kind of tumor from the X-ray picture; other times not. Some of these tumors are not highly malignant and can be cured by X-ray or radium treatment. Others are malignant, and only amputation of the limb will save life. If not treated, the patient has only a short time to live, as the disease does not last more than a year or eighteen months, if untreated.

The Diagnosis of Cancer

The diagnosis of cancer is always difficult and sometimes impossible, as it gives no specific symptoms. In the best hospitals, with every facility for diagnosis, some 10 per cent of cancer patients die with the disease unrecognized. Under the general conditions of private practice, especially among the poor, who do not go to a doctor until they are forced to, this figure of undiagnosed cancer may reach 40 per cent. But these are internal cancers.

Many persons with external cancer watch the growth for months or years, until it is hopeless. The medical profession cannot be held responsible for this, for how can they diagnose cancer if the patient does not come to them? It is obvious that cancer of the brain, cancer of the lung, cancer of the liver and pancreas, kidney and prostate, and many of those of the stomach, and also many of the sarcomas which occur in the bones not a part of an extremity, can be cured only in a small number of cases. The removal of a brain tumor is one of the most difficult operations in surgery, even when the diagnosis of its position has been correctly made. Only a few lung tumors have ever been cured, none of the pancreas or liver, and, as has been said, only 5 per cent of stomach cancers. No bone sarcomas of the spine have ever been saved, so that at the present time the profession has to concentrate on accessible growths and try to get patients to come early when a diagnosis and effective treatment are possible. Cancer, being a growth of cells from our own bodies, causes no change in the serum of the blood, so that no blood tests are of value in diagnosis. As it is a part of our bodies, it gives no symptoms but grows quietly until either it presses on nerves and causes pain, presses on or destroys some essential organ and causes symptoms, fills a passage of some sort, such as the windpipe, the swallowing tube, or the bowels, and causes obstruction, or presses on the covering of the bone until it causes pain. In other words, cancer gives only secondary symptoms. A person with cancer may be in perfect health, apparently, and die within a few months. Especially is this true of cancer of the lung, in which the symptoms of cough, expectoration, and pain in the chest may be mistaken for influenza, tuberculosis, or bronchitis, and cancer is revealed only when an X-ray picture is taken.

Cancer of the internal organs is evidently difficult to diagnose. Where an organ is hollow, like the intestine, and an opaque medium can be administered, to afford a shadow picture by X-ray, then it is possible to do something effective in diagnosis, but a cancer may grow to the size of an orange anywhere in the abdominal cavity and the patient not know of its presence. To diagnose all the internal cancers it will be necessary to find some general diagnostic symptoms which it is hoped will be discovered at some future time by research in the laboratories and hospital wards. This vital test has unfortunately not yet been found. The doctor, therefore, must concentrate on the diagnosis of the accessible tumors, the ones which can be seen or felt easily. One of his greatest difficulties is getting people to come to his office at a time when the growth is small and curable. Every physician knows that intelligence of a high order is not necessary if combined with common sense, yet he sees professors, school teachers, and intelligent persons, men and women, watch a growth develop for months and even years, hoping that it will not prove to be a cancer, and knowing all the time that it is and refusing to consult a physician. On the other hand, he meets with hundreds of nervous persons who one week have a cancer, and the next week have tuberculosis, and the next leprosy. For such people the only thing to do is to make a careful examination, and assure them that they have not cancer.

In the meantime, the education carried on by the newspapers, scientific journals of a more popular variety, such as *Hygeia,* and the efforts of the American Society for the Control of Cancer have brought correct information to those who have intelligence enough to use it. There is not the slightest question that the cancer situation, as regards early diagnosis, is improving. Many people are being saved today who would not have been saved five years ago, but still 3,000 people die of cancer of the skin in the United States every year, all curable in the early stages, while 10,000 women die of cancer of the breast, curable at one stage in 80 per cent.

TREATMENT OF CANCER

The treatment of cancer at the present time lies in the hands of the surgeon and the radiologist. The surgeon may use the scalpel, the electric cautery knife, or any other mechanical means that he chooses to remove a tumor. All he can do is to get outside of the growth and remove it and any possible extensions. If, by any mischance, particles of the tumor have passed beyond the scope of his operation, the patient cannot be cured. The radiologist competes with the surgeon in only two fields: cancer of the skin and cancer of the neck of the womb. X-ray and radium are effective in skilled hands in certain tumors of the mouth, throat, and larynx. Radiation fails in carcinoma of the esophagus; it fails in cancer of the stomach, liver, gall bladder, pancreas, and kidney. It is of little use in cancer of the intestine. It may cure an occasional cancer of the prostate. The more benign types of bone tumors may be treated either by surgery or by radiation. They do not necessitate amputation of the limb, and the patient may be allowed to choose. The highly malignant cancers of the bone have never been cured by radiation, and very few have been cured by surgery. The patient must trust the expert to decide the form of treatment. It may depend somewhat on the skill available within the neighborhood. A good radiologist may be preferable to an incapable surgeon, and vice versa. It cannot, however, be insisted on too often that diet, medicine, serums, organ extracts, various forms of colored lights, including ultraviolet light, have absolutely no curative effect on tumors. No tumor should ever be treated by ointments, plasters, or massage. The plasters and ointments do nothing, while massage or any rough manipulation may rapidly spread the tumor throughout the body.

It is hardly necessary to say that the most competent physician is none too good when he comes to grips with cancer, even if he does his best. If so, why accept a quack or any mental cure? The physician may not cure many cancers, but the quack or the mental curist has never cured any.

THE PREVENTION OF CANCER

If so small a proportion of cures of cancer can be obtained, in comparison with the prevalence of the disease, it may properly be asked, Can medical science offer suggestions in regard to the prevention of cancer? The answer is, Yes. All the industrial types of cancer, some of which have been mentioned previously, such as those which result from handling tar, oils, and aniline dyes, from burns, social habits, such as betel-nut chewing—all are under perfect control at the present time, if intelligent use is made of our information. More careful dentistry will diminish cancer of the tongue and mouth by preventing irritation from rough teeth or ill-fitting dentures. Those who use tobacco should be careful to see that scars or ulcers on the lips and tongue are promptly attended to, and that the white spots which are so often seen on the tongues of smokers are properly treated; chronic ulcers, such as the ordinary leg ulcer, should be promptly healed; moles and warts should be watched, and moles removed if they are in any situation where they are constantly irritated, scraped, or rubbed, or in any way subject to injury. They should be cleanly cut out, and not treated by caustic, electro-coagulation, diathermy, X-ray, or radium. The pigmented spots on the skin of old people are easily removed by small doses of X-ray or radium, and the ultimate development of a cancer may be prevented by this sort of treatment. Those with a family history of cancer of the stomach and intestines should eat simply and keep their bowels open. After the age of forty, they should have an annual examination, supplemented by a radiographic study. It has been said by a famous surgeon that 35 per cent of cancer of the rectum is preceded by chronic inflammatory disease of the lower bowel. Cancer of the cervix is unquestionably correlated with injuries produced in childbirth, and suitable care of such tears should always be had, combined with physical examination after the age of forty. If any evidence of chronic inflammation, such as leucorrhea, or other types of discharge occur, the injury to the cervix should be repaired. The removal of gallstones will prevent the occurrence of gall-bladder cancer.

The careful study of nodules in the breast will permit of early diagnosis of cancer in that region.

The chief things which any person over forty should keep in mind are that only early cancers can be cured; everyone is liable to cancer; diagnosis is impossible by the layman; therefore consult a physician. Inasmuch as the disease is fatal if not promptly and properly treated, see the best physician that you can find, and take his advice at once.

CHAPTER XXIV

The Hazards of Industry
CAREY P. McCORD, M.D.

INTRODUCTION: OCCUPATIONAL DISEASES

Every job on which *anyone works brings with it some degree of exposure to risk from contact with chemical substances, with electric power, with conditions of temperature, humidity or similar changes in the environment that may cause illness. The occupations are now recognized as of first importance as a factor in causing disability.*

The human body has in it certain factors for controlling its own temperature, but sometimes outside conditions become so severe that the body's own thermostatic function will not control. Cold constricts the blood vessels in the skin; heat expands them. Sudden changes of temperature, particularly from extreme heat to cold, result in discomfort and are believed to be associated with pains in the limbs and with catching cold. Excessive heat for long periods of time can produce changes in the body leading to unconsciousness and even to death.

In the article which follows, Dr. Carey P. McCord considers first the general conditions associated with occupational diseases and then classifies them according to the chief factor involved in bringing about the illness. For example, if anyone is exposed to extreme dry heat he can develop heat stroke. This is associated with fever, a rapid pulse, flushing of the skin, profuse sweating, and a fall in the blood pressure. Eventually, of course, exposure to extreme heat may so affect the organs and tissues of the body that anemia, inflammations of the skin, disturbances of the kidney, and breakdown of many of the other organs of the body may follow. There are innumerable occupations in which heat is a factor, particularly such occupations as those of blast-furnace and boiler-room workers, of workers in the chemical and cement industries, of cooks, laundry workers, tinners, and similar occupations.

639

Sudden changes in the temperature are particularly likely to occur to men in the ice industry, to butchers, to candy makers, cooks, drivers, electrotypers, fishermen, florists, miners, packing-house employees, soap makers, and similar occupations.

CAISSON DISEASE

One of the most interesting of all occupational diseases is called caisson disease. It is associated with work under conditions in which the air is compressed. In building tunnels, laying deep foundations for buildings, and in submarines, work has to be done under increased air pressure in order to keep out water. The worker is lowered gradually, and at short intervals the pressure of the air in the tunnel is increased. He first feels the sensation of compression in his eardrums, and this can be relieved by swallowing. If the air is compressed too quickly, bleeding may occur. On account of the compression, the blood and the tissues of the body dissolve an increased amount of air. If now the pressure is suddenly decreased, bubbles of nitrogen are formed which cut off the blood supply from various parts of the body. As a result, the patient develops the condition called the bends, known scientifically as caisson disease. The chief symptoms of this condition are weakness, dizziness, pains in the back and legs, painful constriction of the chest, difficulty with hearing, and occasionally paralysis.

DAMPNESS

Occasionally workers are employed in places which are exceedingly damp. This happens particularly in such occupations as those of the fisherman, leather preparers in the glove industry, laundry workers, packing-house employees, workers in the paper industry, pottery workers, sewer workers, and farmers. Most occupations in which dampness occurs are also associated with high and low temperatures and with high humidity.

There are, however, some conditions in which the wetness alone is the serious factor. Exposure to dampness is usually associated as a contributing factor with coughs and colds, in rheumatic disease, and in changes in the skin. Of course, the human being is not adapted to living in exceedingly damp areas; hence he should endeavor to avoid the dampness by wearing waterproof clothing, rubber boots, and similar protective coverings. Moreover, accumulation of water can frequently be prevented by digging channels or ditches to carry away the excess.

Dust as a Hazard

The most serious hazard today in many industries is dust. The dusts not only block the tissues, but in some cases act as an irritant, so that there are inflammation, swelling, and even destruction. Moreover, the dusts sometimes carry germs with them into the tissues, and once in the body the germs may set up inflammations.

Among the most dangerous of the dusts which affect mankind is silica. This produces a condition known as silicosis. X-ray pictures show the lungs full of nodules following the lodgment of the silica in the lymphatics. When the disease is well advanced, the lungs do not expand, and breathing is difficult, and there may be continuous coughing.

The dust from asbestos produces the same type of inflammation that silica produces, although apparently milder. In order to prevent silicosis, workers in any industry in which silica is much used should avoid inhalation, and the head of the industry can aid the worker with certain simple procedures. Water or oil may be used to wet the dust, thus preventing it from rising and filling the air. Exhaust systems can be applied to remove the dust at the point where it develops. Sometimes the work can be done in an enclosed chamber with the worker outside. Finally, where dust is exceedingly excessive, helmets may be worn by the workers to cover the head and neck, and they can get their air by breathing through pipes from a non-dusty area.

Workers in such an industry should have their lungs X-rayed regularly, and there should be a physician in the plant who is familiar with the changes that take place in the lungs under exposure. Whenever a worker in a dusty trade has a cough, a dryness of the nose and throat, pain on breathing and hoarseness, whenever he coughs or expectorates blood, and develops colds which simply refuse to clear up, he should begin to wonder whether or not the dust is affecting him unfavorably. There are hundreds of industries in which dust is a serious factor. In all of them it is a hazard, but when it is silica or asbestos dust, it is a menace to health and life.

Infections of Industry

Certain industries are associated with the likelihood of special infections of the body. For example: workers with hides and animal hair are constantly exposed to infection with anthrax. This begins as a malignant pustule, an inflamed pimple or a boil, which becomes hard, has a purple center and a deep red zone around it. Gradually this breaks down and discharges a thick, bloody material, and eventually may even become gangrenous. The lymph glands in the neighborhood swell, and the veins become inflamed. Associated with this there may be general weakness, including chilliness, loss of appetite, vomiting, and a high fever.

Anthrax is a dangerous disease, and workers with hides must do everything possible to prevent infection. Foreign skins or hair should never be carried on the unprotected shoulder. All hides and animal hair should be thoroughly sterilized. The workers should wash their hands frequently in antiseptic solutions, and those who sort hair should wear breathing devices to prevent inhalation.

As is pointed out elsewhere, the body may become infected from the tissue of infected rabbit with tularemia, from infected straw with actinomycosis, from a contaminated nail with tetanus, from infected milk with undulant fever, and so on, from various substances. Workers in mines and on farms who walk about barefooted may develop hookworm infection.

Every cut, scratch, or abrasion sustained in any industry should be treated at once with suitable antiseptics, such as iodine, to prevent infection. Industries in which infections of the skin, such as boils, carbuncles, and abscesses, are most likely to develop are those of the butcher, the canner, feather workers, fertilizer makers, garbage workers, glue makers, hair workers, dairy workers, silk workers, soap makers, and veterinarians.

RADIANT ENERGY DISEASES

Among the most serious of the occupational diseases recently developed are those associated with the use of radium, the X-ray, and various radioactive substances. Exposure to X-rays and to the emanations from radium may produce serious burns and irritations of the skin which result in cancer. They also affect the blood and the blood-forming organs seriously, so that deficiencies of both the red and the white blood cells are exceedingly common.

Employees in watch factories who prepare the luminous dials have sustained generalized radium poisoning with disastrous results. Workers must learn to protect themselves against these hazards, first of all, by suitable screening against the rays through the wearing of aprons and gloves infiltrated with lead. Brushes for radium painting should never be pointed with the mouth or lips.

Another type of radiant energy which may produce damage to the human body is that associated with ultraviolet and infra-red rays. These are occupational hazards particularly in welding and cutting. The ultraviolet rays are invisible. They cause intense irritation of the eyes and a burning of the skin. Sun-blindness and desert-blindness represent the type of injury that can be caused to the eye by ultra-violet rays. The infra-red rays are essentially heat rays and can cause all the damage that heat of intensity applied to the human body can cause in other ways.

Workers around ultraviolet or infra-red rays may protect themselves against these rays by wearing goggles, helmets, shields, and masks equipped with colored lenses especially designed to exclude dangerous rays. The rays cannot penetrate ordinary clothing, so that covering of the body with a sufficient thickness of clothing will prevent injury and damage to the skin.

Among the industries in which exposure to ultraviolet and infra-red rays are most common are blacksmiths, cutters who use the oxyacetylene gas, furnace workers, glass blowers, iron and steel mill workers, and everyone working in the motion-picture industry. The welders who use the arc for cutting and welding steel are also constantly exposed to dangerous rays.

In the following article, Dr. Carey P. McCord has presented some of the general considerations associated with occupational diseases, and he presents a consideration of the one hundred and fifty most common hazards likely to be found in industry. Any worker associated with any of the poisons here listed should take steps to protect himself against exposure by inhalation, by contamination of the skin, and by other sources.

M. F.

AN OCCUPATIONAL DISEASE is any abnormal state of the body or mind resulting from work. It differs from an accident in that some time must pass between the first exposure to the causative agent and the development of the symptoms. For example, a painter may be exposed over a period of days to the action of a paint solvent. This slowly irritates the skin, so that in the course of a week a rash appears on his hands and forearms. This is an occupational disease.

Some occupational diseases come on so slowly that twenty years may pass before there are serious symptoms. This is especially true in the production of a disease of the eyes called miner's nystagmus. In this condition, the eyes oscillate rapidly. In silicosis, a disease of the lungs due to a special kind of dust, the time before the disability occurs may be as long as fifteen years if the amount of silica in the dust is low.

In a metal-plating plant, chromium-plating solution may splash into the eyes and cause an injury. This is an accident. The same solution, however, breathed in as a vapor, can lead in time to erosions and perforations of the membrane between the nostrils in the nose. This condition is an occupational disease.

A disease may be occupational in one trade and not in another. A nurse who cares for a patient with scarlet fever may develop the disease. In this case her occupation is the cause of the disease. A worker in a plant who catches scarlet fever on his way home from work does not have scarlet fever as an occupational disease. Among workers in a certain office two developed water in the knee joint. One was a salesman who always sat at his desk; the other was a scrub-woman. In her case, the trouble with the knee joint was certainly occupational.

One of the most common occupational diseases comes on slowly and is often ignored. This disease is the result of an undue loss of chemicals from the body, brought on by sweating. On a hot summer day it is not unusual in many trades for a worker to perspire from four to six quarts within the twenty-four hours. A loss of two thirds of an ounce of salts in this sweat is common. This loss paves the way for various dysfunctions of the body, eventuating in undue fatigue, muscular or abdominal cramps, upsets of the bowels, and acidosis. When induced by work, this state properly may be classed as an occupational disease.

Every person who works incurs, in the course of years, some impairments or decrepitude justly associated with his work. Much of this lies within the domain of the ordinary wear and tear of work. Approximately 10 per cent of workers suffer at some time during their work life from characteristic occupational diseases, immediately and definitely connected with employment as the cause.

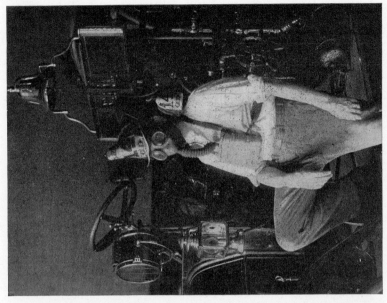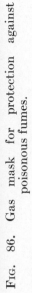

Fig. 86. Gas mask for protection against
poisonous fumes.

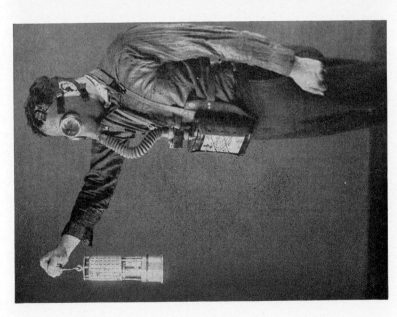

Fig. 85. Mask for miner.
The all-service gas mask devised by Bureau
of Mines chemists and believed to afford protection against more different varieties of poisonous
fumes, gases, and vapors than any other device.

The agents leading to occupational diseases may act on the exposed portions of the body or enter the body through such portals as the breathing tract, the food passages, the skin, or mucous membranes. Manifestly, this necessitates that the offending agent be in such form that it may find entry into the body, or at least be brought into intimate contact with the skin. An ingot of lead is a minimum hazard to workers handling it or sitting on it, but when that ingot is melted and vapors arise, or when it is corroded to produce white lead, a practical and treacherous hazard exists.

The practical hazards of industry commonly include: dusts, gases, vapors, fumes, smokes, odors, toxic liquids, abnormal temperatures, abnormal humidities, abnormal air currents, wetness, oxygen diminution in the respired air, defective lighting, glare, unusual chemical, physical, or light rays, improper seating, postural hazards, vibrations, monotony, speeding, noises, bacterial and other parasitic hazards, unusual air pressures, and explosive mixtures.

POISONING FROM DRUGS AND CHEMICALS USED IN INDUSTRY

Acetanilid, which is well known as a dangerous drug in the treatment of headache, is extensively used in the manufacture of many chemicals, such as paranitranilin. It is commonly taken into the body under industrial conditions in the form of dusts. The action of acetanilid simulates that of aniline oil. An outstanding manifestation is a blue discoloration of the skin, notably of the lips, finger-tips, and ears, which is due to the formation of methemoglobin in the blood.

Acetylene gas is in itself probably nontoxic, except that it may act as a simple asphyxiant; that is, it may displace oxygen in the air to an extent that life may not be supported. However, the use of acetylene may be associated with a number of hazards from impurities or decomposition products. These include sulphur and arsenic compounds, carbon monoxide, and, in addition, from oxyacetylene torch work there may arise the fumes of metals, such as zinc, which are harmful. Chemical rays from acetylene torch work may lead to injury to the eyes, producing such conditions as conjunctivitis or retinitis.

Ammonia gas causes profound local action on the skin, eyes, and respiratory tract. Four hundred parts of this substance per million of air constitute the threshold for immediate irritation of the throat. Prolonged exposure to one fourth of that amount may bring about edema along the respiratory tract. Although ammonia accidents may be severe and fatal, it is unlikely that ammonia as such enters the body.

Coatings, such as lacquers and varnishes, may contain amyl alcohol or related amyl compounds. Toxicity is not great, but it may lead to low-grade irritation of the eyes, nose, and throat.

Aniline oil is a much used chemical in a variety of industries, especially in the manufacture of chemicals. A large number of compounds derived from aniline exert a harmful action similar to that of aniline itself. Aniline is definitely toxic, producing both acute and chronic poisoning. It quickly enters the body through the skin, but poisoning may be brought about by the action of dusts or vapors. In severe acute poisoning there may be observed sudden prostration with blue coloration of lips, nose, and fingers, and unconsciousness with or without convulsions.

Both arsenic and its compounds are highly toxic. Arsenic is widely used in industry, and in addition is present as impurities in many industrial substances unknown to industrial workers. Unsuspected poisonings arise in scores of industries making no direct uses of this substance. It may enter the body in the form of dusts, or vapors, or fluids. Local action may be produced on exposed parts. In constitutional disease the principal systems or organs involved are: gastrointestinal tract, the kidneys, the liver, the nervous system, and the respiratory tract. The loss of hair and of nails, together with bronzing of the skin, are common features.

Asbestos gives rise to a disease of the lungs known as "asbestosis." It is due to the action of asbestos dusts. This disease resembles silicosis, and may in fact be silicosis, since asbestos is principally magnesium silicate. Many years of exposure may be required to establish the disease. Once established, it is permanent. Complication by tuberculosis is frequent.

Asphalt is not a chemical entity but a tarry substance of inconstant make-up, found in nature or resulting from petroleum or coal distillation. Asphalt contains many toxic agents, notably skin irritants. Operations involving the heating of asphalt constitute greater practical hazards than the handling in cold form.

Bakelite is the trade name for a synthetic resin produced from the interaction of phenol and formaldehyde. This resin may be dissolved in benzol. In the manufacture and use of bakelite practical hazards may be found in phenol, formaldehyde, benzol, and "hex" (hex-amethylenetetramine). The latter is a frequent source of dermatitis.

Benzene (benzol) differs from benzine. The former originates in coal-tar distillation. This widely used fluid is one of the outstanding hazards of industry. Concentrations above one hundred parts per million of air are to be regarded as hazardous. Vapors enter the body along with respired air. High concentrations may lead to immediate action, characterized by convulsions, unconsciousness, and prompt death; but the greater number of cases are chronic and center about the results of destruction of several forms of blood elements. Some persons are far more susceptible to the action of benzene than others. Chronic poisoning is characterized by damage to blood-forming organs, kidneys, liver, nervous system, and by increased susceptibility to ordinary infections. Hemorrhage into the skin, from the nose, mouth, stomach, rectum, lungs, and genitalia, are prime manifestations. Benzene in contact with the skin may be absorbed and produce systemic poisoning, or local skin action may take place leading to a dermatitis.

Benzine is a nontechnical term applied to various derivatives of petroleum distillation, such as gasoline, naphtha, etc. The action of this chemical may be local on the skin, or systemic after the inhalation of vapors. This substance is more toxic than commonly believed, and may give rise either to "naphtha jags" (which is an acute disease resembling alcoholic intoxication), associated with respiratory tract irritation, or to chronic forms characterized by profound changes in the nervous system, liver, and kidneys. Chronic benzine poisoning may simulate multiple paralysis.

Bichromates are extensively used in lithography, photography, blueprint work, the dye industry, etc. Their action is similar to that of chromates and chromic acid. Local action may be extensive and intractable. It may produce a dermatitis of unbroken skin, deep burrowing ulcers ("chrome holes"), perforation of the nasal septum, inflammation of the respiratory tract, and a condition akin to sensitization may be instituted by chromium, in which trivial exposures produce profound inflammation of large areas of the skin not in contact with the irritant. Damage from chromium is always slow in healing.

Bisulphide of carbon is much used in artificial silk manufacture and in the rubber industry. Its action is primarily exerted on the central nervous system, causing conditions resembling insanity. It may lead to blindness, paralyses of various groups of muscles, and in addition damage to the kidneys and the gastro-intestinal tract takes place. A highly rapid heart is a rule.

The manipulation of brass in cold form is not known to produce characteristic damage. Brass dust may induce a mechanical dermatitis, and the skin and hair may become green from the copper content of the brass. When, however, brass is in molten state, metal fume fever may arise, which primarily depends on the action of zinc rather than the copper or the brass. The disease produced is variously termed "zinc chills," "brass ague," "foundrymen's chills," etc. In addition, workers about molten brass may acquire lead or arsenic poisoning as the result of these metals being present as impurities in the brass. Workers around molten brass are, as a rule, extensively impaired physically and on the average live a shorter life than workers in general.

Much stated in respect to the hazards of brass work applies to bronze workers. Especially, lead may appear in bronze, and lead poisoning is not a rarity.

Bronze powders is a term extensively applied to the divers metallic powders used in printing and decorating. All such bronze powders are capable of producing inflammation of the skin. Low-grade respiratory tract irritation is common.

Butyl alcohol is a widely used ingredient in solvents. Its toxicity is believed to begin at about one hundred parts of the vapors per million of air. In addition to being a respiratory tract irritant, butyl alcohol may lead to damage to the kidneys, liver, lungs, and to the causation of anemia.

Various compounds of cadmium may enter the body through the lungs in the form of dusts or fumes, and to a lesser extent dusts may enter the stomach. Edema of the lungs may be produced, with or without pneumonia and related injuries. Some scar tissue may be produced. Cadmium likewise injures the liver, kidneys, and intestinal tract. Vomiting may take place, together with diarrhea.

Wherever used, carbolic acid (phenol) is a potential source of severe injury. Harm may be either local, beginning with a slight burn and culminating in gangrene, or may be systemic, following skin absorption, inhalation, or accidental swallowing. Deleterious action is swift, and death may be produced within a few hours. Any portion of the body may be affected. Commonly the respiratory and intestinal tracts, the liver, the kidneys, and blood-forming elements are obviously damaged.

Carbon dioxide is not toxic except as it displaces oxygen necessary in respired air. It is a simple asphyxiant. Deaths in industry from exposure to undue amounts of carbon dioxide are fairly frequent and commonly may be construed as accidents rather than occupational diseases.

Carbon monoxide is one of the most widespread and insidious hazards of industry. Carbon monoxide easily combines with the hemoglobin of the blood and inhibits the oxygen-carrying power of the blood. May be accepted as an accident in the usual case, although a chronic form of poisoning may exist. The characteristic features of poisoning are the bright red discoloration of the flesh, notably of the lips, fingers, nose, and ears, and unconsciousness. The abnormal color mentioned is not always the characteristic cherry red, but may be bluish, greenish, or yellowish red. Prompt artificial respiration after removal from exposure is highly desirable when respiration has ceased.

The action of carbon tetrachloride is characteristic of a group of chlorinated hydrocarbons, including ethylene dichloride, trichlorethylene, and chloroform. The threshold of danger is below five hundred parts of the vapors per million of air. Poisoning may be acute, delayed, or chronic. In acute poisoning the essential manifestations are headache, respiratory tract involvement including pneumonia, vomiting, diarrhea, abnormal pain, sense of moving masses in the abdomen, and irritation of the kidneys. The delayed poisoning may arise twenty-four to forty-eight hours after exposure. Delayed poisoning largely centers about destruction of liver tissues and damage from the subsequently produced guanidine. In chronic poisoning persistent jaundice is a frequent characteristic. Exposure through inhalation is the common source of poisoning. Dry-cleaning establishments using carbon tetrachloride in open systems are believed to afford the most frequent source of exposure. Many cases occur from cleaning of metal parts.

In the manufacture and industrial use of chloride of lime, dusts and gases may lead to asthma, inflammation of the eyes, injury to the respiratory tract, and skin diseases. Harmful action is probably subsequent to liberated chlorine, although impurities may account for some damage.

Chlorine is an irrespirable gas, hazardous in small quantities, leading to prompt swelling (edema) of the lungs and air passages. The chronic form of intoxication, due to the intake of minute quantities over long periods of time, is characterized by severe bronchitis, persistent coughing, and pain in the chest.

Many of the widely used household insecticides consist of ground-up chrysanthemum buds used, as such, as a powder, or are extracted by such agents as ethylene dichloride, kerosene, etc. Both in the manufacture of these insecticides and in their use, extensive skin damage may be occasioned. In the powder form the offending agent may be pyrethrotoxic acid; in liquid forms, this combined with the solvent constitute damaging agents. In industry the disease state is more prevalent in summer months, due to the additional extracting action of perspiration.

Any toxicity connected with the industrial uses of copper is questionable, other than mechanical dermatitis and metal fume fever. Green perspiration and discoloration of hair may lead to an unwarranted degree of apprehension. The copper ion is no less toxic, if, in fact, it enters the body under any circumstance in quantities other than traces.

Creosote is an indefinite term covering various tarry substances from wood, coal, or petroleum. It contains many irritant constituents to the skin, eyes, and respiratory tract.

In the shaping of metal objects with lathes and similar machinery, coolants and other anti-friction agents are in wide use. These agents may be oils or solutions of irritant salts, such as soda ash in emulsions. Irritation to the skin may be produced mechanically by the plugging up of the openings of the skin, sealing in effete materials, or by the direct action of the cutting compounds or their decomposition products. In addition, some harm may be created by bacteria from spitting into containers of these compounds.

Cyanides are extensively used in highly different industries, such as metal plating, case hardening, and insecticidal work. Action may be local, in the production of extensive ulceration, or systemic. The action is that of or related to that of hydrocyanic acid. Cyanides are highly toxic industrial agents.

Dichloro-difluoromethane is a newly developed refrigerant, the toxicity of which is not fully known. From animal experiments it is known to produce tremors and difficulties in walking.

Dinitrobenzene is an intermediate in the manufacture of many chemicals, including dyes. It causes systemic disease, characterized by chocolate-colored blood, jaundice, marked loss of weight, labored breathing, mental sluggishness, impaired vision, and many other changes.

Ethyl benzene is a solvent for paraffins, resins, and lacquers. It causes dizziness, unsteady gait, trembling of extremities, slow, labored breathing, together with local irritation.

Ethylene dichloride is one of a series of chlorinated hydrocarbons with action similar to carbon tetrachloride, as well as its manifestations. The use of ethylene dichloride is increasing in dry-cleaning establishments, in the making of insecticides, in the disinfestation of grain elevators, etc.

Ethyl nitrite is a by-product in the manufacture of mercury fulminate. The latter is employed as detonator in gun cartridges. Exposure to fumes leads to low blood pressure, flushing of the skin, rapid heart, rapid respiration, excruciating headache, and abnormal temperature.

Formaldehyde is a gas, and when this gas is combined with water, formalin is produced. The liquid formalin exerts a destructive action on the skin. Formaldehyde vapors leave the solution. Systemic action is cumulative, leading to the degeneration of the liver and to nephritis. Severe damage may be done to the respiratory tract through irritation and subsequent edema.

Grain itch is a disease of the skin having many names, such as "prairie itch," "threshers' itch," "Texas mange," and "Ohio scratches." This disease is common around threshing operations and hay baling but may appear as a non-occupational disease in bunkhouses where straw mattresses are utilized. This disease is due to an animal parasite, an itch mite technically termed *pediculoides ventricosus*.

Granite is a form of siliceous rock with a high content of free silica. It is a common source of silicosis, to which disease reference should be made.

Heat, or the absence of heat, is the source of a number of specific occupational conditions, such as thermic fever, sunstroke, heat exhaustion, chilblains, etc. Heat is not the source of characteristic occupational diseases, but of ill-defined systemic impairments productive of degenerative diseases and fatigue. The specified conditions, with the exception of chilblains, may, with propriety, be regarded as accidental injuries.

"Hex"—hexamethylenetetramine—is known in medicine as uro-tropin; it was formerly used in the curing of rubber. It is now used in molding plastic objects, such as in bakelite molding. It is a source of severe dermatitis, which occurs more frequently in summer.

Hydrogen is an explosive gas with a low degree of toxicity. It is a simple asphyxiant, causing the displacement of oxygen. It is also a slight irritant to the eyes and is found about plating vats, battery charging, etc.

Hydrogen sulphide, a highly toxic gas widely distributed in industries, such as tanneries, artificial silk mills, and oil fields, is a source of ulcerated eyes. This gas is dangerous in quantities, such as one hundred parts per million of air; one thousand parts per million of air will promptly kill.

Intermediate stages in ink manufacture are prone to produce occupational diseases. Certain inks in finished forms are harmful; for example, phenol ink used in shoe marking, and rotogravure ink. In the melting of composition lead and in the recovery of type metals, adherent inks may give off acrolein and other irritant vapors.

The manufacture of many insecticidal agents designed for use in households and elsewhere involves hazardous exposure. Among others, potentially dangerous agents are chrysanthemum buds, formalin, ethylene dichloride, hydrocyanic acid, etc.

Kerosene is a petroleum distillate with a higher boiling point than benzine. The toxic properties are the same as those for benzine, only less dangerous because of a higher boiling point.

Lead constitutes a foremost occupational disease hazard, with exposure in no less than two hundred different industries. Practically all forms of lead are poisonous, although the less soluble forms constitute less dangerous hazards. This substance may enter the body through inhalation of dust, ingestion of dust, or paste (such as lead in oil), the drinking of fluid, such as lead-bearing drinking water, and some organic lead compounds are absorbed through the skin. Minute traces, such as 1 mg. daily, may produce lead poisoning as a result of cumulative properties. Some persons are far less susceptible than others to lead. The principal lesions are found in the neuro-muscular system, circulatory system, gastro-intestinal tract, and brain.

Lime, chemically known as calcium oxide, may produce local burns of every degree of severity. These burns are deep, leading to tenacious

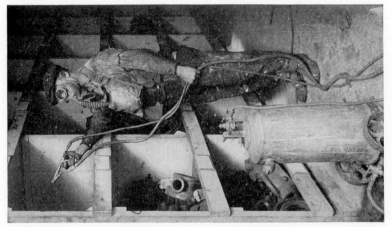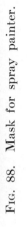

FIG. 88. Mask for spray painter.

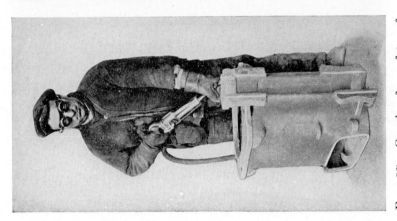

FIG. 87. Goggles for safety of eyes.

eschars, which delay healing. Lime may contain impurities, including arsenic, that give rise to poisoning characteristic of these impurities.

Litharge is a form of lead oxide, much used in storage battery manufacture. The poison that may result from this substance is similar to that caused by lead.

Manganese is a metal associated in the ore form with zinc, lead, etc. Manganese enters the body primarily as a dust through inhalation and ingestion. After several months of exposure those who become affected gradually develop a deterioration of the central nervous system leading to permanent, irreparable paralysis. Patients develop masklike faces, become clumsy in all motions of the body, are unable to stop while in motion, and are permanently disabled.

Meerschaum is a complex magnesium silicate. Mining and the shaping of articles from meerschaum lead to dusts that create a fibrosis of the lung tissues, and lead to clinical manifestations similar to those from silicosis or silicatosis.

Mercury poisoning is one of the oldest occupational diseases, which has been well described by Ramazzini (1700), although he was not the first writer to discuss this subject. Mercury compounds rather than the metal itself are the source of the poisoning. These intoxicants may enter the body through the skin, by inhalation, or by ingestion. No less than two hundred occupations provide exposure to mercury or its compounds or both. Outstanding manifestations are salivation, gastrointestinal inflammation, urinary changes, skin ulceration, neuromuscular lesions, particularly tremors, and mental depression.

Mesothorium is a disintegration product of thorium, between thorium and radiothorium. This term, however, is applied to extensive series of similar bodies, such as thorium X, thoron, etc. Activity of commercial mesothorium is due to the presence of radium mesothorium I and its transformation products, alpha, beta, and gamma emanations.

Methyl alcohol, also designated by such terms as methanol, wood alcohol, Columbian spirits, wood naphtha, and wood spirits, may be made synthetically from the combination of carbon monoxide (or carbon dioxide) and hydrogen, under conditions of high pressure and temperature. The natural product is derived from wood distillation. Both the natural and the synthetic product are highly toxic. The threshold of toxicity is near the concentration of five hundred parts of vapor per million parts of air. Methyl alcohol may enter the body through the skin, by inhalation, and by ingestion. Characteristic lesions are optic atrophy, nephritis, toxic degeneration of the liver, gastro-intestinal inflammation, and pulmonary tract inflammation.

Methyl chloride is employed as a refrigerant and as such has been responsible for a large number of cases of poisoning. Due to the fact that methyl chloride appears to decompose into wood alcohol in the body, the clinical manifestations are the same as those of methyl alcohol poisoning. Gross exposure leads to a primary intoxication, with death from narcosis. Known industrial accidents in hotels, apartment houses, etc., have been of the acute narcotic form. The production of deaths by methyl chloride from refrigerator leaks is well established.

Methyl violet is an aniline dye used in making indelible pencils. There is considerable variation in constituency of dyes termed methyl violet. This agent is especially toxic to the tissues of the eye. Necrosis of the cornea of the eye may readily be produced by flakes of indelible pencil lead material entering the eye.

Mica is the name given various siliceous minerals, and dusts therefrom in any of its forms are siliceous. Silicatosis may be induced if the exposure to concentrated dust is prolonged. Mechanical injury of the skin from mica particles has long been recognized. Among other industrial uses, mica is employed in electrical insulation factories and in stove foundries.

Narcissus bulbs, which so closely resemble onions, contain a deadly alkaloid named narcissin. The eating of narcissus bulbs has caused deaths from the action of narcissin. Industrially, the only harm known to arise is a skin disease, which also is attributed to the narcissin.

The toxicity of nickel is often mentioned but rarely proved. Workers in nickel-plating departments truly develop divers intoxications, but in many instances these may be attributed to the adjuvants in plating departments rather than to nickel itself. The so-called nickel rash is a term covering practically all forms of dermatitis from whatever source arises around nickel-plating works.

Nickel carbonyl is a clear, pale straw-colored liquid which boils at a temperature of 43° C. This salt is quite volatile and possesses toxic properties. In the milder forms of poisoning workers suffer from headache, giddiness, unsteady gait, nausea, and at times dyspnœa, which symptoms quickly disappear upon removal to fresh air. Severe poisoning is manifested by dyspnœa, which after a lapse of 12 to 36 hours is increased, accompanied by cyanosis, a rise in temperature with coughing, and with more or less bloodstained expectoration. The action of the heart is increased but otherwise normal. Delirium of varying types is generally present. Fatal termination of a case takes place usually from the fourth to the eleventh day of illness.

Nitrobenzene (oil of mirbane), an intermediate in the formation of aniline, may produce local skin burns, systemic disease from skin absorption, and intoxication by inhalation. Manifestations are weakness, loss of appetite, burning sensation of skin, abnormal sensation, anxiety state, reeling gait, stammering speech, abnormal reflexes, and convulsions. Later these may be followed by paralyses, amblyopia, brown-colored blood, methemoglobin, and in chronic cases yellow skin. Still later degeneration of red corpuscles and condition of hematoporphyrin are manifested. It is frequently fatal.

Nitrocellulose in its many forms is believed to be relatively harmless. Danger may arise from the many chemicals employed in its manufacture. It is possible that the coatings applied to nitrocellulose for special purposes, such as waterproofing, may be harmful.

Nitrogen peroxide is one of several oxides derivable from nitrogen. This highly irritant gas may lead to a delayed poisoning characterized by pneumonia and pulmonary edema.

Nitroglycerin is responsible for "dynamite head," a condition well known to blasters. The characteristic picture of nitroglycerin action is an intolerable headache associated with a rapid pulse. The keeping of a small portion of dynamite, or other explosive, about the person, perpetuates the tolerance, which apparently is readily established. Enough nitroglycerin may adhere to the clothes of explosive workers to bring about nitroglycerin harm to other persons in their homes. When nitroglycerin explodes, toxicity from the resulting gas is not due to nitroglycerin but to products of combustion.

Nitrous chloride is a highly irritating and asphyxiating gas, possessing insidious delayed action leading to pulmonary edema and respiratory tract inflammation. This gas is highly explosive, notwithstanding which fact it is somewhat extensively used in industry.

Nitrous gases or oxides constitute outstanding intoxicants in industry. Of these, nitrogen dioxide is possibly the most dangerous. As little as sixty parts of this gas per million of air will cause irritation along the respiratory tract, and one hundred parts per million of air may cause death. The action produced may not be immediate.

Phosgene or carbon oxychloride is used as a chemical warfare agent as well as in industry. Its harmful action is apparently limited to the lungs and respiratory tract and the blood stream, with secondary cardiac impairment. Violent lung inflammation develops with edema, later followed by necrosis of the lung tissue. The result is frequently death. Lesser exposure may lead to minor degrees of impairment, as mentioned above, which eventuate in emphysema, bronchitis, bronchiectasis, and dysfunction of the heart. The condition may be accidentally produced in metal industries.

Phosphorus, because of its toxicity, is not employed to any great extent in the United States at the present time. It is utilized, however, in the manufacture of fireworks, in the making of phospho-bronze, and in the chemical industry. White or yellow phosphorus is severely toxic. Susceptibility to poisoning varies. Red phosphorus is essentially free from toxicity. Phosphorus primarily acts upon the bones, leading to necrosis and periostitis. The common site of this bone affection is the jaw, entry of the phosphorus being made by way of carious teeth. Soft tissues in the region of the bone become much involved as a secondary process. Phosphorus necrosis is a continuous process and always results in deformity or death.

Extensive exposure to phosphureted hydrogen leads to prompt death without symptoms indicative of phosphorus poisoning. Symptoms are shortness of breath, marked gastro-intestinal irritation with vomiting and diarrhea, prostration, tremors, and finally active convulsions and death from respiratory failure. Long continued lesser exposure may lead to bone changes, nephritis, etc. Phosphureted hydrogen constitutes an insidious hazard in such work as oxyacetylene welding, the manipulation of ferrosilicon, etc.

Picric acid or trinitrophenol enters the body through skin absorption, by inhalation, and by ingestion of dusts. The commonest lesion is a dermatitis (picric itch). This may be brought about by use of picric acid and picrates. In addition to the dermatitis, there may be yellow pigmentation of the skin suggesting jaundice, gastro-intestinal disturbance with pain, degeneration of the blood, nephritis, and degeneration of the liver.

The ingredients of Portland cement are limestone, shale, silica, and carbon. In this dusty trade, silicosis may arise, and other dusty lung diseases may exist, even though silicosis itself may not be present. The incidence of tuberculosis is high, along with all other respiratory diseases.

Putty commonly contains ground whiting and linseed oil, but frequently lead compounds. Colored putties may contain harmful dyes, such as chromium in green putty. Acrolein may be formed from the decomposition of linseed oil in putty.

Pyrene is a trade name for one brand of carbon tetrachloride. When decomposed by heating, pyrene may give rise to phosgene vapors.

Quinine has been the cause of a dermatitis among pharmaceutical workers; also of edema of eyelids with conjunctivitis and itching. It is a low-grade respiratory irritant.

In the manufacture of rayon and other artificial silks, many harmful agents may be utilized as intermediates and adjuvants. The outstanding objectionable agent is carbon bisulphide. It is possible that rayon is now being weighted with lead and tin as are also natural silks. This practice introduces the lead hazards.

Rotogravure ink has been associated with dermatitis. Paranitraniline red or a similar substance is probably the active agent leading to that type of dermatitis. Readers of rotogravure newspapers may become affected.

Sandstone is a silica-bearing rock with a high free silica content. It is known as a source of silicosis.

Sealing wax of various brands may differ in composition. It may contain resinous materials from coal tar or petroleum or from vegetable matter. At times it is colored with arsenic. Turpentine and other harmful solvents have been employed.

Sewer gas may contain hydrogen sulphide, carbon monoxide, carbon dioxide, any of which may lead to disasters.

Shellac itself, which is an Indian resin, is probably nontoxic. The substances in which it is dissolved may be poisonous, and in the past have caused many scores of poisonings and deaths. As a solvent, wood alcohol has been the source of blindness and death.

Free silica, in any of its many forms, when taken into the body through the respiratory tract, slowly leads to a dusty lung disease known as silicosis. Silicosis is probably the result of chemical action of the siliceous materials, but undoubtedly mechanical action plays some part. Cases may be produced within less than one year of exposure, but the usual case requires several years to develop. Patients complain of difficulty in breathing, of pain in the chest, and of impaired heart function. No treatment is efficacious. Tuberculosis is a common concomitant. This disease is encountered among workers in granite and sandstone quarrying, in stone dressing, in mining, and in city excavation work, etc.

Silver, or its salts, as used in industry, is harmful from just one standpoint, and that is that it produces black deposits within the skin, a condition known as argyrosis.

Sodium cyanide produces muscular weakness, inflammation of the conjunctivæ and pulmonary tract, edema of the eyelids, irregular pulse, loss of weight, painful urination, mental disturbances, etc. In addition, cutaneous manifestations are probable.

Sulphur dioxide is the commonest household refrigerant, with the exception of ice. It is also used extensively in a variety of industries or is the product of other materials. Twenty parts per million of air will produce some irritation; fifty parts per million is dangerous. Action is limited to the respiratory tract and to reflex actions. Contrary to common belief, tolerance for sulphur-dioxide action is not established. Chronic bronchitis and other persistent manifestations are well known. It may also produce acidosis.

Talc is magnesium silicate. As such, it is capable of producing fibrosis of the lungs.

Tannic acid may attack the unbroken skin and may partially tan the skin. A dermatitis is universally present among hide handlers in the tanning yard using the tannic acid process. When the skin is broken, deep undermining ulcers may arise.

Tar is a general term applied to a variety of substances derived from wood, coal, or petroleum. Tar cancer is a rare affection among persons exposed. Skin diseases and irritation of the respiratory tract are common.

Tetraethyl lead is an organic lead compound utilized as an anti-knock substance in motor vehicles. The opportunities for intoxication are largely limited to the manipulation of this substance in its manufacture. It is one of the few forms of lead entering the body through the skin. Apparently this form of lead has a special predilection for brain tissues, leading to encephalitis.

Thallium, a toxic metal, consists of salts which are useful in the making of rat poisons, in the preparation of depilatories and other pharmaceuticals, in disinfectants, in dye manufacture, and in lead alloys. When taken into the body it causes loss of hair, optic atrophy, distorted color vision, lymphocytosis, etc.

The tin industry is attended by many hazards in mining, smelting, and refining, but these are probably due to impurities, heat, etc., rather than to any toxic properties of tin itself under industrial conditions. At the present time scant proof of the toxicity of tin exists.

The tobacco industry is a generally hazardous one. Tobacco workers may acquire acute nicotine poisoning, but the situation is ameliorated by an apparent tolerance for this substance. Tobacco may produce blindness, but genuine incidents are rare. Tuberculosis rates are high in this industry. Arsenic is a potential hazard, from the use of that substance as an insecticide during the growing period. The drying of tobacco may give rise to the formation of carbon dioxide in dangerous concentrations. High temperatures and high humidities characterize certain departments.

Toluene (toluol) is closely rated to benzol. It is advocated as a substitute for benzol, owing to lesser capacity for intoxication. It is more active as a narcotic agent than benzol, but less frequently produces chronic intoxication. When poisoning occurs, the clinical picture is that of benzol poisoning.

Trichlorethylene is a chlorinated hydrocarbon similar in action to carbon tetrachloride.

Pure gum spirits of turpentine is less hazardous than other types. It may, however, produce irritation of the skin and mucous membranes, gastritis, salivation, genito-urinary manifestations, etc.

Vanadium is a metal which is seldom used. Its salts find use in photography and in the manufacture of steels. Toxicity has been attributed especially to the trioxid. The outstanding manifestations are marked irritation of the respiratory tract, eventuating in hemorrhage, rapid loss in weight, nephritis, optic atrophy, and general condition simulating nervous breakdown. This condition is so rare as to be open to question as to its existence.

White damp is a term used by miners for carbon monoxide in mines. Black damp is ordinarily carbon dioxide. Stink damp is usually hydrogen sulphide.

Wood turpentine is unlike gum spirits turpentine, being made by steam or destructive distillation of cut or fallen timber. Steam-distilled wood turpentine earlier was a marked irritant to skin and mucous membranes. Modified processes now obviate some of this irritation.

Destructively distilled wood turpentine is less of an irritant than the steam distilled. All turpentines are somewhat irritating.

Xylene (xylol) is closely related to benzene (benzol). It is more toxic than benzene in producing acute narcosis, and is less toxic in the production of chronic conditions. The clinical disease produced, although rarely, is similar to that of benzene poisoning.

Industrial zinc is probably nontoxic. Recently produced zinc oxide, as in the manufacture of brass or in galvanizing, may lead to zinc chills, also termed brass chills, brass workers' ague, etc. The condition is characterized by great thirst, marked chilling little influenced by heat, with or without elevated temperature, eventuating in deep sleep with profound physical depression. Zinc is not involved in any chronic form of poisoning.

Zinc chloride is much used in wood preservation as a fire repellent and fungicide. It is associated with the production of dermatitis. Zinc sulphate produces marked alimentary tract inflammation, culminating, in severe cases, in ulceration of the stomach or duodenum.

CHAPTER XXV

The Skin
ARTHUR W. STILLIANS, M.D.

T HE SKIN is an elastic membrane perfectly adapted to furnish protection of many sorts to the body without in the least interfering with motion. It is made of two parts, an outer called epidermis, meaning outer skin, and an inner connective tissue foundation. The *epidermis* is composed wholly of epithelial cells in several layers, the cells in the inner layers joined by tiny bridges of cell substance under which flow minute canals. As the cells in the innermost layer multiply and push those above toward the surface, the topmost ones flatten, become horny, and reach the surface tightly cemented together in a protective layer that is made flexible and watertight by being well oiled and covered by a thin film of oil. The horn cells on the surface are lifeless and are constantly being shed from the surface as new cells from below take their place. The pigment or coloring matter of the skin, which plays so important a rôle in protection from light, is produced in the innermost layer of the epidermis. The cells that produce hair and those that do the active work of the skin glands are also derived from the epidermis, really a part of it.

The *inner, connective tissue layer* of the skin is composed of fibers forming a mesh-work support for the blood and lymph vessels, nerves, glands, and hair. As seen under the microscope, the line between the two layers of the skin is not straight, for the lower surface of the epidermis and the upper one of the connective tissue layer dovetail together, conical elevations called papillæ on the inner layer fitting into depressions on the under surface of the epidermis. This serves to fasten the two layers together securely, increases flexibility, and greatly increases the extent of the surface for radiation of heat from the blood, one of the most important functions of the skin. The innermost part of the connective tissue layer is the cushion on which the skin rests, absorbing shocks from without and allowing the skin to move freely upon the underlying parts. It also gives the rounded appearance to the body which adds so much to beauty. As may be supposed, it contains fat, in large cells between the loose mesh work of fibers which carry the larger vessels and nerves and support the bases of large hair follicles and sweat glands.

Several different kinds of *nerves* end in the skin: those that notify of pain, those for touch, pressure sense, and temperature changes, those that control the dilatation and contraction of blood vessels, and, last but not least, those mysterious nerves that control the nutrition of the skin, called the trophic nerves.

The *sweat glands* are simple tubes coiled tightly at the lower end where the sweat is formed. From this coil a wavy tube passes outward to the epidermis, enters it and forms a spiral passageway between the epidermal cells, to open on the top of one of the minute ridges to be mentioned later.

The *sebaceous* or *fat glands* are composed of a number of bag-like structures grouped together, their ducts joining to enter the upper part of the hair follicle. Within the glands the epithelial cells enlarge and turn to a semi-solid fat, which is discharged on the hair and the surface of the skin. It is estimated that the skin contains over two millions of each kind of glands.

Beneath the sebaceous gland a small involuntary *muscle* joins the hair follicle at an acute angle. By its contraction it squeezes the gland and at the same time erects the hair. Thus the hair actually can stand on end. Further description of the hair will be found in the part devoted especially to this structure. Besides the tiny involuntary muscles attached to each of the long hairs, there are special voluntary muscles, the muscles of expression, attached to the skin and fascia of the face and neck.

The skin has *elasticity*—that is, it can stretch, but only so far. It can accommodate itself to moderate stretching, like that accompanying deep breathing, and return to its original smooth condition; but when overstretched, as in pregnancy, its inner layer often ruptures and heals with a scar. Thus are formed the white lines so often seen on the abdomen of a woman who has borne children, on the skin of stout people, or of children who have grown rapidly. However, when the body shrinks quickly, as after a wasting disease or too rapid reducing, the skin cannot contract to fit it; but hangs in folds. Under normal conditions the skin is slightly stretched, as is shown by the gaping of wounds. Its tension is slight, however, for these wounds can be drawn together easily.

The normal *texture* of the skin is fine, because the scales covering it are minute, oiled, and covered with delicate hair. The skin may be coarse, like that on many noses, because of large sebaceous ducts. Often faces that are scarred are referred to as having large pores. This is incorrect. On the skin, as best seen on the palm of the hand and sole of the foot, are many fine ridges arranged in patterns that are characteristic for each individual and that are used for identification. On these ridges the sweat pores open. Coarser, less regular lines are caused by motion, folding the skin along these lines. Still larger lines are caused partly by motion and partly by the attachment of the skin to the underlying fascia, about the joints and under the breasts. Dimples are caused by the attachment of muscles of expression drawing in the skin at this point when they contract.

The *fat* of the skin is mainly sebum, produced by the sebaceous glands; but the sweat glands and the epithelial cells themselves as they turn to horn produce fat which supplements the sebum.

The *color* of the skin is determined by the amount of pigment in the lower layer of the epidermis and by the color of the blood and the size of the superficial blood vessels. Through the epidermis of blondes the red color shows diffusely as through ground glass, with just enough effect of the pigment to make the color creamy. Brunettes have more pigment, and other races than the white race have still more, until in the black race the red color of the blood is largely concealed.

Flushing of the skin is the result of a dilatation of the blood vessels near the surface; *blanching*, a result of contraction of these vessels. A person may be pale because he is anemic, his blood is deficient in hemoglobin, the iron containing coloring matter, or because his peripheral blood vessels, for some reason, have shut out the blood that should be coursing through them.

Tanning and *freckling*, the increase of skin pigment diffusely or in spots, is a reaction designed to protect against the harmful effect of light. The white race has to acquire all but the minimum of skin pigment. The dark races develop it partly before, partly after birth.

The *nourishment* of the skin is obtained from the blood circulating in the inner layer about the glands and hair follicles and in the papillæ. In the latter lymph exudes from the capillaries and passes into the canals of the epidermis, circulating between the cells, giving up nutritive substances and taking up waste matter, then passing out again to the papillæ, where it is taken up by the blood or lymph and carried away. No food for the skin comes through its outer surface. There is really no such thing as a skin food. Its nutrition comes from the blood.

The Functions of the Skin

The chief function of the skin is protection. Besides this, some of its nerve functions are connected with sexual life and other emotional fields, as are the decorative functions of the skin and its appendages, the hair and nails.

Mechanical protection is afforded by the skin and its cushion of fat, freely movable on the parts underneath.

A dry skin is a good insulator against all but high-voltage electrical currents.

Insulation against cold is aided by the contraction of the tiny muscles of the hair follicles, which elevate the follicles to form "goose flesh," supplementing the contraction of the blood vessels of the surface, preventing radiation of heat.

Prevention of evaporation of body fluids is, of course, of great importance. It was this provision against drying out that made it possible, millions of years ago, for living beings to emerge from the sea and risk the drying effect of air, a bitter enemy of life.

Not much less important is the prevention of the entrance of water and other harmful substances from without.

Protection against acids is excellent, against alkalies not so good, for they soften the horn cells, and they and other chemicals that remove fat reduce the resistance of the skin and favor penetration.

Radiation is one of the chief functions of the skin, protecting against the harmful effect of heat. This, in hot weather or during a fever, is accomplished by dilatation of the blood vessels, increasing the amount of blood exposed to the cooling air, and at the same time by increase of the sweat, which, during evaporation, absorbs heat. Thus the production of sweat is one of the most important functions of the skin. Its value as an eliminant of waste products from within the body is slight, for only volatile bodies are eliminated in the perspiration. The odor of the sweat is the chief source of *body odor*, now popularized as B. O., about which so much is said. It is due partly to these volatile bodies from within, partly to the fatty acids in the skin. While sometimes unpleasant, giving the unfortunate possessor much mental distress, cases are on record of a pleasant, violet-like odor of the sweat. Apparently this violet odor in babies is due to carotene. During the time when we may not be aware of perspiration, it is nevertheless going on, but only at a rate at which it can immediately be evaporated. This is called *insensible* perspiration.

Under ordinary circumstances *absorption* through the skin is slight even for fatty substances. By friction, fats may be forced into the hair follicles and absorbed, carrying with them other substances. The quantity of such substances is so small that while it may be valuable in the case of strong medicines, for food it is too slight to be of consequence, and even then must be reworked by the internal organs before the skin can use it. The popular idea that fats applied to the surface can feed the skin is a fallacy. Fats or creams thus applied may serve a useful purpose in keeping the skin supple, preventing scaling and cracking and maintaining the resistance of abnormally dry skins.

The nerves of the skin protect the body against harm, warning of the danger of excessive heat or cold or sharpness; help us to become acquainted with the world about us, and provide one of our sources of pleasure: the feel of smooth surfaces, polished wood, delicate fabrics, flower petals, and the like.

By pigment formation the skin can protect the body successfully from the harm of ordinary sunlight and ultraviolet rays; but against Roentgen rays and the rays of radium its efforts, though often manifested by pigmentation, are of no avail, for these rays penetrate the pigmented skin as easily as they do the nonpigmented.

Besides these more or less obvious functions of the skin, it has the ability to clear its surface of germs within a short time. The mechanism of this action is not understood. There are some bacteria against which the skin is powerless in this way; it cannot rid itself of them. It is important to realize, however, that even against these the normal skin is an important first line of defense. Further, if germs do gain entrance to the skin, whether from without or through the blood stream, the normal skin can produce chemical substances which may inhibit their growth or wholly destroy them. Of course, some agents of infection are too strong to be controlled in this way, and the resistance of the skin may be lowered without warning.

These efforts of the skin to protect itself and the whole organism against infection often take the form of an inflammatory reaction in the skin. This power of reacting against germs and their toxins has been utilized by Von Pirquet, Schick, Dick, and others, to produce the tests for the ability of the body to resist tuberculosis, diphtheria, scarlet fever, and other infectious diseases. Various skin tests have also been devised to show sensitization in asthma, hay fever, urticaria, and eczema. They are all of more or less value in diagnosis. Thus the skin has become a bureau of information, ready to report on the state of affairs in relation to protection against these diseases or on the presence of hypersusceptibility, whenever requested to do so by the physician. It has been characterized as a mirror of the body. In addition to its ability to protect against infection, the skin produces the vitamin that protects against and cures rickets. This explains in part the beneficial effects of sun baths and ultraviolet light baths, particularly for infants.

Marks on the skin, as moles or scars, are often useful in identification. The use of the peculiar patterns of the ridges on the finger tips has become familiar in the identification of criminals. More recently, these patterns have been found useful in obstetrical hospitals, where each new arrival, as his first official act as a member of the human race, leaves a footprint upon the hospital records.

Keeping the Skin Healthy

As has been said, the skin gets its nourishment from the blood and lymph. The importance of general good health to the health of the skin cannot, therefore, be overestimated. Local care of the skin and the use of various cosmetics and so-called "skin foods" is so stressed in advertising at present that one is apt to get the impression that the skin can be fed independently of the rest of the body. This is not true, for the skin is an organ of the body and, like the other organs, is dependent on the health of all for its well-being.

The condition of the blood has a direct effect on the skin. Anemia and other abnormalities of the blood, and defective circulation, deprive the skin of nutrition and proper drainage of waste products and make it pale, too greasy, or too dry, lessening its resistance to irritation and infection. Disease of the liver acts much the same way and in addition may cause damming back of the bile in the circulation and yellowing of the skin, or jaundice, which is often preceded and accompanied by annoying itching. Diabetes lessens the resistance of the skin because the cells are unable to utilize the sugar owing to a lack of insulin. Besides this, the sugar-containing sweat favors the growth of germs, and the diabetic urine irritates the skin with which it comes in contact, and the resulting inflammation offers an easy entrance for infection. This shows how important, for diabetics, is the care of the skin. Joslin says, in the chapter on diabetes, that a diabetic should keep his feet cleaner than his face, because serious infection so often begins in this disease about the toes.

CONSTIPATION

Constipation also has an effect on the health of the skin. Failure to eliminate waste through the bowels and absorption of toxins from the bowels injures the proper sanitation and nutrition of the skin. The irritative effect of cathartics on the bowels may favor the absorption of the toxins which they were intended to eliminate. All this goes to show that beauty is more than skin deep.

The skin needs the general health benefit derived from plentiful, well-chosen, well-prepared, well-digested food, from outdoor exercise, interesting work, and restful sleep, and a definite, not excessive, amount of sunshine.

BATHING

Local care is, of course, of great importance. Besides the removal of grease and dirt, bathing, particularly if the bath is ended with a cold shower, has a beneficial effect on the circulation. This is accentuated by the rubbing necessary to drying, more vigorous because of the feeling of vigor consequent on the cold shower. Frequency of bathing is an individual problem. Some find frequent bathing debilitating, while on others it has the opposite effect. Some people cannot get a good reaction to cold baths and therefore should not take them. Often such persons react better to a mild application of cool water and can train themselves to the cold shower by gradual increase in the duration and decrease in the temperature of the bath. Nervous people and those with dry skins are the ones most apt to object to frequent bathing.

The use of soap in the bath is to be regulated according to the kind of bath and the kind of skin that is being bathed and according to the season of the year. In the summer time soap can be used more freely by most of us, for there is much perspiration that needs removing; more will follow after the bath, and there is no danger of depriving the skin of the oil necessary to its welfare. In winter, however, the skin secretes less sweat and oil, the cold air is dry, and so is the warm air of our steam-heated dwellings. Soap, used freely, is apt to add the unbearable extra burden. The skin resents it by paroxysms of a stinging itch known as winter or bath itch. This can be corrected by limiting the use of soap during the winter months to the hairy parts of the body and those parts that get the dirtiest, the hands, face, and feet. Once a week or so it can be used generally and the bath followed by some sort of inunction or oily rub.

Some women and a few men find that their abnormally dry skins will not tolerate soap on the face at any season. The skin becomes scaly and itches, and if the irritation is carried farther becomes red in patches, the condition known as chapping. For such people cold cream is a justifiable substitute for soap. More refreshing, however, is oatmeal water, made by boiling oatmeal for five minutes in a bag made of several layers of gauze. The water in which it was boiled, plus all the fine material that can be squeezed through the gauze, is cooled and used for cleansing. It must be made fresh every day or two. A handful of oatmeal should suffice for a gallon of water. It removes dirt better than plain water, taking the place of soap to a considerable degree, and can be used on some irritable skins with impunity.

Those with greasy skins, however, must recognize that these methods are not for them; but that their skins are best cared for by vigorous washing with hot water and soap, followed by a cold shower.

Baths are classified according to temperature as follows:

Cold bath	below	60 F.
Cool bath	between	60 and 80 F.
Tepid bath	between	80 and 90 F.
Warm bath	between	90 and 100 F.
Hot bath	over	100 F.

The tepid bath is soothing and quieting and, if long continued, depressing. The warm bath is the best for cleansing. Both hot and cold baths are stimulating, and the greatest effect of this kind is obtained from a hot bath followed by a cold shower, which stimulates the circulation, preventing chilling and increasing resistance against infection. Rubbing the skin with the hands or the washcloth while in the water and vigorous rubbing while drying assist in obtaining this effect. The duration of the bath should be short, unless a soothing effect is desired. A longer warm bath at night conduces to sleep, a short cold shower in the morning stimulates, providing there is the proper reaction to it.

Sweat baths, among which the Turkish bath is the most popular, are not needed as a general thing. If benefit can be derived from them, they should be taken under the direction of the physician. The same rule applies to medicated baths, mud baths, and sulphur baths, for under some circumstances they do harm and should, therefore, not be taken indiscriminately.

Open-air bathing is one of the most popular of the sports of today and of past ages, and deservedly so. Bathing suits have become so abbreviated and sensible that large skin surfaces are exposed to the air and sun between swims. At the beginning of the season care should be used to avoid too long exposure to the sun, and the same warning applies to those who go to the Southern beaches during the winter. The skin, long protected from light, cannot stand much of it at first. Severe sunburn damages rather than benefits and should be avoided. Gradual inuring of the skin to the strong sunlight should be the rule.

SOAP

The so-called wild German tribes introduced soap into what the Romans called civilization. Before that event, bathing among the Romans was done with plain water followed by perfumed oil, or, if the need was urgent, a rubdown with ashes preceded the bath. The place of soap in our civilization is so important that it is hard to picture our lives without it. Those who lived in Germany or Austria during the Great War can realize better than most of us what such a situation means.

When fats are boiled with a solution of an alkali, they are split into glycerin and fatty acids and the latter unite with the alkali to form soap. The glycerin is a valuable by-product. Potassium hydrate forms soft soap, of which the green soap used in the hospital is the familiar example. Sodium hydrate forms hard soaps such as ordinary laundry or toilet soap. The solution of these in water is viscid, that is, it has the power of holding together, illustrated by the formation of bubbles, which are globules of air separated from the rest of the air by a film of soap. This viscid character of soapsuds enables it to emulsify the grease on the skin, carrying with it the dirt, and they both then dissolve in the water and are carried away.

In the making of soap there is always a part of the alkali not combined with the fatty acids, and this is the "free alkali" so often mentioned in connection with toilet soap. It makes the soap strong, loosening the dirt and grease so that it can better be removed. For rough work considerable free alkali is needed; but for skins it is desirable that the free alkali should be reduced to the minimum. Strong soap removes more fat from the skin than is good for its health and leaves it red and irritated, an easy victim to infection. In good toilet soap the free alkali should not exceed one fourth of one per cent. For dry and delicate skins superfatted soap is made by removing as much as possible of the free alkali and adding wool fat. This does not become rancid and leaves a film upon the skin to replace that removed in washing. These superfatted soaps are only a little less efficient as cleansers than the regular soaps and for babies and older persons with dry skins are highly recommended.

Transparent soaps are made by adding alcohol, glycerin, or sugar during the manufacture of the soap, preventing it from crystallizing and becoming opaque. They are generally more apt to contain free alkali than the opaque kind; but there are exceptions to this rule.

Green soap is a strong one; that is, it contains a considerable amount of free alkali. The surgeon prefers it because of this fact, in order to get his hands and arms as free from germs as possible. Not uncommonly, however, he suffers from its irritating quality. Pure green soap is not green but yellow.

Hard-water soaps are often only ordinary soaps with an excess of coconut oil to make them form suds more readily with water containing much calcium. Coconut oil is an ingredient of most soaps and is not harmful as long as the amount is small; but in excess may be irritating to delicate skins.

Soap is not only cleansing in its action, but, as Reasoner and others have shown, soapsuds actually kill most of the ordinary germs. Unfortunately two, the typhoid bacillus and that cause of most of the boils and other skin infections, the ubiquitous staphylococcus, are able to resist it. It would seem desirable to add to soap an antiseptic that would be powerful enough to kill these two also. The danger of this is that the soap is thus made irritating to the skin, and irritation reduces the resistance of the skin, thus defeating the very purpose of the addition. It seems better to maintain the normal germ-killing efficiency of the skin by proper care rather than to attempt direct action upon the bacteria with antiseptics combined in soap.

Good soap need not be expensive. It is made so only by special perfumes, fancy packing, and high-pressure advertising. All toilet soaps contain some perfume, justifiable because it conceals the soapy smell. This need not make it expensive. Choose a soap adapted to your needs made by a reputable firm, and you will make no mistake. It is remarkable how often soap is chosen by the method followed by the doctor's young hopeful, who insisted on having the "smelly" soap.

POWDERS

Dusting powders and face powders are soothing, cooling, and drying, as well as protective and decorative. Each tiny particle of powder acts to increase the surface for the evaporation of insensible perspiration, thus cooling and drying the skin. It also protects against the irritation of cold air or sunshine and the rubbing of clothing. The requirements for a good powder are that it be fine and nonirritating. Talcum is the best known and most widely used powder. It is of light weight, very fine texture, and adheres well to the skin. Zinc stearate is heavier and also a good adherent. The starches, potato, wheat, or corn, are useful but absorb moisture and swell, making them less desirable where much moisture is present. Powdered orris root is a popular ingredient of some of the most expensive and extravagantly advertised face powders but is a frequent cause of dermatitis because the skin so readily becomes sensitized to it. It had better be avoided. Lead salts are often used in face powders of the same expensive and extravagantly advertised class but should be prohibited, for they not seldom cause black spots on the face from a chemical reaction with the sulphur always present in the skin, or even result in lead poisoning from absorption. Boric acid in small amounts is often added to dusting powders for its action in deterring the growth of germs. Stout people and babies are the chief beneficiaries of dusting powders. Without them, they are apt to suffer from irritation in the folds of the skin, known as intertrigo. In applying powder to the infant, great care should be taken to have it in one of the patent containers made to prevent the possibility of the baby getting the open end of the container in its mouth, for several deaths have been caused by the baby's shaking the powder into its mouth and inhaling it.

COLD CREAM

The fat in the skin is an important ingredient. It keeps the horny layer of the skin soft, flexible, and watertight and forms over it a thin protective film. When fat is deficient the skin becomes rough, dry, and scaly, often inflamed, and much more liable to infection. The owner of such a skin is notified of this condition by a feeling of stiffness or even itching or pain. In common words the skin is chapped. This happens most often in the winter, when cold dry winds are prevalent. To counteract it, fat may be supplied to the skin in the form of cold cream, supplementing nature. To avoid the removal of fat by ordinary washing with soap and water, cold cream is rubbed on the skin and wiped off, removing much of the dirt with it. This does not compare, of course, with the cleansing attained by the use of soap but is fairly efficient. Cleanliness may be next to godliness but is not an unmixed good for those with dry skins. It can be overdone, or, rather, it can be done in the wrong way. In those with greasy skins, however, cream is harmful if it takes the place of hot water and soap cleansing. Cream adds to the grease already too plentiful and in cases of acne increases the tendency to form pustules.

Many different fats are available for anointing the skin; but cold cream, ointment of rose water, a perfumed emulsion of fat and water, is deservedly the most popular. There are many formulas for it; but all have about the same effect upon the skin. Light, soft creams are called cleansing creams and are sometimes advertised as "skin foods," which of course is a misnomer and a false claim, for the skin is fed only through the stomach, as the rest of the body is fed. Other preparations advertised as greaseless cold creams and recommended as cleansing creams are not creams at all but soaps made with sodium carbonate. Of course, they cleanse better than real cold cream, but they also defeat the purpose of creams for they take oil out of the skin instead of adding it. Some cold creams become rancid in time. This can be delayed by adding a small amount of boric acid, 5 or 10 per cent, to the cream. Many of the commercial cold creams are now made with petrolatum in place of real fats. Petrolatum, better known as vaseline, a trade name, is not a fat but a derivative of petroleum which has many of the properties of fats but does not become rancid.

A good formula for cold cream that will not turn rancid and that contains some wool fat, one of the fats most beneficial to the skin, is as follows:

Hydrolysed wool fat	2.0
White petrolatum	6.0
Rose water	20.0

Melt the two fats, mix them and allow them to cool, then beat them up with the rose water until white and creamy.

Other substitutes for soap. There are greaseless lotions made with tragacanth that are viscid and therefore remove dirt. An example:

Oil of rose	0.05
Oil of lavender	0.1
Oil of bergamot	0.2
Powdered tragacanth	5.0
Boric acid	15.0
Glycerin	15.0
Water to make	500.0

Shake the tragacanth with the glycerin and oils, then add water little by little, shaking the mixture vigorously each time. Let it stand twenty-four hours, or until it is smooth. This lotion, rubbed on and wiped off, is a fair cleanser. If allowed to dry upon the skin it forms a protective film. It can be used in this way after washing to prevent drying of the skin and for this purpose should be applied before the skin is completely dry. Oatmeal water, bran water, and almond meal are also fairly good cleansers which do not remove fat.

ANTISEPTICS

For application to small wounds tincture of iodine is probably the most widely known. It should be painted on, one coat only. More than this does not add to the good effect and increases the danger of irritation. The bottle must be kept tightly stoppered, preferably with a rubber stopper, for if the tincture is exposed to the air it evaporates and becomes so strong that even one application may cause a severe reaction. After iodine has been applied, no preparation of mercury should be used on the same area for several days for fear of an unpleasant skin irritation. The stain of iodine can be removed by dilute ammonia water.

Boric acid in saturated solution is a deservedly popular household remedy. Though it does not kill germs, it limits their growth and is soothing rather than irritating to inflamed skin. It should be made by filling a clean (boiled or scalded) fruit jar or large bottle one fourth full of the boric acid crystals, then adding boiled water to fill the jar. When this has cooled, it is a saturated solution, and what is needed can be poured off. By keeping crystals at the bottom, water above, a saturated solution is always ready for use. For infections it should be heated and applied on a large dressing covered to retain heat as long as possible. For most acute skin irritations, however, it is best applied cool on a thin compress, allowing for evaporation. The compress should be again wrung out of the cool solution when it becomes warm.

The solution of hydrogen peroxide is a useful household remedy. It does not kill germs, except those that cannot grow in the presence of oxygen, the anerobes. These occur in the mouth and other cavities of the body. More often, peroxide is used for cleansing wounds. It attacks and destroys pus and blood and at the same time gets into small crevices and by forming oxygen gas loosens dirt so that it can be wiped or washed away. Care must be taken not to put peroxide into a cavity from which it cannot easily escape, for under these circumstances the gas may form under pressure and cause great pain and actual damage to the tissues.

Boric acid powder is an excellent powder for open wounds and is also much used combined in ointments.

Carbolic acid, often used in the household, is a dangerous drug, for it does not dissolve well in water, and when the attempt is made to make such a solution, concentrated carbolic acid often comes into contact with the skin and burns it. It should be used only under the direction of the doctor.

Collodion dressings, advertised as "new skin," which were popular some years ago but seem much less so now, are proper dressings for clean wounds but should not be applied to infected ones. A small pledget of sterile gauze applied with a bandage or adhesive plaster is much safer where there is any suspicion that the wound is not sterile, and such suspicion nearly always is justified in accidental wounds. Court plaster moistened with saliva and stuck on a wound is as bad a dressing as could be imagined.

MASSAGE

Massage, including rubbing and kneading, is a well-established means of maintaining circulation in those prevented by disease from exercising, and of restoring circulation to parts in which it is deficient. The face, however, seldom lacks exercise. Our days are full of it, at meal times as we chew our food thoroughly (let us hope), and between meals as we talk and allow the play of our emotions to find expression on the face. The rubbing in of cold cream is not necessary, for it exerts all its benefit on being applied gently. Massage is refreshing, however, and if followed by a good washing, as it always should be, does no harm in most cases. In any active inflammatory condition massage is harmful. In acne it is of doubtful benefit, and the grease that always accompanies it is harmful. In any real infection, such as boils, it is dangerous, particularly on the face. It is just as foolish to expect massage to remove a double chin or wrinkles as it would be to attempt to rub away the nose or the lines in the palm.

STEAMING

Steaming the face or other involved parts of the skin is a valuable measure in greasy skins containing blackheads. It causes increased perspiration and acts more vigorously than washing with hot water. It should not be carried to the point of causing the face to get very red (a paralysis of the small blood vessels) and should always be followed by a cold shower or application of cold towels to restore tone to the vessels. Like the hot bath, if used too frequently it may cause drying or even chapping of the skin.

ELECTRICITY

There is no justification for the home use of electricity in the care of the skin, except under the direction of the physician.

SUN BATHS AND ARTIFICIAL SUBSTITUTES FOR THEM

The use of arc lights and quartz mercury vapor lamps in the home is being popularized. There is no doubt of the beneficial action of these and of the sun's rays under proper conditions and control. Light baths of whatever kind should be given cautiously, allowing the skin to become accustomed to the light and to respond with pigmentation, instead of being burned. Those who are blessed with a blond complexion should exercise particular care to protect the skin from the harmful effects of light. There are some abnormalities and diseases of the skin, as well as some internal conditions, in which light is harmful. Light treatments in the home should be given under the direction of the physician.

On the water or snow the reflected rays should be avoided. Hats are no protection against these rays, which contain the ultraviolet rays that are most active in producing irritation. Particularly at high altitudes, their penetration is great, and the effect of sunlight much greater than its visual intensity indicates. At low altitudes these rays are largely absorbed by the atmosphere, and comparatively few of them reach us.

Care of the Skin at Various Periods of Life

INFANCY

The skin of an infant requires gentle treatment. Soap should be of the mildest superfatted kind, and even this should be employed only when absolutely necessary. After the bath a bland powder should be used, care being taken that the baby cannot get the opportunity to shake the powder into its mouth and lungs. The folds of the body should receive more powder than the rest of the skin. The clothing should be soft, carefully rinsed after washing, and not too heavy. Many infants are kept too warm and suffer from heat rash, which may, as a result of scratching, become infected and eventuate in more serious skin disease.

CHILDHOOD

The same rules apply as in infancy, except that the young child and the older small boy or tomboy girl require for their hands (and too often for other parts of the body) more soap and water. The mother should not, however, let her love of cleanliness carry her too far with the scrubbing process, for it is better that the child be a little less than perfectly clean rather than hampered in its exercise. Precautions against overcleanliness can be safely left to the defensive power of the child in most cases. The little girl sooner or later out-

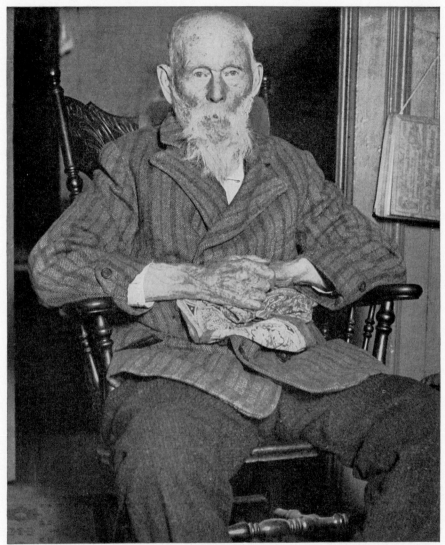

FIG. 89. Skin of the aged.

grows the age of dirt and then may need restraint in the other direction, to prevent her abusing her delicate skin with soap. Both boys and girls, if they have blond skin that freckles, should be urged to wear hats in the sun and to grease the skin before going swimming. This affords some protection. There are several special protective ointments on the market. The present vogue of sun baths is, on the whole, beneficial but, like all fashions, when overdone becomes a harmful craze. Those with blond skins should be taught in childhood that severe sunburn harms them and should acquire the habit of protecting the skin against such harm. Care later in life comes too late to be of much benefit.

ADOLESCENCE

The chief change seen in the skin at puberty is the greasiness which appears in so many skins at this time, often accompanied by blackheads and pimples. The measures to be described later under the heading of acne must be instituted at once, active daily washing with hot water and soap, and insistence on good habits of eating, work, play, and sleep.

MIDDLE LIFE

This is the active, strenuous time, when health is most often neglected for the sake of work or even sometimes for the sake of play. Loss of sleep, irregular meals, worry, all have their effect upon the health of the skin, as well as of the rest of the body, and are seldom necessary. The study of philosophy should be taken up, for it will be needed from now on into old age. Worry, hustle, and impatience hasten the onset of age, which is announced too early at the best by the condition of the skin. The use of cold cream upon the skin becomes more generally justifiable because of lessening fat production.

AGE

Age brings lessened nutrition to all parts, including the skin, and the latter loses fat, becomes wrinkled and rough. Fat should be applied artificially, soap used sparingly, and the skin protected as well as can be done. The same care as specified for the unnaturally dry skin should be given these skins. The special changes of the aging skin will be taken up individually.

Inflammations and Abnormalities of the Skin

CHAPPING

Chapping is one of the simplest forms of inflammation of the skin. It is seen commonly in the winter time, on the tender skin of children. The cold dry air of out-of-doors and the warm dry air indoors conspire with hot water and soap to remove the fat from the skin, causing red, dry, scaly areas. Ordinarily such areas, when spared the irritation of soap and anointed with some fat, will promptly return to normal. If they do not yield at once, have the doctor see them, for all that looks like chapping is not so simple a form of inflammation.

CHAFING

This occurs commonly in babies and stout adults. It is caused by the rubbing together of parts moistened by sweat, offering an excellent opening for infection to take place. The parts should be kept scrupulously clean and well powdered. If this does not suffice, a flat bag made of gauze may be filled with talcum powder and suspended between the opposing surfaces to prevent rubbing. If these simple measures are not successful, have the physician see the case, for some form of infection probably has taken place.

SUNBURN

Sunburn is an inflammatory reaction of the skin to the rays of light, not to heat rays. It occurs on snow fields as well as in the hottest climates. The redness does not appear at once, but several hours after the exposure to light. If given an opportunity, most skins can produce enough pigment to protect themselves against any ordinary exposure to the sun; but when they receive a large dose of light without any preparatory hardening, they react with an acute inflammation. Some skins do not produce pigment in all parts; but freckle instead of tanning, and there are some that apparently cannot produce pigment at all. These are the skins most harmed by light, and they should be protected by large hats, face powder, or one of the special protective ointments now on the market.

When sunburn has already shown itself, the skin may be powdered (face powder will do), or cold cream applied gently, or, if the burn is severe, cold compresses of saturated solution of boric acid may be used. After applying them for some time, dab the skin dry and powder it well. In the early spring or summer the skin should be gradually inured to the sun's rays so that it may become tanned. This is beneficial to a healthy skin, but severe sunburn is harmful.

ECZEMA

Eczema (accent the first syllable) is the commonest disease of the skin and in the minds of many is a serious disease. In fact, the term covers such a multitude of conditions that it should not necessarily convey any such impression. Many cases of eczema are promptly curable. The disease may be caused in many different ways. A number of other diseases of the skin are closely related to eczema and still others imitate it so closely that at times they are hard to distinguish. While eczema is too complicated a problem for home treatment, there are certain things that everyone should know about it.

It is often difficult to work out the cause of a case of eczema. Be patient with your physician; give him time and your enthusiastic coöperation, for in many instances that is the only way in which it can be done.

Do not consider eczema a dirt disease. It is just as often made worse by too much cleanliness. Neither is it a sign of "bad blood" or any disgrace to the family in which it occurs. There is absolutely no stigma attached to it. Of course, it is a fact that eczema, hay fever, asthma, and other signs of hypersensitiveness do occur in some families more often than in others, due to a weakness or to an exaggeration, no one knows which, of the mechanism that protects against infection. It is a family peculiarity, just like a tendency to moles or a greasy skin.

Everyone knows that scratching makes eczema worse. There is one of the close relatives of eczema that is largely the result of constant scratching or rubbing. Of course, it is hard to refrain from scratching when an itch is forcing itself on one's attention; but the itch will return worse than ever if scratched, and the temporary relief scratching affords is paid for dearly by the increase of inflammation it causes. Saturated solution of boric acid, dabbed on and allowed to evaporate, or 50 per cent alcohol used in the same way (provided, of course, that the skin is not broken), will often give temporary relief and act as a substitute for scratching. Even in applying an ointment, there is a temptation to rub with some vigor for the pleasure it gives. This should be resisted as a temptation of the demon that makes eczema worse.

Ordinarily, soap and water irritate acute eczema. They should not be used unless advised by the doctor. The home treatment of eczema may do much harm, for the skin is hypersensitive, and an irritant that would be entirely harmless upon ordinary skin may do great damage to eczema. Many an eczema is maintained and made chronic by wrong treatment, self-prescribed, "counter-prescribed," or even "ad-prescribed."

DERMATITIS FROM EXTERNAL IRRITANTS

The common example of this is the inflammation caused by poison ivy or poison oak or sumac. The plants, chemicals, fabrics, and other substances that may cause this form of dermatitis are as numerous as those causing eczema, and in fact the two are closely related, so that it is at times impossible to say definitely where one leaves off and the other begins. Children should be taught the appearance of poison ivy and poison oak, so that the children may avoid them in their excursions to study nature. Both have glossy foliage, arranged three leaflets on a stem. In the fall, among the first to change color, they turn a beautiful red, and are often collected for this reason by uninformed enthusiasts.

If contact with the plant has been unavoidable, the next procedure should be to wash thoroughly with soapsuds and hot water followed by rinsing with strong grain alcohol. Even after the dermatitis has begun, this will lesson the severity of the attack; but when it has become well established, this treatment comes too late and may irritate.

Among house plants the primrose is a common cause of dermatitis. Tincture of iodine that has been allowed to become strong by evaporation, or the too enthusiastic application of the fresh preparation, often is responsible for it. One coat of a fresh preparation is all that is necessary, and more will not have any better effect but may have a bad one. In bygone days the mustard plaster also was a common cause, but today it is not so often used. It should always be tempered to the kind of skin upon which it is to be placed.

As treatment, the observations concerning eczema apply here equally. Soft ointments should not be used in these acute cases, for they often make them worse.

HEAT RASH

Heat rash (prickly heat) occurs more often in infants than in older persons and is best prevented by avoidance of too heavy clothing and the free use of bathing and dusting powder. After the eruption is present, if it refuses to yield promptly to cooling measures, as dabbing with 50 per cent alcohol followed by dusting powder, the physician should be consulted, for such eruptions afford an excellent opportunity for infection of the skin.

IMPETIGO

Impetigo is the superficial infection of the skin seen so often in children. It is caused by pus germs, the streptococcus or the staphylococcus, and in adults and older children is ordinarily not serious. In infancy impetigo is often dangerous to life. Attacks of this disease may occur at any time; but it is frequently epidemic during the summer in connection with bathing-beach infections. No delay should ensue before consulting the physician, and every effort should be made to prevent others, especially infants, from exposure. Keeping the hands away from the infected parts, and after unavoidable contact promptly washing them, is an important aid in limiting the spread of the infection.

SEBORRHEIC DERMATITIS

Seborrheic dermatitis was formerly confused with eczema but is now known to be a distinct disease. It is manifested by greasy or dry scales, involving first of all the scalp, spreading to the face and upper trunk, clearing up under treatment, but recurring at a later date. It is supposedly an infection spread by means of combs and brushes and should not be neglected; severe attacks are often difficult to treat successfully, and even though mild, the disease commonly leads to baldness.

ACNE VULGARIS

Acne vulgaris, like the disease just discussed, is a disease of the fat glands of the skin. At puberty, along with other changes in the body, these glands develop and frequently take on excessive activity, causing the skin to become greasy and plugs to form in the pores. These plugs of grease and cell débris soon catch enough dirt to show as

black points on the skin, commonly called blackheads and by the doctors comedones. These plugs cause some irritation, as do all foreign
bodies, and nature tries to eliminate them by the formation of pus.
When the pustule breaks, the comedo is forced out with the pus. Unfortunately, if the pus remains too long in the deeper lesions before
being freed, the pressure and dissolving action of the pus destroys
the connective tissue about it. This loss must be replaced by scar
tissue, leaving a permanent disfigurement. If scarring does not follow
the pustule, the process is repeated many times in the same follicle.
Acne tends to clear up as the patient grows older, but the risk of
scarring is too great and the distress of the young person at the disfigurement too acute to justify neglect of treatment. The physician,
opening the pustules with a tiny knife, is not causing scars, as many
think. He is preventing them by releasing the pus before it has time
to destroy tissue.

Since it occurs usually in greasy skins, acne is benefited by the free
use of hot water and soap. Children affected with the disease should
not be accused of causing it by reluctance to use these measures.
No amount of scrubbing can cure a real case of acne. Neither is acne
a sign of sexual irregularity, as some ignorant persons insinuate. The
unfortunates afflicted with the disease are embarrassed enough because
of their facial blemishes without the added cruelty of such insinua-
tions.

In mild cases, pustules may be few and comedones many, forming
small yellowish elevations with the yellow, brown, or black point in
the center. When the horny layer of the skin forms completely over
the surface, the end of the fatty plug cannot become dirty but remains
as a white pearl-like body called milium, or whitehead. These remain
without much increase in size until removed and do not recur as
promptly as the blackheads.

Acne is not always confined to the face but involves also the chest,
upper back, and outer sides of the arms. In persons of low resistance
it becomes a disfiguring, distressing, and indeed serious disease. Cold
cream or other greasy applications should not be used, for the skin
has already too much fat. Massage is apt to do harm because of the
cream employed. Patent medicines called "blood purifiers" are apt to
make acne worse, because many of them contain iodides. The acne
patient does not need a "blood purifier."

Removal of blackheads is beneficial, as can easily be understood when the method of formation of pustules is considered. It should be done with care, however, not to injure the skin by too much force. Many nervous patients increase their disfigurement by too enthusiastic attempts to remove blackheads by squeezing without preliminary loosening. The face should first be washed thoroughly with hot water and soap, hot towels applied for about ten minutes, then the skin sponged with alcohol, and if necessary a needle, sterilized by flaming, used to loosen up the top of the comedo before pressure is applied with a blackhead remover, a small instrument with a hole about $\frac{1}{16}$ of an inch in diameter in one end. The surface about this hole should be flat and smooth. After the blackheads have thus been removed, the application of hot towels should be repeated, followed by a short application of cold water and drying with a towel. This second application of heat lessens the inflammatory reaction to the pressure. Deep pustules, the kind that are most apt to cause scars, should be opened by the physician.

Care of the health is important in all youths, but particularly in those who have acne. Fresh air, good food, proper exercise, and plenty of sleep are essential to good health. Strict dieting never cures acne and may do harm if not properly supervised. Many youngsters with this disease need restraint, however, in the matter of eating and drinking and should be particularly warned against the bad effect of sweet carbonated drinks, candy, and ice cream between meals, and irregularity in the eating and sleeping schedule. Constipation should be avoided by the generous use of vegetables and fruits and by the formation of regular habits of bowel evacuation.

The nervous overenthusiasm in removing blackheads, already mentioned, is not so difficult to cure as the nervous urge to pick at acne lesions, which amounts in some to a habit. This more or less unconscious picking at the lesions causes disfiguring excoriations, resulting sometimes in bad scars.

This somewhat lengthy discourse on acne is not intended to convey the idea that acne can be cured by home treatment. Only the mildest cases can be handled without the help of the physician.

ACNE ROSACEA

Acne rosacea is the disease that reddens the nose and cheeks and in extreme cases causes enlargement of the end of the nose, popularly called "whisky nose" or "grog blossom," appellations that are not justified, for many sufferers from this disease are strict abstainers from alcoholic drinks. The trouble is caused by a nervous reflex dilatation of the sensitive blood vessels of these areas on the face as a response to stomach or pelvic disease or local conditions in the mouth or nose. It must have the care of the physician. The patient can do much, however, to restrain its development by the avoidance of hot foods or drinks, spicy or peppery foods, and particularly alcoholic beverages. Alcohol irritates the stomach and sets up the reflex already mentioned, at the same time that it acts directly to dilate the peripheral blood vessels. After frequent dilatations, the vessels become paralyzed and remain as disfiguring red or bluish lines. The consequent slowing of the circulation is probably the chief reason for the enlargement of the end of the nose. This can be much improved by proper treatment.

EXCESSIVE SWEATING

Excessive sweating annoys some women greatly, and the pads worn in the armpits and the various applications to this area are not fully satisfactory remedies. However, that is all that can be done without consulting the doctor. Sweating is too important a function, particularly in warm weather, to attempt its serious reduction, and it is doubtful whether attempts to do this would be successful, for Nature has great defensive power. Perhaps, in this case, she knows best.

BODY ODOR

Body odor is usually synonymous with the odor of the sweat. It is said that certain European perfumers advise the use of perfume suited to the body odor of the client. Foul-odored sweat is a great affliction, fortunately not common. It occurs most often on the feet and in bona fide cases persists in spite of the most meticulous cleanliness. Baths of potassium permanganate, one part to five hundred of water, are helpful in destroying the odor. The disease is often amenable to treatment for excessive sweating. Talcum powder containing 2 per cent salicylic acid may be used between baths.

RINGWORM

This old name, given because of a misconception of the cause of the ring shape of the patches on the glabrous skin, is a complete misnomer, for the disease, in most of its manifestations, is not in the shape of rings. Of course, worms have no part in its causation. The cause is one of the many varieties of higher fungi related to the common molds which attack bread left in an open moist place. This has been known for many years by the medical profession. Only lately have the doctors realized how important and widespread these infections are. This disease is carried between the toes of a large percentage of those who consider themselves perfectly healthy. The wonder is not that it breaks out in other parts now and then; but that this happens so seldom. So far as is now known, it is spread chiefly by walking on moist, infected floors of bathrooms, gymnasiums, and golf clubs. Other sources of infection will, no doubt, be discovered with continued search.

Lying dormant for months and years, the disease now and then becomes acute and causes great distress and loss of time at work. Still more important is the fact that it offers an excellent opportunity for more serious infection of the feet and hands. These fungi are more active in tropical countries than in our temperate zone, and the name *"dhobie itch"* given to the ringworm infection of the groins is an evidence of this fact, as the more modern name *"athlete's foot"* is evidence of the chief mode of infection in our country.

The treatment of these infections is often difficult and taxes the ingenuity of the physician to the utmost. The hair and nail infections are most difficult of all forms to treat, and the latter is one of the important sources for the spread of the infection. Of recent years much has been accomplished in the prevention of these infections in schools and colleges by the use of pans of one per cent solution of sodium hypochlorite, into which the pupils are required to step on their way to and from the gymnasium. Cleanliness of the feet, particularly care to keep the clefts between the toes clean and dry, is of great importance in preventing infection. It has been shown recently that women students have less ringworm than the men, probably because of better care of their feet. This fact should not be used, however, against any particular case of infection, for there is no doubt a great difference of susceptibility to these organisms, and those afflicted may not be lax in regard to cleanliness but only unfortunate in their susceptibility.

Treatment of most cases of this kind should be kept up for a long time after cure has apparently been obtained. The organisms lurk among the epithelial cells and await an opportunity, perhaps in the

form of simple moisture, to multiply rapidly and cause another outbreak.

LOUSINESS

All three forms of lice infesting man obtain their nourishment from
blood sucked from the hair follicles. In procuring this food they inject
a poison into the skin, which causes intense itching. Among ordinary
folks the best known of this interesting family of parasites is the head
louse, pediculus capitis (Fig. 90). The children of the family too frequently bring home samples of their parasite in the hair. Its eggs,
called nits, tiny white pear-shaped bodies glued to the hair, everyone
knows. Fewer have seen the parent louse, for its semi-translucent gray

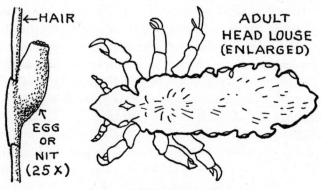

FIG. 90.

body is not easily distinguished through the hair. Scratch marks and
blood crusts, sometimes pustules and matting of the hair are seen.

Thorough soaking of the hair and scalp with a mixture of equal
parts of kerosene and sweet oil is the simplest method of eradicating
the lice. A cap is formed of cloths soaked in the mixture and left upon
the head overnight, extreme care being exercised to keep the child
away from fire. The next morning a thorough shampoo is given, and
after this, hot vinegar applied to loosen the nits, which then are removed with a fine comb.

The body louse, pediculus corporis or vestimentorum (Fig. 91),
lives in the clothing and attaches its eggs to the fibers of the underwear. To obtain blood it reaches over to the skin, and this explains
why the blood crusts and itchy pimples which are typical signs of this
disease are found most plentiful on parts like the waist and shoulders,

where the clothing rests closely upon the skin. Only those who neglect cleanliness of body and clothing can harbor body lice, though it must be recognized that some individuals are much more attractive to the louse than are others. This is proved by the story of four doctors who stood around a table upon which a louse had been placed. Although they changed positions about the table, the louse always traveled toward the same doctor. Body lice are of importance because they carry typhus or spotted fever, a dangerous disease fortunately rare in the United States. Rocky Mountain spotted fever is carried for the

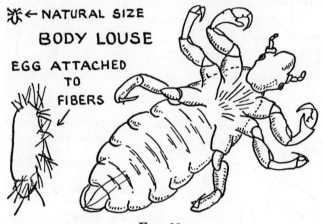

FIG. 91.

most part by ticks, and Brill's disease, a mild form of typhus, is associated with rats, possibly carried by their fleas.

The crab louse, pediculus pubis, is more nearly round and is found clinging to the hairs with its head down close to the skin. It is found most often on the pubic region; but occurs at times in the axillae, on the chests of hairy men, or even in the eyebrows and eyelashes. Shaving the hair to get rid of the nits and thorough washing will eliminate this form of louse. The nits can be picked off the brows or eyelashes.

THE ITCH, SCABIES

The itch mite, a member of the spider family, is very small, as the illustration (Fig. 92) indicates. This shows the female mite. The male is still smaller. Living on the surface of the skin, his only purpose in life seems to be the propagation of his kind. After impregnation, the female burrows into and along the upper part of the epidermis, depositing her eggs as she goes, producing a burrow about one fourth of an inch long. As the eggs hatch, the burrow loses its roof and appears as a dark-colored fine groove, seen most easily upon tender skin between the fingers, on the breasts, genitals, abdomen, etc. Itching is more severe at night, because the female itch mite is a night worker. Only in babies whose faces are kept covered are the tracks of the itch mite seen upon the face.

The diagnosis of scabies is often difficult, as is likewise the treat-

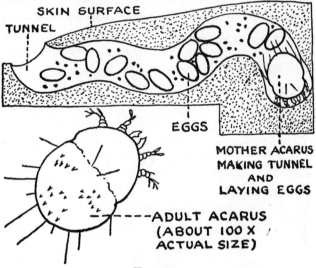

FIG. 92.

ment. A doctor should always be consulted. Much damage can be done by unsupervised home treatment of this disease and the other conditions frequently confused with it.

CORNS

Corns are caused by pressure, as everyone knows, usually that of improperly shaped shoes. The world is slowly becoming more sensible in its dress, but pointed shoes are still much in favor, and corns still flourish. The only effectual treatment is protection from pressure. Removing the central horny plug with a knife, or softening with a salicylic acid preparation followed by soaking in hot water and scraping out the plug is good treatment, but is of no lasting benefit unless the pressure is removed. Anything that does not yield to such treatment over a period of a few weeks is not a corn. Consult your physician.

WARTS

Because they are at first tiny, flat, skin-colored elevations that are inconspicuous, warts are often neglected until they have had an opportunity to show their ability to propagate. The serum or blood from the original wart is allowed to remain on the skin for a time. A month or so later a new wart appears on this spot. This property is called autoinoculability; that is, one can infect himself again and again. In this way whole crops of warts are raised, like dandelions, where they are least desired. It is plain, therefore, that warts should not be picked with the finger nails or pared with the pocketknife. The virus that causes warts belongs to the very interesting group of "filtrable viruses," whose ability to pass through the finest porcelain filter has given them the name. Whether they are infinitesimally small bacteria or jelly-like bodies that can conform to the shape of the openings in the filter we do not know, for they are invisible, and our only way of detecting them is the effects they produce by infection. Because the wart infection is so slow in developing it is often not possible to remember where they were acquired.

Ordinarily warts are painless; but sometimes on the fingers, and commonly on the soles of the feet, they are tender, causing exquisite pain when bumped or walked on.

Ever since prehistoric time warts have been treated successfully by suggestion. Tom Sawyer's method and many others like it which are still used by boys all over the world are survivors of the ancient practice of the witch or voodoo doctor. The modern child is often too sophisticated, even at an early age, to have any faith in such practices, and other methods must be used. The only objection to the faith cures is their encouragement of false beliefs and gullibility, which is even worse than warts. Warts are sometimes difficult to cure by chemical or electrical methods; therefore the treatment is best left to the physician. A popular home treatment is the use of nitric acid. This is mentioned only to be condemned, for it often results in unsightly scars or even keloids.

Seborrheic warts are the brown to black-topped elevations that occur on the trunk, less often on the face or scalp, of people in middle life or later. They are of no consequence except for the fact that they are sometimes hard to distinguish from senile keratoses, which are important lesions.

KELOIDS

Keloids are benign tumors (tumors that never become malignant) which grow in scars. At times there is no history of a preceding scar; but it may have been so slight that it was not noticed. Some people have the peculiar tendency to form keloids in their scars, or these tumors may occur in some of their scars and not in others. They should not be cut out, because of their ability to return, making a larger tumor than before the operation, unless treated at the same time with radium or Roentgen rays which have a very beneficial effect on them.

MOLES

Moles are birthmarks, even though, as often happens, they appear in adult life. The ordinary skin-colored or brown mole, whether covered with hair or not, seldom becomes dangerous except when exposed to chronic irritation. When located so that the clothing rubs upon them, or so that they are frequently cut in shaving or irritated in some other way, they should be removed thoroughly by the physician. If thought disfiguring, they may be removed without fear of evil consequences except a slight scar, which often results because the mole extends so deeply that it cannot be removed without destruction of some of the connective tissue.

Blue moles, much less common than the brown kind, but not rare, are in a class by themselves. They become malignant much more commonly than the ordinary kind of moles, and when they do change, are dangerous tumors. They may, however, last throughout life without any such change. Consult your physician about them.

VASCULAR BIRTHMARKS

Vascular birthmarks may be flat "port wine marks," slightly elevated, flat-topped "strawberry marks," or the deep cavernous dilatation of the veins occurring as skin-colored soft swellings. These are easily compressed, return immediately to their original shape, and tend to become bluish and still larger when the baby cries. Often the skin over such a mark is the site of one of the flat kinds already mentioned. All these should be treated during infancy, when the skin is able to renew itself most readily and resulting scars are smaller.

It is to be hoped that the old superstition that prenatal influences on the mother cause birthmarks is no longer believed by anyone in this day and age. Superstition and error die hard, however, and therefore space is taken here to register definite rejection of such theories. Birthmarks, even those that do not appear until the person is in adult life, are laid down in the early months of pregnancy and cannot, therefore, result from happenings to the mother at other times.

BLOOD VESSEL TUMORS OF OLDER SKIN

In middle age tiny red points appear on the skin of the trunk, less often on the face and extremities, and grow to form soft tumors of large pea size in some cases, bright to bluish red. They are harmless and need no treatment unless they are thought disfiguring. They do not become malignant.

CHLOASMA

Chloasma is the unequal browning of the skin of the face that occurs in women more often than in men and, like all increases of pigment, in dark-complexioned persons oftener than in blonds. Its popular name is "liver spots"; but the liver cannot be held responsible. Pregnancy and pelvic disease, from which, too, it is supposed to result, are also seldom at fault. Diligent search commonly reveals no cause for these unpleasant blemishes. The treatment is apt to be unsatisfactory, for it consists in trying to remove the surface layers of the skin by means of an inflammatory reaction produced by irritants. These, when strong enough to be effective, are hard to control and often cause too great an inflammation with most unpleasant consequences to the patient. Beware of these so-called "freckle removers." They may work well for one person and have a disastrous effect on the next one using them. Rubbing the dark patch with lemon peel at frequent intervals is harmless and some claim beneficial. Peroxide solution, made active by the addition, at the time of using, of about 20 per cent of ammonia water, may be beneficial to some; this is questionable, however, and care should be used to stop before too great an irritation has been produced. All such remedies act by causing scaling, and this is seldom deep enough to affect the pigment without causing an unpleasant inflammatory reaction. Such reactions sometimes result in increase of pigment, as is common following a blistering use of mustard plaster.

FRECKLES AND TANNING

These changes in the skin brought about by light have been discussed already; but they are so important that repetition may be excusable. The natural reaction of the skin to light and some other forms of irritation is the formation of pigment, tanning. Some skins, notably those lacking pigment, are not able to produce pigment as readily as the darker ones and often produce it only in spots. Freckles, therefore, are the indication of a weakness of the skin in this important function. Such skins should not be needlessly exposed to light, for they cannot protect themselves or the owner from its sometimes harmful effects, which do not appear at once, but may come to notice much later as *senile freckles,* liable to change to keratoses and end in cancer of the skin. These are larger and fewer than the ordinary freckles of youth and are more persistent. Such a skin should be protected as much as is possible from direct sunlight; though, of course, this is locking the barn long after the horse has been stolen, for such a skin should have been protected since early childhood. After the damage has occurred its progress may be delayed somewhat by the daily application of a good cold cream. Treatment of senile freckles is usually not necessary unless they are disfiguring or show some tendency to become rough and horny. They should then be eradicated. The freckles of youth are best treated by preventive measures, as already stated. The mild applications already suggested for chloasma may be tried if the freckles are disfiguring; but time and protection from light are the most successful measures.

SENILE KERATOSES

Senile keratoses are horny spots in the skin which may appear slowly or suddenly and remain rough for a certain time, when the horny crust falls off, leaving no mark or a slightly red spot. After a longer or shorter time the horny crust returns, and this may go on for years before signs of cancer occur. They should be removed during this early stage.

CANCER OF THE SKIN

Cancer of the skin enjoys the peculiar advantage over cancer in other parts of the body that it can be seen at its beginning and treated early. Inability to do this is the chief reason why cancer elsewhere cannot be cured as readily. Any unusual growth in the skin should be shown the physician at once, without taking the great risk of home treatment or delaying until ulceration occurs. The idea that cancer always causes pain is another very harmful one, for skin cancer seldom causes pain until it is in the last stage, when it is too late to save the patient's life. Home treatment is worse than simple delay, for it is like trying to put out a fire by pouring on gasoline. If anything will insure the change from a harmless to a malignant growth, or encourage one that is already malignant, the usually irritating home treatment will do so.

Scaly spots or growths on the lips and the hands should have attention early, for cancer occurring on these parts is apt to be more malignant than upon the face. There are many degrees of malignancy in various cancers and this is especially evident on the skin. Nearly all kinds, if attacked early, can be cured, however. Very old people, or persons weakened from other causes, do not respond so well to treatment; but many of these also can be freed from the tumor.

WRINKLES

Wrinkles are caused by loss of elasticity of the skin and often also by loss of the fat which has kept it distended. As the skin grows old its blood supply decreases, with consequent loss of muscular and fibrous tension as well as the looseness resulting from loss of body weight. The surface of the skin also is apt to become dry and rough, adding to the disfigurement. Some benefit can be obtained from the elimination of soap and the assiduous use of cold cream, particularly after washing, to keep the surface of the skin smooth. Massage and steaming the skin may be of some help in prevention, because they increase circulation; but, as already mentioned in regard to freckles, it is too late to gain much by treatment after the change has become apparent. The time to treat effectually is in youth and throughout life, if the ravages of age are to be delayed. Steaming in particular should be used with great caution, for aging skin is more easily damaged than that of youth.

Operative "face lifting" is of only temporary benefit, even when it is done correctly. The skin continues to become more and more relaxed, and the wrinkles return. Stout people who wish to keep their fine, smooth skins should be very careful in reducing. Unless it is done very slowly indeed, the skin is apt to be damaged, becoming loose and wrinkled.

Above all, do not listen to the temptation to have paraffin or petrolatum (vaseline) or anything of this nature injected beneath the skin to fill out the hollows. Many sad cases of the bad results that, years afterward, follow such treatment are seen by physicians, from one to another of whom the victims go, hoping to find help. The presence of this material in the tissues leads, months or years after it is injected, to the formation of tumors that cannot be successfully removed and that in time become purplish and very deforming. No reputable physician will recommend this method. Wrinkling is the first sign of *atrophy* of the skin. Its further progress is shown by further loss of elasticity, and further thinning until it is almost transparent, so that the veins are seen quite clearly through it. All that can be done for such a condition is to protect from irritation as much as possible and to keep the surface well supplied with fat.

XANTHOMA

Xanthoma is the name given yellow tumors in the skin caused by deposits of fats due to inability to dispose of them in the normal way. The only form of this disease seen frequently involves the tissues about the eyelids, most often the inner part of the lower lid, as small yellowish bodies, in plaques or lines. They can be removed by the physician with the production of slight scarring, but they often return, because the internal condition that causes them is still operative, though seldom sufficiently so to cause other symptoms.

The Hair

The hair is formed by a dipping down of part of the epidermis, which forms a pouch, at the bottom of which is a papilla, like that of the epidermis; but this one is a specialist among papillæ in that it is able to build hair. From this a cylindrical body of epithelial cells forces its way up through the pouch, called the follicle, which is now long and narrow. Soon after they leave the parent papilla the cells of this cylindrical body become horny like those of the surface of the skin, and form a spine that extends beyond the surface for a greater or lesser distance. After the cells turn to horn they are no longer alive but form only a mechanical projection. As the hair grows by formation of new cells at the papilla, the part above pushes out until it has attained its destined length. It then ceases to grow, unless cut off, and after a longer or shorter period of rest falls out, leaving the papilla in the skin to form a new hair. As already mentioned, the sebaceous duct joins the hair follicle near its upper end, filling the follicle with fat, which, at the narrow part, somewhat higher, is forced into the body of the hair. Below the gland the erector muscle of the hair joins the outer part of the follicle. During periods of excitement this muscle raises the hair from its normal slanting position to an erect one. Contraction of this muscle also helps to force out the contents of the sebaceous gland, and during excitement or when the body is chilled, puckers the skin into the condition we call goose flesh.

Most of the hair on our bodies is only a remnant of the hairy covering of our ancient ancestors. It is fine and consists of two layers, the cuticle, a layer or layers of tiny flat scales surrounding the hair, overlapping one another like shingles on a roof, and the cortex, the long strands of spindle-shaped horn cells with tiny spaces between them, presumably for oil. These fine hairs are called lanugo hairs, from the word for wool. Coarser hairs, like those of the scalp, contain in addition to the two layers mentioned a third, a fine pith-like center filled with a few larger cells. The cortex contains the pigment of the hair in the form of granules and also as a fluid within the cells.

THE FUNCTION OF THE HAIR

The function of the hair to man is decorative and protective, preventing or moderating the action of cold, light, and mechanical injury. The decorative is by far the more valued function, although fashion at present decrees that it shall be exercised only on the scalp.

The hair changes as the person grows: the fine hair of the infant changes to ordinary scalp hair soon after birth; the axillary and pubic hair and the beards of boys develop after puberty, while in old age the sad thinning and loss of color of the scalp hair takes place.

The color of the hair is due to the pigment in the cortical cells. Blond hair contains only soluble pigment, while the various darker shades are produced by the addition of more or less of the granular pigment.

The form of the hair. Scalp hair may be oval in cross section, and is then straight, while curly hair is flat.

THE CARE OF THE HAIR

Cleanliness, normal growth, and an attractive appearance are the objects of caring for the hair. The necessity of washing the hair and scalp depends on the amount of oil on the hair and the amount of dirt in the environment. Oily hair may need washing every week, while normal or dry hair may be kept in excellent order by washing once a month. For greasy scalps a strong soap such as tincture of green soap is needed, while dry, clean scalps may be washed with mild soap or even with white of egg. Whatever is used, the rinsing should be thorough, and, if possible, the last rinsing should be with cold water, for stimulation. Wetting the hair daily is objectionable, largely because it is a lazy man's method of avoiding the use of the brush. Vigorous brushing of the hair daily is the best method of massaging the scalp, increasing its circulation and stimulating the oil glands. In taking the daily shower, it is best that the hair should not be wet, though this objection can be met by brushing the hair at some other time of day, when it is dry. Applications of oil or pomade or the modern abominable mucilages are harmful in the same way, that they encourage the omission of the daily brushing.

Curling the hair with hot irons or heat with the addition of strong alkaline preparations, as in permanent waving, injures the hair, causing it to split at the ends.

Cutting the hair does no perceptible harm. The fact that men become bald oftener than women is due to their unhygienic hats, not to the cutting of hair. Cut hair grows more rapidly. It is the rule for hair to stop growing when it reaches a certain length peculiar to the individual. When cut, it begins to grow again in the effort to reach its proper length. Cutting does not increase the thickness of hair growth. Shaving makes the hair seem coarser, because the short cut ends, as they grow out, are stiff, owing to their shortness. Singeing the hair is a foolish procedure, due to an old superstition that there is a "vital fluid" in the hair and that singeing prevents this fluid from escaping. Its only real benefit is to the financial depression in the barber shop.

Oiling the hair is necessary in some cases in which insufficient natural oil is produced even under stimulation, but it can often be avoided by proper care of the scalp.

Dyeing the hair is a serious procedure, not to be undertaken lightly. It is to be done only when real necessity exists, for it is expensive, time-consuming, and always associated with some danger of skin irritation due to the chemicals used in the dye. Most skins stand these chemicals well; but every now and then a patron or one of the employees of the hairdresser will become sensitized, and a troublesome dermatitis results. After this, no contact with this particular substance, whether in the same dye or in another, can be tolerated. Not only this, but sensitization to one chemical frequently leads to sensitization to others, causing much trouble. The dyeing process has to be repeated at regular intervals as the hair grows, to prevent the telltale light zone at the root. Of course, this will not deter a woman who has decided to improve her appearance from dyeing her hair. It is a great pity to see beautiful hair spoiled by dyeing, as every skin specialist too often sees, because of a whim or misguided zeal in the unending search for more beauty. Dyed hair is never so beautiful as natural hair. If it must be done, go to the best hairdresser available, for it is a job for an artist.

This same advice is applicable to the purchase of wigs. The heat and interference with the ventilation of the scalp due to the wearing of such an adornment can be compensated by added care, more frequent washing, and the application to the scalp of lotions or creams.

<h3 style="text-align:center">COMBS AND BRUSHES</h3>

Combs and brushes are the tools for the care of the hair. They should be properly made and well cared for to accomplish this purpose. The comb should not be so sharp as to injure the scalp with ordinary use, and the teeth should be smooth and not too closely set. The old-fashioned "fine comb" is fine for only one purpose known to the writer, the loosening of the nits of head lice. The comb should not be made of celluloid, because of the danger of fire. It should be kept clean, and if the owner suffers from excessive scaling of the scalp ("dandruff") the comb should be regularly sterilized by soaking it, after washing in 1 per cent solution of formalin for an hour, then rinsing and drying.

Brushes should be made of stiff bristles, set far apart, and should be kept clean and occasionally sterilized as advised for the comb. After this, rinse thoroughly and dry in the sun if possible. Combs and brushes should not be used in common, for the disease causing dandruff and baldness is supposed to be infectious, transmitted from one to the other through this medium. The barber, of course, uses a common comb and brush, but should sterilize them each time before use. If this is omitted, it is well, after a visit to the barber shop, to use some sort of mild antiseptic, as 50 per cent grain alcohol, most easily obtained as spirits of bay rum.

DANDRUFF

The skin of the scalp, like all the skin, scales constantly in small amounts. Frequently, however, the scalp itches and produces more than the normal amount of scaling. This combination may be the first signal of the onset of *seborrheic dermatitis*, the disease which is the great cause of baldness. If all such cases, in this early stage, were promptly, efficiently, and persistently treated, baldness would be much less common; but neglect of slight scalp disease is the rule, and young men usually come for treatment after considerable loss of hair has occurred. The disease may appear in childhood but most often is first noticed in youth, between twenty and thirty years of age. By active, persistent treatment its progress can be arrested in a large percentage of cases. After itching and dandruff have been present for some time, excessive loss of hair is noticed, often with attacks of real dermatitis, with red scaly patches on the scalp. These lessen or clear entirely, only to recur with further loss of hair over the center of the scalp, which grows again; but finer and shorter. Such attacks and remissions alternate for years.

The treatment should be managed by the physician; but the patient must expect to work hard at the job of applying it. It consists of stimulation of the scalp by shampoos, ointments, or lotions, applied with massage, without neglecting the massage of daily brushing. Some forms of light treatment are also helpful; but the chief points in treatment are patience and persistence. In the intervals between attacks the use of a lotion may be thought sufficient, in the hope of preventing further attacks. The state of the general health has much to do with attacks of seborrheic dermatitis. Overwork, loss of sleep, worry, and many other causes of lowered resistance may operate; but the disease often occurs in those who appear perfectly healthy in every other way and in whom all tests fail to show disease elsewhere than in the hair follicles.

TOXIC BALDNESS

Toxic baldness comes on often a month or more after infections such as influenza or typhoid fever or a number of other conditions. The loss of hair is quite general over the scalp but seldom complete, that is, only severe thinning of the hair occurs, and in most instances, under proper treatment, it is fully restored.

ALOPECIA AREATA

Alopecia areata is a fairly common disease of the hair, occurring oftener in children than in adults but not uncommonly in the latter. Wholly without warning, a bunch of hair may be found upon the pillow in the morning, or a small completely bald patch seen upon the scalp. There may be only one small spot; but frequently others appear and join to form large, queerly shaped areas. In rare cases this progresses until all the hair upon the body has disappeared. Such cases are difficult to cure, but to the ordinary case with a limited amount of baldness of the scalp a much more cheerful outlook can be given, for they usually clear up after some months of treatment. In the bald patches the hair may grow in blond at first, even in dark-haired persons; but this usually changes to the normal color later. In those of middle age or later, the hair may come in white and remain so. The afflicted one need not be frightened if the first growth of hair falls out, for continuation of treatment is usually successful in causing a permanent growth. The cause of the disease is not known.

SENILE ALOPECIA

Senile alopecia occurs in some of those who have not been deprived in youth of their hair by the seborrheic infection. It involves the same areas of the scalp, more often the frontal portion at the sides, and progresses very slowly. The scalp may be found to be losing its fatty cushion and to be tightening upon the skull so as to hinder circulation.

GRAYING OF THE HAIR

Graying of the hair often precedes the loss from senile changes and occurs quite early in some of the members of certain families. Worry and other nervous stress undoubtedly play a part in bringing it on. Prevention of early graying is the same problem as the prevention of other forms of ageing. The preventive treatment, briefly expressed, optimum hygiene, to be successful, must begin early and be carefully followed throughout the lifetime of the individual. Sudden graying of the hair is a rare phenomenon, supposedly due to the sudden entrance of air between the layers of the cortex into the spaces formerly filled with fat. Normal graying, on the other hand, is due to failure of the papilla to form pigment or to the failure of the pigment formed to get into the cells of the hair.

SUPERFLUOUS HAIR

Undesired hair on a lady's face is a greater trial even than the lack of it upon the head of her husband. This common form of irregular hair distribution often begins in early adult life and causes great mental distress. The mild form appears as lengthening and darkening of the ends of the mustache or groups of long hairs on the sides of the chin; but in severe cases the beard is complete and fairly thick. Efforts to relieve this condition have been made since time immemorial, and the old methods are still in use: the razor, the pincette, and the epilating paste. That the resin-wax strip of cloth in which the hair is caught as it hardens is a new method I doubt very much. Shaving and the use of an epilating paste are alike in removing only that portion of the hair which projects from the follicle. After their use the hair grows out stiff. The pincette and the resin-wax method pull out the whole hair, and it grows again only after a considerable time and then as a young hair, pointed at the end.

When the Roentgen rays were first studied it was thought that they might be the long desired means of wholesale removal of hair; but it was soon found that it could not be done by this method without great danger of injury to the skin. That such injury might not make itself known for months or years after the treatment did not make it any less serious. All reputable dermatologists have agreed that this method is unsafe. Only the electric needle is left to give lasting relief to the sufferers from this deformity. It is slow and tedious; but safe, certain, and not very painful.

If fine hairs become dark colored, they can be made less conspicuous by bleaching with peroxide solution, to four parts of which one part of ammonia water is added just before applying it on a cotton pledget. This should not be used often enough to irritate the skin.

SHAVING

Shaving should be done with a clean razor, after the application of clean shaving soap with a clean brush. The modern tendency to shave one's self, promoted by the safety razor, is beneficial in that the danger of infection at home is less than in a shop frequented by others. After shaving, bay rum or another strong alcoholic solution may be used as an antiseptic. The razor should be carefully wiped with a clean cloth, and it and the strop put away where they are protected from accidental infection. If the brush has been exposed to infection, it can be sterilized as directed for the hairbrush. Bleeding can be stopped by pressure with a clean towel wet with clean hot water. The styptic pencil used in barber shops is at times a dangerous source of serious infection. Blood crusts can be removed with hydrogen peroxide. When infection is present upon the bearded region, this area should not be shaved over; but the beard may be closely clipped with scissors. Metal instruments may be sterilized in formalin or by boiling.

SYCOSIS (BARBER'S ITCH)

Sycosis (barber's itch) is a deep infection of the hair follicles in the bearded region. It is not always acquired in the barber shop, but may originate in many other ways. The organisms are the ordinary pus germs, and only people with a particularly low resistance to these germs are liable to the disease. When once established, it is very slow and difficult to cure. To prevent it, every small infection should be treated when first noticed, perhaps best by touching the spot with tincture of iodine. When infection has become established, the physician must not be expected to cure it quickly, but the patient must exercise much patience and give the doctor full coöperation if a cure is to be accomplished. Another form of sycosis, less common, is caused by ringworm fungus, usually acquired from some animal. It also is very stubborn.

Acne vulgaris often involves the back of the neck, and often, without its being present elsewhere, there is a follicular eruption in this region, causing scars which sometimes form keloids, called acne keloid.

THE NAILS

The nails are horny plates designed for protection of the ends of the fingers and toes and also for weapons of defense and offense. These latter uses have to some extent gone out of style. These plates are produced by the epidermal cells much as are the hairs. Normally they are smooth, curved from side to side and very slightly curved in the long axis. At the base is a light colored oval area called the lunula, where the active growth of the nail is going on, and over it, next the fold of skin under which the nail grows, is a special membrane, the eponychium, popularly called the "cuticle." As the nail grows, the free end wears off in those doing rough work, or in those who have itching skin disease and keep their nails worn short and highly polished from constant scratching. When protected from friction and injury the nail may grow several inches long, as used to be the fashion among certain classes in China.

HYGIENE OF THE NAILS

They should be kept cut fairly short. Fashion decrees at times that they should be trimmed so that they are pointed. This does them no harm. Neither does the polishing, if it be done in a way to avoid infection, nor the colored enameling which is now popular. Careful pushing back of the eponychium is also harmless if gently done with a smooth, clean instrument, preferably of wood. Cutting this membrane is harmful. The manicurist should understand something of surgical cleanliness and should sterilize her instruments by boiling after each use of them. The polishing pad has gone out of style, and the present-day use of a liquid polish is much more sanitary. After trimming off hangnails, the little tags of skin that become loosened along the sides of the nails, the spot should be touched with tincture of iodine, being careful not to apply too much and cause a disfiguring stain or irritation. Do not bite or pick hangnails, for these methods favor infection. Cleansing of the nails should be done after thorough washing, that the dirt under the free edge may be well loosened. A sharp instrument should not be used for this, because it will roughen the inner side of the free portion, dirt will adhere more tightly, and more scraping will be necessary to dislodge it. If the skin of the hands is dry the nail folds should receive special attention in applying cold cream, for deformities of the nail may result from lack of oil.

Transverse grooves appear in the nails commonly after illness, sometimes after so trivial a disorder as seasickness, and disappear by growing out to the free end. Any disturbance of the nutrition of the nail may cause this deformity or overenthusiastic care of the nails—pushing down the cuticle too roughly, cutting it, or injuries received in other ways. The same is true of other deformities of the nails—*longitudinal ridges, pitting, splitting*—and often it is impossible to find the cause of these irregularities of growth because they are so slight that the nail changes are the only evidence. *Loosening of the nails* at the sides of the free border occurs in children without any other sign of disease; but is usually only temporary. *Spoon-shaped nails* and other malformations may be hereditary, with accompanying hair and tooth deficiencies, or may result from malnutrition. Shedding of the nails results from some severe diseases of the skin, and there have been reported queer cases in which the nails were shed repeatedly.

White spots on the nails, "gift spots," may be caused by general disease or local injury. They are the result of imperfect formation of the horny plate as the nail grows.

Thickening of the nails may be caused by nutritional disorder, skin disease, or more frequently by ringworm infection of the nail. It occurs most often on the nail of the big toe and if not due to infection may be kept in order by paring and scraping. *Ringworm of the nails* is important because, owing to the fact that it is unobtrusive in its manifestations, it is often not noticed, and if treated, is very difficult to cure. Therefore it is likely to remain long as a focus of the disease from which infection is spread to other parts.

Ingrowing toe nails are caused by short or tight shoes and can be cured, before they become severely inflamed, by carefully cutting out the ingrowing part at the sides of the free border of the nail.

Whenever, in cutting the nails—the toe nails in particular—there is any suspicion that the skin has been injured, a mild antiseptic, as tincture of iodine, should be applied.

CHAPTER XXVI

Eye, Ear, Tongue, Nose, and Throat
MORRIS FISHBEIN, M.D.

DISEASES OF THE EYE

THE EYES are used constantly almost from the moment of birth to the time of death, except for the hours spent in sleeping. Good eyesight is necessary to an enjoyable existence, and the handicap of blind-

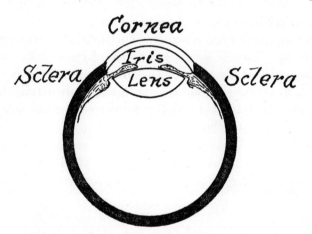

FIG. 93. Section of eye from before backwards. Clear cornea. Colored iris with hole the pupil. Lens and sclera or white of the eye.

ness one of the most serious that can affect a human being. Although the human eye is one of the finest instruments of which mankind has any knowledge, even a normal eye has certain defects. The visual field of a human being is not nearly as great as that of many other species of living organisms. A bird or a fly has a much wider range of vision than does the human being.

The mechanism of vision is complicated and difficult to understand, except by those who have some knowledge of the construction of the eye. The chief factors involved in seeing are the optic nerve and the center in the brain for vision; the retina, which is the portion of the eye that acts to convey things seen through the optic nerve; the lens, which is the focusing tissue; the muscles, which control the lens; the iris, which makes the pupil and which controls the amount of light entering the eye, and, of course, the associated fluid material, which is necessary to the proper working of the mechanism.

The eye is one of the most adaptable of organs. The distinctness of vision varies with different parts of the retina. For example, as one goes from a bright light into darkness, the vision is, at first, very bad, but after some minutes improves rapidly. The retina has the power to adapt itself to correspond with variations in the intensity of illumination. The various parts of the retina vary in this manner.

SPOTS OR SPECKS IN VISION

Because of the nature of the construction of the eye, there are several visual disturbances which do not represent actual defects but are the result of the construction. As one looks up at the blue sky or as one looks suddenly at a white ceiling, one notices a number of minute specks that move in front of the eye. These specks are the blood corpuscles moving in the smallest blood vessels of the retina. As will be shown later, such specks constantly seen may be a sign of changes in the fluid material of the eye. If the heartbeat is increased by exercise, the corpuscles will move faster, and the specks, which represent the corpuscles, move faster.

SEEING COLORED LIGHTS

Bright lights seen at night, as for example street lamps, may appear to be surrounded by areas of color or colored rings, blue inside and red on the outside. These are due to the tissue of the lens and of the cornea, which is the membrane over the eye. These tissues are ordinarily not seen.

BLACK EYE

One of the most common disturbances of the eye is injury caused by a blow of some type. Indeed, these injuries are so common that they have become common material for the cartoonist. Anyone who shows up at the office with a black eye is sure to be the victim of several presumably comical remarks as to marital conflicts. Actually, it may merely be the result of running into an open door. Anyway, that's an alibi if one sticks to it. The immediate effect of a blow on the eye with a blunt instrument may not be serious, but the later effects may be extremely serious. It is, therefore, best to treat every severe blow of the eye as a serious condition until sufficient time has passed to indicate the extent of the damage. Sometimes there is merely bleeding of the small vessels in the white of the eye. An X-ray picture may show that the bones of the skull which surround the eye have been broken.

It is safe, whenever one has had a blow on the eye, to go to bed immediately and to put an ice-bag on the eye and to have competent medical attention as soon as possible.

PENETRATING INJURY

Much more serious than a blow with a blunt instrument is the penetrating injury, such as may be brought about by a sharp probe, or by flying particles of glass, steel, or similar material. If any of the fluid material of the eye has escaped through the injury, the condition is especially serious. Fortunately, the X-ray is now of great aid in indicating whether or not a substance has actually penetrated the eyeball.

The removal of the foreign substance from the eyeball is a most difficult process, and one of which only trained physicians are capable. The use of a magnet is sometimes helpful. There are many substances which are not attracted by a magnet and which may cause great harm if they remain in the eye. Sooner or later destruction of the tissue occurs around the foreign substance. Sometimes there is infection, and not infrequently complete loss of vision.

Flying particles of hot steel are usually free from infection. However, even when germs are not carried into the eye with the foreign substance, they may be brought to the eye by the blood and localize in the spot which has been damaged by the irritation.

SYMPATHETIC OPHTHALMIA

Most serious in connection with any penetrating injury of the eye is the serious inflammation of the other eye, known as sympathetic ophthalmia. This occurs some fourteen days after the injury to the first eye, most frequently in from four to six weeks, but may occur many months or even years later. The appearance of the eye first injured helps the physician to determine the possible onset of such an inflammation in the other eye. In the majority of cases, proper preventive measures are taken immediately. If the first eye is severely damaged and inflammation is serious, it is customary to remove the injured eye promptly before any signs of inflammation have appeared in the second eye.

No one knows yet just why sympathetic ophthalmia occurs. It is such a serious condition, however, inasmuch as it means loss of both eyes rather than of one, that the physician must give the benefit of the doubt to the patient. If the vision of the eye first injured is destroyed, if the eye is soft, if it is painful, and if the condition seems to be progressive, the physician will feel that to remove the eye immediately is safest for the patient.

CARE OF EYE IN INDUSTRY

Another fairly common type of injury to the eye is the burn by caustics of one type or another, such as lime or acids. In industry, it is well to follow certain rules for all workmen who happen to suffer injuries to the eye:

1. Under no circumstances should an untrained or inexperienced employee attempt to remove any foreign body from the eye.

2. Immediately after an accident, the eye may be bathed with suitable mild aseptic or sterilized solutions, preferably a weak solution of boric acid made with sterilized water.

3. The eye should be covered with a sterile bandage moistened with this solution.

4. The person whose eye is involved should be sent immediately to the physician who is in charge of such cases. If the factory or workshop does not have a first-aid department, arrangements should be made with some near-by hospital or medical institution to give prompt attention to such cases. This will mean the avoidance of a great deal of unnecessary blindness and furthermore a much shorter period of disability than is otherwise the case.

FOREIGN BODIES IN EYE

This brings up the question of removing foreign bodies from the surface of the eye. There are hundreds of superstitions as to how this is best done. They concern sneezing, rubbing the other eye, and similar methods. It is much safer to rub the other eye than to rub the one in which the foreign body has lodged. In most instances, rubbing tends to push the foreign substance farther into the eye.

People who understand how to remove foreign bodies are exceedingly careful to make certain that their own hands are clean and that every instrument or other material used in the process is clean or sterilized. The eye itself must be handled with the utmost delicacy. The person first looks upward so that the lower lid of the eye may be pulled down and carefully studied. He then looks downward while the upper lid is turned back. It is impossible to turn the upper lid back safely while the person is looking up or moving the eyeball constantly. With practice, skill can be developed in turning back the upper lid. This is then carefully studied. If the foreign substance is not seen, the physician then looks at the surface of the eyeball, changing the light so as to catch the reflection of any foreign substance which may be imbedded in the cornea.

Of course, the competent physician has means of anesthetizing the surface of the eye and of avoiding injury to it in the removal of foreign substances. He is careful not to introduce infection, and to follow up the removal by later inspection to make sure that no untoward results are occurring. Secondary infections may bring about ulcers which will destroy the sight of the eye.

CONJUNCTIVITIS

The most common form of infection of the eye is conjunctivitis, which means an inflammation of the conjunctiva, the covering which lines the eyelids and runs onto the eyeball. This may become infected by any one of several different germs. Generally there are burning and smarting of the eyelids, formation of pus, intense reddened appearance of the lids which may spread to the eyeball, and, usually associated with this, sensitivity to light, and the pouring out of tears.

PINK EYE

The treatment given by the physician varies according to the character of the germ that produces the infection and according to the extent of the infection. One germ produces the condition called "pink eye." Shortly after this germ gets into the eyes they become reddened, the lids will be found glued together in the morning, and there will also be swelling and puffiness. Sometimes this disease is transmitted by the use of a common towel, and in other cases by soiled hands. In

RUPTURE OF THE CHOROID

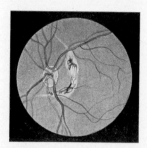

INTRAOCULAR HEMORRHAGE WITH GREATLY INCREASED TENSION

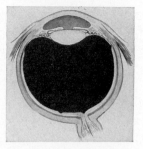

RUPTURE OF IRIS AND MONOCULAR DIPLOPIA

This is to be left alone.

This may require enucleation on account of pain.

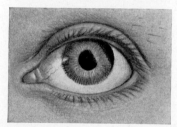

TRAUMATIC CATARACT

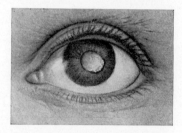

This requires very delicate operative measures. Under a conjunctival flap the cornea must be entered, the root of the iris grasped and a most delicate thread passed through it. This is anchored to the corneoscleral junction.

Its management requires expert opinion based on considerable experience. An eye physician should be seen at once.

DISLOCATION OF THE LENS

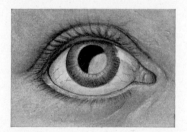

DETACHMENT OF THE RETINA

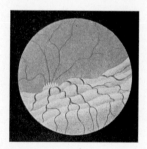

Often no treatment at all is necessary. If the eye becomes irritable or double vision results, an eye physician should be consulted. Treatment requires very delicate operative procedure.

This also requires very precise operative interference. New technic recently developed has improved the prognosis considerably.

FIG. 94.

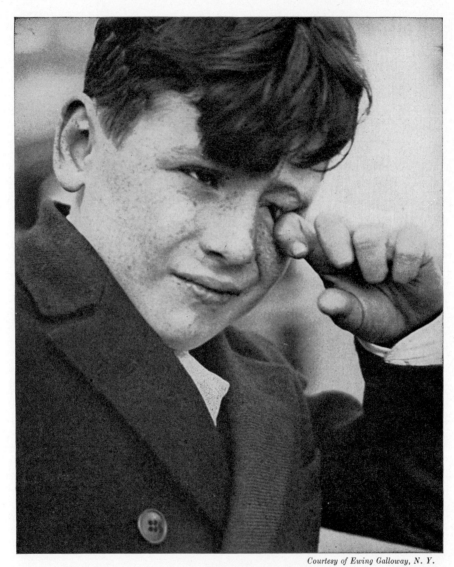

FIG. 95.

Wrong method of removing foreign body from eye.

treating such infections the doctor usually advises hot fomentations which are put on the eyes for five minutes at a time; sometimes recommending that boric acid or witch hazel be added to the hot water. It is not well, however, to take such infections lightly. It is safer to be certain of the exact nature of the condition.

TRACHOMA

For instance, trachoma is a serious infection also affecting the eyelids, and there are infections by the same organism that produces venereal diseases. These infections are so serious that they may spread to the cornea, causing large ulcers, with partial or complete loss of eyesight. In the case of such infections of the eye, it may be necessary to use treatment that is practically constant day and night, in order to save the eyesight. Indeed, most physicians recommend, under such circumstances, that the patient be put in the hospital.

STYES

There are also numerous small glands in the eyelids which secrete oily material so that the eyeball is lubricated when the eyelid passes over it. When one of these glands becomes infected it is filled with pus. This is the common condition called stye, also known scientifically as hordeolum. In a few days the stye, like any ordinary pimple, comes to a head and breaks; then the pus escapes. If the stye is not properly treated and the source of the infection eliminated, one stye will follow another, and they persist for a long time. If the stye does not open itself, and if it is not opened, it will tend to be cleared up from within, in which case a hard lump may be left which is filled with scar tissue. This tends to enlarge, and it is best under such circumstances to have the lump, called chalazion, removed by a physician. Repeated formation of styes indicates that the body has little resistance against infection. Under such circumstances, it is well to guard the general health by suitable diet and cleanliness.

TEAR DUCTS

A chemist said to his wife, "Your tears have no effect on me; they are simply salt and water." Tears keep the eyes moist so that the delicate tissues, of which they are made, are preserved. If the eyes are not constantly kept moist, the tissues dry and are much more easily attacked by bacteria.

In a little bony notch on the inner side of the eye there is a gland called the tear gland or lacrimal gland. From this, six or more little tubes carry the tears to the eyes. There is another tube, which is known as the nasal duct, which carries fluid from the eyes to the nose. Hence, whenever a person cries or his eyes water, his nose runs simultaneously. When the amount of moisture is so great as to overflow, the excess comes down through the nasal duct until there is so much that it falls on the cheeks. Most of the time there is just enough moisture to keep the eye in the proper state of softness and luster.

Occasionally a tear duct becomes blocked because of the presence in it of a cinder or a hair. Under such circumstances, it is necessary to open it up. This requires special instruments and the care of a physician who knows how to do the unblocking correctly.

In other instances the gland and the duct become infected. Then there is a reddened swelling in the inner corner of the eye and the discharge of a small amount of pus. Pressure over the swelling will force out most of the pus. It is sometimes possible to get relief by treatment, but in other instances it may be necessary to cut into the gland, and there are instances in which it has to be removed surgically.

Tears have always had a romantic interest. In 1581 a Latin writer described a girl sixteen years old whose tears resembled blood. More recently a similar case was described in Pennsylvania. Apparently in such cases there has been a leaking of red blood cells out of the blood vessels into the tear gland. In some instances in which bloody tears appeared, the women concerned had not experienced the normal changes that occur to girls. In other cases there were tumors of the eyelids.

ULCER ON EYE

The most dangerous infection of the eye is the ulcer on the eyeball. This may be due to any kind of infection, but the worst forms are those due to the germ that causes pneumonia, the pneumococcus, and the one that causes gonorrhea, the gonococcus. In both of these types there is rapid destruction of the tissue of the eyeball. If there is penetration or perforation due to such destruction, the interior of the eyeball is also infected, and then there is complete loss of vision.

There is another type of infection of the cornea or covering of the eyeball which occurs most frequently in young children who are undernourished and have frequent colds, and particularly in those who have tuberculosis. In such cases there is an excessive flow of tears and a great aversion to light. This symptom is called photophobia. Because of the aversion to light, which produces blinking and pain, the person is likely to keep the eyelid shut on the inflamed eye. If the eye is studied, it will be found full of little flecks of material deposited by the inflammation.

Another type of inflammation of the cornea is due to the second great venereal disease, syphilis. This is a most serious condition when it affects the eye, as well as when it affects any other part of the body. For this reason, the physician who treats the disease treats not only the eye but also the infection as it concerns the rest of the body.

It must be remembered that there are various ways in which germs can attack the eye. They may come in from the outside or from the inside. The same germs that cause inflammation in the joints or in the nervous system, coming from infection in the tonsils, or the teeth, or the throat, may also be carried by the blood to the eyes and bring about serious infection there. Under the circumstances, the mere healing of the condition in the eye is not sufficient. It is necessary to find the systemic cause responsible and to take care of that as well.

People with tuberculosis, infections of the teeth, the tonsils or the sinuses, with high blood pressure, kidney disease, or diabetes may have symptoms affecting their eyes directly related to the other diseases that have been mentioned, and the diseases of the eye will not be improved until the other conditions are brought under control.

INFLAMMATION OF THE IRIS

The iris is the colored circle surrounding the pupil. Any condition which affects the surface of the eye may also attack this tissue. The condition is likely to come on insidiously. Then there are persistent redness of the eye, pain, dimness of vision, and aversion to light. Such an infection is dangerous because there is a tendency for adhesions to form between the edge of the iris and the lens. This will produce a deformity of the pupil and interfere with vision. It is, of course, necessary for a physician to find out as soon as possible the cause of the infection and to control it.

CATARACT

The lens does not have blood vessels or nerves but receives its nourishment from the fluid material in the eye. The lens is entirely surrounded by a capsule which acts as a filter, keeping out undesirable material. Should this capsule be broken, the lens is infiltrated with material from the fluid of the eye; then it becomes cloudy, and the person has what is called traumatic cataract. As people get very old, the capsule gradually becomes less efficient, and the nutrition of the lens is interfered with. As the lens becomes clouded, it gradually becomes cloudy from the outside toward the center. When finally the center becomes clouded, it is exceedingly difficult for the person to see. This condition is called senile cataract.

It must be remembered that the human eye is like a camera. It has a lens; it has a shutter, which is the iris. The pupil is the hole in the shutter through which the light enters. At the back of the eye is the retina or sensitized plate on which the image is cast.

Most cases of cloudiness or cataract of the lens, such as have been described, occur in people between fifty and seventy years of age. The only treatment for senile cataract is surgical. There are no drugs, no drops of any kind, no exercise or treatments which are successful in stopping the slow development of a cataract. Nevertheless, such methods of treatment have been used by vast numbers of quacks to get money from people who fear approaching blindness because of cataract.

There are numerous operations now developed which are relatively simple and which are quite safe in the majority of instances. Moreover, good vision follows in 97 per cent of the operations for cataract. After the cataract is removed, the person wears what are known as cataract glasses. These are made so that they help in focusing the image properly on the retina.

The person who has been unable to see for some time because of the development of clouding, who has been unable to play golf or get about, and who then recovers his sight by a simple operation that any competent specialist in diseases of the eye can perform, is one of the most appreciative of all the people benefited by modern medical and surgical science. When the cataract is removed, the result is like defrosting a window or raising the window shade: the light comes in without obstruction, and the individual is able to see.

INFLAMMATION OF RETINA

The tissues of the eye behind the lens are also subject to infections and inflammations. There are the delicate membranes of blood vessels and pigments, the rigid outer coating, and the retina or membrane of light perception. The large cavity is filled with vitreous, the fluid of the eye. Normally, rays of light pass through the vitreous without any hindrance, but occasionally there are small pieces of tissue in the vitreous which cast a shadow on the retina, such shadows being seen constantly as specks. Inflammations which affect the retina and the delicate membrane associated with it may be associated with the changes that take place in the blood vessels or tissues in old age, with infections elsewhere in the body, and with specific damage to the tissue itself.

The physician uses an instrument called the ophthalmoscope to look into the eye and to observe any changes that have occurred in these tissues. When the vision of the eye becomes diminished, and without any pain, without any redness or inflammation, the physician looks for the cause. Sometimes he sees changes in the retina which indicate a systemic disorder, such as diabetes, tuberculosis, and high blood pressure. Obviously that condition must be taken care of before any attempts are made in relationship to the eye itself.

DETACHMENT OF RETINA

Sometimes the retina itself is loosened, so that the condition called detachment of the retina occurs. As soon as any part of the retina becomes detached from its bed, the vision controlled by that part is disturbed, and unless it is reattached in a short time the vision is lost permanently. The person who has had detachment of the retina should go to bed immediately. Sometimes competent control of fluid intake helps the situation. In other instances operations have been developed which appear to be useful in aiding reattachment of the retina. Several competent authorities say that reattachment with recovery of vision occurs in about 15 per cent of the cases.

GLAUCOMA

One of the most dangerous of all of the diseases of the eye is glaucoma, a condition responsible for a large proportion of blindness that exists today. The cause of this disease is unknown. Its principal manifestation is an increase of pressure inside the eye. Glaucoma causes about 15 per cent of all the blindness that occurs, and about one half of all the blindness that occurs in adults. The blood that comes into the eye to nourish it must pass out, or the fluid accumulates, in which case there is a sense of pressure with pain, the eye gets hard and red and, from the front, appears gray and cloudy.

In other cases, the fluid goes out partially but not completely, so that the increased pressure and the loss of sight take place gradually. A competent physician can actually measure the pressure in the eye by means of a special instrument called the tonometer. He can also look into the eye with the ophthalmoscope to see whether there has been sufficient pressure to cause a depression in the optic nerve tissues as they come into the eye.

As the glaucoma develops, the individual can see in front of him but not so well on the sides. Gradually his field of vision becomes narrow, with final loss of sight. The expert can determine the narrowing of the field of vision by the use of the apparatus called a perimeter. If untreated, glaucoma leads certainly to blindness. It is difficult to control. Excessive pressure on sensitive tissue, such as of nerves, produces degeneration.

Physicians treat glaucoma by use of drugs which lower pressure in the eye and contract the pupil. Such a condition cannot be treated by the use of glasses. If medical methods fail, it is customary to use surgery to establish proper drainage and to keep the pressure in the eye permanently low.

No condition of the eye should be neglected, because prompt diagnosis and treatment are necessary to take care of the condition before permanent changes occur.

THE EAR AND ITS DISTURBANCES

The outer ear differs but little from other external portions of the body in the things which may disturb it. It may be the subject of small tumors which, of course, must be removed if they show the slightest tendency to growth or irritation. Sometimes cysts form which are nonmalignant tumors but which continue to swell or grow as long as the opening is blocked. These should be opened and the wall of the cyst removed, if there is not to be a recurrence.

ERYSIPELAS OF EAR

In erysipelas the ear will swell to tremendous size. Obviously it must be protected to prevent breaking down of the tissue due to the swelling and irritation. In frost bite of the ear it should be gradually warmed until the circulation returns. Then the skin must be protected to prevent infections with ulcers.

TIN EAR

One of the most common forms of injury to the ear is what is commonly called "tin ear" of the pugilist. Repeated blows on the ear result in the pouring out of blood between the cartilage of the tissue and its surrounding membranes. At first such swellings are bluish-red; they feel like dough, and they are opaque, so that light will not pass through. In some instances, it may be advisable for the surgeon to open the tissue and to remove the clot of blood, and, in that way, to prevent permanent thickening and swelling. It is sometimes necessary to plan the use of bandages which mold the ear and hold its shape while such surgical treatment is being undertaken.

Modern ideas of beauty demand that the ear lie fairly close to the head and that it be relatively small. Hence the plastic surgeons, particularly the bogus plastic surgeons, are likely to induce people to try all sorts of operations to hold the ears back or to lessen their size. Such operations are in many instances of doubtful value and may result in permanent changes which are harmful. They should never be undertaken unless the person's occupation is such as to make slightly protruding or large ears a menace to earning a livelihood.

INFECTION OF EAR CANAL

In addition to the diseases that may disturb the outer ear, there are disturbances which affect the canal up to the point of the eardrum. Almost any infection may involve the outer canal of the ear. Under such circumstances it is necessary to remove the infection and to prevent its recurrence by the use of proper antiseptics which a physician can supply and which should be used only after he has given proper instructions.

There is a good rule in medicine: namely, never put anything in the external ear any smaller than the elbow. The tissues are most delicate and may be seriously harmed by the use of wires, toothpicks, ear-spoons, or similar irregular or unsterilized devices. A scratch of the lining of the canal may result in the formation of a boil, which is exceedingly painful and which is difficult to handle in such an inaccessible part of the body.

HARD WAX

The cerumen or wax of the ear is easiest removed, when it becomes hardened, by the use of a syringe with slightly warm water. This need not be done often, and harm can be done by needless or too frequent syringing. The syringe should always be sterilized by boiling before using, and the water should be previously boiled and then used warm. Before a person attempts to syringe an ear for himself or for a child, he should learn the technic.

The person whose ear is to be syringed usually sits in good light. It is customary to put a towel or cape around the neck and tuck it in over the collar to prevent soiling of the clothing. A kidney-shaped pan is held at the edge of the ear so that the fluid returning will run in the basin and not down the neck. In an adult the ear is pulled up and backward in order to straighten out the passage. Then the nozzle of the syringe, which has been filled and had all the air expelled, is placed just inside the outer opening. The water is then projected along the back wall slowly and without too great pressure, so as to permit return of the flow as the water goes in.

After the ear has been washed, the head may be turned on one side and the extra fluid allowed to run out. A person who understands the technic may then wipe out the canal with a small wisp of cotton. If a permanent antiseptic, softening material, or lotion is to be used, the physician can prescribe the proper one, and this is held in place with a little wisp of cotton, never inserted under pressure.

A foreign body in the external ear will seldom cause much discomfort unless it is a living insect. Cases are on record in which living insects have entered the ear and remained for many years, gradually being surrounded by hardened wax or cerumen, to the point at which a person lost his hearing entirely. The damage from foreign bodies in the external ear lies in rough attempts to remove them. If a living insect gets into the outer ear, a physician can destroy it by the use of a little chloroform vapor, under which circumstance the insect will either come out of its own accord or be killed, when it can be removed by a syringe.

It is not well for anyone to attempt to remove a foreign body from the outer ear if it cannot be syringed out, unless he has had special training in this type of work. Several interesting technics have been developed for removing foreign objects, one being the use of a device

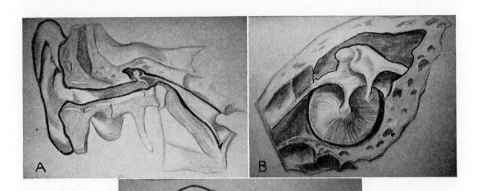

A. The outer ear, the middle ear and the eustachian tube. The sound waves, caught by the shell-like outer ear, are carried through a canal to the drum in the middle ear, where the eustachian tube equalizes the pressure on the drum.

B. In the middle ear are located the drum and the ear bones, the entrance to the mastoid, and the eustachian tube, which leads to the back of the nose. Closure of the eustachian tube and infection of the middle ear are common causes of impaired hearing.

C. The inner ear is a spiral organ, lined with different sized hairs like piano strings, for receiving the different pitches of sound. Connected with this organ (see diagram), are three small semicircular canals by means of which we maintain our balance.

FIG. 96.

with an adhesive material at the end which sticks to the body that is to be removed. It is then gradually withdrawn.

A foreign body that is infected may produce irritation and serious infection with the formation of boils or abscesses which, in the external ear, are a menace frequently to life itself. A boil in the external ear demands the immediate and competent attention of an expert, who can arrange to open it in such a manner as to permit the infectious material to escape, to withdraw the pus, to relieve pain by a prescription of proper remedies, and to prevent the spreading and recurrence through the use of suitable antiseptic preparations.

EARACHE

When there is an infection of the nose or throat the bacteria sometimes get into the ear behind the eardrum through the eustachian tubes, the passages leading from the mouth and nose cavities into the ear. Therefore, many infections of the ear may be prevented by properly cleansing infected noses and throats with mildly antiseptic and alkaline sprays and washes.

Emphasis must be placed on the word "properly" because such washes, as generally applied, force fluid, pus, and bacteria into the ear. These nasal douches should never be taken with any but the most gentle pressure, perhaps slightly snuffling the warm, alkaline fluid into the nose.

The early diagnosis of infection of the ear is important, if inflammation of the mastoid bone, behind the ear and contiguous to the brain, is to be prevented. The ears should always be examined if a child is ill and has fever. The presence of fever, a bulging drum, and the symptoms mentioned are sufficient reasons for the physician to incise the eardrum to save the hearing of the child and to prevent burrowing of the infected pus into the mastoid region. When the diagnosis and the proper treatment of an infected ear are delayed, the results are likely to be extremely serious.

The first symptom of an infection in the ear is usually pain in the ear, and in some cases this is the only symptom. It must be remembered, however, that pains in the ear also are found in connection with presence of boils in the ear canal. Sometimes a pain in the ear may be associated with an unerupted wisdom tooth and inflammation of the joints of the jaw and severe tonsillitis or an infection of the sinuses around the nose.

The doctor makes up his mind as to the presence of an acute infection of the ear by taking the temperature, which in these cases usually is high. However, special examinations in such cases of acute infections of the ear are made by direct inspection of the eardrum, using a magnifying device and a light. This device is called an otoscope, meaning a device for seeing the ear.

In most instances, a physician called to such a case and making a diagnosis of severe infection within the ear will arrange to open the eardrum promptly. This not only relieves the pain, but also makes it less likely that the infection will spread to the mastoid.

Sometimes the pain may be relieved in the early stages by dropping into the ear some warm eardrops, usually composed of glycerine with a small per cent of phenol. Strength of this solution is, of course, to be determined by the doctor in charge of the case. Sometimes mere application of heat to the ear brings relief.

MASTOIDS

If the condition spreads into the mastoid, mastoiditis develops and constitutes a much more serious condition than infection of the internal ear alone. When the infection spreads to the mastoid, great tenderness will be found in that region, and also pain on pressure. The physician watches carefully this development. From the very first, the mastoid bone may be tender on pressure because of the swelling on the inside. Whenever pain is severe and there is fever, the physician knows that the infection is serious, and he is likely to recommend immediate incision of the eardrum. The operation is not difficult and, if performed soon enough, is likely to prevent more serious complications.

People have strange notions about perforation of the eardrum, believing that this will interfere with hearing and cause other damage, whereas actually the eardrum heals promptly after the infection disappears, and hearing is likely to be just as good as it was previously. It is far less dangerous to hearing to incise the eardrum than to postpone the incision too long.

The Tongue and Its Disorders

The tongue is an organ which has always aroused the interest of the medical profession. Doctors of an earlier day used to pay a great deal of attention to the appearance of the tongue because of the relationship of such appearances to disturbances of the rest of the digestive tract.

Occasionally the tongue is abnormal in its construction at birth so that the condition of tongue-tie is produced, and there are other cases in which that portion of the tissue holding the tongue is abnormally long, permitting actual swallowing of the tongue with occasional asphyxiation. In some conditions the tongue becomes too large for the mouth and protrudes beyond the lips. This is particularly the case in the large tongue of the child that has deficient thyroid secretion with the development of cretinism.

GEOGRAPHIC TONGUE

Sometimes the surface of the tongue is marked by long, deep furrows instead of being smooth. There is a common condition called "geographic tongue" because the surface of the tongue looks like a relief map. In this condition there are grayish thickened patches on the surface. Apparently it is a mild inflammatory disorder which tends gradually to improve, the treatment usually including merely the washing of the mouth at fairly frequent intervals with mild antiseptic and alkaline mouth washes.

INFLAMMATION OF TONGUE

The tongue may be suddenly inflamed from a number of different causes, such as injuries, burns, insect bites, and occasionally association with such serious infectious diseases as scarlet fever, typhoid fever, or smallpox. Whenever the tongue is infected, the lymph glands in the region also become infected and swollen. In very serious cases death may result from such inflammation of the tongue, but in the vast majority of cases mild treatment tends to lead to recovery.

There are many nervous disorders or conditions affecting the nervous system in which there is pain in the tongue or burning of the tongue without any visible evidence in the neighborhood of the tongue itself. This condition sometimes occurs in locomotor ataxia, in hysteria, and in all sorts of nervous upsets of one type or another. Under such circumstances a physician may make sure that the condition is functional and not due to any destruction or inflammation of the tissues concerned. If he discovers actual disease of the nervous system, the case is treated by the well-established methods. If such disease is not discovered it may be necessary to use psychologic methods in controlling the symptoms, not only as they affect the tongue, but probably as they affect other parts of the body as well.

The tongue is primarily responsible for the sense of taste which is, at the same time, a composite of the sense of smell and the feel of food on the tongue. Loss of the sense of taste may result from inflammation or swelling of the tongue; it may be associated with hysteria. In the same way there may be exceeding sensitivity to tastes so that a person is constantly tasting sweet, sour, salt or bitter; and in other instances foods taste different from what they should.

In every such case it is necessary to make a most careful study of the entire patient, his surroundings and environment, and particularly his emotional condition.

THE NOSE

The nose is, in general, the least ornamental of the features of man. It is the mark for more insults and injuries than any other adornment of the human countenance. It is unnecessary to locate it geographically, since it presents itself. Remarkably, however, modern living conditions have made the nose, in more ways than one, a center of interest.

Actually, there is not much to the organ itself. It is composed of some small bones and cartilages and certain soft tissues which go to surround the two cavities. Of equal importance with the nose and inevitably to be considered with it are the nasal sinuses. These sinuses are cavities in the bones in the head which connect with the inside of the nose by means of small openings. There are, of course, nerves which take care of the motor and sensory functions of the tissues and which may be involved in any condition affecting the nose.

The most important of the structures in the nose from the point of view of disease is the mucous membrane or tissue which lines the cavities. It is one of the most sensitive tissues in the body, and when bruised or hurt in any way may respond with considerable trouble for the possessor. Not infrequently, minor infections occur, particularly in the hair follicles or in the roots of the hairs which are in the nose. These hairs have the purpose of filtering out dust or infectious material which comes into the nose with the air.

It is now generally well known that common pus-forming germs, such as staphylococcus and streptococcus, are widespread and easily get into the human body whenever they come in contact with a tissue that has been damaged in any manner. They may set up an infection which eventually may spread throughout the body. The pernicious habit of picking the nose, pulling out the hairs, or trying to squeeze out pimples or other infections may result in most serious inflammations or other disorders.

HYGIENE OF NOSE

The right way to take care of the nose is to remove carefully, by proper use of a handkerchief, such materials as can be reached easily. Those which cannot be reached may be washed out by the use of a mild spray, without pressure. There are now generally available all sorts of mild sprays of inert oils and small amounts of camphor, eucalyptus, or menthol, which serve this purpose conveniently. Under no circumstances should such materials be put in the nose under high pressure. If a spray is not convenient, the simplest method is to drop one or two drops into the nose.

An infection in the lining of the nose manifests itself by redness, swelling, discomfort, and pain, which increase steadily. The tip of the nose becomes swollen, and sometimes the swelling may even extend up to the eyelids. In the presence of any serious swelling involving the nose, it is well to have an inspection by a physician, who will determine the presence or absence of a localized spot of infection such as a boil or pimple, who can arrange to cause the infectious material to be released, and who will provide suitable dressings of warm antiseptic or saline solutions tending toward recovery.

When for any reason the nose is lost entirely, the facial expression naturally suffers. When the bridge of the nose disappears, as sometimes occurs in certain forms of disease, a saddle nose is caused which is anything but beautiful. The frequency of automobile accidents has resulted in damage to many a proboscis. Falls, industrial accidents, railroad wrecks, and gunshot wounds also produce damages that require medical attention, and the results of pugilism are a constant source of income to specialists in nasal reconstruction.

Mother Nature brings many a break into prominence by bestowing upon it a hump, a knob at the tip, or a deviation to one side or the other. In street fights anything can happen to a wayfaring nose, and medical literature records several instances in which the tip of one has been bitten off by an agitated opponent—male or female.

Forms of the nose have been described as long and short, upturned and downturned, humped and flat, wide and narrow, pointed and saddle-shaped. It is just as well that people do not worry too much about their particular type of nasal appearance. As soon as they get their minds fixed on this, they look into the looking glass until it gets tired of reflecting their appearance. The experts find that almost any

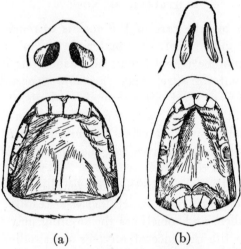

(a)   (b)

FIG. 97.   (a) Normal jaw and nasal cavity. (b) Effect long-standing nasal obstruction.

amount of repairs and reconstruction is never satisfactory to the person who once embarks on the paths of nasal improvement.

PLASTIC SURGERY OF NOSE

If the loss of tissue or destruction of tissue causes damage to the health of the person concerned, the case certainly demands surgical attention. There are many ways of building up a broken-down or absent bridge. Some surgeons transplant bone and cartilage, some use celluloid, and others use ivory. Humps are removed by dissection and scraping or cutting. The best way to take care of a deformity from an accident, however, is to give it the best possible attention immediately after the accident. It is much easier to secure a good result if such care is given at that time than to attempt a complete rebuilding operation when tissues have healed in the wrong manner.

FOREIGN BODIES IN NOSE

Children not infrequently push all sorts of things into the nasal cavity. The character of things pushed into the nose is limited only by the size and the possibilities. Insane people also occasionally indulge in a similar performance. Among some of the common substances that have been found by physicians are chalk, buttons, seeds, and pieces of wood.

Occasionally the nasal cavity becomes infected with worms. Among others are maggots and screw worms, and indeed almost any of the worms which can live in the human body. Worms are seldom found in a normal nose. However, in the presence of any disease with an associated odor, flies are attracted which may lay eggs or in other ways convey the larvæ of the worms to the nasal cavity. Among the first signs of infestation of the nose by worms are irritation, sneezing, and an increased amount of discharge usually streaked with blood. The removal of worms from the nose is not a serious matter. The nose may be washed repeatedly with solutions containing proper antiseptic substances.

The removal of inanimate foreign bodies not infrequently requires the greatest skill of a competent specialist. It may be necessary to use an anesthetic, to apply various solutions which will constrict the tissue of the nose, to employ the X-ray to localize the foreign body exactly. Once this is done, the doctor merely grasps the foreign body with a forceps and withdraws it, endeavoring to cause as little damage to the soft tissue as possible.

POLYPS IN NOSE

Sometimes growths in the nose, like polyps, are difficult to distinguish from foreign bodies. Usually the discharge coming from the nose as a result of the presence of a foreign body comes only from one side. Sometimes the removal of polyps or similar tumors is followed by the disappearance of chronic infection in the nose and sometimes also by the removal of asthmatic symptoms. It is not possible for the average person to diagnose the presence of nasal polyps for himself. The condition can, however, be diagnosed by a physician following an examination of the nose, in which he looks directly into the nasal cavity.

NOSEBLEED

There are many causes of bleeding from the nose, because the blood supply to the tissues is generally rich and the tissues themselves quite delicate. In many diseases in which the tendency to bleed is great, such as hemophilia and purpura, two conditions in which the elements of the blood are so altered that bleeding occurs frequently and coagulation of the blood takes place with difficulty, bleeding from the nose is a common symptom.

In the presence of severe infection and in the condition called scurvy, which is due to a deficiency of vitamin C, bleeding of the nose also occurs with a fair amount of frequency. In practically all of the conditions which produce severe anemia, nosebleed is not unusual. In cases of hardening of the arteries with exceedingly high blood pressure there may be rupture of a small blood vessel in the nose with severe nosebleed for some time. The bleeding from the nose and the loss of blood serve to lower the blood pressure.

Of course, any blow on the nose or any bruise which breaks a blood vessel will result in bleeding. There are also cases in which tumors within the blood vessels cause hemorrhage. In ordinary cases of nosebleed, if the person is at once placed in a horizontal position so that the blood pressure is lowered, and if he is kept cool, he tends to recover, since in most instances the bleeding will stop promptly.

There are many superstitions about stopping nosebleed, such as dropping a key down the back, pressing on the hard palate, and similar performances. However, there is no efficacy in such measures, except that they serve to distract the attention of the person whose nose is bleeding and keep him from being too much frightened during the short interval that usually elapses before the bleeding stops.

In more serious cases, however, physicians use measures which have a greater degree of certainty, such measures including packing of the nose with sterilized gauze, direct inspection with pinching of the bleeding vessel, cauterization with some substance like silver nitrate or chromic acid, and the use of various solutions which temporarily constrict the blood vessels, giving the blood opportunity to clot. In general, physicians avoid leaving packing in the nose for long periods of time because of possible dangers to the ears through blocking of the tubes that pass from the nasal cavity to the ears, and because of possible effects from blocking the nasal sinuses.

It should be borne in mind that the bleeding from the nose is not in itself a disease, but rather a symptom of disease; that it may be the warning sign for the onset of a serious disorder, such as a change in the blood, or even a tumor of the adrenal glands. On the other hand, it may merely be due to increased mental or physical excitement or any other condition that suddenly raises the blood pressure. In most cases the amount of blood lost is small, but if the person has repeated hemorrhages the amount lost may be sufficient to cause anemia and to demand special treatment for restoring the blood.

Sometimes hemorrhage from the nose in children is overlooked, because the blood goes back in the throat and is swallowed. In most cases of bleeding from the nose, even severe cases, the hemorrhage stops of itself in approximately ten minutes. If the hemorrhage continues longer, or if it is repeated, the condition is most serious and demands efficient attention. It is especially important to remember not to blow the nose after the bleeding has stopped, because that will dislodge clots and start the bleeding over again.

SINUS DISEASE

The public has learned that there are sinuses or air spaces surrounding the nose, and, associated with this knowledge, according to Dr. Lee M. Hurd, there has developed among neurotic types a fixation on the sinuses in which there is not only headache and pain, but also a slight mucous discharge to lend strength to the picture.

On the other hand, there are some phlegmatic individuals with obstructed breathing in the nose and a profuse discharge who wonder why they always feel tired, have no appetite, who wonder why they have pains in the joints and limbs, and who have not realized that the nasal condition is primarily responsible for the trouble.

According to Dr. Hurd, the mucous membrane of the nose becomes deranged either by a bad diet which is deficient in vitamins, by sensitivity to various protein substances, or by some disorders of the glands of internal secretion.

The changes that take place in the mucous membranes make it possible for germs to invade them easily, and then the infection has begun. If rats are put on a diet that is deficient in vitamin A, the mucous membranes change, and infection of the sinus occurs. In cases when there is sensitivity to various food substances, the mucous membranes swell and are much more likely to be invaded by germs. In the same way, disorders of the glands of internal secretion are reflected by changes in the mucous membranes.

If the underlying cause is removed, the infection may be brought under control, but in the vast majority of cases correct treatment involves not only control of the underlying cause but also treatment of the infection. If the vitamins are insufficient, they may be supplied through giving a well-balanced diet. For the sensitivity, it is necessary to make diagnostic tests, which will indicate the special substance to which the person may be sensitive.

Disorders of the glands of internal secretion must be carefully investigated. There are some cases, for instance those in which the thyroid is deficient, in which it is possible to supply the deficiency through proper preparations.

Persons who work indoors in crowded rooms where the air is bad and the temperature too low or too high are more likely to develop infection of the sinuses than those who spend a good deal of time outdoors.

A constant discharge from the nose, particularly a discharge of pus, is one of the most certain indications of infection in the sinuses. Sometimes when discharge from the sinus becomes blocked there is swelling of the forehead, dizziness, and even ringing in the ears. There are several sinuses, each of which must be studied individually by the physician in order to determine the extent and nature of the infection. Such a study involves a thorough examination through the nose of the openings of the sinuses into the nose, washing of the sinuses to obtain the discharge, transillumination in a dark room which indicates whether or not the sinuses are clear, and the use of the X-ray, which indicates whether or not there is thickening of the walls of the sinuses or any amount of material present in the cavity.

A person with chronic infection of the sinuses is likely to wonder what the possibilities are for his relief. Dr. Lee M. Hurd is convinced that individuals with chronic sinusitis never recover without treatment. Many of them have low-grade infections in which surgical treatment is not advisable, and these patients can be helped by drainage, frequent washing, and the application of various antiseptic substances.

In other cases, however, the infection of the sinus persists to such an extent that it involves danger to surrounding tissues. Cases are known in which the sight of an eye has been lost because of infection in a neighboring sinus. There are other instances in which the infection extends from the eustachian tubes to the ear and thus involves the mastoid process. The constant inhalation of pus may set up bronchitis or pneumonia. The continuous slight fever results in a loss of vigor and in disturbances of digestion.

There are even cases in which loss of memory or neurosis has occurred because of the constant infection and irritation. It has been well established that an infection in the nose may be carried by the blood to other parts of the body, resulting in serious inflammations of joints, infection of the heart and the kidneys, and even meningitis.

In children, chronic infection of the sinuses may be associated with enlarged adenoids and tonsils. The removal of the adenoids and tonsils may eliminate the source of the infection and end the trouble. At the same time, it should be emphasized again that correction of the diet to include a proper amount of vitamins A, B, C, and D is of importance.

There are, of course, cases in which the same child may have an enlargement of the tonsils and adenoids, and associated with this a sensitivity to various protein substances. Obviously attention to both conditions is necessary if complete recovery is to be secured.

In older people, when the antrum is involved, the large sinus on each side of the nose, it may be necessary to remove all infected teeth in relation to the antrum and to clean out the infected bone at the roots of the teeth. An opening into the antrum from the mouth permits drainage and the healing of the diseased membrane. If such measures fail, it is possible to employ a surgical procedure, which involves a wide opening of the sinuses or even complete obliteration; such methods are, however, so delicate that they should be undertaken only by those especially competent, and then after the most careful consideration.

THE SENSE OF SMELL

Everyone knows that there are some odors that are pleasant and others disagreeable. In many instances the sense of pleasure or of discomfort is associated with some previous experience of the person concerned. For instance, the perfume called attar of roses is generally much more pleasant than that of asafetida. There are persons, however, to whom the smell is not altogether pleasant. Some odors seem exceedingly pleasant at the first whiff and then tend to become more unpleasant the longer they are present. This is because of their intensity.

In the University of Edinburgh, Dr. J. H. Kenneth has undertaken a series of researches, including twenty-nine men and thirty-four women who were examined as to their response to odors of many different substances and combinations of substances. The state of health of the person concerned seems to have something to do with the enjoyment of odors or with disagreement.

Psychological study was also made of associations with various smells. One man who was given camphor to smell immediately felt distressed and visualized the odor of a wardrobe and then a feeling of suffocation or being in the dark. It appears that the odor reminded him of an incident in 1892 when he was placed in a closet because of some youthful misdemeanor. In the closet were clothes which had been supplied with camphor as a moth preventive.

A girl who smelled xylol visualized herself on board a vessel in a harbor in Ceylon. The odor of xylol resembles that of benzol which comes from harbor launches. The odor of cedar-wood oil was associated with a summer evening on the Norwegian coast, with a cigar box in which money had been placed, with a road in the country. Later investigation indicated that the person had been in the habit as a child of walking along this road chewing the end of a cedar-wood pencil.

To one woman the odor of cedar-wood oil brought up the idea of spring cleaning and the cleaning of floors with a cedar-wood mop. Another girl told of the playing of the music of Chopin when she smelled vanilla; another thought of Ireland's song, "Sea Fever," when smelling pine oil.

The usual thought associated with asafetida was garlic or onions. One person thought of a street car in Edinburgh, and it was discovered that these cars were formerly lighted by acetylene gas which gives off a similar odor. The odor of orris root brought to one girl the idea of smelling an elephant at a distance. These investigations are of the greatest importance as an aid in the psychologic studies of the human reaction. They seem to offer further opportunity for more of the interesting home psycholgical games in which so many people now indulge.

The nose, like many other organs of the body, is lined with tissue called mucous membrane that secretes mucus. Sometimes these cells, over-grow, and when they do, little tumors are formed which hang down into the nose and interfere with breathing; also by the obstruction they cause they may aid in setting up infection. Hence, it is desirable that they be removed. Sometimes even after they are removed they return, and since the exact cause of such tumors is not known, there is nothing to do but keep on removing them.

In general, the causes of tumors are not definitely known, although certain contributory factors are recognized. Several observers believe that polyps never occur except in the presence of infection, although others are convinced that the infection follows the polyps.

It is generally well established that the use of radium following the removal of tumor cells may prevent the formation of additional tumors. Hence, it has been suggested that the removal of nasal polyps be followed by mild treatment with radium element in order to prevent their return. The radium is usually applied in the form of a screen container several days after the polyps have been removed, when the inflammation due to the surgical procedure has subsided. Sometimes the polyps form in the sinuses rather than in the nasal cavity itself. Under such circumstances, a physician can detect their presence by injecting into the sinus a substance which is opaque to the X-ray, such as lipiodol. Then an X-ray picture is taken, and this reveals the presence of the tumor or growth inside the sinuses, preventing their filling completely.

THE THROAT

There are general inflammations of the throat associated with redness, swelling, and excessive discharge of mucus due to many different causes. Most common, of course, is exposure to cold, an extension of inflammation from the tonsils, the adenoids, or the nose. Excessive use of tobacco; excessive exposure to dust, smoke, irritating fumes, and sudden changes in temperature; excessive dryness, and similar atmospheric conditions may cause irritation of the throat. People who are sensitive to certain food substances sometimes react with blisters on the tissues of the throat, which become secondarily infected and produce irritations and inflammation.

There may be severe pain associated with swelling and inflammation of the throat, including pain in the ears because of blocking of the tubes which lead from the nose to the ears; there may also be a sense of fullness or obstruction, with much hawking and spitting.

The first thing to know about any inflammation of the throat is its cause. If the condition happens to be due to diphtheria, prompt action is necessary, including the giving of diphtheria antitoxin. If, however, it is due to some other type of germ, other methods of treatment are employed.

SORE THROAT

The pain of an inflamed throat is best relieved by use of an ice bag filled with cracked ice. Most doctors are now convinced that gargles seldom go deep enough in the throat in sufficient quantity or strength to permit them to have much effect in killing germs or in curing disease. They have the value of washing out everything they reach. They serve to relieve some of the dryness of the mouth and throat that is usually present with inflammation. They sometimes substitute a good taste in the mouth for a bad one, although some of the gargles themselves taste so bad that they make a bad taste worse. To have a definite effect from any antiseptic in the throat, it is necessary to apply it directly to the infected or inflamed part. This is best done by spreading material with a cotton swab or by using an atomizer properly. In order to get the antiseptic into the back of the throat, it may be necessary to hold the tongue or to use a tongue depressor.

MOUTH WASHES AND GARGLES

The primary purpose of a mouth wash or throat wash is to clean and soothe. A good cleaning mouth wash is merely salt solution made by adding a fourth of a teaspoon of salt to a half glass of warm water. If there is much mucus, the addition of a quarter of a teaspoon of bicarbonate of soda or ordinary baking soda may be beneficial. Most mouth washes and gargles sold in drug stores contain water, salt, baking soda or boric acid, with flavoring material and dye substances of various kinds. Many of them contain alcohol. Alcohol is astringent, cleansing, and somewhat antiseptic. Ordinarily, mouth washes may contain one part of alcohol to four or five parts of water.

There are innumerable lozenges now available which can be dissolved on the tongue. These have a soothing effect or slightly anesthetic effect. They also serve to moisten the mouth, but their antiseptic value is little, if any. The dryness that occurs in the mouth during any inflammation of the throat may be alleviated by drinking some effervescing water, such as ginger ale or vichy, or by chewing gum, or by the use of lozenges.

The most serious form of sore throat, next to diphtheria, is called epidemic septic sore throat. This is spread frequently by infected milk. When the milk supply is properly pasteurized, virulent organisms are destroyed. If, however, there is any carelessness whatever in

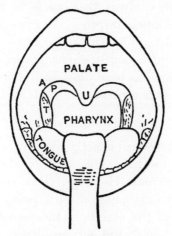

FIG. 98. Diagram showing palate, uvula, tonsils, pharynx, and tongue.

the process of pasteurization, the germs causing septic sore throat may get by and infect considerable numbers of people.

This germ is a streptococcus. It is found on the udders of the infected cows and infects all the milk that comes from the infected cow. Sometimes the udder of the cow may not be infected, but the milker may have a sore throat. The milk that has become infected is then mixed with the general milk supply, and anyone taking part in the consumption of the infected milk supply is likely to develop septic sore throat.

Milkers should invariably wash their hands thoroughly before milking cows, and it will do neither the milk nor the milker any harm if the hands of the milker are washed frequently during the whole milking process. This will protect not only the milk and the consumer, but also the cow.

Infections of this type in the throat may spread gradually through the throat, involving the rest of the body. Septic sore throat usually begins with fever, chills, and a rapid pulse. These, however, are equally the symptoms of numerous other disorders of an infectious character. The fact that there are numerous other cases in the community at the same time helps to indicate the epidemic character of the disease. In most instances, investigation by the health department will serve to indicate that practically all the cases occur on the route of one distributor of milk. The study is then made to find which of the employees concerned is himself infected. An examination is also made of the herds of cows to determine whether or not any of the animals have infected udders. Not infrequently epidemic sore throat is mistaken for influenza. One epidemic has been described in which the condition was traced to infected ice cream rather than infected milk.

TONSILLITIS

No one has ever determined exactly why we have tonsils. Apparently they serve some purpose in taking care of the infectious organisms that come into the throat. However, their response to infection is prompt swelling and inflammation with pain, soreness, difficulty in swallowing, swelling of the glands in the throat, high fever, a rapid pulse, a general weakness, and serious illness generally. Not infrequently the germs which develop in the tonsils are carried by the blood to other parts of the body and there set up inflammations, the regions particularly affected being the joints, the heart, and the kidneys.

The germ that is most frequently responsible for tonsillitis is the streptococcus, which is also responsible for various forms of heart disease, for erysipelas, and for similar conditions. When the tonsils have once been seriously affected, they apparently are likely to become infected again and again.

In children particularly it is exceedingly important to make sure that the condition is tonsillitis and not diphtheria. Tonsillitis produces a throat that is purplish-red and swollen, whereas diphtheria produces a grayish-white membrane. The special importance of the distinction lies in the fact that the control in diphtheria depends on early diagnosis and the prompt administration of a sufficient amount of suitable antitoxin.

The patient with tonsillitis should go to bed promptly. A physician will usually apply directly to the place of infection suitable antiseptics to destroy the germs that are on the surface. He will also control the fever and provide medication which may be helpful. The applica-

:ion of an ice bag or hot packs will give relief from the pain and soreness. A gargle with a small amount of baking soda helps to clear out the adherent mucus.

Chronic tonsillitis is especially dangerous because of the secondary effects. For this reason, physicians advise surgical removal of the tonsils in all such cases. Tonsillitis itself is seldom fatal, but the possibility afterward of an infected ear, or infected joints, or heart disease is so serious that a sort throat should never be neglected. Many years have passed since the medical profession first recognized the importance of removal of infected tonsils because of their relationship to disease. Tonsils are sometimes removed simply because they are so greatly enlarged as to interfere with swallowing and breathing. Between this simple enlargement and the severe states of infection in which the tonsils are filled with pus there is a wide variety of possibilities.

Much investigation has been done to prove that the infection in the tonsils may be carried by the blood to other parts of the body and there set up secondary infections which threaten life. There are well-established cases in which infection of the tonsils was followed by infection of the heart, of the kidneys, and even of the peritoneum, resulting finally in fatal peritonitis. There is also considerable evidence to indicate the relationship of infected tonsils to colds, infected ears, fatigue, nervousness, and rheumatic symptoms.

If it could be definitely proved that removal of the tonsils early in life would entirely prevent or greatly diminish these diseases, routine removal of the tonsils would be advised by all physicians. Unfortunately absolute proof of this fact cannot be provided.

There are many other possibilities for the production of colds, of nervousness, and of fatigue besides infection in the tonsils. Furthermore, the tonsils are not the only glandular structures involved in the upper respiratory tract. The adenoids, which lie in the postnasal cavity, may also be seriously infected and transmit infection to other parts of the body. Hence the combination "tonsils and adenoids" is just as well known as are the combinations of ham and eggs and Amos 'n' Andy.

Investigators in the University of Cincinnati have recently made a controlled study of the relationship of removal of tonsils and adenoids to various diseases. They are convinced that the removal of these structures early in life decreases greatly the incidence of colds, nasal obstruction, and sore throats. On the other hand, they feel that infection of the sinus, headaches, and growing pains were more frequent after tonsillectomy than before.

Anyone who understands the difficulty of evaluating scientific evidence will realize that much more observation must be had before the

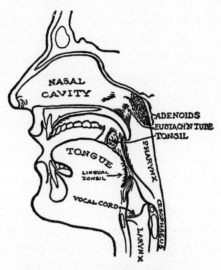

FIG. 99.   Lateral diagram of head showing relation of adenoids, tonsils, nose, ear, and larynx. Observe how close to the ear the adenoids are. Again observe that the floor of the nose and the adenoids are in the same horizontal plane. Also, discharge dropping down from the adenoids could easily fall on the vocal cords causing such disturbances as laryngitis and croup.

final decision in this case can be made. At present there is plenty of evidence to warrant the prompt removal of tonsils that are infected or that are seriously enlarged.

In two of the common diseases that affect children, namely, scarlet fever and diphtheria, many, if not most, of the symptoms relate to the throat. For this reason, the question as to whether or not removal of the tonsils is of any help in preventing scarlet fever cr in making it less severe is of importance.

Children who have diphtheria, and who have large tonsils, frequently suffer more than those whose tonsils have been removed. Frequently those who have diphtheria continue to carry the germs in their throats after recovery from the disease. Apparently the presence of infected tonsils is likely to encourage the development of a carrier rather than to discourage it.

Recently, Dr. William L. Bradford studied all of the children in the schools in Rochester, N. Y., who had had their tonsils removed and compared them with children who had not had their tonsils removed so far as concerns the relationship to scarlet fever. Of 600 children with scarlet fever, 122, or 20 per cent, had had their tonsils removed previously.

The degree of severity of the disease was about the same in those who had had their tonsils removed as in those who had not. About the same percentage of both groups developed complications, and the rate of disappearance of the germs from the throat was about equal in children with and in those without tonsils.

However, the children who had had their tonsils removed had a few less organisms in the period of convalescence than did those who still had their tonsils. Apparently, therefore, removal of tonsils is not extremely important so far as relates to the severity of scarlet fever or inability to recover from the condition completely and without complications.

Dr. N. G. Shaw studied particularly the relationship of removal of the tonsils to the prevention of diphtheria. A study of a large number of children, using the Schick test as a means of determining their immunity from diphtheria, did not indicate that removal of the tonsils served in any way to give the children better resistance to diphtheria than was had by children who still had their tonsils.

These studies are an indication of the way in which medical science continues to test and retest its procedures. They do not in any way indicate the desirability of keeping enlarged or infected tonsils in the throat.

Such tonsils are a menace and should be seen by a physician who will determine when and how they are to be removed. The studies do indicate that the tonsils are not particularly associated with the prevention of scarlet fever or diphtheria or with the occurrence of complications in these disorders.

Ten years ago, 1,000 children in Rochester, N. Y., had their tonsils removed at the age of five or six years. They were examined at that time and complete records of infections previous to the operation were noted.

Ten years ago the parents of an equal number of children were recommended to have the children's tonsils removed, but the operation was not performed for various reasons. These two groups of 1,000 children each represented children in the same schools and from the same homes, living under similar conditions.

Now, Dr. Albert D. Kaiser has looked into the records of these children, who are just of high-school age, and his information affords definite evidence of the value of the operation in those children operated on for the control of certain conditions studied in both groups. In order to make the comparison, the complaints usually associated with infection of the tonsils were tabulated, the history of infections of each child was obtained, and any physical defects in any way related to the tonsils and adenoids were recorded.

The figures show that sore throats, a common childhood complaint, do not occur as frequently or as severely in a child whose tonsils have been removed as in one whose tonsils have not been removed. Only 10 per cent of the children whose tonsils were removed had any complaint of sore throat, whereas 35 per cent of the others had such a complaint.

Frequent head colds occurred in 45 per cent of the children before operation. Ten years after the operation, 22 per cent of those operated on still have head colds, whereas 30 per cent of those not operated on have head colds.

It was found that measles occurred with equal frequency in both groups of children. Diphtheria occurred in 28 cases among those children operated on, and in 42 cases among those not operated on. Scarlet fever occurred in 73 cases of those operated on and in 102 cases of those not operated on.

One of the chief reasons why the tonsils are removed is to prevent rheumatic manifestations, including St. Vitus's dance, rheumatic fever, and infections of the heart. Apparently St. Vitus's dance was not affected by removal of the tonsils, occurring just as often in those children who were operated on as in those not operated on. There was a lessened amount of rheumatic fever in the children whose tonsils had been removed, and a lessened amount of infections of the heart. However, the difference in the figures was slight.

Dr. Kaiser is convinced that the removal of the tonsils influences appreciably the incidence of sore throats and renders children less susceptible to scarlet fever and diphtheria. It does not appear to be especially important for the prevention of head colds and infections of the ear, and it influences unfavorably the occurrence of bronchitis and pneumonia.

The wholesale removal of tonsils, whether diseased or related to disease, is not warranted. In certain conditions they may be removed for definite effects, which experience has shown may certainly be secured. At present, the vast majority of physicians are convinced that the correct method for removal of the tonsils is complete surgical removal rather than the use of slow destruction by electricity or any other recently introduced method.

CHAPTER XXVII

The Venereal Diseases
MORRIS FISHBEIN, M.D.

THE VENEREAL DISEASES are among the most common that afflict mankind. They spread from person to person in response to satisfaction of the biologic demand of the glands of man, but also occasionally through perfectly innocent sources, such as contaminated utensils, towels, and other appurtenances intimately used by human beings.

One fact must, however, be constantly kept in mind: both major venereal diseases, syphilis and gonorrhea, are caused by germs. The germs must be transmitted in order to transmit the disease. Every case of either one of these diseases comes from another case. Until a patient with one of these diseases is satisfactorily treated and his infection brought under control, he is a menace to everyone around him, including his wife—if he is married—his children, his friends, or associates.

The diseases are not new with man. They have probably existed since the earliest times, certainly since the Middle Ages. Everyone should have knowledge of the nature of these diseases and means of transmission, means of prevention, and correct method of treatment. Proper dissemination of such knowledge seems to be the only hope for their ultimate control.

SYPHILIS

Whether or not syphilis existed previous to 1493 is not established with certainty. About that time it appeared in Barcelona among Spanish sailors who had returned from Haiti. It reached Italy with the army of Charles VIII, and from Italy spread throughout Europe. At first it was called "Neapolitan disease" or the "French pox." The name syphilis was given to it in 1530 by a writer named Fracastorius. Since that time, physicians have studied the disease constantly. Even before the modern era doctors had learned to treat syphilis with a fair degree of success with mercury. However, it was the discovery of the organism of the disease, and later the discovery of specific methods of treatment, that offered the first promise of complete control. The organism of syphilis, known as "spirochaeta" or "treponema," was definitely established as the cause of the disease by the investigator Schaudinn in 1905. The organism is seen only with the microscope, and is found in the sore which is typically the first sign of infection with this disease.

TRANSMISSION OF SYPHILIS

In the vast majority of cases syphilis is transmitted from one human being to another during sexual relations. There are, however, records of accidental infection, such as those which occur on the hands of surgeons and midwives who have not properly protected their hands during their work; such as occur on the lips from infection through kissing, and such as occur occasionally on the breasts of wet nurses. Occasionally also the child may be infected before birth from its mother, in instances even when the mother herself is not actively diseased.

These facts should not frighten anyone into a phobia or constant fear of syphilis, since the disease is not transmitted as easily as the description may seem to suggest. Hotel beds, public lavatories, bath-tubs, door knobs, books, utensils used in public eating places are not easily infected. Moreover, the germs do not live easily in the presence of dryness. Finally, it is necessary for the organism to get into a sore or an easily infected spot in order to invade the body. In most instances, thorough washing with soap and water does much to re-move danger of infection. When it seems likely that one has been directly exposed to the development of the infection with syphilis, the rubbing of mercury ointment into the exposed area has been proved to be a protective measure of great value. It is well, however, to emphasize again that syphilis is rarely acquired by those who observe the elementary laws of personal hygiene and who have sexual relations only with those who are free from the disease.

FIRST SIGNS OF SYPHILIS

The first sign of syphilis is usually the appearance of a sore on the genital area or on the finger or wherever the germs gain entrance into the tissues. These sores develop slowly. At the same time the lymph glands in the region near by become swollen. A physician who sees such a sore makes his diagnosis certain by taking some of the fluid from the sore and studying it under what is called the dark field microscope. By reflected light he is thus able to see the spirochaetes wriggling in the fluid. He may also spread some of the secretion on a glass slide and stain it with suitable stains which make the organisms visible with the ordinary microscope.

The healing of the primary sore or its removal will not, however, prevent syphilis from invading the body. Usually, by the time the organisms are found freely in the sore, the body has already been quite fully invaded and it is necessary to give general treatment to control the condition. If immediate treatment is given before the appearance of the secondary symptoms, these are not likely to appear. Hence, the physician urges emphatically that every case of syphilis be treated at the earliest possible moment; in fact, that every case diagnosed from the symptoms be treated even before getting the results of the Wassermann test, so as to be certain that the control will be brought about at the earliest possible moment.

The test known as the Wassermann test, and a similar test, known as the Kahn test, are means of examining the blood so as to determine whether or not it contains a substance opposing syphilis, which is present only if syphilis has invaded the body. These tests are positive in more than 95 per cent of cases in an early stage. By their nature they enable the physician to determine whether or not improvement is taking place, and later whether or not the patient has been cured.

Venereal diseases can be cured, provided treatment is given sufficiently early and with sufficient intensity and for a long enough period of time.

The secondary symptoms of syphilis appear about the time when the first sore is disappearing. These symptoms represent invasion of the body as a whole. Now the person is usually sick, he may be jaundiced, and eruptions may appear about the body. Frequently the hair falls out in spots, and occasionally serious sores develop on the skin. There may even be inflammation of the eyes, of the mouth, of the joints, or of the nervous system in this stage of syphilis. Because these symptoms may come and go, some patients are inclined to neglect treatment in the second stage of syphilis. This, however, should never be done. It is easier to treat the condition in this stage than in the third stage, in which the brain and nervous system become involved.

In the secondary stage there has seldom been destruction of the tissues of the body, so that treatment in this stage is more likely to be effective. Under no circumstances should the patient believe that the gradual disappearance of the symptoms represents cure of the disease. He should have a definite statement by a competent physician after that physician has made sufficient laboratory tests to venture an opinion with reasonable certainty.

In the third stage of syphilis, there occur not only destruction of tissues, but growths within various organs of the body, inflammations of the blood vessels, hardening of some of the organs, and other serious changes. In fact, the lesions of this disease are so varied that Sir William Osler once said that one who knew all of syphilis really knew all of medicine. The third stage grows constantly worse unless sufficiently treated. Fortunately, the third stage of syphilis is not likely to be as dangerous to other people as are the first and second, because in this stage the lesions are buried deeper within the body, so that the organisms are not so easily transmitted outside the body.

In the later stage of syphilis, it affects the nervous system. As a result come those two exceedingly serious diseases which are responsible for much disability and death: locomotor ataxia or tabes dorsalis, and paresis, also called general paralysis of the insane and dementia paralytica. In these conditions, other methods of treatment are required besides those commonly used for syphilis in the early stages. It may be necessary to apply treatment directly to the spine or to the brain. It may be necessary to infect the patient with malaria, which has been found to have special virtue in the attack on general paralysis, or to use the heat treatment, which has come to be well established as a useful method.

FACTS ABOUT SYPHILIS

Among certain facts which should be known to everyone relative to syphilis are the following:

This disease does not cause pimples.

It does not cause itching conditions of the skin.

It may cause ulcers of the legs, but more frequently these are due to varicose veins.

It may be responsible for failure to produce children, but there are also other conditions which may produce such failures.

It is not a form of blood poisoning, but testing of the blood will show whether or not the patient has syphilis.

It is not responsible for the vast majority of cases of baldness, but some cases of loss of hair not only of the head but of the entire body may be due to syphilis.

It has not been established in any way that syphilis is the cause of cancer or that these two conditions are in any way related.

INSTRUCTIONS FOR THOSE WITH SYPHILIS

At the time of the World War, the United States Army Medical Department issued certain definite instructions to those with syphilis, which, somewhat modified, may be advised today since they are just as accurate now as they were in 1917:

If you have any sore on your genitals, no matter how small, or if you think you have syphilis, consult your physician. Do not under any conditions rely on the "blood medicines" that promise to eradicate syphilis, and do not be caught by advertising doctors—quacks—who try to get your money by promising to cure you quickly. Do not let druggists prescribe for you; they are not qualified to treat syphilis.

Do not hesitate to tell your doctor or dentist of your disease. Later in life if you get sick at any time, you should tell your doctor that you have had syphilis, since this fact may furnish a clue to treatment on which your cure depends.

Live temperately and sensibly. Do not go to extreme in any direction in your habits of life.

Try to get a reasonable amount of sleep—eight hours is the amount needed by the average person. And as a safeguard to others, sleep alone.

You should not smoke or chew tobacco.

Absolutely do not use alcoholic liquors. All experience shows that drinking—even moderate drinking—is bad for syphilis.

Take good care of your teeth. Brush them two or three times a day. If they are not in good condition, have them attended to by a dentist. But when you go to him, tell him that you have syphilis.

Do not have sexual intercourse until you are told by your physician that you are no longer contagious. It will interfere with the cure of the disease, and it is criminal, for it is likely to give the disease to your wife.

You must not marry until you have the doctor's consent, which cannot be properly given until at least two years have passed after cure seems complete. If you do, you run the risk of infecting your wife and your children with syphilis.

Early in the course of syphilis, while it is contagious, the greatest danger of infecting other people is by the mouth. Because of this danger, do not kiss anybody. Particularly, do not endanger children by kissing them.

Do not allow anything that has come in contact with your lips or that has been in your mouth to be left around so that anybody can use it before it has been cleaned. This applies to cups, glasses, knives, forks, spoons, pipes, cigars, toothpicks, and all such things. It is better to use your own towels, brushes, comb, razor, soap, etc., though these are much less likely to be contaminated than objects that go in your mouth.

If you have any open sores—you will not have any after the first week or two, if ycu are treated—everything that comes in contact with them should be destroyed or disinfected.

To live up to these instructions will only require a little care until you get used to them; after that, it will be easy. If you do live up to them, there is a good prospect that syphilis will not do your health permanent harm or cause injury to others; and you will have the satisfaction of knowing that, after your misfortune, you have acted the part of an honest man in your efforts to overcome it.

One of the difficult things about syphilis is that to cure it often requires a long time—two years or more. In two or three weeks after you begin treatment, you will not know from any symptom that you have syphilis, and you will, therefore, be tempted to neglect further treatment. This is the great mistake that many persons with syphilis make. To insure future safety, treatment must be continued long after all evidence of the disease has disappeared. For your own good, you must see to it that you do not neglect your treatment after the first few months.

In the treatment of syphilis, the competent physician has available today many remedies that were not at his command until the last few years. Previously, as has already been mentioned, he was largely dependent on the use of mercury, which was given in the form of rubs, pills, injections, and by various other methods. Then came the newer methods of treatment, involving the famous discovery by Paul Ehrlich of "606" or salvarsan, which is found to have a specific effect in clearing up the lesions of this disease. More recently bismuth has been developed as a remedy of special merit. For years iodides of one type or another have been used to control various symptoms.

The man who treats a patient with this disease is guided not only by the results of the Wassermann and Kahn tests, which are made repeatedly, but also by frequent studies of all of the symptoms affecting the various tissues and organs in the body. It is particularly important before he makes his final decision as to whether or not the patient is cured or whether or not the patient should marry that he check his decision by tests of the blood, tests of the spinal fluid, and similar investigations.

WHEN PEOPLE WITH SYPHILIS MAY MARRY

One of the questions most frequently asked by a patient with syphilis is whether or not he may marry. Most physicians are convinced that a patient should be free from all syphilitic symptoms for at least one year before marriage should be contemplated. In some American states the bridegroom is compelled to furnish a medical certificate to show that he has been examined and found free from venereal disease. This is, for instance, the law in Alabama, Louisiana, North Carolina, North Dakota, Oregon, Wisconsin, and Wyoming. However, none of these states requires a certificate from the prospective bride. The marriage of a person who has a contagious venereal disease is forbidden in Delaware, Indiana, Maine, Michigan, Nebraska, New Jersey, Oklahoma, Pennsylvania, Utah, Vermont, Virginia, and Washington. However, there does not seem to be any good evidence that any of these states secures adequate evidence from those applying for a license to marry.

The treatment of this condition is one of the most intricate problems that can confront a physician. He must use his remedies in relationship to the reaction of the patient and the response of the patient to them. No one with the disease should ever discontinue treatment until he is pronounced by a competent physician free from danger of transmitting the disease and cured to the extent that the condition is brought absolutely to a halt in his body. Persistence in the use of the new remedies that are available under proper control will yield a successful result in the vast majority of cases.

Gonorrhea

Gonorrhea has existed certainly since Biblical times. Although it is a widespread and serious disease, it is not a killing disease. As a cause of ill health, it ranks among the leaders, but as a cause of death it is not especially prominent. Many people believe that gonorrhea concerns only the sex organs, whereas the germ which causes it, described by the investigator Neisser in 1879, may invade any part of the human body. Like syphilis, it is spread mostly by sexual contacts. However, there are infections of the eyes sustained during childbirth or in other ways which attack mostly infants at birth. There are infections of the tissues in women associated with the use of bathtubs and toilet devices not properly cleansed, which are accidental infections with this disease. Little girls are occasionally infected by soiled hands of mothers or nurses.

Gonorrhea is responsible for a considerable percentage of all cases of blindness. It is one of the common causes of infection in the female abdomen, resulting in necessary surgical operations and occasionally removal of the female organs. It is responsible for a considerable amount of sterility in men due to infections of the various parts of the sex tracts. It is found not only among the poor but in all classes of society.

FIRST SIGNS OF GONORRHEA

From three to five days after a sex contact with a person who is infected the first signs of the disease may appear. These usually are a feeling of burning or stinging at the time of urination, associated with redness and soreness, and associated also with the formation of pus or matter which drips from the sex organ. This material is highly infectious and should not be allowed to come in contact with the eyes or sex organs of any other person.

If a physician is consulted immediately, he may be able to stop the disease in these early stages, when it is confined to the lower portion of the sex organs. If, however, it is not stopped at this time, the germs get farther back into the glands of the male and into the organs and tissues of the female. To the extent to which these organs and tissues are involved, gonorrhea is a serious disorder. The physician may make his diagnosis by an examination of the matter under the microscope, in which case he can actually find the germs, and also by tests of the blood. Occasionally the condition affects the joints, and it is also largely responsible for painful heels, causing outgrowths on the large bone of the heel.

TREATMENT OF GONORRHEA

In the treatment of this condition, the physician uses many types of remedies, including antiseptics which are injected directly into the tissues and the application of various other remedies by mouth and by injection into the veins or under the skin. The hygiene of this condition is the same as that for any infectious disease, including the use of good food, fresh air, and proper attention to the bowels.

ADVICE TO THOSE WITH GONORRHEA

During the time of the World War a distinguished committee set forth some regulations which are well to repeat as basic advice for those who have this condition. This advice follows:

Persist in treatment until your doctor tells you you are cured.

Do not try to treat yourself.

Do not use a patent medicine or some "sure shot" that may stop the discharges but will not cure you.

Do not let an advertising doctor—a quack—get your money, and do not let a drug clerk treat you.

If you have had gonorrhea and you suspect that it is not cured, report to your medical officer.

During the acute stages keep quiet and take little exercise. As long as you have any discharge avoid violent exercise, especially dancing.

In order to avoid chordee, while the disease is acute, sleep on your side, urinate just before going to bed, and drink no water after supper.

Never "break" a chordee. To get rid of it wrap the penis in cold wet cloths or pour cold water on it.

Except at night, drink plenty of water—eight or ten glasses a day.

Do not drink any alcoholic liquors; they always make the disease worse and delay its cure. Also avoid spicy drinks such as ginger ale.

Do not eat irritating, highly seasoned, spicy foods, such as pepper, horseradish, mustard, pickles, salt and smoked meats, or fish.

Always wash your hands after handling the penis, particularly in order to protect your eyes. Gonorrhea of the eyes is very dangerous; it will produce blindness if not at once treated, and the infection is easily carried to the eyes on the fingers.

Keep your penis clean. Do not plug up the opening with cotton or wear a dressing that prevents the escape of the pus from it. Wash the penis several times daily.

Burn old dressings, or drop them into a disinfecting solution.

Never use anybody's else syringe or let others use yours. While you are using a syringe keep it clean by washing it in very hot water, and, when you have finished with its use, destroy it.

Avoid sexual excitement. Stay away from women. Do not have intercourse. It will bring your disease back to its acute stage, and it is almost sure to infect the woman. Sexual intercourse while you have gonorrhea is a criminal act.

You are likely to obey instructions while your gonorrhea is acute, because it causes so much pain. Persist in them after pain is gone; by so doing you will prevent relapses, make your cure much easier and more certain, and expose no one else to the disease.

MARRIAGE AFTER GONORRHEA

As regards marriage after an attack of gonorrhea, the patient should be examined at weekly intervals to determine whether or not any infection is present following treatment. The results should be negative three consecutive times before he can be considered definitely cured. It should be remembered that self-treatment with drug-store remedies is just as dangerous as complete neglect of treatment in this condition.

Prevention in gonorrhea is far better than cure. The chief factor in prevention consists in the avoidance of sex contacts when infection is present, and infection is likely to be present in any promiscuous woman, either commercial or private. There are various methods of protection against the possibility of infection, such as the use of rubber devices and injections of various antiseptics immediately after sex contact, these antiseptics being held in the organs until the antiseptics have sufficient amount of time to act.

CHAPTER XXVIII

The Care of the Teeth
MORRIS FISHBEIN, M.D.

THE CARE OF BABY'S TEETH

THE IMPORTANCE OF TEETH for health and long life is beginning to be more and more realized. Few mothers realize that the first attention to the teeth of the child must begin before it is born. The mother should visit the dentist early, keep her teeth clean and well cared for, and eat the proper food so that the child's teeth will be properly developed. The proper foods include plenty of milk, fresh vegetables, eggs, fresh and cooked fruits, the coarser cereals, and a sufficient amount of calories to provide energy. Foods to be avoided are the sweets in excess, meat in excess, pastries, and highly seasoned foods.

During the early months it is not necessary for the expectant mother to eat more than her usual amount of food, but during the last four months the amount of food must be increased slightly in order to provide a sufficient amount of material for building the tissues of the child.

There used to be a notion that it was not safe for a prospective mother to visit her dentist, but it is now realized that the dentist can do the necessary dental work without serious harm or shock, and that it is better to take care of the teeth immediately than to permit bad conditions to go on for months.

Of special importance for building sound teeth are vitamins C, D, and A. Vitamin C is found plentifully in orange and tomato juice and in the fresh vegetables; vitamins A and D particularly in cod-liver oil and egg yolks. The physician should see the prospective mother just as soon as she knows that she is going to have a child and advise her regarding the taking of cod-liver oil or of excess vitamins in the form of concentrates.

The baby that is nursed by its mother gets the best food a baby can get. If it is not nursed by the mother, it will have to have a diet arranged so as to include the necessary substances. The basis of all baby diets is milk, but milk is deficient in certain necessary substances, and these the doctor can provide for through modifications of the diet. He will tell the mother when the baby is to have orange and tomato juice and cod-liver oil and the amount of each it should have. The vegetables are the first foods to be added to the baby's diet, and they should be started slowly in very small quantities. By the time the child is one year of age it can eat most vegetables; it can also be having fresh milk, fruit, and Zwieback or toast.

Many physicians and dentists believe that coarse foods strengthen the jaws and help in hardening the gums. When a new tooth is about to come in, the coarse foods serve as a resistance against which the gums may work in order to permit the tooth to cut its way through. If the child is excessively irritant when the teeth are coming in, it is wise to have the advice of the dentist or family physician.

The first teeth come in at the front of the mouth between the fifth and eighth months, as a rule. If they happen to be a little early or late, there is no cause for worry. The next teeth come in between the eighth and tenth months, and the others about the time of the first birthday. Until the first teeth appear, the mouth of the child does well if let alone. After the first teeth appear, the gums and teeth may be wiped daily with a soft clean cloth dipped in water to which a little salt has been added. It is well to be exceedingly gentle.

About the eighteenth month a soft toothbrush may be substituted for the soft cloth, and as soon as the child is old enough it should learn to brush its teeth for itself. If the child likes the taste of toothpaste, it may have toothpaste. If it prefers the water with added salt, it may have that. Most physicians and dentists are convinced that a toothpaste is of service only in cleaning and polishing the teeth and has little, if any, special value for preventing infection or counteracting acid.

The chief reason for preserving the baby teeth is to keep the mouth in the right shape for the second teeth. All of the twenty teeth that are called temporary teeth are usually in the mouth by the time the child is three. Behind the first set is the second set. In order to have the second set properly developed, the food must be right and the mouth free from infection. The only certain way to control infection is to have dental care when it appears.

The most important permanent tooth comes in between the fifth and sixth year of life and is known as the six-year molar. It comes in six teeth back from the one in the front of the mouth in the center.

There are four six-year molars, one on each side of the upper and lower jaws. They should have the most careful attention. Once gone, they are not replaced except with artificial teeth. If they decay and are removed without proper dental attention, the entire expression of the face and of the mouth may change. In the absence of the proper molars, food is not sufficiently ground before entering the stomach.

Every child should see a dentist following the appearance of the six-year molars. Only a generation has passed since dentists first began to give special attention to the teeth of the child. Now the subject is so important that there are many dentists who specialize exclusively in children's teeth. They are concerned with seeing that all of the teeth are straight, that they fit properly against the opposites in the other jaw, that they do not grind off surfaces that are meant to stand, and that they remain firmly and are not pushed into the wrong positions.

With the help of the X-ray, the dentist is able to see that the teeth are sound at their roots. By personal inspection he finds tiny spots which indicate the beginning of decay. These can be filled and polished and their decay stopped. The additional cost of the X-ray pictures means future saving. Preventive dentistry done early is cheap. Curative dentistry, done after decay has proceeded far, after the teeth have gotten into wrong positions, after some teeth have been lost, may be expensive and can be prevented.

Orthodontia

Within recent years a new specialty has arisen in dentistry and in medicine called orthodontia. The word means "straight teeth." As explained by Dr. Frank A. Delabarre, it means literally to arrange crooked teeth in a more harmonious and symmetrical curve so that they will function better and improve the facial appearance. It is, of course, necessary to realize that back of all health are proper nutrition and growth. Unless the child has a diet which contains a sufficient amount of calcium, phosphorus, vitamins A, C, and D particularly, it is not likely to have good teeth.

Unless the baby teeth have been suitably controlled and well taken care of, the teeth that come in thereafter will not be properly developed and distributed. Dentists are convinced that there are a con-siderable number of bad habits that are associated with development of malocclusion, which means improper closing of the teeth and jaws. Breathing through the mouth, sucking the thumb, and similar bad habits may be associated with bad formation of the teeth, the bones of the jaw and the muscles which control them.

The twenty baby teeth of infancy begin to disappear around the age of six, at which time also the four big six-year molars appear. Unless there is a full number of healthy teeth in the mouth at each age, they will not be properly arranged nor will they close properly. Each tooth depends on the one next to it for support. If any groups of teeth are pushed out of position, the whole set becomes irregular.

The orthodontist is a specialist in producing regularity of the teeth. Through gradual changes exercised at certain points the teeth are brought into proper position. This is done by the use of wire and of gold, and must be done slowly and carefully so as not to de-stroy the teeth in the process. It is a specialty within dentistry which concerns the ordinary care of the teeth. It is no longer necessary for any girl to appear in public after she has grown to mature age with teeth crossing over one another or with the protruding snaggle teeth that gave so many women a comical appearance in the past. Science in this way does much for human happiness.

THE CARE OF ADULTS' TEETH

The care of the teeth in the adult involves not only a suitable diet, but also a certain amount of simple dental hygiene. The popular slogan that a clean tooth never decays is probably correct if associ-ated with the right definition of a "clean tooth." It is equally true that millions of unclean teeth never decay. Of course, unclean teeth are not desirable, because they permit the growth of bacteria that are usually associated with foul breath, they are unesthetic in appearance, and they are associated with irritations of the gums, cheeks, and tongue that may be serious.

About 1890 it was shown that certain acids formed by the action of mouth bacteria on a substance containing sugar when held in con-tact with enamel of the teeth for a certain number of hours would cause the enamel to fall apart and open the way to destruction of the softer dentin substance beneath. Since the acid must exist in con-centrated form in order to do such work, the process usually goes on only in the tiny pits, fissures, or other defects in the enamel, or in the spaces between the teeth. The exposed surfaces of the teeth seldom decay because the natural movements of the lips, cheeks and tongue help to keep them clean.

Associated with the cause of tooth decay are errors in the diet. It is useless to take in large amounts of calcium unless the calcium is assimilated. Apparently phosphorus, the products of certain glands, ultraviolet rays, and the vitamins are involved in the use of calcium by the body and must be taken in the diet in order to permit the process to go on satisfactorily.

Once decay begins, once the enamel of the tooth is broken down, bacteria, constantly present in the mouth, aid the destruction. Chemical changes occur that are disastrous. The most that anyone can do is to keep teeth clean by the best methods possible, to overcome acids by the use of proper alkaline washes or pastes, and to see that the diet is of the proper nature to keep the teeth in a state of satisfactory nutrition.

TOOTHBRUSH

In cleansing the mouth a good toothbrush is necessary. Most of the toothbrushes sold today are too large for efficient brushing. There are all sorts of shapes available with many strange distributions of bristles, but so far as is known it is impossible to make a toothbrush that will conform exactly to the shape of the dental arch inside and outside. Some toothbrushes are made with bristles higher in the center and low at the ends, some with the bristles high at one end and low at the other end, some with bristles lower in the middle and high at both ends.

This seems to make little difference, the only necessity being that the brush be small and that the handle be such that it can be manipulated so that the bristles will reach the front, back and sides of every tooth. The toothbrush demands proper care to give it long life and to prevent its acting as a carrier of infections rather than as a preventive.

When a toothbrush is split, when bristles begin to break off and come out, the toothbrush should be thrown away. A new toothbrush should be put in a strong salt cold-water solution for two hours before using. Cold water should be used to moisten the brush before using and to rinse it thoroughly after the teeth are brushed. The brush

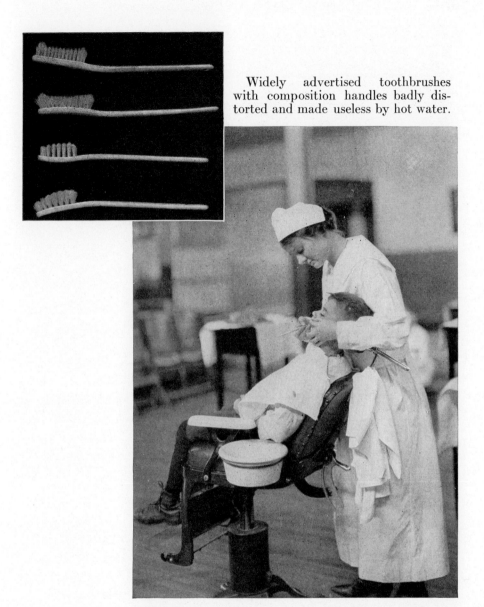

Widely advertised toothbrushes with composition handles badly distorted and made useless by hot water.

Every child should have its teeth cleaned regularly.

FIG. 100.

should then be hung in the open air in such position that the bristles will not come in contact with anything else for twenty-four hours before the brush is used again.

Obviously, therefore, persons should have two brushes, one for morning and one for evening use. If a toothbrush is kept moist for too long a period of time or kept in an airtight container, the bristles are quickly destroyed. Most important, however, is the fact that bacteria grow on warm, moist toothbrushes, and that the use of the brush before it has dried thoroughly will merely add new bacteria to those taken from the mouth in the previous washing.

TOOTHPASTE, MOUTH WASHES, AND TOOTH POWDERS

One of the most debatable questions in medicine and dentistry today concerns the exact value of toothpastes, mouth washes, tooth powders, and similar mixtures for the health of the mouth and the teeth. Many physicians and dentists are convinced that the most any toothpaste can do is to keep the teeth clean and polished, and that therefore any good soapy preparation that tastes well serves the purpose. However, the preparations that are available are complex in their formulas and extraordinary in their claims.

Some toothpastes are widely advertised because of their alkaline content, since it is urged that alkalis tend to counteract the tendency of the mouth to become acid. It has not, however, been proved that there is any serious tendency in this direction, nor that an opposite tendency is especially valuable.

Another preparation is sold with the argument that it duplicates normal saliva and that the presence of normal saliva prevents tooth decay. It has been argued that sugar helps to cause decay of the teeth and that food particles between the teeth increase dental caries. The disadvantage associated with food particles and sugar is that these provide mediums on which bacteria grow and that bacterial products are injurious to the teeth.

Some toothpastes are sold with the special claim that they kill the germs in the mouth on contact, but most physicians realize that the first mouthful of food or the first breath of air will bring new germs into the mouth. Some toothpastes contain abrasive substances which scratch the enamel, and this is bad, since anything that makes a scratch or an abrasion may produce a spot in which germs may enter more easily.

Another toothpaste is sold with the claim that it contains a substance which digests away food particles and mucus, and another is sold with the claim that it contains enough of certain antiseptic to sterilize the gums and keep them sterile. The important thing for the average person to remember is the fact that most of these preparations are kept in the mouth not longer than a few seconds and that any effects which they may accomplish are quite temporary.

The exact causes of tooth decay are not known. There is evidence that the lack of certain vitamins in the diet tends to encourage diseases of the gums and tooth decay. There is evidence that insufficient amounts of calcium in the food may be associated with tooth decay in the young. Unquestionably, diseases affecting the mouth, with the presence of bacteria, encourage decay in the adult. Hence, it is advisable to have the mouth clean for this reason. There exists an equally important reason for the regular use of cleansing preparations in the mouth. The person with a dirty mouth and with a bad breath is a social misfit.

Pyorrhea

Pyorrhea means a flow of matter. However, the flow of matter or, to speak of it scientifically—pus—is not the most significant thing about this disturbance of the mouth and teeth. The important fact is that the condition becomes chronic and that as a result of this the tissue of the gums separates from the roots of the teeth. When they have once separated they are not likely to become attached again. Moreover, a constant presence of infectious matter leads to secondary disturbances in the body which may be exceedingly serious.

The blood picks up the germs from the pus pockets around the teeth and carries them to other parts of the body, where they set up new infections. Because the teeth are loose and the mouth is foul, the person with pyorrhea is likely to lose his appetite. He is unable to chew food satisfactorily, his digestion is interfered with, and he becomes in general much sicker than he would be with a clean mouth cavity.

Because the mouth is easy to get at, because the gums are tough, and because the saliva keeps the mouth constantly lubricated, the tissues stand a great deal of punishment before the condition becomes so severe that it is impossible to delay attention. For this reason, pyorrhea is usually a chronic rather than an acute disease.

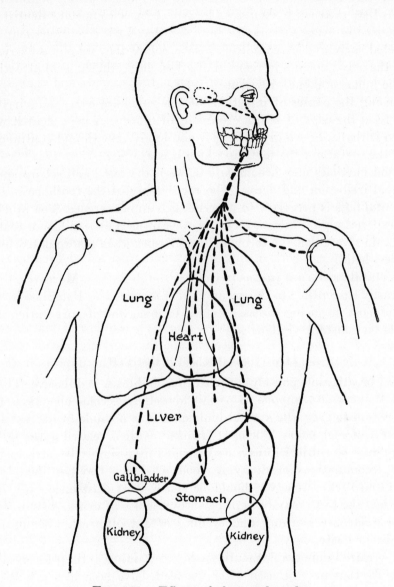

FIG. 101. Effects of abscessed teeth.

For this reason also it is necessary to remind people again and again that the mouth should be looked at by a competent dentist at least once in every six months in order that such conditions may be detected early and given adequate care before they become so serious that the only hope lies in removal of all of the teeth, surgical attention to the gums, and the provision of artificial plates.

Among the causes of infections of the gums are continuous irritation from the edge of rough crowns or of fillings. A good dentist will see to it that a crown or a filling is absolutely smooth and continuous with the surface of the tooth to which it is applied.

Food particles may accumulate between the teeth and set up spots of local irritation and decay. The regular use of the toothbrush and of dental floss is necessary to prevent such an occurrence. Toothpicks, and especially pins, knives, forks, or other objects used in lieu of toothpicks, do severe damage to the delicate tissues when manipulated by a careless hand.

Tartar deposits are just as irritant as rough fillings. Moreover, they are easily susceptible to the accumulation of bacteria. Pyorrhea is one of the most menacing diseases known to man, and its prevention depends on constant vigilance.

HALITOSIS OR BAD BREATH

Bad breath, now politely referred to as halitosis, is offensive. There is little excuse for anyone to permit himself to become obnoxious for this reason to everyone around him, since it is possible to prevent the presence of such odors. The most frequent cause is related to the teeth, which may be subject to cavities or which may simply be surrounded with accumulations of decaying food products. Cavities should be filled and tartar deposits should be removed at least once every six months. The teeth may be kept clean by the use of dental floss and by the regular use morning and evening of a toothbrush with proper powder or paste.

There are innumerable mouth washes containing antiseptics, alkalis, or acids, that may be used after the teeth have been brushed. Weak hydrogen peroxide solutions are sometimes of value. It is best to use strong solutions only on the advice of a competent physician or dentist.

After the teeth as the cause of bad breath have been eliminated, the tonsils must be examined as to the presence of infection. Another frequent cause of bad breath is infection in the nose or in the space behind the nose. The formation of crusts and of accumulations of infected material is bound to produce foul odor of the breath. Halitosis may also result from chronic disturbances of the stomach and of the intestines. If the tongue is constantly coated, if there is eructation of sour material from the stomach, the person concerned should consult a physician in order to find out exactly what form of disease is present, so that it may be relieved with appropriate treatment.

FALSE TEETH

The person who is compelled to wear any form of removable appliance in the mouth to replace natural teeth has special problems to which dentists have been giving concern. False teeth, artificial teeth, removable bridges, and plates are included in this category.

The person who is going to lose his natural teeth by extraction because of infections or due to any other cause should have a thorough study by the use of the X-ray before any natural teeth are removed. The dentist who is going to make the artificial denture can then advise intelligently which teeth may be saved and which should be extracted. This is particularly important because he wants to restore the patient's natural appearance, and he wants to retain everything possible to permit the making of the most suitable denture.

To do this, he takes impressions of the mouth, makes a record of the patient's profile and facial contour, studies the natural color of the teeth and similar factors. It is sometimes possible in making an artificial denture to correct deformities or abnormalities of the lower portion of the face. When a person is fitted with an artificial denture his experience is similar to being fitted with a suit or a dress. It may not be exactly right the first time, and some adjustments may be necessary.

When the work is completed the patient should not assume that it is permanent. The human body is a growing and changing organism which differs from year to year. This means that dentures should be studied from time to time if they become uncomfortable so that old ones may be refitted or new ones substituted. If this is not done there actually may be changes in the appearance of the face, deep lines and wrinkles being associated in some instances with the constant wearing of unsuitable dentures.

Artificial plates and teeth must be given even more care than natural teeth. They should be brushed carefully and thoroughly after each meal and on going to bed at night. In this cleaning, cold or luke-warm water should be used—never hot water. It is just as important to be careful about handling dentures as handling expensive eye-glasses. The dentists suggest that when removing the dentures from the mouth the wearer should lean over a washbowl filled two-thirds full of water and hold the plates close to the water when brushing them. Then the water will break the fall if he happens to drop the artificial plate.

It is not advisable to try to crack nuts with artificial teeth. Biting threads, eating hard candy, and chewing on bones are sometimes re-sponsible for ruining expensive dentures.

Just as soon as the teeth are secured, the person will do well to go into a private place and practice reading aloud in order to get used to the feel of the teeth and to their weaknesses. When the false teeth are first inserted, the facial expression may seem to be changed, but this is due to the effort of the muscles to take care of the plates. Just as soon as the false teeth become properly adjusted, the effort will disappear, and the expression will become natural again.

Naturally, the hardest thing to do with the false teeth is to eat. The person who has the teeth thinks that he has to manipulate both the teeth and the food. He will, therefore, do well to begin with food that requires little chewing and to avoid steaks and chops for the first few days. Small bits of food chewed slowly will easily be taken care of. Big masses of food may cause trouble. Until one learns to manipulate the teeth, and until the gums and the ridges have become hardened, one need not expect to eat everything and anything that is offered. If there are spots in the gums and the ridges have become ex-cessively sore, the dentist should be consulted immediately to make the necessary changes and to prescribe the necessary treatment.

Artificial teeth, when out of the mouth, should be kept moist. The best arrangement is to put them in a salt solution, boric acid, or some favorite mouth wash.

CHAPTER XXIX

Advice on the Diet
SOLOMON STROUSE, M.D.

INTRODUCTION

AN OLD-FASHIONED PROVERB *says, "Tell me what you eat and I will tell you what you are." Modern medicine has learned both the truth and the fallacy of this proverb. Our modern knowledge of nutrition has eliminated a great many of the fads in diet of an earlier day. It has, at the same time, brought to light the importance of diet for the control of disease as well as for the maintenance of the body in health. The questions of deficiencies of the human diet in their relationship to specific diseases are fully discussed in the chapter on deficiency diseases.*

The following chapter by Dr. Solomon Strouse calls attention to the important constituents of an average diet; the relationships between proteins, carbohydrates, fats, mineral salts, and vitamins; the importance of the relationship of acids to alkalis, and similar topics. It traces the progress of food through the digestive tract and then discusses specifically the value of such substances as meats, fish, sugars. milk, cereals, fats, fruits, vegetables, and other substances.

The chapter is supplemented by some tabular data, indicating the protein yield of various foods, the caloric yield of various foods, and the distribution of protein, fat, and carbohydrates for food used in normal diets. These diets are still further supplemented by other tabular data, describing the essentials of a normal diet as well as diets for special purposes.

M. F.

The Development of the Normal Diet

WHEN ADAM AND EVE first walked in the Garden of Eden, some unconscious power led them to pick and choose the proper herbs and vegetables. When the children of Israel wandered through the desert, they too found what they needed. It seems rather a remarkable coincidence that the selective power has been such as to permit man to survive.

There is a sound basis for most of the Mosaic laws of food (now about three thousand years old). The first law, which prohibited the use of animals that did not chew the cud and had cloven hoofs, ex-cluded all but herbivorous animals. The reason was that the carnivora ate flesh which might not be good, and therefore the flesh of the carnivora itself would become polluted. The second law restricted the eating of sea food to that with fins and scales. This, of course, excluded the mollusks, which were soft meat and which easily went into decay. The third law, restricting birds, especially enumerated all regarded as carrion eaters, the reason being obviously the same as for the law of animals. The fourth law, regarding blood, was based on the belief that blood potentially was the carrier of any pollution of the animal. The kosher method of killing simply removes blood from the animal as completely as possible. Others of the Mosaic laws which were developed during the later years of the history of the Jews cannot be explained either on the basis of modern knowledge of nutrition or on what was known of the Jews at the time. Probably many of these were mere superstition and taboo. Certainly they cannot be explained on the basis of our present knowledge of foods. Yet on the whole the remarkable historical continuity of the Jews indicates that their laws of living were based on sound concepts. This history is perhaps the most outstanding tribute to the trial-and-error method of which there is knowledge.

No formulation of a normal diet can be considered fairly without the realization of this and similar historical facts. Traditional, racial, and hereditary factors are of importance. Despite all that science has taught in recent years regarding the value of balanced diets, such knowledge alone is insufficient for the formulation of a normal dietary. The experiences of the human race might have been quite different, the result might have been much better, if modern dietary knowledge had been correct procedure five thousand years ago. Not as many infants would have died; people would have lived to a riper age; and the whole history of the world might have been different. Yet the fact remains that the world has survived.

The basis of the survival has been the old adage that the appetite is the guide to nutrition. This adage is, of course, only partially true. Given an abundant food supply, it is probable that appetite will guide the individual to a normal diet. However, the appetite easily becomes perverted. Whereas the infant who has not tasted sugar may pick out the best foods for his or her development, later in life, when the appetite has already been changed by poorly selected foods, it no longer is a guide.

Just at this point the truly marvelous contributions made by experimental nutritionists and physiologists come to help. The lessons of history cannot be excluded in constructing a diet, nor is it possible to achieve the optimum result without knowledge of the nutritional studies. The dietary aim naturally is an ideal, an ideal of perfect health for everybody, an ideal which aims to save the lives of infants and prolong the lives of adults, to prevent illness, improve general health, and to increase the store of human happiness. This ideal of course cannot be realized; practical considerations stand in the way. Just as the physician cannot send the stevedore with heart disease to California for the winter, so he cannot always prescribe an ideal diet on a limited budget. However, the task of prescribing an ideal diet is not nearly as difficult as it might seem to the uninitiated. In this chapter an attempt is made to simplify and clarify the situation and to show how a few fundamental facts and procedures make it possible for any person of average intelligence to eat fairly normal food.

FOOD FADS AND FANCIES

One of the great troubles with the tremendous interest in food has been a willful ignorance or malicious effort on the part of faddists and propagandists to obscure the issue. It might be just as well to start this discussion of food with comment on some of the present-day fads and fancies which seem to have an all too powerful hold on the imagination of many individuals. The propagandist spirit of the American advertiser, coupled with the gullibility of the reading public, at least up to 1930, made it possible to flood the world with all kinds of foolish dietary advice, practically never founded on scientific experiment, usually completely erroneous, at times dangerous, and inevitably useless. The public has certain ideas on food; individuals or groups follow dietary regimens as they would worship idols.

It is high time for authority to throw the light of truth on some of these absurd and unfounded fads. It is, however, rather strange that some of the so-called dietary principles which have gained vogue seem to have the backing of "medical authority (?)." Consider the roughage habit. According to the adherents of the roughage school, it is necessary to load the intestines with all kinds of indigestible and unassimilable substances like bran, which form an irritating bulk in the large intestines, and which may, although not always, lead to irritation of the intestines. Whereas a certain amount of indigestible residue is necessary to normal action of the bowels and evacuation, this is a long step removed from the rather violent loading of a weak bowel with a mass of unnecessary work.

Another current fad concerns flour. Partly as a result of the roughage theory, partly as a result of fear of the depleting effect of the milling process in making white flour, many people have the impression that to eat products made of white flour is to incur danger. There is no scientific evidence which has ever proved that statement. Yet the various kinds of whole wheat, bran, and other substitutes for milled flour have received a vogue entirely out of proportion to their value. There are certain cases in which it is advisable to add the whole of the wheat, but this is no argument for its widespread, unfounded use as a general panacea for all ills.

Certainly, in America in the last decade, there has been a tendency towards the lessening of the meat intake, with a resulting theoretic possibility at least of considerable danger to the organism. The fear of meat is difficult to explain; perhaps it is the result of a rather widespread restriction of animal protein in the diet of people with high blood pressure. "Blood pressure" is a common complaint, made much of by physicians, insurance examiners, and the public in general; for years meat was taboo to such an illness. The apeing mannerism of following one's neighbor perhaps caused Jones to follow Smith and Brown to follow Jones in lowering the meat intake. As a matter of fact, there has been some scientific work to prove that this tendency actually results in protein deprivation and a resulting condition that does not make for the best health.

From a scientific point of view, a decade ago pioneers tried to show that meat in moderate doses was rarely harmful even to a person with high blood pressure. Then the pioneers were not listened to, but today scientific medicine accepts their conclusions as proved. Two dangers of protein restriction are: protein edema and poorly balanced diet. It is a common observation of physicians that a person who is not permitted sufficient protein in his diet makes it up in either fat or carbohydrate. This may result in an unbalanced diet, of which more will be said later, or in an increase of weight which might not be advisable for that particular person. In people with high blood pressure, it is known that increase of weight is an undesirable burden, yet this extra trouble may immediately follow protein restriction. The intake of protein, from whatever source, may vary within wide limits, and healthy life can continue on an intake varying roughly from two ounces up to as high as five ounces of pure protein daily. The meat habits of a group are determined by the original habits of their ancestors, the environment in which they live, the quantity of meat in comparison to other foods, and other extraneous factors. The dangers of either over- or under-indulgence are grossly exaggerated.

Perhaps another important basic reason for the development of food fads and fancies lies in the well-established fact that certain people have idiosyncrasies or may be sensitive to certain foods. One of the best known physicians in the United States tells this story of one of his early patients, a charming young lady who had been sick for many weeks and who had already had several medical advisers. As he walked into her room he was greeted with the question, "Doctor, would you mind if I asked you a question before you started on me?" He replied, "Of course not." Whereupon the young lady said, "Tell me confidentially what foods you dislike." When the doctor informed this patient that he had no particular dislikes for food, he naturally inquired the reason for her question. He was then told that each one of the previous doctors had restricted the particular article of diet which, as far as the young lady was concerned, disagreed with the particular doctor.

Physicians no longer prescribe diet on this basis, but the rocking-chair brigade of the hotel summer resorts and the ubiquitous lay medical adviser is only too apt to give free instruction to anyone who will listen. There is such a thing as food idiosyncrasy. There are individuals to whom bananas or strawberries or cabbage or any other perfectly normal food may act as a poison. This is not due to the food but is due to a state of "sensitization" of that particular individual to that particular food, and has nothing whatever to do with the construction of a normal diet for normal persons. It is not always known why a person becomes "sensitized"; the fact that he is compels him to avoid certain foods.

Food Poisoning

At this point food poisoning can be discussed. There have been serious epidemics of food poisoning, usually due to some error in the transportation or handling of the food. This may occur in canning, in improper icing, or in numerous ways, but when food poisoning occurs it affects everyone who eats this lot of food. Individual cases of poisoning by food are so extremely rare as to be negligible. The old diagnosis of "ptomaine poisoning" is no longer made, and from the standpoint of diagnosis the last thing to think of in the presence of a "bellyache" is the food. It is of greatest practical importance to realize that most abdominal pains are caused by something wrong in the insides of the person and are not the result of the ingestion of food. Rare instances of green-apple bellyache or similar insults to the stomach which occur as the result of a debauch are usually clean cut, but even in such instances it is not safe immediately to assume that the food and not the body of the person concerned is at fault.

Extraneous Factors in Diet

To return to the fundamental considerations which must be borne in mind in the development of the normal diet, certain extraneous factors which lie beyond the field of actual digestion, assimilation, or scientific food values must be recognized. The three most important "outside" influences are the source of the food supply, heredity, and tradition. A study of dietary habits of a people living in the midst of plenty shows that such persons are apt to eat more of their local supply. For instance, in the tropics, where fresh fruits and vegetables are abundant and cheap, those foods form the major part of the dietary of the tropical races. On the other hand, in Alaska, where fat is the most available food, fresh fruit and vegetables are rarely, if ever, seen in the dietary. Whereas, in the more temperate zones between the two extremes, where the source of food supply depends only on the rapidity of transportation, a more generalized diet will be found in common use. It is not difficult to bring California and Florida fruit and vegetables to the New York market in midwinter. but it would be difficult to carry them to Alaska. During the seasons when local truck farms and orchards are producing, local districts will be found to consume the products of the local markets. It is rather interesting to find only occasional disturbances of nutrition resulting in groups of people, although naturally an occasional bad result is seen.

The ability to buy food is also important in establishing a normal diet. Even in the midst of plenty, availability of food has little interest for the man who cannot buy it. Such a condition exists during any economic depression, when terrific unemployment results in insufficient budgetary allowance and inability to purchase proper food; with consequent effects on nutrition standards. How malnutrition will be reflected in the history of the world in the next two or three decades is a problem about which one fears to speculate.

Heredity and tradition cannot be discounted in the consideration of normal diet. The tradition of certain of the Italian localities to take their carbohydrate in the form of spaghetti and ravioli forms a contrast to the Slavic tradition of coarse rye bread. Yet both spaghetti and rye bread furnish an excellent source of cereal carbohydrate. The same is true, for instance, of certain of the Orientals in whose diet fresh fish is a staple, whereas to the average Occidental such food is so distasteful as to be practically impossible of assimilation. Inconsistently, however, raw oysters and clams are well tolerated. From the standpoint of food value, the fresh fish is probably as good as a fried pork chop. In a population with as mixed an origin as the American people, it would be quite natural to anticipate such wide ranges in dietary construction. It would be obviously ridiculous to demand that the American citizen of Russian, Scandinavian, or Italian descent be compelled to consider a piece of white bread as the standard form of starch.

THE NEED FOR FOOD

The body needs food for two purposes: as fuel to supply energy, and to repair the waste of body tissues which goes on in the daily wear and tear of life. Considering the fuel aspect of food first, one starts with a discussion of the significance of the word "calorie." This word seems to be shrouded in mystery, yet there is no mystery attached to it. Calorie is simply the name given to the fuel value of anything that is burned up. Large establishments using a great deal of fuel do not buy coal by the ton but by the number of heat units or calories furnished per dollar. Food plays the same rôle in the human machinery as does coal in the furnace or gas in the motorcar. The first purpose of food is to furnish fuel; if this fuel in the form of food were not available to the body, the body would naturally immediately start to consume itself. Starvation is the result of the fires of human life burn-

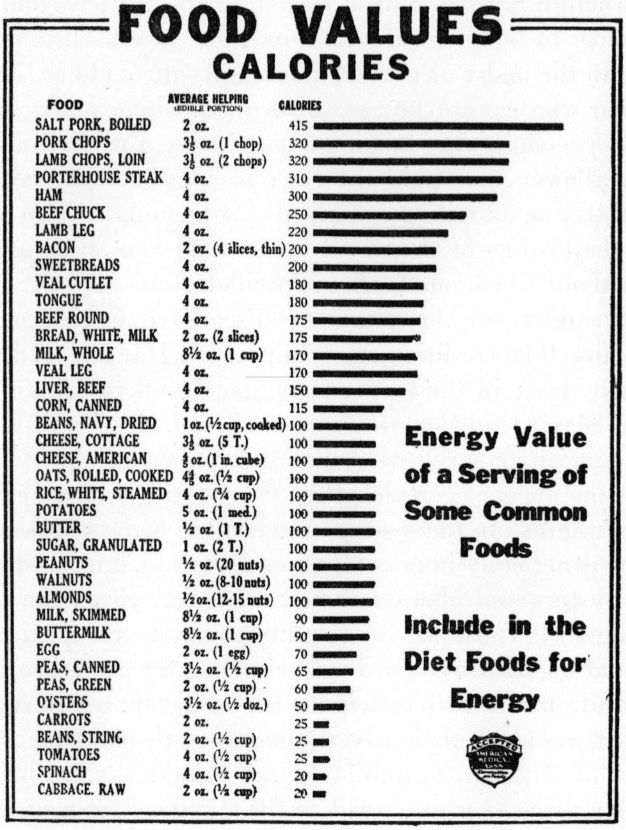
FOOD VALUES
CALORIES
FOOD | AVERAGE HELPING (EDIBLE PORTION) | CALORIES
SALT PORK, BOILED | 2 oz. | 415
PORK CHOPS | 3⅕ oz. (1 chop) | 320
LAMB CHOPS, LOIN | 3⅕ oz. (2 chops) | 320
PORTERHOUSE STEAK | 4 oz. | 310
HAM | 4 oz. | 300
BEEF CHUCK | 4 oz. | 250
LAMB LEG | 4 oz. | 220
BACON | 2 oz. (4 slices, thin) | 200
SWEETBREADS | 4 oz. | 200
VEAL CUTLET | 4 oz. | 180
TONGUE | 4 oz. | 180
BEEF ROUND | 4 oz. | 175
BREAD, WHITE, MILK | 2 oz. (2 slices) | 175
MILK, WHOLE | 8½ oz. (1 cup) | 170
VEAL LEG | 4 oz. | 170
LIVER, BEEF | 4 oz. | 150
CORN, CANNED | 4 oz. | 115
BEANS, NAVY, DRIED | 1 oz. (½ cup, cooked) | 100
CHEESE, COTTAGE | 3⅕ oz. (5 T.) | 100
CHEESE, AMERICAN | ⅘ oz. (1 in. cube) | 100
OATS, ROLLED, COOKED | 4⅘ oz. (½ cup) | 100
RICE, WHITE, STEAMED | 4 oz. (¾ cup) | 100
POTATOES | 5 oz. (1 med.) | 100
BUTTER | ½ oz. (1 T.) | 100
SUGAR, GRANULATED | 1 oz. (2 T.) | 100
PEANUTS | ½ oz. (20 nuts) | 100
WALNUTS | ½ oz. (8-10 nuts) | 100
ALMONDS | ½ oz. (12-15 nuts) | 100
MILK, SKIMMED | 8½ oz. (1 cup) | 90
BUTTERMILK | 8½ oz. (1 cup) | 90
EGG | 2 oz. (1 egg) | 70
PEAS, CANNED | 3½ oz. (½ cup) | 65
PEAS, GREEN | 2 oz. (½ cup) | 60
OYSTERS | 3½ oz. (½ doz.) | 50
CARROTS | 2 oz. | 25
BEANS, STRING | 2 oz. (½ cup) | 25
TOMATOES | 4 oz. (½ cup) | 25
SPINACH | 4 oz. (½ cup) | 20
CABBAGE. RAW | 2 oz. (½ cup) | 20
Energy Value of a Serving of Some Common Foods
Include in the Diet Foods for Energy
ACCEPTED
AMERICAN MEDICAL ASSN

FIG. 102.

ing human life itself. Therefore, in constructing a diet it is always essential that sufficient calories be given to maintain body weight and to supply fuel for the energy consumed by the body.

Frequently the human body is compared to a machine. This analogy must never be allowed to go too far, because the machine, built of non-inflammable material, simply goes out of commission when the necessary fuel is withheld. The fundamental concept, however, of the use of food for fuel in the human body is exactly the opposite. As soon as insufficient fuel is furnished in the form of insufficient calories, the machine continues to work, using its own material as fuel, and if the procedure is allowed to continue too long, death inevitably results. The main difference, then, between the human body and a machine of metal is that the machine of metal is a thing apart from the substance fed to it as fuel, whereas the human body is of the same substance as the fuel, and therefore its life depends entirely on sufficient outside fuel being furnished to prevent its consuming itself.

The practical importance of this idea extends not only into the life of normal human beings, but is of particular importance in the life of overweight or obese persons. Loss of weight means loss of body tissue, and this in turn is equivalent to the burning of a percentage of one's own body as fuel. Therefore, all reduction methods are based on a restriction of caloric intake. It makes no difference under what guise this insufficient caloric diet may travel or what it contains, anybody who eats less than he burns up will lose weight. Again attention is called to the fads and fancies which have made a spectacle of this simple law.

CALORIES

There are two general ways of figuring out the fuel needs of a person. One method is the statistical, which may be called the mass method of study. By an analysis of the food intake of large groups of soldiers, schoolmistresses, or miners it is possible to obtain an average for that group. As a matter of fact, if it is known that such a group of persons is maintaining life, activity, and health, it is fair to assume that the average diet obtained in this statistical study would be a safe diet. Plenty of statistics are available from all countries and from almost all groups of persons to give a basis for the average diet for any given group. For instance, it has been demonstrated that tailors use approximately 2,700 calories daily, whereas woodsawers may use 5,000 to 6,000 calories per day. A seamstress working by hand uses approximately 2,000, and a washwoman 2,900 to 3,700 calories. Farmers in various countries have been estimated to use approximately 5,000 calories, whereas lumbermen in Maine use 8,000. Obviously the amount of food taken by anyone depends practically entirely on the nature of his work. The more work, the more energy consumed, and the more fuel needed to supply the energy.

The other method of determining fuel value of food is by the study of individual needs. A person of certain build, height, weight, age, and occupation is in general similar to another person with the same qualifications. Mere existence, which includes the act of breathing, the beating of the heart, the involuntary movements of the body—activities which continue even during sleep—consume energy. All interchanges of energy are grouped under the general name of metabolism. And the energy of mere existence is called basal metabolism.

Today basal metabolism can be estimated for any person by means of a simple breathing machine. In this machine the patient is allowed to breathe oxygen for a certain length of time. The amount utilized is carefully measured, and on the basis of some comparatively simple calculations the rate of energy consumed by this individual can be estimated. This is all that is meant by basal metabolism, and it is comparatively easy to find out just how much any person of a given age, height, and weight will need to sustain mere existence. Many thousands of control experiments of the nature of the one just outlined have given standards of comparison. The results are expressed in terms of either plus or minus variations from the standard. In other words, if the report reads "basal metabolism, plus 15 per cent," it means simply that that individual is consuming 15 per cent more energy than the normal.

It is further known that every activity of the body, whether it is walking, talking, eating, playing golf, or mining coal, increases the amount of energy consumed by the body. Such increases can be estimated either by individual study or by the mass method already discussed. Therefore, having found the basal requirements of an individual, the doctor can, by the addition of the demands of the individual's other activities, compute what his total needs for the day will be.

CLASSIFICATION OF FOODS

However, in addition to the fuel value of food there are certain other demands that food must fill. The need to repair body waste is one of the most important; there must be a sufficient supply of mineral salts and vitamins and water. Protein supplies the material to replace tissue waste and, to a certain extent, energy. The main source of energy, however, is in the fats and carbohydrates of the diet.

The main food elements are grouped under several big headings:

Height (inches)	5	6	7	8	9	10	11	12	13	14	15	16	17	18	19
								Years							
38	34	34													
39	35	35													
40	36	36													
41	38	38	38												
42	39	39	39	39											
43	41	41	41	41											
44	44	44	44	44											
45	46	46	46	46	46										
46	47	48	48	48	48										
47	49	50	50	50	50	50									
48	----	52	53	53	53	53									
49	----	55	55	55	55	55	55								
50	----	57	58	58	58	58	58	58							
51	----	----	61	61	61	61	61	61							
52	----	----	63	64	64	64	64	64	64						
53	----	----	66	67	67	67	67	68	68						
54	----	----	----	70	70	70	70	71	71	72					
55	----	----	----	72	72	73	73	74	74	74					
56	----	----	----	75	76	77	77	77	78	78	80				
57	----	----	----	79	80	81	81	82	83	83					
58	----	----	----	83	84	84	85	85	86	87					
59	----	----	----	----	87	88	89	89	90	90	90				
60	----	----	----	----	----	91	92	92	93	94	95	96			
61	----	----	----	----	----	----	95	96	97	99	100	103	106		
62	----	----	----	----	----	----	100	101	102	103	104	107	111	116	
63	----	----	----	----	----	----	105	106	107	108	110	113	118	123	127
64	----	----	----	----	----	----	----	109	111	113	115	117	121	126	130
65	----	----	----	----	----	----	114	117	118	120	122	127	131	134	
66	----	----	----	----	----	----	----	119	122	125	128	132	136	139	
67	----	----	----	----	----	----	----	124	128	130	134	136	139	142	
68	----	----	----	----	----	----	----	----	134	139	137	141	143	147	
69	----	----	----	----	----	----	----	----	137	139	143	146	149	152	
70	----	----	----	----	----	----	----	----	143	144	145	148	151	155	
71	----	----	----	----	----	----	----	----	148	150	151	152	154	159	
72	----	----	----	----	----	----	----	----		153	155	156	158	163	
73	----	----	----	----	----	----	----	----		157	160	162	164	167	
74	----	----	----	----	----	----	----	----		160	164	168	170	171	

FIG. 103. Height and weight at various ages.

protein, fat, carbohydrate, water, mineral salts, and the so-called accessory food factors, vitamins. Usually food as it is eaten is composed of a mixture of these main food elements, frequently with one predominating. A study of food analyses will show, for instance, that beef or the meat of any animal, including fish and poultry, consists mainly of protein with a varying amount of fat. Protein is the one element of food that contains nitrogen and for that reason is the only food that can replace tissue lost in the body. Many foods contain small amounts of protein, but not in the proportions available in animal matter. Proteins are chemically complex substances made up of a number of so-called amino acids. The nature of a specific protein depends on the kinds and amount of amino acids and the manner in which they are combined. For this reason all proteins do not have the same nutritional value. Some of the basic components (amino acids) are necessary for metabolism and are not supplied by all of the proteins. The most common and important proteins and their sources are: albumin from egg, the protein of wheat and corn, the protein of milk, of meat, and the glandular organs. Some of the other cereals, vegetables, and nuts also contain available and utilizable protein.

The carbohydrates are the starch or sugar parts of food; they are indispensable for rapid use as fuel. They are found in fruits, vegetables, cereals, and milk. Ordinary sugar is the most concentrated type of carbohydrate available. Sugar is found in pure form in fruits and to a lesser extent in some of the vegetables. Starch is a higher combination of sugars and furnishes the main ingredient of the various cereals. Bread contains a large amount of starch. From the standpoint of actual utilization of sugar, it makes no difference whether the carbohydrate is obtained in the form of starch or of the simpler sugars. The simpler sugars are absorbed as such or after slight chemical change, whereas starch needs a longer process of digestion to make it available. This is of importance particularly in the treatment of diabetes mellitus. Vendors of certain artificial food products advertise them as being free from sugar, which is partially true; but when such articles of food contain liberal amounts of starch, they must be classed in the same category as straight sugars.

Fats of course are known as such: meat fats, oils, and butter fat being the most obvious members of this family. They are found both in animal and plant life, and whatever their derivation are potentially equal energy producers. The same amount of fuel value is attached to

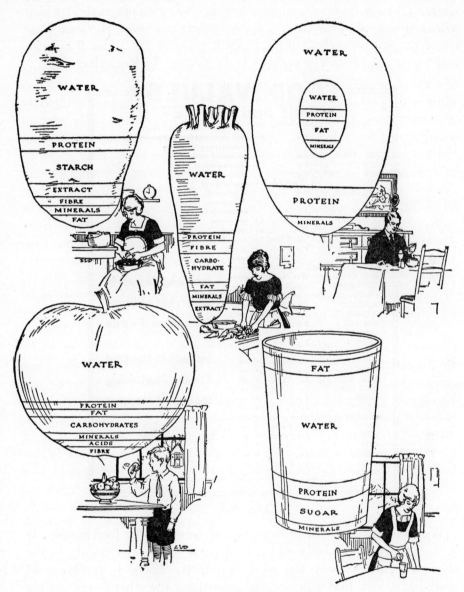

Fig. 104. Facts about foods.

771

an ounce of butter fat, olive oil, cottonseed oil, or oil derived from maize. There is, however, a difference in their vitamin content which will be discussed subsequently. As a fuel, fat is twice as valuable as either protein or carbohydrate, since 1 gram of fat yields 9 calories and 1 gram of protein or carbohydrate yields only 4 calories.

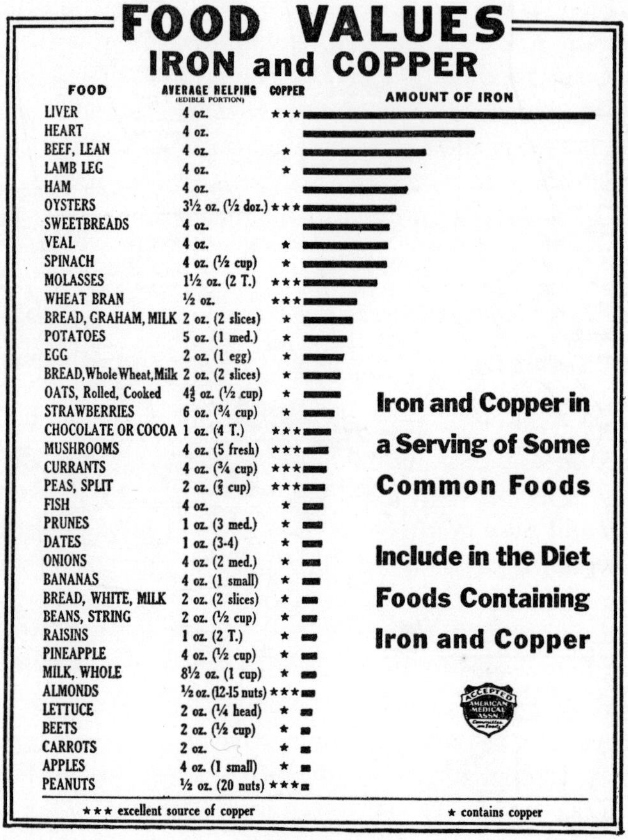

FOOD VALUES
IRON and COPPER

FOOD	AVERAGE HELPING (EDIBLE PORTION)	COPPER	AMOUNT OF IRON
LIVER	4 oz.	★★★	
HEART	4 oz.		
BEEF, LEAN	4 oz.	★	
LAMB LEG	4 oz.	★	
HAM	4 oz.		
OYSTERS	3½ oz. (½ doz.)	★★★	
SWEETBREADS	4 oz.		
VEAL	4 oz.	★	
SPINACH	4 oz. (½ cup)	★	
MOLASSES	1½ oz. (2 T.)	★★★	
WHEAT BRAN	½ oz.	★★★	
BREAD, GRAHAM, MILK	2 oz. (2 slices)	★	
POTATOES	5 oz. (1 med.)	★	
EGG	2 oz. (1 egg)	★	
BREAD, Whole Wheat, Milk	2 oz. (2 slices)	★	
OATS, Rolled, Cooked	4½ oz. (½ cup)	★	
STRAWBERRIES	6 oz. (¾ cup)	★	
CHOCOLATE OR COCOA	1 oz. (4 T.)	★★★	
MUSHROOMS	4 oz. (5 fresh)	★★★	
CURRANTS	4 oz. (¾ cup)	★★★	
PEAS, SPLIT	2 oz. (⅔ cup)	★★★	
FISH	4 oz.	★	
PRUNES	1 oz. (3 med.)	★	
DATES	1 oz. (3-4)	★	
ONIONS	4 oz. (2 med.)	★	
BANANAS	4 oz. (1 small)	★	
BREAD, WHITE, MILK	2 oz. (2 slices)	★	
BEANS, STRING	2 oz. (½ cup)	★	
RAISINS	1 oz. (2 T.)	★	
PINEAPPLE	4 oz. (½ cup)	★	
MILK, WHOLE	8½ oz. (1 cup)	★	
ALMONDS	½ oz. (12-15 nuts)	★★★	
LETTUCE	2 oz. (¼ head)	★	
BEETS	2 oz. (½ cup)	★	
CARROTS	2 oz.	★	
APPLES	4 oz. (1 small)	★	
PEANUTS	½ oz. (20 nuts)	★★★	

Iron and Copper in

a Serving of Some

Common Foods

Include in the Diet

Foods Containing

Iron and Copper

★★★ excellent source of copper   ★ contains copper

FIG. 105.

Water is one of the most important elements in the food supply. It is the carrier in the body which transports the food elements to the cells and carries away the waste products. There is fundamental truth in the idea that a person can go without the other foodstuffs for a long period of time but life after deprivation of water is of comparatively short duration. Under common conditions human beings control their water intake by a simple mechanism; for that reason water, although essential to proper nutrition, does not become an important item in the construction of a menu. It is, of course, recalled that most solid foods contain water.

Various mineral salts are also vital to the body, and this phase of diet and health is still the subject of much investigation. The common use of ordinary table salt is a direct result of the need of man for this material. Other elements, however, are just as vital, and among the most important are iron, calcium, iodine, and phosphorus. Each one of these in some combination or another is vital, particularly to the growing child. A deficiency of some of them is associated with disease. A carefully balanced dietary régime concerns itself with the salt content of foods which, as might be anticipated, varies greatly. However, the variety of articles seen at an ordinary well-balanced meal, which will include milk and vegetables, usually contains sufficient mineral salts to take care of the body needs.

ACID-BASE RATIO

Recently, considerable attention has been paid to the question of the so-called acid-base ratio of food. Chemically the body maintains a rather constant level of mild alkalinity. It is known that acidity of the body tissues is inconsistent with life, but variations in the alkalinity are possible and may even result from marked imbalance of the diet. All foods, when the processes of digestion and absorption are finished, yield an ash which is either acid or alkaline. Food may be classified as acid-producing or alkaline-producing food. A tendency towards the acid side of the chemical balance of the body may result from excess ingestion of some of the acid-producing foods of which meat, egg yolks, and fish are the most prominent members. Not a great deal is known regarding the clinical significance of these conditions, although certain disease conditions are recognized which are alleviated by a diet balanced towards the alkaline side. Generally speaking, the fruits and vegetables are alkaline-producing foods.

Body alkalinity is quite different from stomach acidity. The layman frequently confuses these two states. The fruit juices which when they enter the stomach are acid, are usually poor food for a person who has already too much acid in his stomach, but such stomach acidity may have nothing whatever to do with the general body reaction. The fruit juices, acid in the stomach, become valuable alkali when they reach the blood stream and the tissues.

In health, true acidosis does not occur. In certain diseases, such as in some phases of diabetes, there is a chemical poisoning known as acidosis. This is due to the actual accumulation of organic acids resulting from the incomplete chemical utilization of certain food substances. There is another state of acidosis seen in some diseases such as nephritis or inflammation of the kidneys, where, owing to the inability of the kidney normally to excrete, certain acid products accumulate. Usually these are of the inorganic type, and frequently alkalis of the inorganic type are used to combat such a state. Neither one of these conditions has anything to do with normal diet.

VITAMINS

The name vitamin is applied to a group of food elements found in certain fresh natural foods. Nutritional failure and disease result from the exclusion of these foods from the daily diet. The action and characteristics of vitamins have been definitely established, and recently much has been learned about their chemical structure and chemical action. As important dietary factors and necessities of a health-promoting diet, they rank with carbohydrates, proteins, fats, mineral salts, and water. The dietary need for what we now know as vitamins was first brought to the attention of scientists by reports of the ill effects resulting from a lack of fresh food in the diet of sailors. The deficiency diseases are discussed in another chapter in this book.

DIGESTION, ASSIMILATION, ABSORPTION

In order to understand how the body uses food for its own purpose one must have a basic knowledge of the processes of digestion, assimilation, and absorption of the material eaten. Before such a complex substance as a piece of meat or such a comparatively simple one as a glass of milk can be utilized by the body, profound chemical changes are initiated. These changes start as soon as food passes the lips. The mouth actually "waters" when food is brought near, and this watering process is due to the secretion of juices by the digestive glands surrounding the throat. These juices perform two functions, first, to moisten the food, and second, to take part in the breaking down of some of the starches.

The teeth are a definite part of the digestive system. Proper chewing of the food, which is constantly being moistened by the salivary juices, means a better preparation of such food for the work of the stomach and intestines. These two initial procedures in the use of food are frequently considerably underemphasized. Food then passes into the stomach, where digestion and mixing continue further. The stomach digestion is not extensive, being limited in the main to a

FOOD VALUES
VITAMINS

Common Foods as Sources of Vitamins

FOOD	A	B	C	D	G
BEEF	✠	✠✠	— to ✠	— to ✠	✠✠
BACON	— to ✠	✠ to ✠✠✠	?		✠✠
PORK	— to ✠	✠✠✠	—		✠✠✠
HAM	— to ✠	✠✠✠	—		✠✠✠
LAMB	✠	✠✠✠	—		✠✠
VEAL	— to ✠	✠✠?			✠✠
LIVER	✠✠✠ to ✠✠✠✠	✠✠✠	✠	✠	✠✠✠
HEART	✠	✠✠✠	✠?		✠✠
KIDNEY	✠✠	✠✠✠	✠?		✠✠✠
BRAINS	✠	✠✠✠			
FISH, LEAN	— to ✠	✠		— to ✠	
OYSTERS	✠✠	✠✠✠	✠	✠✠	✠✠
COD LIVER OIL	✠✠✠	—	—	✠✠✠✠	—
EGGS	✠✠✠	✠ to ✠✠	—?	✠✠✠	✠✠✠
MILK, WHOLE	✠✠✠	✠✠	✠ variable	— to ✠	✠✠✠
MILK, SKIMMED	✠	✠✠✠	✠ variable	—	✠✠✠
BUTTERMILK	✠	✠✠✠	✠ variable		✠✠✠
BUTTER	✠✠✠	—		✠	—
BREAD, WHITE, MILK	✠	✠	— to ✠	— to ✠	✠
BREAD, WHOLE WHEAT, MILK	✠✠	✠✠✠	— to ✠	— to ✠	✠✠
PEANUTS	✠	✠✠✠			
WALNUTS	✠	✠✠✠			
BEANS, NAVY, DRY OR CANNED	✠	✠✠✠	—		
BEANS, STRING	✠✠	✠✠✠	✠✠	— to ✠	
PEAS, GREEN	✠✠✠	✠✠✠	✠✠✠	— to ✠	✠
PEAS, DRY	✠	✠✠✠	?		✠
POTATOES	✠	✠✠	✠✠	—	✠✠✠
CARROTS	✠✠✠	✠✠✠	✠✠	— to ✠	✠✠
CELERY	— to ✠	✠✠✠	—		
LETTUCE	✠ to ✠✠✠	✠✠✠	✠✠✠		✠✠
SPINACH	✠✠✠✠	✠✠✠	✠ (cooked)	— to ✠	✠✠
TOMATOES, RAW OR CANNED	✠✠	✠✠✠	✠✠✠	—	✠✠
CABBAGE, GREEN, RAW	✠✠	✠✠✠	✠✠✠	—	✠✠
APPLES, RAW	✠	✠ to ✠✠✠	✠✠	—	✠✠
ORANGES	✠✠	✠✠✠	✠✠✠	—	✠✠

✠ contains vitamin ✠✠✠ excellent source of vitamin — no appreciable amount
✠✠ good source of vitamin ✠✠✠✠ extraordinary source of vitamin ? doubtful

Fig. 106.

partial attack on protein by the pepsin of the stomach and to the coagulation of milk. Yet stomach digestion is an important second step, in some respects the most important. It is the stomach which responds most to stimulations from outside the body. Appetites may be made or broken by the smell of food that is distasteful. Hunger pains can be stimulated in the stomach by the sight or smell as well as taste of the food.

From the stomach, food is passed on into the intestines, where more ferments, especially those from the pancreas, continue digestion. The intestines also have the function of continuing the forward movement of the food. During the passage of foodstuffs through the intestines chemical processes have changed them into a condition in which they are now suitable to be absorbed into the body. Absorption of these simplified end products of digestion into the lymph and blood streams is followed by a rebuilding process in the body. This rebuilding process involves the construction of new units which can be assimilated as part of the body or can be burned as fuel by the body. What is left of the food passes along the intestinal canal, and the unusable remnant, in addition to a certain amount of secretions of the large intestine, forms the feces, or material that is excreted. The feces may be considered analogous to the clinkers in the furnace, while the rest of the food substance which has been absorbed and assimilated is the same as that part of the coal which goes actually to make the fire.

PREPARATION

Frequently the food question is approached too scientifically. The same group of protein, fat, carbohydrate, mineral salts, vitamins, and calorie units may be assembled into a meal which when presented to a normal or particularly a sick person becomes almost useless. If the meat is burned, the eggs are stale, the vegetables are tasteless, or the tray dirty, few people care to eat. It is not only the appeal to the taste and sense of nicety that concerns us in the preparation of food; there is also a sound physiologic principle involved. The digestion and assimilation of food substances depend to a large extent on the so-called psychologic effect. The mouth watering and the stimulation of the stomach at the sight of food, already mentioned, actually mean better utilization of the food. It may be perfectly true that an extremely hungry person will eat because he is starved, but it is certainly not true of people when they are not starving, and the preparation and appearance of food are decidedly important when they are sick.

BUILDING THE DIET

In considering the need of the body for food, the most important factor involved is the one already mentioned: namely, the need of fuel to supply energy. Without a sufficient supply of fuel the body will burn itself up; therefore, the amount of food consumed by the body must at least furnish enough energy to equalize the amount spent by the body. In addition, however, there is always a certain amount of wear and tear on the body tissues which must be replaced by food. This wear and tear can only be made up by protein, and therefore every normal diet must contain sufficient protein to equalize the amount lost in the daily body activity. When sufficient calories are furnished in the diet, no matter by what kind of food, wear and tear is considerably diminished, but when the total amount of calories furnished is insufficient, there is increased destruction of body tissue.

The adult human body is pretty well stabilized, but the growing body of childhood or adolescence represents a constantly increasing demand to keep pace with growth. In feeding children, therefore, the amount of protection that is required to prevent loss of body tissue is greater than it is in adult life. It is an accepted principle of infant and child feeding to use comparatively large amounts of protein in the normal diet. In adult life, however, provided sufficient total food is given, there is apparently a wide variation possible in the protein intake. There are, in fact, two schools of thought, the one following the principle of the physiologist Voit, giving a normal protein intake of approximately 125 grams, and the followers of Chittenden, who give a protein intake as low as 50 grams. Recent work done in America on the explorers **Stefánsson** and Anderson indicates that high protein-fat mixtures, to which these explorers were accustomed in their sojourn in the Arctic regions, when continued under experimental conditions in America did no demonstrable damage to the organism. Something has already been said about the need of having certain groupings of amino acids in the protein molecule, but even this is subject to wide variations. Among the latest food fads in modern life is the fear of protein. Yet there is little scientific evidence to show the dangers involved in comparatively high or low protein intakes.

During the war there was a definite clinical picture of disease developed as a result of insufficient protein, the so-called protein edema or watery swelling of the tissues. In countries where there was not sufficient protein available to meet the needs, otherwise normal human beings developed anemia and edema or dropsy, both of which disappeared subsequently when sufficient protein was given. Perhaps the tendency towards too little protein is more dangerous than towards too much. In general, if a mathematical protein requirement has to be fixed, it is perfectly safe to say that a minimum of from 0.6 gram to 1.5 grams of protein per kilogram or two pounds of body weight should be sufficient protection against either under- or over-indulgence in this necessary article of diet.

VARIETIES OF MEAT IN THE DIET

A cursory study of any food tables will indicate that a large supply of protein is found in animal products, dairy products, and vegetables. The protein from all meats, including fish and fowl, is essentially the same. There is certainly no difference between the red meat of steer and the red meat of lamb. Nevertheless, there are many wild ideas regarding variations in the meats. Individuals who think they are eating too much meat stop at beef and take lamb, fish, chicken, or even eggs. There can be no more absurd contradiction in fundamental ideas than this all too common practice. There is one slight difference between red meats and white meats, and that is in the so-called extractives found in the uncooked red meat. This refers as well to the meat of veal, lamb, and pork as it does to beef. It is a pretty good assumption to consider all meats in the same classification. The food charts show minor variations in quantity content of protein and fat, but from the standpoint of body economy, both in health and disease, they are potentially identical.

An effort to explain the widespread belief in the essential difference in meats leads nowhere to a scientific basis. This idea represents one of the erroneous unfounded traditions current in much thinking on diets. When one tries to analyze traditional tendencies, one soon gets into a maze of unexplainable, somewhat mysterious byways leading nowhere.

Another source of protein is the organs of animals. These differ from muscle protein in their chemical structure, but in the normal diet they can replace other perhaps more expensive portions of the animal. In certain diseases the doctor will advise against the use of these organs because of the difference in their chemical structure. Since the use of liver in the treatment of anemia and of pancreatic extract or insulin for diabetes, the price of these two organs has risen so as to make them no longer economical articles of food. There remain, however, heart, spleen, brain, and kidneys as easily utilizable portions of the animal.

In neighborhoods where fresh fish are abundant and cheap they frequently replace other forms of animal protein in the normal diet. They have exactly the same value qualitatively and practically the same quantitively, and therefore can well replace meats which have to be

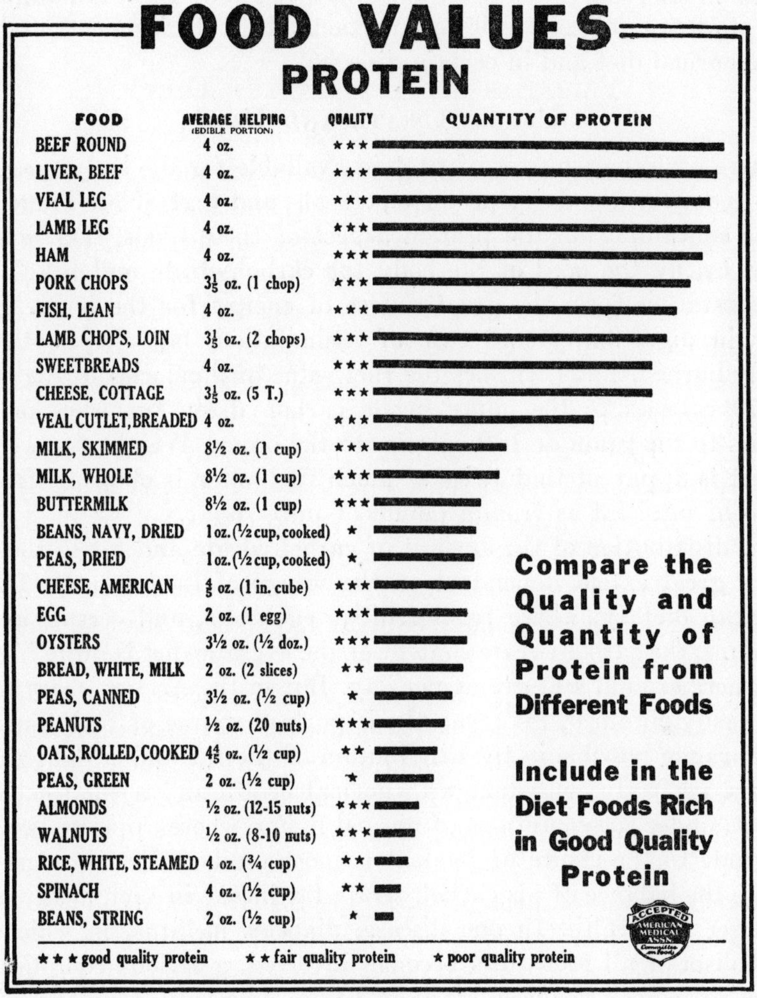

FOOD VALUES
PROTEIN

FOOD	AVERAGE HELPING (EDIBLE PORTION)	QUALITY	QUANTITY OF PROTEIN
BEEF ROUND	4 oz.	★★★	
LIVER, BEEF	4 oz.	★★★	
VEAL LEG	4 oz.	★★★	
LAMB LEG	4 oz.	★★★	
HAM	4 oz.	★★★	
PORK CHOPS	3⅕ oz. (1 chop)	★★★	
FISH, LEAN	4 oz.	★★★	
LAMB CHOPS, LOIN	3⅕ oz. (2 chops)	★★★	
SWEETBREADS	4 oz.	★★★	
CHEESE, COTTAGE	3⅕ oz. (5 T.)	★★★	
VEAL CUTLET, BREADED	4 oz.	★★★	
MILK, SKIMMED	8½ oz. (1 cup)	★★★	
MILK, WHOLE	8½ oz. (1 cup)	★★★	
BUTTERMILK	8½ oz. (1 cup)	★★★	
BEANS, NAVY, DRIED	1 oz. (½ cup, cooked)	★	
PEAS, DRIED	1 oz. (½ cup, cooked)	★	
CHEESE, AMERICAN	⅘ oz. (1 in. cube)	★★★	
EGG	2 oz. (1 egg)	★★★	
OYSTERS	3½ oz. (½ doz.)	★★★	
BREAD, WHITE, MILK	2 oz. (2 slices)	★★	
PEAS, CANNED	3½ oz. (½ cup)	★	
PEANUTS	½ oz. (20 nuts)	★★★	
OATS, ROLLED, COOKED	4⅘ oz. (½ cup)	★★	
PEAS, GREEN	2 oz. (½ cup)	★	
ALMONDS	½ oz. (12-15 nuts)	★★★	
WALNUTS	½ oz. (8-10 nuts)	★★★	
RICE, WHITE, STEAMED	4 oz. (¾ cup)	★★	
SPINACH	4 oz. (½ cup)	★★	
BEANS, STRING	2 oz. (½ cup)	★	

Compare the Quality and Quantity of Protein from Different Foods

Include in the Diet Foods Rich in Good Quality Protein

★★★ good quality protein   ★★ fair quality protein   ★ poor quality protein

FIG. 107.

brought from other districts. The same thing, of course, is true of farm lands where poultry is easily accessible. In such neighborhoods poultry will form a cheaper protein than would be obtained from other kinds of animal life. Like fish, it has the same value as has beef protein.

Eggs, consisting as they do of protein and fat, can likewise replace meat in the dietary. The white of the egg is almost pure protein, and the yolk is almost pure fat. Two eggs will contain approximately the same amount of protein and fat as will a piece of round steak 3 inches $\times$ $3\frac{1}{4}$ $\times$ $\frac{3}{4}$ inch, and can be substituted in that way. The high fat content of egg yolk makes it not an exact substitute for meat products in the normal diet and in certain diseases.

CARBOHYDRATE AND FAT

There are other sources of protein available for the body, particularly in some of the dairy products, cereals, and vegetables. Therefore, before continuing on the protein aspect of these foods, it is wise to review briefly the need of the body for carbohydrate and fat. These two substances form the great source of energy for the body. They differ in digestibility and ease of assimilation, but they both are readily burned. Fat furnishes the fuel value of 9 calories to the gram or 270 calories to the ounce, while carbohydrate furnishes only 4 calories to the gram or 120 calories to the ounce. Weight for weight, then, it is apparent that twice as much fuel value is obtained from 1 pound of pure fat as from a pound of pure sugar.

The distribution of the amount of carbohydrate and fat in the diet is to a great extent dependent on the source of food supply. In the American dietary, where fresh fruits, vegetables, and cereals are so abundant, the carbohydrate content of the average diet is quite high— somewhere around 400 grams per day. But in the Arctic, where fat is more easily obtained, fat forms the important source of fuel. There is a wide range possible in the distribution of the fat and carbohydrate, a range perfectly consistent with normal health and normal activity. In fact, under the conditions of normal living, where appetite becomes the guide to the choice of food, it is most unlikely that anyone will change the balance of his carbohydrate-fat intake in such a way as to endanger his health. In one disease, diabetes mellitus, in which the metabolism of all foodstuffs becomes involved, a serious complication known as acidosis has been attributed to an uneven distribution of fat and carbohydrate. Some of the newer ideas of this disease do not accept this theory as true.

In analyzing the average food supply one notes that the source of fat in the American dietary is to a great extent from butter, cream, eggs, meat, olive oil, vegetable oil, and nuts. Carbohydrates are derived to a large extent from sweets of all kinds. In America the consumption of sugar is greater than in any country in the world; in 1925, about 110 pounds per person per year; in 1932 about 99 pounds per person per year. The cereal grains, fruits, and vegetables also all supply carbohydrate in different amounts.

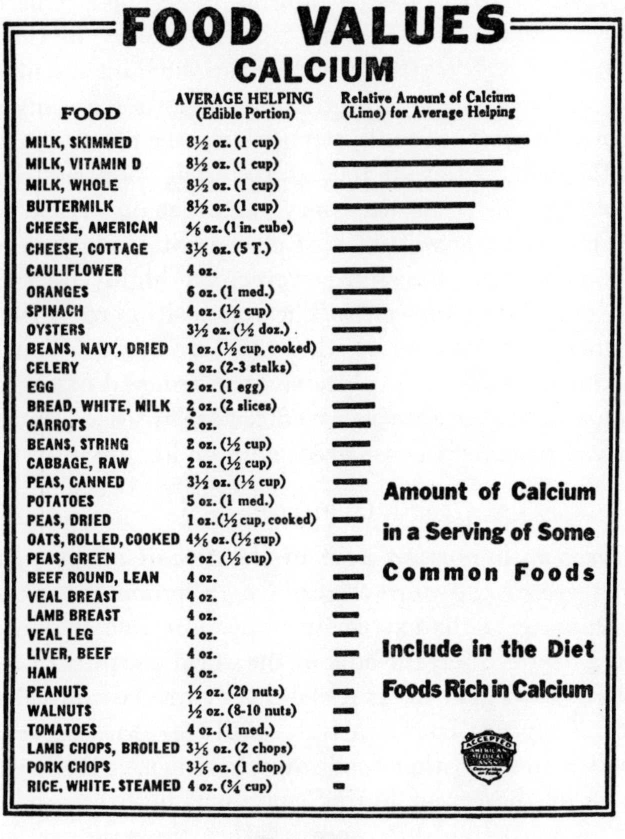

FIG. 108.

MILK

Milk, which is such a stable article of diet for the growing child, is not used as extensively in the dietary of the American adult as it should be. Milk is a natural food, and it occupies the unique position of being almost a complete food. It contains protein, fat, carbohydrate, salts, some vitamins (A, B, C), and serves in the ordinary dietary, both of the child and the adult, as the most constant source of calcium. In children calcium is necessary for the healthy development of normal bones and teeth, and in adult life it is also of value in the preservation of the teeth and in the regulation of the nervous system and heart. The milk proteins supply all the amino acids necessary, and for that reason milk may replace meat in the diet. Carbohydrate is present in the form of lactose or milk sugar, which is easily assimilable and utilized by the organism. The same is true of the fat constituents in milk. *Cream* differs from milk only in the increased amount of fat present. *Butter*, which forms such an essential part of the diet, is consumed perhaps in greater amounts than any other fat.

The various products of milk, particularly the *cheeses*, play a varying rôle in the composition of food in different countries. In America cheese is more apt to be an accessory than a main article of diet for the average citizen; a small block of cheese with his pie is considered to add zest to the meal. Cheeses, however, are highly nutritious food, 'rich in fat and mineral elements. The composition of various cheeses of course depends entirely on whether they are made from whole milk, cream, or skimmed milk. The proteins of cheese and of all milk products are valuable in the treatment of certain diseases, such as gout, where the meat protein is considered more or less toxic to the system.

CEREALS

Cereals form an important part of the diet of all people. The old time-honored use of the word "bread" as a synonym for all food is eloquent testimony to the extremely important rôle that bread plays in life. As a matter of fact, the bulk of the world's supply of food is furnished by the cereal grains. As a class, they are rich in carbohydrate and protein. They are comparatively easily grown and transported, and in comparison with other foods are economical. Before the milling process, most of the cereal grains contained both mineral salts and vitamins. This makes no difference whether the grain is wheat, rye, barley, oats, or rice. There are minor differences in the composition of these various grains, but from the broad standpoint of their use as sources of food they are practically equal. They contain a very high carbohydrate, varying usually around 75 per cent and protein varying from 7 to 15 per cent. The fat content is relatively small. However, when one stops to consider that bread is almost always eaten with butter, when butter is available, and the cereals as such are supplemented by milk or cream, the deficiency in fat is soon made up.

The protein of cereals is not considered as complete a protein as is that of milk or meat, because it does not contain all of the necessary amino acids. There is considerable variation in the quality of proteins found in the various grains. Usually each cereal grain contains some but not all of the necessary amino acids. Of the vitamins, B is contained in abundance in the whole grain, but it is almost entirely removed in the process of milling. A is present only in small amounts. The mineral salts are not present in the cereal grains to a great enough extent to be of real value in the diet. There is present, however, cellulose, which, while without food value, has a rôle in digestion in that it produces peristalsis and assists in the evacuation of the bowels.

Of recent years various processes have been developed for the commercial production of oils from grains. These oils are having a wide use because they are cheaper than butter and olive oil, which formerly were used almost exclusively. Oils are also being made from vegetables. Except for the difference in vitamins, there is no essential difference between the newly developed vegetable and cereal oils and butter. They are practically identical in fuel value and may be used interchangeably if supplemented by vitamin-containing foods, such as fresh fruits, vegetables, and milk.

From what has already been said regarding their essential similarity, it must be evident that there is no necessity for standardizing the kind of cereal grains that form the basis of diet. As a matter of fact, history and current international practice clearly demonstrate the equal efficiency of American white bread, German rye bread, Russian black bread, Italian spaghetti, and Oriental rice.

SUGARS

The common table sugar is cane sugar or sucrose. This may be derived from most fruits, from the sugar cane, the sugar beet, or from various other sources. By the time sugar is refined, there should be no practical difference in its composition or its value as food. Milk sugar is somewhat different, but from the standpoint of the body use, is practically identical. The simpler sugar known as grape sugar or glucose is usually commercially derived from corn syrup. It has practically the same value as has cane sugar, since cane sugar is split by the body into glucose before it is absorbed.

Other forms of sugar are molasses, which contains cane sugar, maple syrup, and honey. From a standpoint of body chemistry, these are equally valuable.

Sugar is the most concentrated form of fuel available for the body. It is burned up more quickly than fat, and for that reason it is sometimes known as a stimulant. Tired athletes or weary soldiers frequently go out of their way to obtain candy. This is physiologically sound because exercise results in the quick burning up of the sugar available in the body, and the need for replacement is made evident by fatigue.

The carbohydrate of the cereal grains, which has already been discussed, is, however, in a more complicated chemical structure, which requires considerable treatment by the body before it can be utilized. Such digestion by the body requires a longer time to make starches and higher carbohydrates ready for absorption. This is the only essential difference between such higher carbohydrates and plain sugar. Potentially a cereal contains 75 per cent carbohydrate, exactly equivalent to an equal amount of 75 per cent sugar solution. This fact is of particular importance in dealing with the disease diabetes. In this disease the gullible patient reads that a certain patent food product contains no sugar—and gets into all kinds of trouble because of the high content of starch. When manufacturers or retailers deliberately sell such food at high prices to an innocent public they are guilty of a neglect that is almost criminal.

FRUITS

Among the common sources of carbohydrate are fruits and vegetables. The fruits are practically a mixture of water, sugar, certain of the vitamins, minerals, and indigestible residue. From a practical point of view, they are fat free and protein free. Their main use in the dietary is in the supply of vitamins A, B, and C. As late as 1885 the disease scurvy was a common threat of long sea voyages, when the diet was lacking in all fruits. There is no more striking episode in the history of food than the discovery by Takaki that the addition of orange and lemon juice to the diet prevented the appearance of this disease. Fruits are also mild laxatives. Nowadays the stabilization of the fruit industry is such that fresh fruits are available almost throughout the year, and the process of canning has reached such perfection that there is no excuse for any diet at any time to be without fruit of some sort.

Vegetables

The vegetables have the same value as the fruits in their supply of vitamins and cellulose. In addition, most of them have an important mineral content, and many are much higher in food value than the fruits. The leafy vegetables, such as spinach, lettuce, cabbage, are not

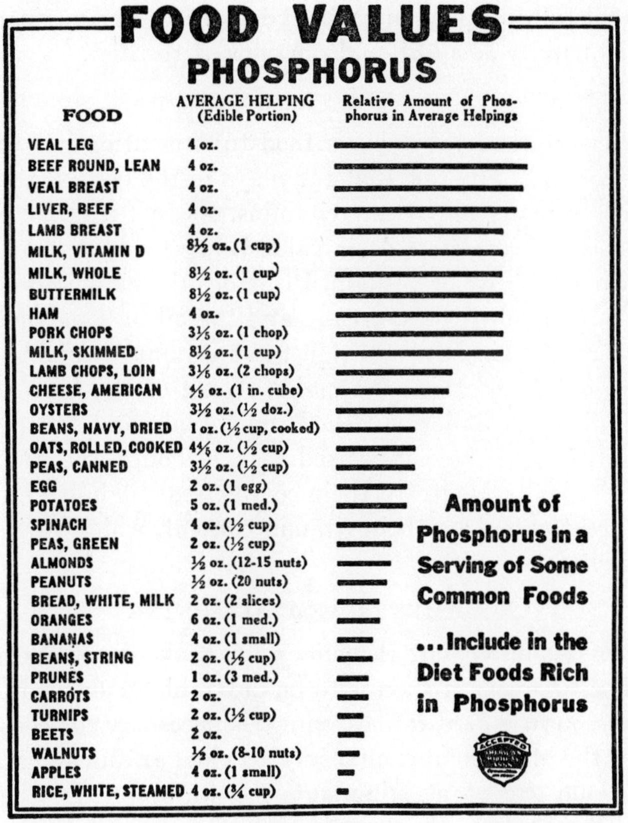
FOOD VALUES
PHOSPHORUS
FOOD
AVERAGE HELPING (Edible Portion)
Relative Amount of Phosphorus in Average Helpings
VEAL LEG 4 oz.
BEEF ROUND, LEAN 4 oz.
VEAL BREAST 4 oz.
LIVER, BEEF 4 oz.
LAMB BREAST 4 oz.
MILK, VITAMIN D 8½ oz. (1 cup)
MILK, WHOLE 8½ oz. (1 cup)
BUTTERMILK 8½ oz. (1 cup)
HAM 4 oz.
PORK CHOPS 3⅕ oz. (1 chop)
MILK, SKIMMED 8½ oz. (1 cup)
LAMB CHOPS, LOIN 3⅕ oz. (2 chops)
CHEESE, AMERICAN ⅘ oz. (1 in. cube)
OYSTERS 3½ oz. (½ doz.)
BEANS, NAVY, DRIED 1 oz. (½ cup, cooked)
OATS, ROLLED, COOKED 4⅘ oz. (½ cup)
PEAS, CANNED 3½ oz. (½ cup)
EGG 2 oz. (1 egg)
POTATOES 5 oz. (1 med.)
SPINACH 4 oz. (½ cup)
PEAS, GREEN 2 oz. (½ cup)
ALMONDS ½ oz. (12-15 nuts)
PEANUTS ½ oz. (20 nuts)
BREAD, WHITE, MILK 2 oz. (2 slices)
ORANGES 6 oz. (1 med.)
BANANAS 4 oz. (1 small)
BEANS, STRING 2 oz. (½ cup)
PRUNES 1 oz. (3 med.)
CARROTS 2 oz.
TURNIPS 2 oz. (½ cup)
BEETS 2 oz.
WALNUTS ½ oz. (8-10 nuts)
APPLES 4 oz. (1 small)
RICE, WHITE, STEAMED 4 oz. (¾ cup)
Amount of Phosphorus in a Serving of Some Common Foods
...Include in the Diet Foods Rich in Phosphorus

Fig. 109.

important as sources of energy or of protein; but some of the seed vegetables, such as beans and peas, are valuable for their protein and carbohydrate. Some of them contain a small amount of fat. Potatoes are in a class by themselves, containing mainly water and about 20 per cent carbohydrate. There are a negligible amount of protein and a valuable ash. Potato peel contains a large amount of cellulose, which is helpful to peristalsis. The main value of potato, particularly the white potato, is that it furnishes an abundance of carbohydrate and mineral salts at a low cost. Most of the other vegetables fall somewhere between the descriptions of the leafy vegetables and the seed vegetables, and their actual composition can be seen in any food table.

NUTS

Nuts vary a great deal in their food content and as a rule are rich in protein and fat and poor in carbohydrate. In the American dietary they are used mainly as additional portions of the diet.

FATS

In the discussions of the various foodstuffs mention has been made of their fat content. The rôle that fat plays in the body is that of fuel and a carrier of many important vitamins. As fuel it is the most concentrated food we have, its caloric value being twice that of an equal portion of carbohydrate or protein. Probably the most important fats are butter, butter substitutes, cream, and the oil of some of the vegetables and cereal grains. In addition to supplying available fuel, the concentrated nature of this food makes it one of the best articles of diet for building up undernourished individuals and for preventing loss of weight. It must be emphasized that, although the fuel value of all fats is practically identical, their complete availability as food depends to a great extent on their vitamin content, which varies greatly in the different fats.

CONDIMENTS AND SEASONING

Some other less important elements go to make up the normal diet. Seasoning is a necessity if food is to be palatable. Table salt, which is the commonest article used for seasoning, is necessary for complete living. Some of the other condiments, such as vinegar and spices, have no particular value except as stimulants to the appetite. The various caffeine and theobromine drinks such as coffee, tea, cocoa, and chocolate are stimulants, which in the case of tea and coffee are without food value. Cocoa has slight food value, but since it is usually made up as a milk drink, it forms a very nourishing and substantial article of diet. None of these beverages is necessary. In many instances they add to the zest and joy of living and for the average healthy individual are certainly without danger when taken in moderate amounts. Taken to excess it is possible that the amount of stimulant may have a deleterious effect.

ALCOHOL

As a food, alcohol has a caloric value of 7 to the gram, is easily oxidized, and therefore is a valuable fuel. Without wishing to enter into the questions involved in the prohibition issue, it can be said from the medical point of view that alcohol in moderate amounts has never been shown to do any harm. Excess of alcohol, like excess of any other article of food, must be avoided. The only difference between the danger from excess of alcohol and that from other food products lies in the fact that alcohol, in addition to being a food, has a definite toxicological influence when taken in larger amounts. Its sociological implications need not be discussed in a medical book.

The necessary basic considerations of normal diet are few and simple. First, there must be enough fuel to supply the energy expended by the body. This fuel is furnished by the three major elements, protein, fat, and carbohydrate, but more efficiently by the fat and carbohydrate. Second, sufficient protein must be supplied to replace tissue waste. Third, water, mineral salts, and vitamins come in as of major importance qualitatively but of minor importance quantitatively. The proportions of the different foods may vary within comparatively wide limits. Certainly the amount of protein needed is an inconstant factor. The carbohydrate and fat may be distributed according to the source of supply and their availability. The necessary vitamins and usually the mineral salts are furnished by milk, fresh vegetables, fresh fruits, butter, and cereals.

For the past ten years considerable prominence has been given to vitamins and the deficiency diseases through popular scientific literature and commercial advertising. Because of this recent emphasis people are apt to gain the erroneous impression that vitamins are the most essential principle of the normal diet. However, any general discussion of human nutrition must include the consideration of other equally important dietary factors. The aim of all scientific food research is to determine the diet for the individual that will create and maintain the highest degree of health. It is true that the majority of the people of the past survived in spite of their ignorance of all the facts of modern dietary science; but it must be added that their survival was dependent upon the selection by the trial-and-error method of those foods which today modern scientific investigation has definitely established as the constituents of the normal diet. This so-called normal diet is a very simple one, consisting of a palatable mixture of common foodstuffs. In fact, it is the typical diet of a prosperous community under normal conditions. To be specific, all of man's nutritional needs will be met if he will plan his daily diet to include: one quart of milk per day, two fresh salads, two servings of leafy green vegetables, one serving of meat, and liberal quantities of butter, fruits, cereals, bread, and water.

PROTEIN YIELD OF VARIOUS FOODS

Food	Amount*	Protein, Gm.
BEVERAGES		
Whole milk	6 oz.	6
Skimmed milk	6 oz.	6
Buttermilk	6 oz.	5
Evaporated milk	6 oz.	12
SOUPS (canned—diluted as directed)		
Asparagus	6 oz.	2
Bean	6 oz.	11
Beef	6 oz.	10
Bouillon	6 oz.	5
Celery	6 oz.	3
Chicken	6 oz.	3
Chicken gumbo	6 oz.	7
Clam chowder	6 oz.	7
Consummé	6 oz.	6
Julienne	6 oz.	5
Mock turtle	6 oz.	11
Mulligatawny	6 oz.	5
Mutton	6 oz.	9
Oxtail	6 oz.	7
Pepperpot	6 oz.	8
Printanier	6 oz.	8
Pea	6 oz.	9
Tomato	6 oz.	3
Vegetable	6 oz.	6
Home-made cream	6 oz.	6 to 10
Split pea	6 oz.	19
FISH		
Codfish	2 by 2 by ¾ in.	5
Haddock	2 by 2 by ¾ in.	5
Halibut	2 by 2 by ¾ in.	6
Salmon	2 T.	7
Sardines	4 small	7
Tuna	2 T.	7
Clams	6	9
Crab meat	¼ cup	7
Lobster meat	¼ cup	8
Oysters	7 medium	6
Shrimp	12	15

*In the tables, t. indicates teaspoonful; T. indicates tablespoonful.

Food	Amount	Protein, Gm.
MEAT		
Roast beef	Av. serving	12
Tenderloin steak	Av. serving	17
Bacon	3 strips 5 in. long	5
Corned beef	....	9
Dried beef	....	6
Lamb chop	1 chop	14
Mutton chop	¾ in. thick	19
Pork chop (lean)	....	31
Veal chop	....	24
Fowl	3 by 3 by ¼ in.	6
Frankfurter	....	8
Ham (boiled)	4 by 3 by ¼ in.	10
Beef liver	4 by 3¼ by ⅜ in.	16
Calves' liver	4 by 3¼ by ⅜ in.	16
Chicken liver	Average size	12
Pork roast	2½ by 2 by ¾ in.	13
Pork tenderloin	4 by 3½ by ¼ in.	19
Round steak	2 by 1 by 1 in.	13
DESSERTS		
Gelatin cream desserts	Av. serving	7 to 10
Cornstarch puddings with egg	Av. serving	7 to 10
Rice tapioca with egg	Av. serving	8 to 11
Fruit gelatins	Av. serving	4
Ice cream	Av. serving	4 to 7
FRUITS	....	1 to 2
VEGETABLES (fresh)	....	1 to 4
CHEESE		
American	1 cubic inch	6
Cottage, dry	2 T.	6
Cream, Philadelphia	⅓ cake	2
Limburger	1 cubic inch	5
Roquefort	1 cubic inch	5
Swiss	1 cubic inch	6
Pimento	2 T.	4 to 7
MISCELLANEOUS		
Breads	Av. slice	3
Egg	1	6
Cereals	Av. serving	1 to 4

CALORIC YIELD OF VARIOUS FOODS

Meal	Amount	Protein, Gm.	Fat, Gm.	Carbohydrate, Gm.	Calories
BREAKFAST					
Stewed prunes	6	2	..	34	144
Sugar	2 t.	..	..	10	40
Farina	½ cupful	2	..	14	64
Sugar	2 t.	..	..	10	40
Whole milk	¼ cupful	2	2.5	3	43
Soft egg	1	6	6	..	75
Butter	1 t.	..	4	..	36
Toast	1 slice	3	..	16	78

Meal	Amount	Protein, Gm.	Fat, Gm.	Carbohydrates, Gm.	Calories
Butter	1 t.	..	4	..	36
Coffee					
Cream	1½ T.	7	4.5	0.7	46
Sugar	2 t.	..	..	10	40
Milk	6 oz.	6	7.5	9	128
LUNCHEON					
Vegetable soup	Av. serving	1	11	9	139
Crackers	2	2	2	10	66
Crisp bacon	3 strips 5 in. long	5	11	..	119
Fruit salad	Av. serving	..	15	16	199
Entire wheat bread	1 slice	..	..	14	64
Butter	1 t.	..	4	..	36
Milk	6 oz.	6	7.5	9	128
Caramel pudding	Av. serving	3*	3	52	247
Sugar	1 t.	..	..	5	20
Milk	¼ cup	2	2.5	3	43
DINNER					
Chilled tomato juice	3 oz.	..	..	3	12
Broiled steak	3½ by 3 by ¾ in.	17	25	..	293
Stuffed baked potato	Av. size	5	2	28	150
Squash	Av. serving	2	4	10	84
String beans	Av. serving	1	4	3	52
Hard roll	1	3	..	16	76
Butter	1 t.	..	4	..	36
Cucumber and radish salad ..	Av. serving	1	..	4	20
Orange ice	Av. serving	..	..	66	264
Black coffee					
		71.7	123.5	354.7	2,818

DISTRIBUTION OF PROTEIN, FAT, AND CARBOHYDRATE

Meal	Amount	Gm. or Cc.	Protein, Gm.	Fat, Gm.	Carbohydrate, Gm.	Calories
BREAKFAST						
Stewed prunes	6 t.		2	..	34	144
Cream of wheat	½ cupful (20 Gm. dry)		2	..	14	64
Sugar	2 t.	10	..	..	10	40
Cream	¼ cupful	60	2	12	2	124
Soft eggs	2	100	13.4	10.5	..	150
Toast	1 slice	30	3	..	16	78
Butter	½ t.	2½	..	2	..	18
Coffee						
Cream	1 T.		0.5	3	5	31
Sugar	2 T.	10	..	..	10	40
Milk	6 oz.	180	6	7.5	9	128

Meal	Amount	Gm. or Cc.	Pro-tein, Gm.	Fat, Gm.	Carbohy-drate, Gm.	Calo-ries
LUNCHEON						
Cream of corn soup	Av. serving		5	9.5	18	178
Crackers	2	14	2	2	10	66
Crisp bacon	3 strips 5 in. long	23	4.5	7.5	..	86
Fruit salad without dressing	Av. serving		..	..	16	64
Entire wheat bread	1 slice	30	2	..	14	64
Butter	1½ T.	2½	..	2	..	18
Milk	6 oz.	180	6	7.5	9	128
Prune custard	1		8	7	56	316
DINNER						
Chilled tomato juice	3 oz.	90	..	..	3	12
Roast chicken		120	24	20	..	268
Stuffed baked potato	1		5	2	28	150
Squash (½ teaspoonful butter)	Av. serving		2	2	10	66
String beans (½ teaspoonful butter)	Av. serving		1	2	3	34
Hard roll		30	3	..	16	76
Butter	½ t.	2½	..	2	..	18
Cucumber and radish salad ..	Av. serving		1	..	4	20
Orange ice	Av. serving		..	..	66	264
Black coffee						
Crackers	2	14	2	2	10	66
American cheese	1 cubic in.	20	6	7	..	87
			100.4	107.5	358.5	2,798

ESSENTIALS OF A NORMAL DIET

1. Calories—
   a. Bed rest .... 1000 – 1200 c. Light work ....1800 – 2500
   b. Invalidism .... 1500 – 2000 d. Moderate work ....2300 – 3000
   e. Heavy work ....3000 – 4000
2. Water—6 to 8 glasses
3. Carbohydrate .... 250 – 325 Gms.
4. Protein .... 60 – 75 Gms.
5. Fat .... 125 Gms.
6. Roughage—6 to 10 servings of bulky food
7. Vitamins—adequate amounts of A, B, C, D, E, and P. P. factor
8. Salts or minerals

	Adults		Children
Calcium	.68 to 1 gm.		1 gm.
Phosphorus	1.32	gms.	1 gm.
Iron	.015	gm.	.015 gm.
Sodium chloride	2	gms.	

CONSTIPATION

Constipation is most frequently the result of taking a diet of foods which have little or no undigested residue in the intestines. The three types of constipation are:

1. Atonic.   2. Spastic.   3. Obstructive

1—Atonic Constipation is the usual type and one in which there is lack of muscle tone, resulting from lack of exercise and incorrect diet.

To correct.

1. Regular daily bowel movements should be established.
2. Six to eight glasses of water a day.
3. Enemas and cathartics should be avoided.
4. A diet with 800 grams bulk of fruit and vegetables may be taken daily which is equivalent to:

    ½ cup of 9 per cent vegetables.
    3 cups of 3 to 6 per cent vegetables.
    2/3 pounds of fruit.

5. Vitamins B and C are of great importance in any disease of the gastro-intestinal tract, so it is advised that an abundance of food containing these vitamins be included in the diet.

SAMPLE DIET

BREAKFAST

Fruit—2 large servings.
Whole grain cereal if cereal is used.
Egg, bacon, ham, or similar food.

Whole grain bread—butter.
Hot beverages.

LUNCHEON

Cream soup, cottage cheese, or other protein food.
Vegetables—2 or 3 servings.

Fruit—1 large serving.
Whole grain bread—butter.
Milk.

DINNER

Fruit cup, grapefruit or melon.
Meat, fish, or fowl.
Potato.
Other vegetables—2 or 3 servings.

Salad.
Fruit or any dessert made with fruit.
Whole grain bread—butter.
Any beverage.

Additional Suggestions:

1. Fruit or fruit juice may be taken between meals and before retiring.

In giving a diet with considerable bulk care should be taken to supply sufficient protein.

2—Spastic Constipation is characterized by irregular spasms accompanied by severe pain. It may result from continued use of condiments, excessive use of tea, coffee, or tobacco.

The diet should

1. Avoid irritation which would increase spasm.
2. Assist in evacuation.
3. Improve general nutritive condition of patient.

SAMPLE MENU

BREAKFAST	LUNCH	DINNER
Strained orange juice.	Vegetable broth.	Cream potato soup.
Cream of wheat.	Soft boiled egg.	Cottage cheese with cream.
Dry toast.	Dry toast.	Dry toast.
Cocoa or milk.	Plain jello.	Baked custard.
	Milk.	Milk.

If milk is not thoroughly digested, it may be peptonized or boiled.

Puréed vegetables and soft cooked fruits may be added when condition is relieved.

3—Obstructive Constipation—Obstruction may be caused by cancer, tumor, or adhesions.

1. The diet should omit all foods with an indigestible residue.
2. Avoid gas-forming foods.
3. Omit meats which putrefy easily.
4. Avoid serious underfeeding if patient is to be operated upon.
(Compiled from various sources.)

BLAND DIET

DIETETIC PRINCIPLES

1. Weak peristaltic stimulants.
2. Sub-acid foods.
3. Moderately low and smooth residue foods.
4. Regular and simple meals.
5. Avoidance of:
   a. Coarse, raw foods.
   b. Stimulating condiments and spices.
   c. Gas-forming foods and mixtures.
   d. Extreme temperatures in foods.

FOODS ALLOWED

Soups—Strained.
Meat—fish or fowl with short fiber.
Milk and milk products—in all forms including cream cheese.
Eggs—soft cooked, eggnogs.
Vegetables—mild, sieved, and potatoes.
Fruit juices—pear, blueberry, peach—sub-acid.
Cereals—without bran; and Italian pastes.
Breads—without bran.
Dessert—custards, simple puddings, jello, blanc mange.
Beverages—weak tea, coffee.

FOODS NOT ALLOWED

Meat sauces, pickles, highly seasoned foods, excessive use of condiments, salads, coarse
raw vegetables, fried foods, acid fruits and fruit juices, hot breads, strong tea,
coffee and cocoa.

DIET

BREAKFAST
Bland fruit juice.
Cooked cereal (without bran).
Soft cooked egg.
White bread (toast)—butter.
Weak coffee, tea or cocoa.
Small amount sugar.

LUNCH
Cream soup strained.
Cottage cheese or other cheese or
   entrée—starchy food.
Sieved vegetable.
Simple dessert.
White bread toast—butter.
Milk.

MENU

BREAKFAST
Pear juice.
Strained oatmeal.
Poached egg.
White toast—butter.
Weak coffee.
Small amount sugar.
(10:00 A.M., eggnog.)

LUNCH
Cream asparagus soup.
Cottage cheese.
Sieved carrots.
Custard.
White bread toast—butter.
Milk.
(3:00 P.M., milk.)

DIET	MENU
DINNER	**DINNER**
Cream soup or clear soup.	Chicken broth.
Meat.	Lamb chop.
Potato or starchy food.	Baked potato.
Sieved vegetable.	Purée peas.
Simple dessert.	Tapioca cream.
White bread toast—butter.	White melba toast—butter.
Milk or weak tea.	Milk.
	(8:00 P.M., weak cocoa.)

NOTE: Milk may be given at 10:00 A.M., 3:00 P.M., and 8:00 P.M.

DIET FOR HYPERACIDITY

DIETETIC PRINCIPLES

1. Sub-acid fruits and fruit juices.
2. Weak secretory and peristaltic stimulants.
3. Moderately bland and nonirritating foods.
4. Adequate nonstimulating proteins.
5. Foods which bind acids.
6. Low salt and moderately high fat.
7. Regular meals.
8. Frequent feedings in some cases.
9. Avoidance of:
   Stimulants, condiments and highly seasoned foods, meat extracts, uncooked foods except tender lettuce, very hot and very cold foods.

FOODS TO USE

Soups—cream.
Meats—tender.
Milk and milk products—all milk modifications and cheeses.
Eggs—soft cooked.
Vegetables—all cooked and easily digested.
Fruits—sub-acid fruits and fruit juice, such as pears, apple sauce, etc.
Salads—cooked with bland dressing.
Cereals—in small amounts.
Breads—white and whole wheat.
Dessert—simple puddings and ice creams.
Beverages—weak tea, coffee, and cocoa, and alkaline mineral waters.

FOODS TO AVOID

Strong meat stocks; rare meat; coarse raw and cooked strong vegetables; acid fruits and fruit juices, coarse fruits; sour or lactic acid milk; hot breads; concentrated sweets, condiments, spices, stimulants; fried foods; and strong tea and coffee

DIET	MENU
BREAKFAST	**BREAKFAST**
Sub-acid fruit.	Apple sauce and pear juice.
Cooked cereal, cream.	Cereal, cream.
Soft cooked egg, or bacon.	Soft-boiled egg.
Toast, butter.	Toast, butter.
Milk or weak cocoa.	Milk or weak cocoa.

DIET	MENU

LUNCHEON

Cream soup.
Cottage cheese or meat.
Vegetable.
Salad—cooked fruit or vegetable.
Simple pudding or cooked fruit.
Bread, butter and milk.

LUNCHEON

Cream of mushroom soup.
Lamb chop.
Carrots and peas.
Pear and cheese salad.
Rice custard, whipped cream.
Bread, butter, and milk.

DINNER

Meat, tender, well cooked.
Potato, butter.
Vegetable, two or cooked fruit or vegetable salad.
Simple dessert.
Toast, butter.
Rich milk.

DINNER

Steak or fish.
Baked potato, butter.
Squash.
Asparagus, hot or as salad.
Custard.
Melba toast.
Rich milk.

FEEDINGS BETWEEN MEALS

10:00 A.M., 3:00 P.M., 8:00 P.M., milk and cream drinks.

DIET FOR HYPO-ACIDITY

DIETETIC PRINCIPLES

1. Natural acid foods.
2. Strong secretory stimulants.
3. Low residue, smooth foods.
4. Restrict liquid intake if motility is impaired.
5. Thorough mastication.
6. Regular and preferably small simple meals.
7. Rest after meals.
8. Avoidance of:
   a. Bacteria-carrying foods.
   b. Extremes in hot and cold foods.
   c. Foods containing sodium bicarbonate, carbonated waters.
   d. Fermentable sugars and sweets.
   e. Excessive use of fats and proteins.

FOODS TO USE

Soups—clear meat or vegetable broths.
Meats—broiled or roasted chicken, lamb, beef, fresh-water fish, raw oysters.
Milk and milk products—sweet and sour.
Eggs—soft cooked.
Vegetables—sieved beets, carrots, celery, peas, potatoes, sweet potatoes, tomatoes, asparagus tip, and squash.
Fruits—cooked and all fruit juices.
Cereals—cooked or dry cereal, rice.
Breads—plain bread or toast.
Dessert—simple puddings, jello, and cooked fruits.
Beverages—weak tea, coffee, cocoa, lemonade, and all sour fruit juices.

FOODS TO AVOID

All raw, coarse fruits, vegetables, fried and greasy foods; pork and all smoked and preserved meats and fish, all iced drinks, frozen desserts, and all very hot foods or drinks. All fermentable sugars and sweets, hot breads, candies, nuts, pies, and all cheese except cottage cheese.

DIET

BREAKFAST
Sour fruit juice.
Cooked fruit.
Cereals.
Egg or bacon.
Toast—butter.
Coffee or tea—cream and sugar.

LUNCH
Meat broth.
Cottage cheese or meat.
Sieved vegetable.
Bread and butter.
Simple dessert or cooked fruit.
Tea with lemon, lemonade, grapefruit
    juice, or fruit juice.

DINNER
Soup or broth.
Meat.
Vegetable.
Salad.
Bread and butter.
Cooked fruit or simple dessert.
Tea, coffee, lemonade, or fruit juice.

MENU

BREAKFAST
Grapefruit juice.
Apricots.
Puffed rice—cream.
Poached egg.
White toast—butter.
Coffee or cocoa.

LUNCH
Beef broth.
Creamed sweetbreads.
Sieved beets.
Melba toast—butter.
Lemon gelatin with whipped cream.
Tea with lemon or lemonade.

DINNER
Roast beef.
Mashed squash.
Sieved spinach.
Cooked grapefruit salad.
Boiled dressing.
Peeled baked apple.
Tea, coffee, or lemonade.

CHAPTER XXX

Posture
R. TAIT McKENZIE, M.D.

Good posture is the cure of some evils and certainly a preventive
of many. In infancy its preventive value has the greatest influence on
the ensuing life of the baby, though much can be done, by means of
persistent exercise, to overcome faults of posture in later life.

The home and school can coöperate effectively in training children
to observe the rules of correct posture. In the school, however, most
can be done in providing desks and seats of correct height and size, as
well as the instruments for gymnastic exercises.

The need for proper seating cannot be too greatly emphasized,
because of its direct effect on the spine. Desks should be designed to fit
the abnormally large or small, as well as the normal-sized child. The
seated pupil should not use a seat so low that his shoulders perforce
become rounded, his head droops, and his chest is flattened. The elbows
should be able to rest on the desk without stooping or unduly elevating
the shoulders, and the edge of the desk should overlap the edge of the
seat. Many schools have a certain number of specially adjustable desks
and seats for the express use of children who are above or below the
average size.

Perfectly fitting seats are not everything. No child can sit still long.
It is not in his nature to do so. He will become weary unless sufficient
opportunity is allowed for exercising and changing the posture during
school hours. If he sits too long, the upper part of the body leans forward on or against the desk, constricting the chest, crowding the
abdominal organs, and impeding the circulation in the veins. The
weight is supported by the arms, and the head, neck, and spine hang
by the muscles of the shoulder blades in abnormal curves. To relieve
this overstrain of the back and shoulder muscles the pupil slumps

back until his weight rests on the shoulder blades and lower end of the spine, leaving the center of the back unsupported. The back sags down in a single long curve, the chest contracts, the breathing is made shallow, and the circulation slows up. This position stretches the muscles and ligaments of the spine, rounds the back and shoulders, and shoves forward the chin.

CORRECT SITTING POSTURE

The correct sitting posture is one in which the pupil sits erect, the pelvis resting equally on the seat, with the arms beside the hips and the head poised so as to bring the center of gravity within a line joining the seat bones. This posture makes a minimum demand on muscular energy, and is most conducive to correct carriage. But the demands of school life do not permit the pupil to keep it long. Reading, writing, and drawing are exercises that require deviations from the ideal. If we add to these requirements ill-fitting desks and long periods of sitting, in which bad posture becomes habitual, the mischievous result cannot long be in doubt. The work of the school day should be arranged with these things in mind. The first year of the child's school life should not have more than one third of the time in confinement at the desk.

KINDERGARTEN TRAINING

Short periods of sitting, followed by double that time spent in muscular activity out of the seat, should be the rule. This activity may in most cases consist of movements correlated with intellectual exercise. In the kindergarten exercise is admirably combined with mental culture by the teaching of imitative games in which the large muscle groups are exercised in hopping, jumping, and running, and in imitating with the arms the flight of birds and insects. The circulation is stimulated and postural faults are prevented, while at the same time the child is taught valuable lessons in natural history in which his interest never flags.

TRAINING IN HIGHER GRADES

The school day of children in the higher grades should have two five-minute periods of corrective exercise at least, in addition to the games of the recess, previously described. These exercises should be designed to promote quick, strong, muscular control; to expand and enlarge the chest by deep breathing; to bring the blood from the abdomen out into the extremities; to correct spinal fatigue, and to teach the proper carriage of the body.

It is not possible for a child to remain long at rest with the weight equally on both feet, because the tension on both legs being the same, the muscles rapidly tire. The pupil instinctively rests his weight on the right, placing his left leg with bent knee out to the side as a prop. This resting position lowers the right shoulder, curves the spine, and may start the first stage of a permanent scoliosis. The best resting pose to teach is that recommended by Dr. Eliza Mosher, in which the inactive foot is placed in front instead of at the side. In this the feet can be changed as the weight-bearing leg tires.

Bad Posture

In order to decide on what may be the best rules and exercises for correct posture, bad posture must first be described. There is a test now widely used by which even the untrained teacher may form an accurate estimate of a child's posture. The first part of the test is designed to find the pupil's ability to take the erect attitude. The long axis of the trunk should continue the long axis of the head and neck. To assist the eye of the observer, a vertical line may be dropped from the front of the ear to the forward part of the foot. In poor posture the axes of the head, neck, and trunk will form a zigzag instead of a straight line.

Another simple way to estimate the extent of the deformity is to stand the child beside an upright pole or rod. The variations from correct posture are three: the so-called fatigue, or gorilla type, in which the head is thrust forward, the chest sunken, and the abdomen protruded; the round-back posture, in which the hollow at the small of the back is obliterated, a posture cultivated by faults of seating already described; and the bantam, or pouter-pigeon type, in which the chest is pushed forward and upward, and the lower spine overextended, forming a marked exaggeration of the natural lumbar curve. This posture is always the result of faulty teaching and is an exaggeration of the correct standing posture caused by the mistaken efforts on the part of the teacher to overcorrect the first two faults.

Endurance Test

A child who can assume a good posture may not be able to sustain it. Some kind of endurance test is therefore an aid whereby faults of posture may be discovered and eliminated by having the children march. As the march proceeds, old muscle habits reassert themselves, and many pupils who could hold the correct posture for a few minutes fall back into habitual faults. Heads will drop forward, shoulders droop, and chests sink, as they march. As these faults appear, the child is taken out of the marching line. Those who pass the standing and marching tests are then put through the third test, designed to show the action and endurance of the muscles of the spine and shoulders that are usually the first to yield to fatigue. When the arms are raised upward these postural muscles, if weak, allow the chin to come forward and the chest to sink backward, so that a few minutes spent in raising the arms forward and upward fully extended, lowering them sidewise and downward to the position at the start, will bring this weakness to the surface.

PHYSICAL TRAINING

Physical training is not only a matter of health. It is necessary for the education of the fundamental nerve centers of the body and the building of character. During the whole of childhood these centers are developing, and their growth is not completed until adult life. For this reason not less than one hour in five should be devoted to training the motor area of the brain, in addition to the time allowed for free play. This should take the form of both gymnastics and athletics. Gymnastics, in addition to their corrective or medical character, have a value in discipline and also in the accurate application of exercise for a given purpose; they are less diffuse than athletics, more concentrated, and for this reason they cannot be applied closely or for long to the very young, except in the guise of play. For girls, the exercises most popular are the peasant dances of Ireland, Scotland, Spain, and Sweden, in which good posture is an integral part of the dance, and agility and grace are developed.

POSTURE OF STUDENTS OF COLLEGE AGE

The necessity for good posture at college age is a logical sequence to the valuable habits learned in childhood. The college student's remediable defects must be corrected, and his physical powers trained to the highest point of efficiency. He must be taught that graceful carriage characteristic of the well-bred man. His powers of self-preservation and efficiency must be increased. If he has not learned

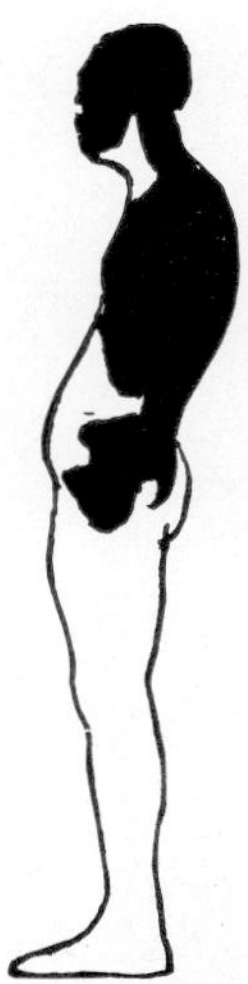

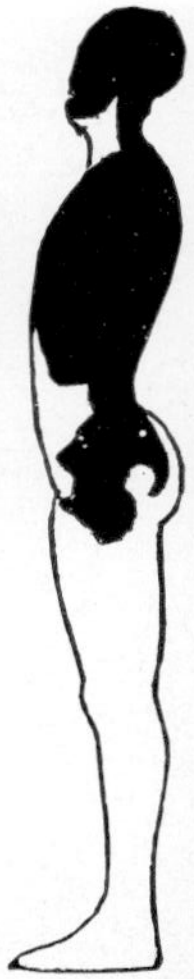

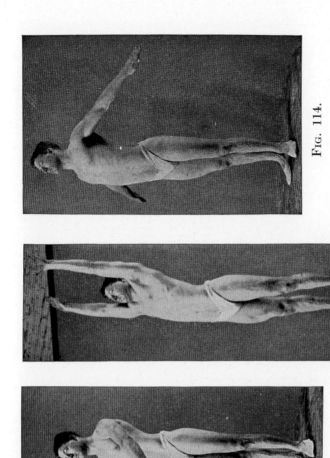

Fig. 114.

Fig. 113.

Fig. 112.

Fig. 110.   Fig. 111.

Fig. 110 shows the relation of the head, thorax, and pelvis in the incorrect standing position.   Fig. 111 shows the relation of the head, thorax, and pelvis in the correct standing position.

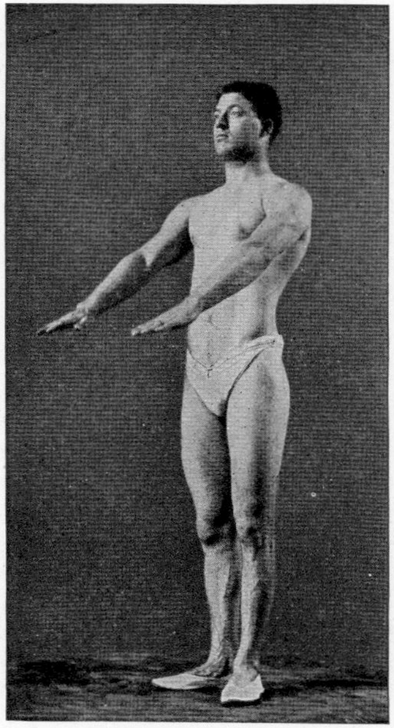

Exercise 2: Arms forward raise; upward stretch; rise on tiptoes; inhale; sideward lower; slowly press arms back and exhale.

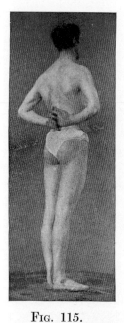

Exercise 3: Standing position; arms downward and backward; fingers interlocked; palms outward; extend neck; roll shoulders backward and forearm into supination, palms being first in, then down and then out; reverse to starting position; relax.

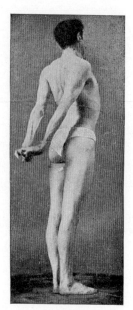

FIG. 115.

FIG. 116.

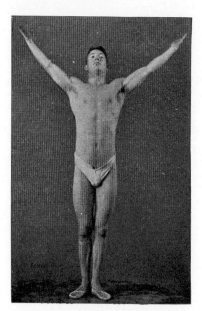

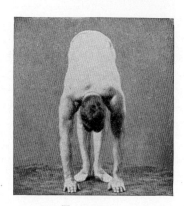

FIG. 118.

FIG. 117.

Exercise 4: Standing position; arms at sides; arms sideward raise; upward stretch; inhale; forward bend; rise; arms sideward lower; exhale.

it already, he must be given the opportunity for physical recreation through a knowledge of sports and games, for athletic activity should be the safety valve of a sedentary life, and should also teach, in addition to those social and moral qualities which can be cultivated so well in no other way, the lesson of gracefully carrying the body. That is why a university course in physical education should begin with a careful examination to find the exact bodily condition of the student and so to give an intelligent foundation on which to base advice and instruction. Nor is the examination of the student complete without a test of his ability to accomplish certain muscular feats that cover the main activities of the body, in exercises of maximum effort and of endurance.

Physical Education for Women

Physical education for women too often follows slavishly the scheme planned for men, not because it is best for women, but because it is the same. This is a deplorable mistake, because bodily training of the two sexes must differ radically in order to fit each for its own future life and environment. It cannot, with impunity, ignore the psychologic and physiologic differences between the boy and the girl and between man and woman.

In these days of professional freedom for women, with its consequent demand on their efficiency and endurance, there is much reason for women to practise good posture. Many women suffer from the effect of faulty attitude with its direct relation to pain, like backache and headache.

The first twelve years of a girl's life need differ little from that of a boy's in physical activity. She may lead the same outdoor life, climbing, swimming, running, playing ball, and nothing will prepare her so well for the great physical and mental change which takes place with the attainment of puberty. Outdoor games and exercises establish nervous stability and poise and give the best possible foundation on which to build her future womanhood.

GAMES FOR WOMEN

Women cannot stand prolonged physical or mental strain as well as men, but with frequent rests they can in the end accomplish almost as much. Certain games, such as football, boxing, pole vaulting, and heavy gymnastics, are obviously unsuited to them; but in dancing, swimming, calisthenics, archery, skating, and fencing they come much nearer to competing with men on equal terms. While they are less adapted to arduous muscular work, their vital endurance is better; so that the disadvantage they have in other activities is made up for by this greater tenacity to life. With a few exceptions, girls accustomed to athletics and gymnastics can continue exercise without detriment during menstruation, though they should refrain at that time from too exhausting contests or competitions.

Swimming is one of the best exercises for women, calling into action most of the muscles of the body, but sparing those of the back so generally overworked in standing and sitting postures.

Finally, it is quite as important to take occasional hours of absolute rest, in the recumbent position, as it is to exercise, especially when the nervous and muscular system is overwrought.

POSTURAL EFFECT OF CLOTHING

The importance of proper clothing for men, women, and children has a high place in the promotion of good posture that cannot be overemphasized, although in these days of greater freedom and simplicity in dress there is not so much need to belabor the point as there was a few generations ago. Any tendency to return to the constricting, overweighted, and too numerous garments of a few decades past should be greatly deplored.

Proper shoes have a definite effect on posture, in both children and adults. It has been found that the ground plan of the human foot varies so that it may be straight, inflared, or outflared; therefore, no one type of shoe will be suited to all types of feet. Deformities of the feet, either from the construction of the footwear or from the breaking down of the longitudinal and lateral arches of the feet, have a vital influence on posture. The balance of the foot, either flat or on a high heel, also affects the posture, although this is not so serious as was formerly supposed, if the shoe is so made that the weight rests on the heel instead of slipping forward and crowding the toes into the forward part of the shoe.

The advantage of the upright position is somewhat offset by the frequency of deformities due to a yielding of the structures concerned with support. The body may yield at the spine, at the knee joints, or at the arch of the foot, which becomes broken down and flattened, causing the deformity known as flat-foot. A typical case of flat-foot shows a turning out of the line of the heel, a convexity of the inner contour of the foot, and a concavity of its outer margin. A tracing of the foot would show no instep. The great majority of such cases are what might be termed static and are found in nurses, clerks, waiters, barbers, motormen, and all others whose long hours of continued standing keep the muscles and ligaments of the foot constantly on the strain. The pernicious habit of standing with the toes turned out always makes it worse. Flat-foot is also found in the very fat, whose weight is too much for their ligaments. Bernard Roth, in his series of 1,000 cases of twisted spine, found flat-foot in 76 per cent of them. In an examination of 1,000 supposedly normal students I have found it in 217 cases. Lovett has found many cases among hospital nurses, who are peculiarly susceptible to it. The symptoms are varied. A considerable degree of flat-foot may be present without causing much irritation, and again great pain may be caused by a comparatively slight degree of this deformity. In any case, the close association between footwear and posture must always be kept in mind. The Posture League has designed shoes of the straight, inflared, and outflared types, providing for this natural variation in the normal foot, and at the same time correcting or preventing a position which would tend to drop the arches and produce pain or deformity.

Clothing and Round Shoulders

Another frequent postural deformity caused or aggravated by improper clothing is round or uneven shoulders. Clothing which is supported by suspenders bearing on the points of the shoulders tends to pull them downward and forward. It is a common deformity among school children, and occurs in almost 20 per cent of university students uncomplicated with other postural defects. It is frequently discovered in girls about the age of puberty, when especial attention is apt to be paid to their figure and carriage. Round shoulders are not likely to be outgrown, and patients usually become permanently and structurally set in the faulty posture, with flattened chest walls and distorted figure.

The clothing should be examined, and when found to be supported from the tip of the shoulders the garments should be altered to bring the pressure in toward the root of the neck, instead of out on the shoulders. It has been pointed out that the cut of most ready-made clothing causes pressure on the back of the neck and tip of the shoulders, constantly tending to produce this deformity. Such clothing, especially men's and boys' suit coats, and men's, women's, and children's top coats, should be bought with particular care that the shape of the shoulders and backs of these garments do not have a tendency to encourage poor posture.

EXERCISES FOR FAULTY POSTURE

The following six exercises are recommended for the correction of the ordinary case of faulty posture:

1. With the patient standing in his habitual faulty position, place the hand about one inch in front of the sternum and tell him to raise the chest and shove it forward to touch the hand without swaying the body. He will at first try to draw the shoulders back, but this fault must be overcome at the very beginning, and the shoulder muscles must be kept relaxed. Gradually increase the distance to which he can bring the chest forward, repeating it again and again until he can take the position without difficulty and without contracting the muscles of the back. While in this position make him breathe deeply five times and then relax. This should be done before a mirror, so that he will recognize the feeling of the correct posture and associate it with the proper attitude as seen in the glass. He should then try to take it without looking at the mirror. This posture should be drilled into him until it becomes habitual and until he can maintain it without discomfort. R. J. Roberts, of Boston, used to tell his young men to press the backs of their necks against the collar button, considering this as the keynote of the position. In whatever way it is accomplished, the object is to get the proper relation between the thorax and the pelvis.

After repeating Exercise 1 twenty times, take:

2. Arms forward raise, upward stretch, rise on tiptoes, inhale. Sideward lower, slowly press the arms back, and exhale. This exercise, when done correctly, expands the chest, bringing in all the extensors of the back and levators of the shoulders.

3. The patient stands, arms downward and backward, fingers interlocked and palms outward. Extend the neck, roll the shoulders backward and forearms into supination, the palms being first in, then down, and then out. Reverse to starting position and relax. This exercise is valuable for projecting the chest forward, stretching the shortened ligaments, and drawing in the abdomen. Care should be taken to have the chin pressed backward when the arms are brought downward and

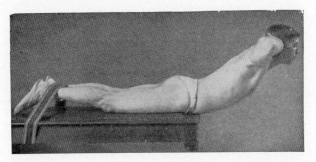

FIG. 119.

Exercise 5: Lie prone on couch with feet strapped; clasp hands behind head; raise head and extend spine, pressing elbows backward.

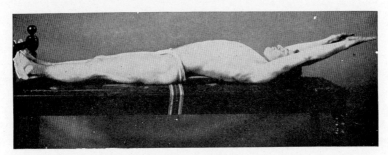

FIG. 120.

The above photograph illustrates a deep breathing exercise, which should be taken to relieve the severity of exercise 5.

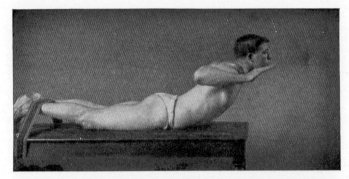

FIG. 121.

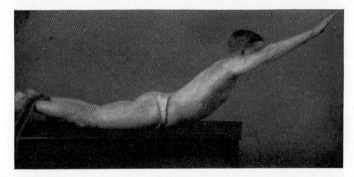

FIG. 122.

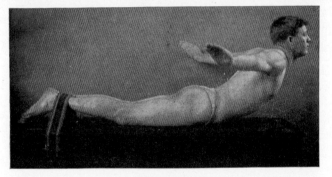

FIG. 123.

Exercise 6: Position similar to that in exercise 4; arms at sides; raise head, bringing arms forward; imitate breast stroke in swimming.

turned outward. In resistant cases, where this exercise cannot be done with the fingers interlocked, a handkerchief tied in a loop may be substituted and held in the fingers.

4. Patient stands with the arms at the sides. Arms sideward raise, upward stretch, inhale, forward bend, and rise. Arms sideward, lower, exhale. In this exercise the lungs are filled when the chest is in the most favorable position for expansion. The breath is retained when the trunk is flexed, forcing the air into the cells of the lungs under pressure. The bending and rising bring into powerful action the extensors of the back and neck and the retractors of the shoulders.

5. Patient lies prone on a couch with the feet strapped, or upon the floor with the feet caught on the edge of a bureau or other article of furniture. Hands clasped behind the head. Raise the head and extend the spine, pressing the elbows backward. This exercise is a severe one on the extensors of the back and the retractors of the shoulders, and should be followed by a deep breathing exercise.

6. Patient lies in similar position as in Exercise 5, arms at the sides. Raise the head, bringing the arms forward. Imitate the breast stroke in swimming.

In this exercise the spine is kept in static contraction, while the retractors of the shoulders are alternately contracted and relaxed.

CHAPTER XXXI

The Foot

PHILIP LEWIN, M.D.

THE FOOT MAKES CONTACT in the majority of cases between man and the world in which he lives. Because the human being formerly walked on four feet he is relatively unstable on two. It is important, indeed, that his feet and ankles be so constructed that he has stability when standing, that he moves easily, that there is comfort both in standing and in walking, and that the tissues themselves are healthy. This requires good circulation of the blood and adequate nerve supply. It is surprising how comparatively small the degree of motion in the ankle joint may be consistent with adequate walking. However, some degree of painless, free motion is essential, particularly if one desires grace and spring to the step. It is only necessary to compare the beautiful stride and grace of movements about the stage of leading actresses with the awkward motion of hands, limbs, and feet of less accomplished performers to realize how significant a graceful gait may be for a general impression of beauty.

The conditions which affect the feet include those which are present at birth, deformities which are acquired due to accidents, diseases of the bones, joints, muscles, and nerves, and disturbances of the circulation of blood to the feet. Many children are born with absence of certain toes, with webs between the toes like a duck, with extra toes, with overgrowth of the leg and foot, and sometimes with one toe lapping over another. Some of these disturbances are of slight importance, but they make it difficult to secure suitable shoes or to walk satisfactorily, in which cases surgical attention may be necessary.

There may be deformities of the feet due to tuberculosis, syphilis, infantile paralysis, other infections, breaking down of the arches, and turning inward or outward of the foot, each of these conditions demanding special consideration. If one falls heavily on the foot, or if the foot is given a hard blow, the bones may fracture. If the foot is suddenly twisted, there is dislocation or a sprain, and sometimes portions of the bones pull apart. Then, too, the surface of the foot may be subjected to the occurrence of warts, small tumors, the development of corns due to either infection or excessive rubbing, and similar disturbances.

The foot is so definitely associated with the posture of the body generally and with the jarring of the tissues within the abdomen and skull, that any interference with its function may affect the whole body. Many disturbances in the leg, the knee, the back, the hip, and disturbances of health generally are associated primarily with deficiencies of action of the feet. When man walked on four feet he was a dweller in fields and meadows. With the development of the city have come hard floors, cement sidewalks, and asphalt streets; with the growth of civilization have come shoes and stockings; with changes in transportation, automobiles and street cars. All of these affect the use of the feet and may be partially responsible for some of the difficulties which are commonly seen by orthopedic surgeons and other specialists in diseases affecting locomotion.

FUNCTIONS OF THE FEET

As has been previously mentioned, there are two chief functions of the feet: (1) To bear the weight of the body; (2) to permit easy walking. The weight-bearing line is determined by dropping a plumb line from the middle of the kneecap; this falls through the middle of the mortise bone of the ankle and through a point between the first and second toes. The two large bones of the foot are this mortise bone, between the leg and the foot, and the heel bone or os calcis. The heel bone serves as the attachment for a tendon known as the Achilles tendon. It will be remembered that in the Greek mythology the weak point of Achilles was in his heel. The heel bone furnishes the initial bearing surface of the foot as it strikes the ground in walking.

SHOES

Millions of words have been written about shoes, and everyone who manufactures them seems to have his own ideas. There are shoes with flexible shanks and shoes with rigid shanks, as well as shoes with semi-flexible and semi-rigid shanks. People without any foot troubles may do well in flexible shank shoes. Those who have foot trouble, however, and who require both exercise and support, will sometimes feel much better with shoes with a rigid shank. It is believed that the best type of shoes have round toes, medium-width shanks, and are made over a last with a straight inner border. Extremes in the height of heels are undesirable, and a good heel is neither too low nor too high, nor set too far forward or too far backward.

Few people understand how to take care of their shoes properly. Shoes will last much longer and give much better service from the

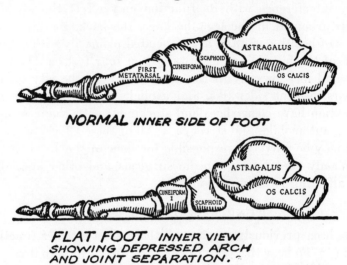

NORMAL *INNER SIDE OF FOOT*

FLAT FOOT *INNER VIEW*
SHOWING DEPRESSED ARCH
AND JOINT SEPARATION.

FIG. 124.   Showing what happens in case of a fallen arch.

point of view of protecting the feet if they are changed at least once daily, and if the pair that is not in action is kept on a suitable shoe tree or shoe form. The rubber heel has proved so well its advantage in minimizing shock to the feet and thereby to the other organs of the body that there is no longer need to emphasize its virtues.

It is now well established that the circulation to the feet must be well maintained if the toes are to be healthful. Such circulation is not maintained when the upper leg is too greatly constricted by tight garters or by rolling the stockings in a hard ridge or knot. Such constriction causes interference with the regular flow of blood and tends to break down the valves in the veins, resulting in varicosity. A recent improvement is the development of stockings with a slight flexible top, thus preventing constriction and making garters unnecessary.

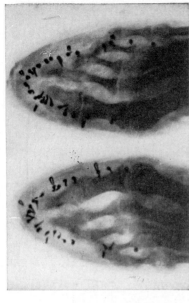

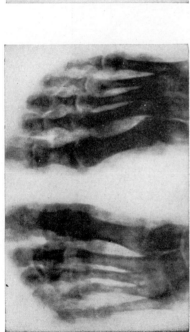

FIG. 126. Effect of too narrow, too short and pointed toed shoes showing cramped position of bones in feet.

FIG. 125. Natural position of the bones in normal foot.

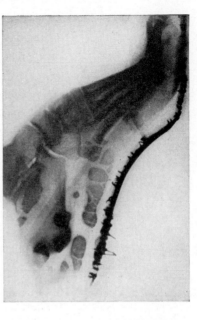

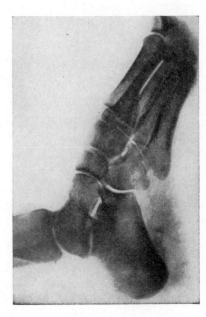

FIG. 128. X-ray normal foot wearing high heel.

FIG. 127. X-ray normal foot.

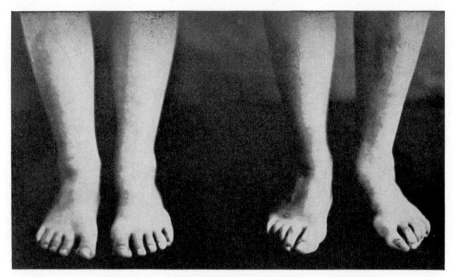

FIG. 129.

Left: Normal Feet. Right: Defects apparently caused by wearing a shoe too short and too narrow.

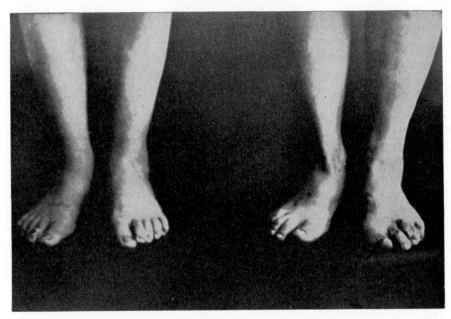

FIG. 130

Left: Defects apparently caused by wearing tight shoes. Right: Deformities apparently caused by wearing short and poorly constructed shoes.

HYGIENE

If they are to be preserved in a good state of health, feet must be kept clean. Certainly they should be bathed once daily, preferably with nonirritating soap. After being dried, the foot may be dusted with a simple talcum powder. In exceptional conditions it may be desirable to have other types of dusting powders, but these should be selected by a physician according to the nature of the condition for which these special dusting powders are to be used. These powders frequently contain salicylic and boric acids. Long applications of medicaments of this kind to the feet may result in maceration, or softening and destruction, and burning of the skin.

A simple measure for aiding to maintain the circulation of the legs and feet in health is the use of the so-called contrast bath. Two large buckets big enough to hold both feet and perhaps to reach up halfway to the knee are needed for the purpose. In one bucket warm water is placed, about 110 degrees F., or sufficient to feel distinctly hot. It is useful if this bucket is in relationship to the hot-water faucet so that additional hot water may be added to keep up the temperature. The other bucket is filled two-thirds full of cool water. The person who is taking the contrast bath sits between the two buckets. He first places both feet in the warm water for one minute, then removes the feet and places them in the cool water for one minute. This procedure is alternated for ten minutes. The alternating dilatation and contraction of the blood vessels is helpful exercise and induces circulation in the tissues. The same effects may be secured by spraying alternately with hot and cold water for one minute each.

There is nothing so restful as massage of the feet, particularly after a tiresome day. The feet may be kneaded with rotary movement of the fingers. If the skin is easily macerated, cold cream, olive oil, cocoa butter, or similar suitable ointments, may be used to lessen irritation. In many instances, when the foot is inflamed because of excessive walking or standing, hot applications in the form of moist dressings of saturated solutions of epsom salts may be helpful to bring about relief.

Most feet get enough exercise simply by walking. For the abnormal foot with weakness of the arches, many special exercises have been developed which are exceedingly useful in strengthening the tissues. These are adapted particularly to the treatment of flat-feet.

FLAT-FEET

The feet of the baby should be examined soon after birth, perhaps not later than at six months, and then again each year to make certain that they are developing properly, and that corrective measures in the form of suitable shoes, supports, or braces are not needed. The exact cause of flat-feet is not known, but it is believed that there is a hereditary tendency, since they tend to run in families. Moreover, some races tend to be more flat-footed than others. When the feet grow rapidly, especially in young adolescent girls, and when improper shoes are worn at the same time, flat-feet are likely to develop.

Flatness of the feet appears most commonly in fat people: first, because the feet carry excessive weight and there is a disproportion between the weight carried and the size of the feet; second, because there are usually associated disturbances of the glands of metabolism in children who are overfat. Such disturbances are likely to be associated with deformities in the growth of the bones and ligaments.

In many instances, flat-feet may be the result of accidents, such as falling suddenly from a height, or similar disturbance, but these are' easily determinable. The child with flat-feet is generally found to be under par so far as its general muscular condition is concerned. These children frequently have knock-knees, the back is rounded, and the mother says that the child is awkward. The shoes are run over in unnatural ways along the borders. The foot is usually not painful in the child because it is still flexible, but the child manifests a disinclination to run and to play.

A competent study of the feet by one who knows how to measure the arch and to determine its functional condition will usually reveal the character of the disturbance. A mere print of the foot, the type of examination frequently given in shoe stores which promote "health" shoes on a pseudo-scientific basis, is not sufficient examination to indicate the real nature of flat-foot. The specialist in care of the feet first determines the extent of the disability and then applies his treatment specifically to the causes and the conditions found. His purpose is to teach proper walking, to increase the power of the supporting structures, to stimulate the circulation of the blood, and to correct conditions associated with flat-feet, such as knock-knees and bowlegs.

Children who have flat-feet must be taught to walk with the feet parallel or toeing in slightly. In walking, the weight comes down on

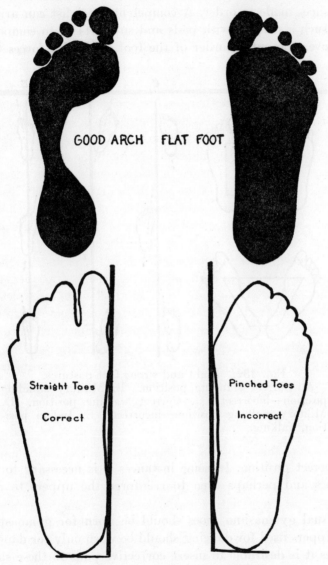

GOOD ARCH   FLAT FOOT

Straight Toes   Pinched Toes

Correct   Incorrect

FIG. 131.   Footprints indicating quality of the
arch.

the heels and is tilted toward the outer border of the feet, coming up
on the toes with a spring. In few instances of flat-feet is it necessary
to have shoes made to order. A competent specialist can arrange the
heels in such a manner with pads and supports as to compel a child
to walk over the outer border of the foot. This also forces the ankle

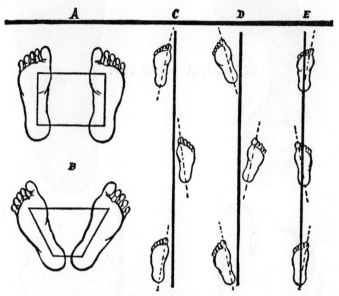

FIG. 132.   Right and wrong foot postures.
A. Correct standing position. B. Military standing
position—incorrect. C. Correct walking position. D.
Military walking position—incorrect. E. Indian position, walking.

into a correct position. In some instances it is necessary to insist on
high shoes and perhaps even to reënforce the uppers to aid weak
ankles.

The usual gymnasium shoes should be worn for gymnastics only.
Ballet slippers used for dancing should be worn only for dancing, and
sometimes it is desirable to insert corrective pads in these shoes also.
Children with flat-feet should not go barefoot, except in the sand, nor
should they wear bedroom slippers around the house, since the shoe is
a corrective measure and should be worn at all times when the feet are
in use.

Most authorities recommend a series of exercises helpful in cor-

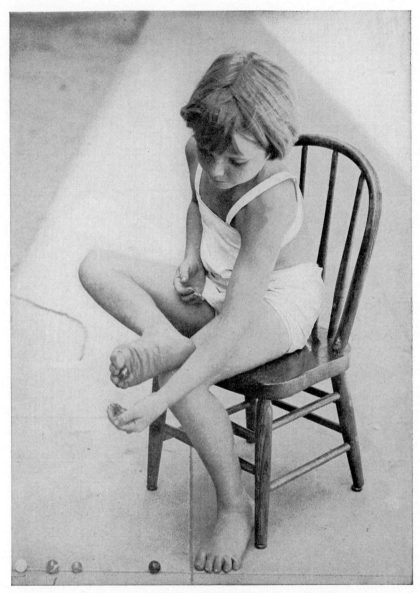

Fig. 133. Picking up marble with one foot and placing it in opposite hand is good corrective exercise for flat-foot.

recting flat-feet. It is difficult frequently to get children to use these exercises, but if they are taught as a game, the child is likely to participate with enjoyment. The list of exercises includes:

1. Stand barefooted with the feet parallel and about two inches apart, straddling a seam or a line in a rug. On the count of one, force the feet apart without really letting them move apart, thus throwing the weight on their outer borders; on the count of two, let them roll in slowly, but not all the way. This is repeated ten times at first, with a gradual daily increase that may run up to one hundred.

2. Same as number 1, except that the two big toes are held together and on the floor.

3. Straddling a seam in the rug or a line on the floor, walk across the room with all the weight on the outer borders of the feet, and the toes curled downward and inward. Make the round trip five times.

4. This is the same as number 3, except that you lift one foot so that it is opposite the other knee, and walk across the room in that way, using the so-called "ostrich step." Weight must at all times be borne on the outer border of the foot.

5. The feet are held parallel, and the knees are maintained in a straight position. The knees are then rolled outward, which automatically causes the longitudinal arch to rise (Lowman). This is repeated from ten to twenty-five times.

6. Rise on the toes, tilt the weight to the outer borders, and come down in two counts. This should be done ten to twenty-five times.

7. Use a supination board, about six inches high and eight feet long, its sloping sides being at the angle of an isosceles triangle. The child walks the length of the board three or four times as one would walk on the ridge of a house-roof.

8. The subject is seated on a chair with legs crossed, so that the raised foot can relax. He then holds the foot at right angles with the leg and not turned in or out. The exercise is done in four counts. On the count of one, the foot is allowed to relax into the position of toe-drop. On the count of two, it is swung in; on the count of three, it is forcibly pulled upward; and on the count of four, it is brought back to the starting position, describing a half circle. This is performed ten times at first, and may gradually be increased to twenty-five times.

9. This is a resistive exercise. The subject sits on a table, and a second person sits on a chair. The subject forcibly swings his foot inward and upward, and holds it in this position with all his power. The second person attempts to swing the foot outward and downward. This effort on the part of the second person is resisted by the subject.

The exercise is carried out from ten to twenty-five times. At no time should the second person use as much power as the first.

10. Older children and adults can perform this exercise as follows: The right foot is turned inward and upward and held in that position firmly. The left foot is placed against the right, and attempts to force the right outward, which effort the right foot resists. Then the feet are reversed. After each of these exercises the subject relaxes his foot.

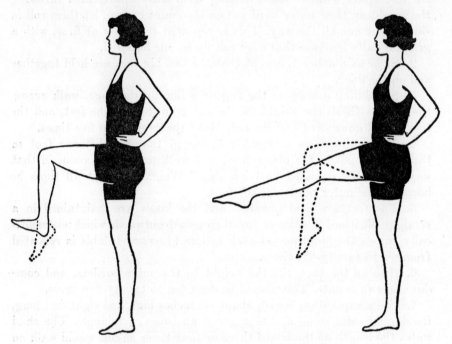

FIG. 134.   Exercise to strengthen the foot.

In addition to these exercises, which are helpful in flat-feet, the circulation may be benefited by the use of the contrast baths previously described. Occasionally operations are necessary to lengthen heel tendons in muscle-bound feet, but in the majority of cases of flat-feet a surgical operation is seldom indicated. A few special exercises have been developed for stretching the Achilles tendon of the heel:

1. Simply walking on the heels across the room five times.

2. From the standing position with the feet parallel, the patient squats down to the position of sitting on the heels, maintaining the heels and toes on the ground. This is done in two counts.

3. The patient stands facing the wall with the toes twenty-eight

inches from it. The toes are placed together and the heels as far apart as possible. With the hands placed against the wall and the heels maintained on the floor, the entire rigid body is allowed to fall forward as far as possible by bending the elbows, and to remain in this position a few seconds before returning to the starting position. This is done in two counts, about ten times.

4. The apparatus for this exercise consists of two handles fastened to the wall and a heavy wooden block three and one-half inches high, twelve inches wide and seven inches in depth, fastened to the floor. The patient faces the wall, standing with the forward parts of both feet on the block, and holding onto the handles. On the count of one, the heels are allowed to touch the floor, the body being kept parallel with the wall. On the count of two, the return is made to the starting position. The exercise is carried out from ten to twenty times, this number being attained gradually.

5. The patient stands with the forward half of each foot on a stair, facing upward and holding the balustrade, and allows the heels to drop. He then returns to the starting position.

FALLEN ARCHES

In many instances, feet are exceedingly painful because of a condition affecting the main bone of the foot, the astragalus. This is particularly the case in the condition commonly called fallen arch, a condition which occurs more often in women than in men. When there is a general infection of the body with rheumatic disorders of one type or another, the bones of the foot may be involved. Obviously, such infections are associated with inflammation and, therefore, exceedingly painful. Tailors, people who stand long hours on their feet, such as motormen or saleswomen, are especially likely to be disturbed by painful feet due to extraordinary stress on the arches. There are pain and rigidity of the tissues and at times even spasms of the muscles in the effort to overcome the pressure.

A study of 97 workers in a department store, who had never complained of foot trouble, revealed the fact that 37 had foot trouble or foot strain; 43 wore shoes that were too short; 40 had heels which upset the body posture; 19 wore heels so high that they were injurious, and in 5 per cent of the cases the shoes were so badly fitted that they produced distortion of the feet.

In case the arch has fallen, a groove, indicating a depression, is visible in a side view or an X-ray plate. Relief frequently occurs when the person is able to stay off the feet, but in the vast majority of cases this interferes with occupation and earning power, and few people are willing to follow such a course repeatedly.

Hot applications and massage of the feet are helpful. The padding of the shoes in such cases is very comforting. The shoes must be fitted so as to aid in supporting the arch with a rigid shank of medium

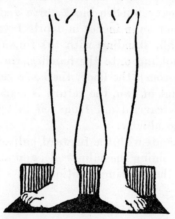

FIG. 135.   Example of rigid
flat-feet.

width. A competent authority usually will insert felt pads to support the depressed structures.

A series of suitable exercises has also been developed for the purpose of building up the tissues that support the metatarsal arch. The following exercises have been found of special value:

1. *Door-stop Exercise.* Two old fashioned door-stops, obtainable at the hardware section of one of the 5-and-10-cent stores, are prepared for use by removal of the rubber tips with a pair of nippers. Then they are screwed into a board about fourteen inches long, eight inches wide and two inches thick. The centers of the door-stops should be six inches apart. A heel rest two and three-eighth inches high is attached.

The board is placed on the floor, and the patient sits on a chair in front of it. Each foot is placed on a door-stop with slight pressure just behind the metatarsal bones. On the count of one, the toes relax slowly. This is continued until one has counted two hundred. (This number should be attained gradually.)

2. *Towel Exercise.* The patient sits in a chair. A large hand towel is spread on the carpet, with the narrow edge facing the patient. Both

feet are placed on the towel so that half of each foot is on the towel. The towel is grasped with the toes of one foot, then with the toes of the other. As the toes of one foot grasp, those of the other foot relax. This is continued until the entire towel is under the feet.

3. *Golf-ball Exercise.* A golf ball is placed on the rug and rolled under the metatarsal arch for one minute. Then it is picked up with the toes of one foot and placed under the toes of the other foot, and the exercise is repeated for another minute. The patient alternates in this manner six times.

4. *Marble Exercise.* Marbles of various sizes are placed on a rug. The patient sits on a chair and picks up the marbles with the toes and throws them forward.

5. *Pencil Exercise.* A round pencil is placed on a hard floor, and by means of the toes curled downward the patient pushes and pulls the pencil around the floor with short, quick movements.

Feet that are badly fitted with shoes are frequently subject to other conditions such as corns, calluses, bunions, hammer toes, and occasionally excessive perspiration and infections with ringworm or so-called athlete's foot.

Sprained Ankle

A sprained ankle is one of the most common injuries affecting human beings, again chiefly because they were not intended to walk originally on two feet. A slight failure of complete support throws the weight of the body unnecessarily on a group of tendons never planned to bear that much weight, and a sprain frequently follows. A sprain represents stretching or tearing of the tissues of the joints. It must not be confused with fracture, which is a breaking of bone. In many instances fracture is overlooked and the condition diagnosed simply as sprain, with the result that healing may take place very slowly.

It is, therefore, exceedingly important to have an X-ray picture taken in every doubtful case, and sometimes several pictures will be necessary to determine the presence of very small fractures in the surface of bones. Sometimes authorities treat sprains by putting on a plaster cast for a few days, elevating the foot and leg, and then applying suitable adhesive straps to give the foot complete rest.

After some seven to fourteen days, when inflammation has subsided and healing has begun, an elastic anklet may be worn. These anklets may be removed each morning and evening for contrast bath—that is, alternating baths of one minute each in hot and cold water, until the feet have been in the water ten minutes. A recent development is the application of heat through the passing of electric current through the tissues, or so-called diathermy. This tends to hasten subsiding of inflammation and recovery.

A simple outline for the treatment of sprained ankle follows:

1. Put the patient at rest promptly, assuring freedom from bearing weight on the feet.
2. Elevate the leg and ankle.
3. Apply ice bags.
4. Call a physician.

When the physician arrives, he will probably arrange to have X-ray pictures made, if necessary. He will arrange for strapping the ankle with adhesive, or, if the sprain is severe, put on a plaster-of-Paris cast. In less severe cases he is likely merely to apply a snug bandage of gauze or cotton. Under no circumstances should the feet be allowed to hang for long periods, since this will tend to accumulate fluid and produce inflammation with more pain and swelling.

PAINFUL HEELS

A painful heel may be due to many causes; sometimes there is inflammation of the heel tendon. Under such circumstances, it is desirable to prevent at once all bearing of weight on the heel bone and to apply suitable bandages or casts so as to make certain that there is a relaxation of the pull of the tendon on the muscles of the calf and on the heel bone. In addition, there must be suitable baths and massage to stimulate the tissues and aid recovery. If the condition is very slight, elevation of the heel by the use of pads of felt or sponge rubber takes off some of the strain.

In certain infections within the body, such as infection of the teeth, tonsils, or other portions, there may be associated secondary infections in the feet. Associated with this there may be injury to the tissues due to falling on the feet or the wearing of improper shoes. As a result of the continued irritation there may be a growth of bone on the lower, inner surface of the large bone of the foot, the heel bone, and the production of what are called spurs. Occasionally the development of these spurs is associated with infection, with venereal disease, but this is by no means constant.

It is, of course, exceedingly important first to determine the presence of any infection and to control that. Associated with the growth of the spur and infection there are pain, tenderness, swelling, and a tendency to limp. These come on gradually, and the pain and tenderness usually seem to be felt first along the inner border of the heel. Since painful heel may be due to a wart, to inflammation of the covering of the bone, or to an injury, it is well first to inspect very carefully the outside of the foot, and then, if the cause cannot be found, to have an X-ray picture which will promptly reveal the presence of so-called spurs with certainty.

If the foot is then placed at rest and suitably treated with heat, the pain and sensitiveness will disappear. The use of felt pads tends to relieve pain in the weight-bearing portions of the foot. In a considerable number of instances, however, operative removal of spurs of bone may be necessary.

Club-Foot

About 75 per cent of club-feet, which are present at time of birth, are of the type in which the toes point downward and inward. This occurs once in a thousand births; 65 per cent are in males, and in 57 per cent of cases the deformity is present only on one side. The exact cause of club-foot is not known, but it is said to be due sometimes to wrong position of the child previous to birth. In previous centuries such children were permitted to go crippled through life. Nowadays this is not tolerated, because it is realized that early and sufficient treatment by a competent physician will bring about cure. The chance of cure depends on the age of the child when first seen, the type and degree of the deformity, the persistence of the treatment, and similar factors. Active treatment may be necessary for months, and care and supervision for years.

The first treatment for club-foot is usually applied at birth or during infancy. The object is to correct the deformity as soon as possible and to maintain the correction until proper use of the foot has made the correction permanent. In curing club-foot, the competent orthopedic surgeon is likely to manipulate it so as to get it in proper position and to hold it in place by suitable bandages, adhesive straps, plaster-of-Paris casts, or braces.

After the correction is once established, massage, exercise, and modification of the shoes tend to hold the feet in proper position and to maintain suitably the healthful condition of the tissues. In some instances, it is impossible to control club-foot by manipulative measures and the use of casts and braces alone. In these cases it may be necessary to perform surgical operations for readjustment of the tissues or even complete reconstruction.

Ingrown Toenails

The feet are among the most abused portions of the human body and are probably responsible for about as much agony as human beings can sustain. Fashion takes no account of foot comfort or foot health. Modern shoes, particularly for women, bring about extraordinary malformations. Hiking crazes cause large numbers of people to undertake long walks with poor equipment. Motorcars keep most people from walking enough to give the feet even adequate exercise.

When a foot which has been largely neglected from the point of view of hygiene develops a complication like ingrowing toenails, the owner of that foot is in for an exceedingly painful time. The large toenail is the one usually concerned in the ingrowing procedure. Almost everyone thinks himself competent to advise on the handling of ingrown toenails. Therefore, the patient usually has tried all sorts of poultices, antiseptics, and ointments on his toe before coming to the physician. When he finally does come, the nail and the toe will be found red and swollen, with pus not infrequently exuding from under the nail. Not infrequently the infection is brought about by the practice of clipping the toenails with sharp scissors that are seldom sterilized before use.

Some simple suggestions for treatment include:

1. Stop all attempts at the use of poultices, liniments, and soaking of the foot in baths.

2. Apply tincture of iodine daily, but in relatively small amounts, to the infected portions of the nail where it comes in contact with the skin.

3. Do not attempt to manicure the nail in anything like the intricate technic used for finger nails.

4. Use a pair of surgical scissors with rounded ends, which will not lacerate the skin or do much damage if the scissors slip. Cut a shallow "v" or "u" in the middle of the nail.

5. A rolled-up wisp of cotton should be carefully tucked under the edges of the nail and saturated with castor oil.

As dressing for an ingrown nail, it is merely necessary to use a piece of surgically clean gauze, to wear stockings thick enough to afford protection, and shoes loose enough to prevent pressure but not so loose as to cause rubbing. If this procedure is followed repeatedly the ingrown toenail gradually becomes normal, and proper hygiene thereafter will keep it in that condition.

WARTS

Among the most common growths on the human skin are warts of all types. Almost everybody has a "cure" for warts and some rather foolish idea of how they originate. Warts sometimes disappear spontaneously, but the disappearance is usually credited to the fact that someone has murmured a potent charm at midnight in a cemetery or buried a string containing as many knots as there are warts. A wart causes little trouble, but it can grow awfully large in the sight of the person who owns it. The only time warts cause trouble is when they are situated in places where pressure makes them painful.

There seems to be some evidence that the wart is an infectious condition caused by a filtrable virus, or an organism so small that it cannot be seen under the microscope. However, it cannot be easily infectious, since there are many people who are in contact with warts but never get them.

The ordinary wart can be removed by many methods: sometimes merely through softening by the application of corrosive chemicals; sometimes by cutting or sandpapering, and sometimes by the application of an electric current which kills the blood supply and causes the wart to fall off. This last process is painful, but the pain may be eliminated through the use of local anesthetics. The X-ray sometimes is used to cause the disappearance of a wart. Nitric acid, glacial acetic acid, and chromic acid are also used. There is always the danger, however, that the burning will extend deeper than the wart, and as a result an unsightly scar will be left.

One of the most painful types of warts is that which occurs on the sole of the foot. There seems to be plenty of reason for believing that these are infections, since they occur particularly in young people in schools and gymnasium classes who go barefoot around the gymnasium or the swimming pool or wear each other's stockings. Such warts may become so painful as to interfere with walking. Their treatment demands the most careful consideration of a competent physician. The hard skin on the bottom of the foot must be softened, the wart removed, and the damaged tissue protected by proper bandages and antiseptics during the process of healing. Sometimes electrical methods are used for destroying these warts, but this also demands the most careful help of an expert. Operation may be necessary.

BUNIONS

During the period from 1917–1924 about 300 operations were done in a New York hospital for the relief of bunions. In this work some 25 surgeons coöperated and one of them has recently reviewed the results of 200 operations performed on 108 patients. Ninety per cent of the patients were women. Pain was the chief reason for operation in more than half the cases, but one fourth of them had the operation because the foot was badly deformed by the bunions. Indeed, one of the patients had had bunions for thirty-five years, and five of them had had them for more than twenty years.

Most of these patients had tried wearing broad shoes, arch supports, and other devices, fitted by none too competent chiropodists, before they finally decided to have the bunion removed by an operation. While the operation is simple, it is necessary for the patient to stay in the hospital in bed for from twelve to eighteen days in order to permit good recovery before an attempt is made to walk on the foot. In most instances the operation consists in the removal of part of the overgrown bone that is responsible for the pain and the deformity. After the operation patients were able to move the great toe freely in most instances, and were free from pain.

In many instances the bunion may be associated with a chronic inflammation of the joints that has localized to a certain extent in the great toe. When this is the case, operative removal of the bone does not always insure complete elimination of the condition. A physician who is thoroughly informed as to the general condition of the patient is therefore able to decide whether or not the operation may be indicated in any case. The proper selection of the operative procedure in each individual case is conceived to be of the greatest importance.

CORNS

A corn is a circumscribed thickening or hardening of the skin occurring usually on the outer side of the little toe, less often on the second toe. It is roughly cone shaped with the base looking outward and the apex extending inward and pressing on the nerves of the skin. Layers of skin become like dry scales or shells with a central point of hardening, which is called the core. This little point dips down and presses on the nerves beneath and produces pain. The cause of corns is abnormal pressure, which may be continuous or intermittent, as a rule produced by improper shoeing.

Corns are of two varieties: hard corns which occur on the exposed irritated surfaces, and soft corns which occur between the toes, usually between the fourth and fifth. The conditions necessary to produce a soft corn are, first, the approximation of the skin surfaces; second, the production of heat; third, perspiration. Often a little prominence or spur of one of the near-by bones is the cause of a soft corn.

TREATMENT OF A SOFT CORN

The horny rim should be pared down about the center, or the center itself, if it projects, and then a corn plaster applied so as to protect the corn from pressure. The parts should be kept as dry as possible by the frequent use of a lotion of salicylic acid, 1 to 3 per cent in 95 per cent alcohol, followed by a dusting powder. If the corn has become infected, one should use hot wet dressings of saturated boric acid solution before trying to treat the corn itself. In paring, one should be careful not to cut through the skin, and of course use regular surgical precautions against infection. Unless pressure on the site of the corn is prevented, it will recur. If it is impossible to get an ordinary corn plaster to remain in the proper place, one can be built up with adhesive plaster, or the adhesive plaster may be laid evenly over the whole surface of the corn and the skin immediately about it.

In order to understand the treatment for soft corns, it is important to remember that they occur only between the toes, usually between the fourth and fifth, and that the conditions necessary are contiguity of skin surfaces, moisture, and heat. There is often an opening through the skin and usually a fetid odor. Simple chiropody of itself is usually not curative. The various points under treatment are as follows: A proper straight-last, medium-shank, round-toe shoe; second, in these shoes a small felt pad, exerting pressure behind the heads of the metatarsal bones; third, special exercises to strengthen the supporting structures of the metatarsal arch; fourth, a simple dusting powder between the toes three or four times a day (bismuth formic iodide is excellent) ; fifth, the preparation of a stocking, making a stall for the fifth toe, as a thumb in a mitten; sixth, X-ray treatment; seventh, radium treatment; eighth, electrical treatment; and ninth, operation, consisting of removal of the soft corn and the opening in the skin, if present, and the removal of a bony spur from the phalanx.

Soft corns should be kept clean and dry. They should be washed frequently with alcohol, dried, and powdered. The application of concentrated nitric acid or the solid stick of nitrate of silver may be effective.

The treatment of an ordinary hard corn is in most cases unsatisfactory, as after removal it recurs when pressure is again applied. A time-honored remedy is salicylic acid in collodion or ointment. The most important prophylactic measures are correctly fitted proper shoes and hosiery. Palliative treatment consists of immersion in hot water and soap, after which the lesion is pared and covered with adhesive strips or a protective ring-shaped pad.

Perspiring Feet

Hyperhidrosis or excessive perspiration of the feet is a common and troublesome condition. It is most commonly found in overweight individuals—both children and adults—in whom there seems to be a glandular disturbance of some kind. The treatment consists in local applications of 25 per cent of aluminum chloride solution painted on the surface of the foot three nights in succession. The patient should discontinue the treatment for about a week, when he should resume the application for three nights in succession again. Washing the feet two or three times daily is helpful. Chromic acid, grs. 2 to the ounce, may be used as a foot wash, this to be followed by dusting powder on the foot and in the hose. This powder to contain salicylic acid, grains 2 in 1 ounce of talcum powder.

X-ray treatment is usually successful.

CHAPTER XXXII

Nervous and Mental Disorders
GEORGE K. PRATT, M.D.

W<small>E COME NOW</small> to that part of the book which deals with nervous and mental disorders. Readers will find it rather different from other chapters, dealing with physical illness, since in mental disease we are not concerned with a single condition like typhoid fever or appendicitis, but with many conditions, each different in a way from the others, and each of its own degree of severity and curability. Moreover, in nervous and mental diseases we are required to look to a great number of rather complicated causes in order to explain these conditions. But while it will prove a little more difficult for the reader to understand the complexities of nervous and mental disease, the fascination of the subject may more than make up for any difficulty encountered in this chapter.

In the first place, abnormal mental conditions were not always regarded as forms of sickness. As a matter of fact, departures from average mentality in bygone centuries were usually considered to be religious or legal problems, and it was not until well into the seventeenth century that official medicine acknowledged responsibility for including "insanity" as a variety of sickness coming under its province. At first, the physicians of that day hardly knew what to do about this newcomer to the medical sciences. Not very much was known about its symptoms (except a few of the more violent, spectacular ones) and still less was known about what caused it or how to cure it. So for a long time the best medicine could do for mental patients was to see that they were given humane care in suitable institutions and were no longer maltreated or subjected to the abuse that formerly was the lot of the insane in practically every country

825

of the world. For this reason these institutions very suitably were called "asylums."

Gradually, however, physicians here and there came to be interested in these mentally sick people and to engage in various pieces of scientific research with regard to different aspects of their condition. First of all it was discovered that mental disease was not just one sickness, but was, instead, a term that applied to a large number of sicknesses; secondly, that these various kinds of mental disease often had quite different symptoms; and thirdly, that some cases always seemed mild while others were severe. As a result of these observations it became possible at last to classify the different kinds of mental disease and to pin labels on them. This was a great advance over the previous state of scientific ignorance that had shrouded the whole subject, and for a long time afterwards physicians devoted most of their attention to describing, classifying, and diagnosing the many divisions and subdivisions and sub-subdivisions that were coming, with a slow increase of knowledge, to be recognized.

Unhappily for the patients, however, while all this describing and classifying was a necessary step forward to a more scientific understanding of their difficulties, it failed to do very much in a practical way toward getting them well. At last some of the doctors themselves rebelled against what they said was the outmoded practice of trying to understand human behavior on a basis of *what* it was (a basis of description only), rather than *why* it was, and so research was begun in some other directions. These doctors called to their assistance certain other sciences, particularly psychology and philosophy, and between them they commenced to study the problem of *why* people acted as they did and what it was that made them say the things they said.

One group of physicians attacked the problem from the conventional angle of physical medicine. They began to search in the physical make-up of the patient's body for the motives that underlay human behavior. In quite a few mentally disturbed people they were able to find physical diseases—or at least disorders of physical functions—that seemed to account for the symptoms. Thus, in that type of mental disease known as general paresis they found it possible to see with the microscope and often with the naked eye certain areas in the patient's brain where the consistency of the tissue was altered and partially liquefied. They also discovered (much later) that the cause of all the trouble in these particular cases was the tiny micro-organism of syphilis which had invaded the brain and central nervous system. This same group of physicians also were able to point out that certain other types of mental diseases were associated with other un-recognized areas of infection in teeth or intestines. But when all was said and done by this group, there yet remained to be accounted for a majority of all the known abnormal mental conditions for which the most scientific study failed to find any adequate physical cause.

Thereupon a second group of doctors began to attack the problem from what they called the functional rather than the organic point of view. If, reasoned this second group, there are many unusual displays of behavior that do not seem to have a physical cause, then let us begin with some of the cases of insanity in institutions that seem free from any organic disease and see what we can learn by studying, not just the structure and physiology of their organs, including their brains, but also their psychology. In other words, let's study man as a *whole*. This was somewhat of a novel medical idea in those days, for up to that time most physicians had devoted their efforts to studying anatomical fragments of the patient such as heart or liver or lungs, and what these fragments did and how they acted. Now it was pro-posed to study, not so much what these special organs did, but what *the whole patient did* who owned these organs. This method finally became known as the study of "total reactions" and is the method that is being given increasing attention today.

One of the first discoveries resulting from the application of this "total reaction" method was one so obvious that it had been usually overlooked heretofore. This was the realization that the symptoms exhibited by men and women with various types of mental disorder bore a close (if slightly disguised) resemblance to the basic person-alities and traits of character that had marked these persons for many years before they became mentally sick. In other words, the mental disease symptoms, when properly interpreted, were seen to be but exaggerations of similar symptoms in evidence, perhaps, from child-hood, but milder, of course, at that earlier age, and unrecognized then as anything more significant than "queer" or annoying or fussy habits of personality. This discovery, as might be anticipated, led quickly to the formulation of an axiom to the effect that there usually is a close connection between adult mental disorder and the development of unhealthy "patterns" (or habits) of personality during the plastic years of childhood, when personality is in the process of being molded. By applying this axiom it is often possible today to predict with a fair degree of accuracy whether a given child will grow up to become an adult who develops some form of mental disease, or whether he will go through life with his mental health unimpaired. Thus, a child whose "patterns" of personality are so sound and sturdy that they enable him to meet in a healthy manner disappointment in life, failure, or frustration is the child who will probably become an adult free from mental disorder. But another child may develop patterns that prove feeble reeds on which to lean when disappointment or failure confront him. As a consequence, he is unable to adjust himself in a wholesome manner to these trying experiences and is forced instead to flee into some form of mental disease as a sort of compromise adjustment.

Causes of Mental Disorders

Which brings us to one of the most important of all the discoveries made by this group of scientists searching for the answer to the question of why people behave as they do. This discovery had to do with the causes for unusual behavior, of which mental disease is, of course, one example. It was learned, for instance, that one patient was supposed to have become mentally sick because he lost his job and all his money. Another's mental disorder was attributed to a disappointment in love, and so on. But as knowledge of psychiatry (which is that branch of medicine dealing with nervous and mental diseases) began to grow, it finally became evident that many of these alleged causes were not the real basic causes at all but merely *precipitating* causes. That is, the loss of money or the disappointment in love were only the last straws to break the camel's back—the final strains on an adjustive capacity that had never been very strong in the first place. Otherwise, everyone who lost his money or was disappointed in love might be expected to develop mental disease as a result. This would be contrary to the facts, for, as we all realize, the great majority of men and women faced with similar difficulties manage to adjust to them without having to take recourse to mental disorder. And so there grew up the belief among modern psychiatrists that so far as most functional mental disorders were concerned (those in which it is not possible to find a physical cause) the true and basic cause went back to a failure on the part of the patient to adjust himself to certain of the mental conflicts that beset him. Before going any farther with this story of mental disorder, let us stop for a moment to examine some of these mental conflicts and see why it is so hard to adjust to them.

It is necessary first of all to accept the view that when a child is born into the world he brings with him a variety of psychological baggage. Part of this consists of his intellectual endowment, but at the moment we are more concerned with another part which might be called certain emotional tendencies inherited from his immediate ancestors—parents and grandparents. Still a third part—one that is beginning to receive a great deal of serious attention nowadays—consists of an assortment of primitive, savage instincts and "drives," which he also inherits as his share of the heritage of all mankind. These might be thought of as racial tendencies which the whole human race inherits from its ancestors of millions of years ago. These primitive instincts or "drives" include the instinct of self-preservation as well as that of race-preservation and many others. In those days, countless ages ago when man was first beginning his long painful struggle toward his present stage of development, we may imagine there were few niceties. People did about as they pleased. If one caveman was hungry and his neighbor had a fresh piece of bear meat, the first man killed him—if he could—and took what he needed to keep himself alive. If a second cave man took a fancy to the woman of a third, he seized her—if he could—and henceforth she was his, at least until a still stronger caveman took her away from him in turn. And so it went. Life probably was a pretty simple, crude (according to present standards), direct sort of affair. Men and women did what they wanted to whenever they felt like it with little to hinder them except the one restraint of superior physical strength, and there was scant place in the tribal code of that day for those more civilized feelings of altruism and unselfishness.

But slowly man came to be civilized. Slowly he came to realize that the first stirrings of finer needs within him could not always be satisfied by brute force alone, and that it was to the broader interests of that new, finer part of him, as well as to the interests of his group as a whole, to make a place in his scheme of things for regulations, prohibitions, and self-imposed restraints. This was not accomplished, however, without protests from the other part of him that longed for the "good old days" when there were no restraints and man did as he pleased unless someone stronger prevented. Here, then, developed mental conflict—a conflict between desire versus duty; between the savage, primitive instincts that formerly were expressed in crude, direct form with no pretense at disguising them, and the dawning realization that the demands of individual and social progress called for the repression or the transformation of some of these primitive instincts into more socially acceptable ones.

In the tens of thousands of years that have elapsed since this conflict first began, one might suppose that advancing cultural development has succeeded in annihilating these raw, primitive "drives" whose direct display had become, by this time, quite taboo. But here is where another discovery of modern psychiatry throws an interesting light on human behavior. Doctors know that the human body today harbors several vestigial remains or remnants of organs that have no known function in a 1935 model body, but which are believed to have served a vitally necessary purpose in the human body of millions of years ago. Thus, the human appendix as well as the tonsils have no known useful function in this day and age, unless, as some wag once remarked, it is to enable surgeons to ride in limousines. Anatomists likewise tell us that transformed remains of gill slits, dating back to the time when man was emerging from the amphibian stage of his upward development, can still be found in people today. But in the psychological field something of the same thing is believed also to have occurred, and psychiatrists insist that modern man carries with him in the unconscious part of his mind certain vestigial remains of ancient instincts and impulses that once served a useful purpose when given frank, direct expression, but which thousands of centuries of civilization now demand be modified.

This is what is meant when we say that a child is born into the world with psychological baggage that includes—'way down deep in his unconscious—the carry-over of some of these primitive "drives." And this is why every modern nursery school teacher will tell you that the very young child is completely selfish (selfish, that is, when viewed from our adult standards) and completely antisocial as well. In other words, for the first two or three years of his life the child wants to do what he wants when he wants, without any interference. His tiny mental life for this period is much nearer that of his primitive caveman ancestors than it is of his immediate generation, and at first he tries to act accordingly. He demands immediate gratification of all his desires. If he is hungry for food, he demands to be fed—

instantly. If he is hungry for attention, he insists on being cuddled. If he is uncomfortable from a full bladder, he wets himself at once and in any place. He has no consideration for the feelings of others, and his chief aim in life is to get pleasure and avoid pain.

But as he grows older his mother begins to train him in food and toilet habits. She tries to teach him to control his wants, to wait for more appropriate times for their expression. She also, lovingly but firmly, gets it across to him that he can't always have his own way; that self-gratification is only possible through some consideration of others, or is dependent on the will of someone who is stronger. And so gradually he is required to submit to that process known as the "civilization of instinct," and he becomes a more socialized creature. But do not make the mistake of thinking that because he gradually checks some of his primitive desires and shows a willingness to give in to others, he has lost these desires or that he has become altruistic all of a sudden. To be sure, he has learned it is to his advantage to make concessions to this mother-person who has the power to bestow or withhold pleasure; who can approve or punish. And he likewise comes to the conclusion that gratification of his pleasure needs often must come in a roundabout manner, after first placating mother, who stands in the rôle of authority. That is how genuine unselfishness and altruism have their beginnings. The child learns that full gratification requires the coöperation of others, and he becomes altruistic only as he comes to realize that it pays to be altruistic because one gets the most pleasure out of life that way. Nevertheless, while he may submit gracefully to the "civilization of instinct" with a minimum of protest, the savage instincts are always there under the surface of conscious- ness, and the individual, no matter how old he grows to be, is forever trying to shape his mental life in accordance with what the followers of the school of dynamic psychology call the "pleasure principle." But opposed to this pleasure principle is another called the "reality prin- ciple." Both are pulling, in the unconscious mind of the person, in different directions. Swayed by the pleasure principle, he seeks to act in a way that will insure immediate gratification of primitive desires but avoids as much unpleasantness in the process as possible. In the opposite direction he experiences a pull from the reality prin- ciple which tends to shape his mental life according to the demands of necessity as personified at first by the stronger power of the parents and later by the customs of society. Dr. Abraham Myerson, a distinguished psychiatrist in Boston, writing about these conflicts, has this to say about them:

> Every human being is a pot boiling with desires, passions, lusts, wishes, purposes, ideas and emotions, some of which he clearly recognizes and clearly admits, and some of which he does not clearly recognize and which he would deny. These desires, passions, etc., are not in harmony with one another; they are often irreconcilable, and one has to be smothered for the sake of the other. Thus, a sex feeling that is not legitimate, an illicit forbidden love has to be conquered for the purpose of being religious or good, or the desire to be respected. So one may struggle against hatred for a person whom one should love—a husband, a wife, an invalid parent, or child whose care is a burden —and one refuses to recognize that there is such a struggle. So also one may seek to suppress jealousy, envy of the nearest and dearest; soul-stirring, forbidden passions; secret revolt against morality and law which may (and often does) rage in the most puritanical breast.
>
> In the theory of the subconscious these undesired thoughts, feelings, passions and wishes are suppressed and pushed into the innermost recesses of the being, out of the light of conscious personality, but nevertheless, acting on that personality, distorting it, wearying it.

It is for these reasons that we say the real task of childhood is to bring about a balance between primitive, biologic desires on the one hand, and the demands of society as symbolized by mother and father, on the other. If a child can bring about such a balance, we say he is well adjusted and has good mental health. But if he cannot, then the degree of resulting maladjustment depends on the strength of the primitive impulse that grips him, as well as on the severity of the social demands made on him.

Now it should be clearer why we say that the modern conception of mental health may be summed up as the adjustment of one's self to both inner and outer demands in a manner that will be reasonably satisfactory to the individual and to the customs of the society in which he lives.

Adjustment of Behavior

This ability to adjust one's self to experiences that thwart one's desires or primitive "drives" is an ability partially acquired during childhood. This may sound strange to those brought up to believe that mental disorders or emotional disabilities were a sort of curse visited on the patient through the processes of inheritance by an indiscreet ancestor. There *is* such a thing as heredity figuring in the causation of certain types of mental disorder, of course, and it would be incorrect to assume that the modern psychiatrist wholly disbelieves in heredity. Nevertheless, it has been too great a temptation in the past to attribute practically every display of human behavior we don't happen to like to this factor, and scientists have been forced in recent years to admit that, after all, while considerable knowledge exists about the laws of heredity in laboratory white mice and guinea pigs, the same knowledge is not necessarily applicable to human beings. Indeed, there are very few *facts* about human heredity known to science, and a vastly greater amount of research will be necessary before we will be in a position to say definitely what traits man inherits and what ones he forms after birth as imitations of or reactions to similar traits displayed by his parents.

Modern opinion, therefore, is veering around to the belief that the type of training a young child receives from its parents during the flexible years when its personality is in the process of being shaped determines pretty much how successful he is going to be in harmonizing the conflicts we have just mentioned, and how well he adjusts. For this reason increasing attention is being paid today to problems of mental hygiene and child guidance among normal boys and girls. It has been found quite possible in many instances for mothers, fathers, school teachers, and others to help the child form habits or "patterns" of personality so staunch and sound that these will aid him in meeting and adjusting to the inevitable frustrations in life that come sooner or later to each of us.

The formation of sturdy patterns of personality in these early years helps to explain why one person is able to adjust in a reasonable, healthy way to some distressing experience such as the loss of a loved one, loss of job, or the inability to attain some cherished ambition, while another, faced with a similar experience, cannot adjust to it and expresses his resulting maladjustment in terms of symptoms of some kind of mental disorder. Thus, a boy, let us say, of six is taught by his parents to develop the healthy pattern of making his own tiny decisions and of finding his childhood security in the products of his own accomplishments rather than in having to depend for success on the personal favoritism of others. As this boy grows older and passes into adolescence these patterns remain with him, and he is able to cope with the mixture of adolescent emotions (made up of the desire to grow up and be independent, versus the wish to remain in the sheltered, protected state of childhood) with a minimum of difficulty. This ease of adjustment will likely be true also of his adult years when he will find himself able to meet adult responsibilities, disappointments, and rebuffs without having to run away from them by developing neurotic symptoms.

On the other hand, another boy of six may have a mother whose own emotional satisfaction in life can be gratified only by realizing that someone needs and depends on her. As a result she may develop what has come to be called an overprotective, oversolicitous attitude toward her child which keeps him emotionally tied to her and fails to allow him to become normally independent. As the physical and intellectual growth of such a child continues apace, his emotional growth tends to remain stunted. He reaches the physical age of adolescence, but because his principal patterns of personality are still the dependent childish ones of an earlier age period he is unable to adjust to adolescent demands and produces a variety of symptoms to express his maladjustment. Symptoms of this sort sometimes take the form of quarrelsomeness, defiance, or rebellion; or they may express themselves in the quieter but more ominous form of causing the youth to withdraw into a seclusive, shut-in, and solitary existence in which he forsakes the discomfort of trying to adjust to the world of reality in favor of retreat into a daydream world of fancy and imagination.

MENTAL TRAINING IN CHILDHOOD

Proper mental hygiene training in childhood, therefore, becomes extremely important if good mental health is to be maintained and mental disorder avoided. One of the most vital things of all in the process of helping a child form healthy patterns of personality is to assist him in creating a feeling of security for himself. By this is meant, not so much a feeling of physical or economic security as of *emotional* security. To feel emotionally secure a person must develop at least two firm convictions: first, that he is recognized as a person valued by others, and that he really belongs to and is accepted and needed by the group of which he is an intimate part. This means, first of all, by his family, then by schoolmates, next by the neighborhood in which he lives, and lastly, by society in general. The second conviction is that he can be confident of success in doing at least one thing really well. It matters little what this thing is providing the person is able to do it by means of his own efforts and is not dependent for success on the favoritism of someone else. To be able to do this gives a legitimate feeling of accomplishment and provides that poise and self-confidence that are the external signs of security.

So much for the connection between childhood patterns of behavior and adult maladjustment. It may be helpful at this point to gain a clearer idea of what kinds of different mental disorders maladjustment produces.

Imagine a straight line. Better still, let's draw one across the page. Like this:

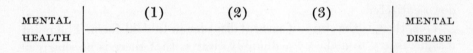

MENTAL   (1)   (2)   (3)   MENTAL
HEALTH   DISEASE

At the left-hand end of the line suppose we imagine there exists a condition of normal or average mental health such as most of us enjoy. As we travel toward the right side of the line some interesting changes begin to appear. For example, somewhere in the vicinity of the point on the line marked (1) we may find that average mental health begins to show a flaw or two in its soundness. This may be manifested by nothing more unusual than the habit of temper tantrums or perhaps of chronic timidity in a child, or possibly by habitual irritability or a feeling of "touchiness" in an adult.

But as we journey farther along the line toward the right, departures from average mental health become more marked. Now, at the point labeled (2), for instance, an individual may come to be thought of by his neighbors as "queer" in some way. Perhaps he shows a fanatical streak about religion or politics or some of the healing cults. If it happens to be a woman, maybe she is "queer" about keeping such an immaculate house that everyone in it is uncomfortable; or else she may go around with a perpetual chip-on-the-shoulder attitude, complaining that everyone else is trying to get the better of her. While still retaining more or less of the good mental health they started out with, such persons nevertheless show by their "queerness" that they already have traveled some distance from the left-hand end of our line.

At the point marked (3) mental health becomes unmistakably impaired, and the efficiency of the individual becomes correspondingly lessened. Now the symptoms are much exaggerated. If, previously, these individuals may have complained that the world has not given them a square deal, now they may develop definite delusions of persecution and arm themselves against their "enemies." Or it may be that other curious notions have crept in. They can't go into closed places or mix with crowds, or else they grow panicky when required to ride on the subway, or are obsessed with distressing ideas that they are going to faint or die.

At last the right-hand end of the line is reached. Here is where mental health vanishes completely and mental disease reigns supreme. Now the individual is "insane," his patterns of adjustment broken down entirely.

This, then, is the story of mental disorder in tabloid form. The point it is necessary to make unmistakably clear is that there is no sharp or clear-cut line that divides mental health from mental disease. Mental health may be thought of as excellent, good, fair, or poor, grading imperceptibly to the right of this line toward the point where mental disease may be said to enter the picture. This point is extremely difficult to locate on the line because standards differ in different groups, and what might pass for merely a poor or even fair degree of mental health among one group of people or in one section of the world, might well be labeled a mild degree of mental disorder in another. Moreover, it is only when mental disease has progressed from mild to extreme that we are justified in calling a person "insane."

INSANITY

"Insanity" is purely a legal term. It has no medical standing. It simply means that a given person's symptoms of mental disorder have grown so serious and his sense of judgment has become so faulty that the law steps in and makes it possible for others to decide for the patient what measures are necessary for his proper treatment and the safeguarding of his property. Although in this country alone there are more than three hundred thousand such "insane" persons in mental hospitals, there are doubtless twenty to thirty times as many others who display some signs of maladjustment or mental disorder of such lesser types as probably will never bring them to a mental hospital. While not in good mental health and often "queer" and hard to get along with, the great majority of these persons are never thought of by their fellow citizens as mentally sick. And yet, according to modern psychiatric conceptions of what constitutes mental disorder, the fears, worries, spells, and what not of these men and women are made of precisely the same stuff, although of course in lesser degree, as that from which definite mental disease is made.

This modern psychiatric conception of what constitutes mental disorder is explained admirably by Dr. C. Macfie Campbell, professor of psychiatry at Harvard Medical School, in the following:

> *A disorder is a mental disorder if its roots are mental.* A headache indicates a mental disorder if it comes because one is dodging something disagreeable. A pain in the back is a mental disorder if its persistence is due to discouragement and a feeling of uncertainty and a desire to have a sick benefit instead of putting one's back into one's work. Sleeplessness may be a mental disorder if its basis lies in personal worries and emotional tangles. In fact, many mental reactions are indications of poor mental health, although they have not usually been classed as mental disorders.
>
> Thus, discontent with one's environment may be a mental disorder if its causes lie, not in some external situation, but in personal failure to deal adequately with one's emotional problems. Suspicion, distrust, misinterpretation are mental disorders when they are the disguised expression of repressed longings into which the patient has no clear insight. Stealing sometimes indicates a mental disorder, the odd expression of underlying conflicts in the patient's nature. The feeling of fatigue sometimes represents, not overwork, but discouragement, inability to meet situations, lack of interest in the opportunities available. Unsociability, marital incompatibility, alcoholism, an aggressive and embittered social attitude; all these may indicate a disorder of the mental balance which may be open to modification.

How different is this conception from the older one that held there were only two varieties of people; the sane and the insane!

MENTAL DEFECT

Before going any further it is important that we digress for a few pages to explain about another kind of abnormal mental condition. This is not a condition of mental *disease,* but instead, of mental *defect.*

After talking with someone who is seriously mentally sick or "insane" many people are astonished to discover that the patient remembers things, knows what they are talking about, and that in general his intellectual faculties are usually not affected by his illness. This is due to the fact that most kinds of mental sickness are disorders of the patient's feeling or emotions and not of his intellect. To be quite accurate, there are a few kinds of mental disease (especially those associated with physical changes in the brain) in which the more advanced stages are accompanied by a lessening of intelligence, but for the most part patients ill from mental disease tend to retain much of whatever original intellectual ability they once possessed.

Feeble-Mindedness

With mental defect, however, this is not true. A person who is mentally defective ("feeble-minded" is another term meaning the same thing) is one whose intelligence has never developed properly. Mental defect and mental disease, therefore, are two quite different things and should not be confused with each other. The illustration of two balky automobiles might be used to explain this difference. One auto balks and falters because the driver does not know how to manage its complicated machinery. This might be compared to mental disease where in most instances the auto itself (the human machine) is sound enough, but where the driver has not learned how to coördinate the use of brake, clutch, and gas throttle. On the other hand, a second auto may balk and falter despite excellent driving because there is a defect or flaw somewhere in the original machinery. This is comparable to a person with a condition of mental defect whose intellectual processes have been deficient since birth because of faulty heredity, birth injury, or the onset of infectious disease (measles, scarlet fever, "sleeping sickness," etc.) early in childhood.

In a very simple little pamphlet the late Dr. Walter Fernald, one of the great pioneers in this country in the study of mental deficiency, describes the symptoms of feeble-mindedness as follows:

The symptoms of mental defect vary according to the degree of defect. In extreme cases the defect is observable in early infancy. The baby does not "take notice" or follow sounds or bright lights, or smile, or grasp objects with his fingers, or have vigorous muscular movements, or nurse properly, and so forth. As he grows older his teeth may not appear at the usual age, or he may learn to walk late and with an awkward, shambling gait, or he may be late in using his hands, or his untidy habits may persist for a long time. He is very apt not to talk until he is three or more years old. In general he remains a baby for a long time.

In less severe cases the above symptoms may be less marked or absent and the defect may not be recognized until the child is found to be unable to learn in school at the usual school age, and cannot be promoted from year to year like other children.

He usually shows his defect in other ways. He may not be able to get along with other children in games and sports. He is often teased and picked on by playmates of his own age, but since they do not regard him as an equal he usually associates with children younger than himself. He is usually easily influenced and shows poor judgment and reasoning power. In general he is not able to meet new situations.

As he grows older he is apt to be led into mischief, since he finds it hard to resist temptation. If neglected or allowed to assocate with evil companions they are rather more likely than normal persons to acquire immoral or vicious habits, although this tendency has probably been overstated. Some mental defectives seem innately vicious and troublesome from early childhood, but the majority seem about as amenable to proper associations and proper bringing up as do normal children.

In mental deficiency, whether the cause be inherited or acquired, medical science knows of nothing to do to repair the damage to brain tissue that is responsible for the condition. Consequently, it can never be cured. In this respect, also, mental defect is not like mental disease, where cure is often accomplished. But if mental defect cannot be cured, at least there is much that can be done to help the feeble-minded person make a reasonably satisfactory adjustment to life with whatever limited intelligence he possesses. In the higher grades (there are three recognized degrees of feeble-mindedness: the *moron* who is next to the normal in intelligence; the *imbecile*, who is next lowest on the scale, and lastly the *idiot*); in the higher grades early recognition of the defect will enable parents and teachers to avoid making too many demands that the child keep up to the standards of normal children. This will help him to maintain his morale and prevent him from developing feelings of inferiority as a result of encountering nothing but failure in life. Likewise, he can be trained in good habit formation that will stand him in good stead when his impulsive judgment threatens to fail him. Later, training in simple trades and occupations within their capacity of accomplishment is possible for children of the moron and upper imbecile groups. But like all people with unaverage mental conditions, the mental defective needs *individual* treatment. What works with one fails with another, and each case must be dealt with as a special problem requiring individual methods.

PREVENTION OF MENTAL DISORDER

What can be done about mental disorders? If this were an old-fashioned book of its kind here would be the place to insert a long list of names of the different kinds of mental disorders and illustrate them with a still longer array of symptoms. No doubt this would be mildly interesting, and it certainly would be in keeping with the methods of those physicians we mentioned in the opening paragraphs who spent most of their time in describing and pinning labels on the symptoms of their patients and letting treatment go pretty much at that.

But this is a modern book. And modern psychiatrists are far more interested in learning why the patient had to take recourse in mental disease, and what his symptoms mean, instead of merely what they are. And so, instead of talking about the differences in symptoms of dementia præcox, or hysteria, or epilepsy, or some of the many other mental disorders, suppose we review briefly some of the important points already brought out and then proceed to a final discussion of what can be done to prevent or cure mental disorders.

The following outline of important viewpoints already mentioned may help to clarify the situation:

1. Mental health and mental disease blend into one another like the colors in the rainbow, with no sharp line of separation.

2. Since mind affects body, and vice versa, the *whole* patient must be studied, not just one detachable part of him.

3. Mental disorders never come suddenly. Except for those caused by an organic physical disease they have been in the process of making for many years before finally appearing.

4. Symptoms of mental disorders usually are but exaggerations of attitudes or traits of personality present in the patient for many years previously.

5. While there are thousands of different precipitating causes for mental disorders, most of them have one basic cause in common in an inability to adjust to certain inner conflicts or to the demands for conformity of the outside world.

6. This basic cause is practically always in the unconscious part of the patient's mind, and he is, therefore, unaware of what it is about.

7. Mental *defect* should not be confused with mental *disease*. The first has to do with impaired intelligence. The second with mismanaged emotions.

TREATMENT OF MENTAL DISORDER

Now for something about prevention and treatment. To do this it will be necessary to make a rough division in our material between children and adults, but with some inevitable overlapping. In childhood the job has two aspects. One is to help the child's parents help him to build up sound and sturdy mental health. The other consists in helping parents to nip in the bud before they get well established certain traits and attitudes which experience has taught will grow into some kind of mental maladjustment in later years. Please note the difference in the nature of these jobs. The first has to do with insuring mental *health*, while the second is concerned with preventing mental *disease*. One is like building a fireproof house from the ground up. The other is comparable to calling the fire department early before the fire gets completely out of control. The mental hygiene movement in this country has performed a valuable service to parents and teachers in the past with the second aspect of this job, but until very recently no one in the mental hygiene movement has attempted the more difficult task of building health in contrast to preventing disease.

By the time adult years are reached, there is relatively little that can be done by way of preventing mental disorders, except, perhaps, to keep milder ones from growing more serious. The treatment task also grows more difficult as the mental disorder becomes more deeply entrenched.

But to return for a moment to the maladjustments of children. These are expressed in a variety of ways. Temper tantrums, fussy, dawdling food habits, timidity, shyness, overconscientiousness, bedwetting (in older children), bullying and aggressiveness, stealing, lying, truancy; all these should be regarded as danger signals pointing to some underlying conflict which must be sought out and discovered before anything practical can be done by way of permanently remedying the condition. But unlike the methods of treatment in other branches of medicine, the treatment of behavior disorders and undesirable personality traits in children can seldom be successfully undertaken by directing treatment to the child alone. His annoying behavior is a symptom of maladjustment somewhere within his emotional apparatus and is invariably bound up in some manner with the attitudes and emotional reactions displayed toward him by his parents. The treatment of the behavior problem, therefore, will require that these parental attitudes be taken into account. Indeed, so thoroughly is this believed by mental hygienists that they have created an axiom to the effect that "you cannot change the child's behavior until you first change the parental attitude that caused the behavior." Treatment primarily, then, *is directed toward the parents*, and this treatment consists largely in endeavoring to get them to modify the undesirable attitude that unwittingly and with the best of intentions they have adopted.

But what about the adult? And what kind of treatment is indicated for his mental disorder? Obviously, the answer must depend on the nature of his problem. In general, however, adult treatment can be thought of as comprising two main varieties: treatment of the basic emotional difficulty whenever this proves possible, and treatment of symptoms. One should never be satisfied with restricting treatment of mental disorders to symptoms alone unless there is nothing else to be done. Unhappily, in numerous cases of serious mental disease or "insanity," the case has progressed so far before psychiatric assistance is called that there remains little to do except to treat the symptoms. But with less severe cases—the psychoneuroses, for example, with their many fears, compulsions, anxieties, etc.—it is often quite possible to get at the roots of the trouble and effect a cure by means of a special type of treatment known as "psychotherapy." This method does not make use of medicines or physical kinds of treatment like massage, baths, etc., but relies for its effectiveness instead on a special emotional relationship between patient and psychiatrist. There are several different kinds of psychotherapy. One in particular is called "psychoanalysis" about which a great deal of misunderstanding exists. Only a comparatively few kinds of mental difficulty are suitable, at this stage of our knowledge, for psychoanalytic treatment. Moreover, as yet there are not many psychiatrists in this country who have had the indispensable special training that is necessary before one is competent to use psychoanalysis. But for the particular cases it is suited for, and in the hands of a well-trained psychiatrist, psychoanalysis enables us to explore the unconscious mind of the patient and, after locating the source of the conflict, is a most helpful procedure in the process of emotional reëducation which, if successful, restores the patient to an improved degree of adjustment.

PSYCHOTHERAPY

Other forms of psychotherapy are used for cases that do not re- .juire so deep an exploration into the unconscious. Thus, various kinds of suggestion are sometimes made use of, and occasionally even hypnosis, although most psychiatrists have come to the belief that hypnosis at best is of value only in the temporary relief of symptoms and is powerless to bring about a lasting cure. For this reason it is very little used by capable physicians.

The treatment of more serious conditions of mental disorder, like "insanity," where institutional care is required, is very complicated. Suppose we trace the treatment of an imaginary case of "insanity" and see what happens in an up-to-date hospital for mental disease. First of all, the patient has been, in all probability, behaving queerly for some months before the family has gotten courage to seek medical advice. He may have been depressed, or he may have been excited. Perhaps he has had delusions that others are following him, or that something has been placed in his food, or that "voices" speak to him, or what not. It makes little difference. The point is that the family at last recognize he is "not right." The family physician is consulted. He makes a careful examination, both physically and mentally, and either recommends that the patient be treated in a suitable public or private hospital for mental diseases, or, if the case is an unusually puzzling or obscure one, he may ask that the family authorize him to call into consultation a capable psychiatrist.

Some cases of this kind can be cared for at home, but in an overwhelming number of instances it is far better for patient and family alike if the former is removed to a hospital. This is a hard decision for relatives to make, for there still exists a great deal of cruel and unwarranted stigma about people who require mental hospital care. But it is almost certain that much of the patient's underlying conflict —the reasons for his becoming mentally sick—are tangles up in family relationships, and if he can get away from the well-meaning but unwholesome family atmosphere for a time his chances of early cure are improved.

So we will assume that the family agrees to hospital treatment. Next is the matter of commitment. This is merely a legal device to safeguard the interests of the patient. It consists in making application to a court for an order to have the patient admitted to a hospital in order that he can receive the special treatment available at such a hospital. In most states commitment can be made without undue publicity, the judge (unless he be vindictive or a stickler for the letter of the law) waiving the right to have the sick man haled before the court, and accepting the legally sworn-to certificate of the committing physicians who give their professional opinion that the patient is mentally sick and needs mental hospital care.

The patient arrives at the hospital. In modern, well-equipped state hospitals for the mentally sick he is first taken to the receiving ward, where he remains for ten days to several months, depending on the nature of his condition. While in the receiving ward he is examined very carefully by a number of physicians, and treatment for his immediate needs is prescribed. This may be rest in bed, plenty of nourishing food, and an occasional sedative, if sleepless or restless. But sometimes the patient is wildly excited on admission. Then it is likely that a special kind of treatment known as the "continuous bath" will be ordered by the doctor. This consists in greasing the patient's body with vaseline and then placing him in a specially constructed tub through which flows a gentle stream of water heated to whatever temperature is indicated. Usually it is just above body heat. A canvas sheet is placed over the tub to prevent the patient from getting out and an attendant or nurse is stationed near by to see that the sick man or woman does not hurt himself or slip under the sheet.

After a time the patient relaxes under the influence of the warm water. His excitement begins to subside, and he may even go to sleep. The continuous bath is a far more humane method of controlling excitement and violence than any other kind of restraint known, including hypnotic drugs and the straitjacket. All up-to-date hospitals have them, and in better hospitals of this kind straitjackets, camisoles, and similar devices for confining the arms and legs of patients have been abandoned. Indeed, in many modern hospitals the only place a straitjacket can be found is in the hospital museum.

But perhaps the patient is depressed instead of excited. Possibly he has no appetite and refuses to eat, or maybe he has delusions that he has committed all sorts of fantastic crimes. He may accuse himself of having brought ruin on the family, or of being responsible for all the misery in the world, or of having committed the "unpardonable sin," whatever that may be. At any rate, he is deeply depressed, and the doctors understand that the chances are in favor of his contemplating suicide, if, indeed, he has not already expressed the intention of taking his own life. It is necessary, therefore, to safeguard him from self-injury. Such patients are usually very clever in managing to evade the nurse or others who are on the watch for attempts at suicide, and this is another reason why home care is dangerous, especially for depressed patients. Even under the most constant attention a patient may elude his nurse and dash through a window, or cut himself, or in some other way do away with himself. Eternal vigilance is the price of safety in such cases.

Sometimes the patient won't eat, and then another method of treatment is necessary. If he gets to the point where his refusal to take food threatens to retard his recovery, or if, as not infrequently happens, it comes down to a question of actual starvation, the doctor inserts a soft rubber tube through the patient's nostrils into his stomach and slowly pours down it a mixture of milk and eggs at necessary intervals.

But gradually the patient improves. Now he is transferred from the receiving ward to another. Here he will find other patients whose behavior is like his own and in various stages of recovery. Seeing other patients whose condition has improved is an incentive for our patient to make further progress. Presently he is encouraged to take walks on the ground outside and in company with a nurse or a group of others. He is given an opportunity to visit the occupational therapy department at frequent intervals, where, under skilled supervision, he can get his mind off his troubles and reëstablish habits of concentration and industry.

At last he is well enough to go home. And modern science has another victory to its credit. Unhappily, the hospital course of some patients is not as successful as the one we have described. Some mentally sick men and women are not allowed by their relatives to come to the hospital until their illness has reached such an advanced stage that little but kindly custodial care can be given them. Moreover, some kinds of mental illness seem to be of such a stubborn nature from the beginning that the case is almost a chronic one from the start. Nevertheless, it is astonishing to observe how the rate of recovery is steadily increasing. At the present time about 25 per cent of all first admissions to mental hospitals are completely cured, while an additional 15 per cent are able to return home, after a time, well enough to live in the outside community even though they are not completely recovered.

This recovery rate, however, depends to some extent on the kind of hospital the patient is treated in. Modern, up-to-date hospitals have no difficulty in maintaining this rate, but less progressive ones are usually able to do little more than provide custodial care for their patients. This is why there has come about a technical distinction between *treatment* hospitals and *custodial* ones. In the former every modern form of medical and psychiatric treatment is used to cure the patient. The staffs of doctors are recruited from alert, progressive men and women; the scientific equipment is the last word in efficiency, and the laboratories allow no promising method of treatment to go untried.

COMMUNITY HOSPITALS FOR MENTAL DISORDER

It must be confessed, however, that not all our state hospitals for the mentally sick are of this variety. There still exist backward hospitals where the superintendent is a political appointee whose professional skill has not advanced since his early medical training. In these institutions scientific apparatus is meager, and little or no advantage is taken of recent psychiatric discoveries.

In the last analysis the responsibility for backward mental hospitals rests on the community. It is an axiom as true in this field as in any other that a community gets just about what it is willing to pay for, in the way of public service. If citizens of a community are too negligent to insist on a high quality of psychiatric service, then they must be willing to take what is possible. A well-equipped and modern mental hospital costs money to run, but it also restores a much higher percentage of its patients to health. Any community can have this high quality of service if it wants to.

And now, just a word in closing about state hospitals in contrast to private hospitals or sanatoriums. Any generalizations are sure to do an injustice to certain institutions, but so far as generalizations are permitted, it may be fair to say that a modern *treatment* state hospital is likely to be a more effective place for a mentally sick patient than a *custodial* private one. There are a few private sanatoria not run primarily for commercial profit where some of the best scientific work in the country is being done. These hospitals are at least partially endowed by private funds, so that they are not wholly dependent on patients' fees for support. But if we except these (as well as a handful of commercial ones), then most of the others cannot afford the elaborate and expensive equipment or the legitimately higher salaries commanded by physicians of superior skill.

The modern state hospital, on the other hand, deals with several thousand patients instead of fifty or a hundred or so. It receives its funds from the state government and is thereby enabled to equip itself in the most effective manner. Furthermore, while the salaries of its staff are often lower than those of some private sanatoria, the progressive scientific spirit permeating the whole atmosphere and the opportunity to use adequate equipment tends to attract to it the better medical men and women in the psychiatric field. On the whole, therefore, if expense is a serious matter for the family to consider, it will be well for them to consider the state hospital (but *only* if it is a modern, progressive one) in favor of a small, inexpensive but custodial private one.

This story of mental disorders comes now to a close. Mankind has traveled far since those days, centuries ago, when sufferers from "insanity" were regarded as being afflicted with demons and evil spirits and chained in dungeons. The mystery of mental disease has been stripped away, and now we are able to recognize it as a kind of sickness, often amenable in some measure to psychiatric treatment and curable in an increasingly large number of cases. The stigma that formerly surrounded mental patients is rapidly disappearing, and the general public is taking to heart the advice of the mental hygiene movement, that the earlier the symptoms of mental disorder are noted and treatment begun, the better the chances for recovery.

The final eradication of mental disorder will come when more effective methods are devised to build sound and positive mental *health* in our children. This will require medical leadership of a high order; a leadership that recognizes the task is not alone a medical one, but one requiring the assisting services of the forces of education, sociology, psychology, and practically all the social sciences. It will be a coöperative job with victory as the reward of research and infinite hard work.

CHAPTER XXXIII

Old Age

MORRIS FISHBEIN, M.D.

ALTHOUGH ONE HUNDRED YEARS of life is possible to human beings, only 30 people in 3,000,000 reach that age. And more than two thirds of the persons who do reach that age are women. The reason for this latter fact is that women are usually less exposed to accident and infection and, what is more important, are more apt to lead temperate lives.

Census figures from Great Britain show that the average number of persons more than 100 in the British Isles is about 110, and that 80 of this number are women.

These figures are not absolutely accurate, since most old people are proud of their age and tend to exaggerate. For example, in nearly every census, more people who give their ages as over 91 are found than people who give their ages as between 85 and 90. British health authorities assume that many jump from 85 to 91 in a year or two.

THE SPAN OF LIFE

However, the span of life is gradually increasing. And in time we may expect to have more and more people above 90. The chief reason for this remains the rapid decline in death rates for infants. Thus, a man born in 1854 had a life expectancy of 40 years. Now he may reasonably expect to live to be 59. Having reached the age of 60, a man's expectancy of life is now 14½ years, and a woman's 16 years.

Since heredity seems to play a large part in longevity, it is conceivable, according to Sir Humphry Rolleston of England, that encouragement of intermarriage between families that tend to live long would produce stock that tended to live long. However, such experi-

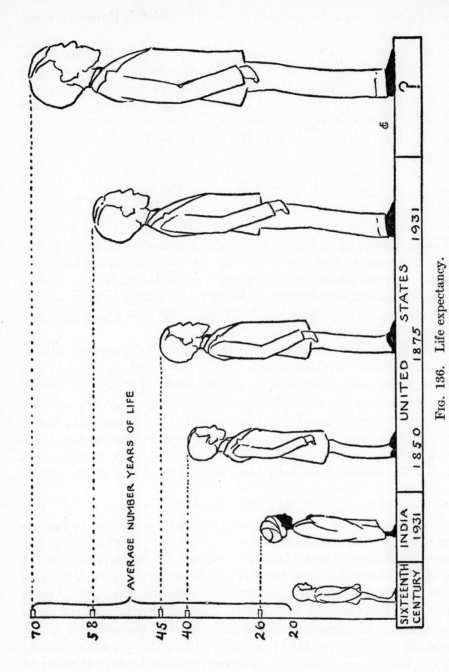

70

58

AVERAGE NUMBER YEARS OF LIFE

45

40

26

20

| SIXTEENTH CENTURY | INDIA 1931 | | UNITED STATES 1850 1875 1931 | | |

FIG. 136. Life expectancy.

ments among humans are almost impossible, and this theory must remain largely a matter of conjecture.

One of the real problems we have to face is to make the lives of the aged happier and healthier. They must realize their own shortcomings in regard to strength and ability to throw off disease, while those around them should always take into consideration the changes which come with advanced age. If older persons observe the simple rules of health, there is no reason why their declining years should not be happy.

CHANGES IN OLD AGE

One of the things which every person over sixty must realize is that his organs are functioning more slowly than in his youth and that allowances must be made for this change. The glands tend to function less in old age, so that the skin becomes dry. Even the gastric juice carries a lower percentage of hydrochloric acid, and for this reason there is difficulty with digestion. Moreover, the mucus in the intestines becomes less, so that there is a tendency to dryness of the intestinal contents and therefore to constipation.

One of the significant changes in old age is the blunting of sensibility to pain. This is very important, because the breaking down of the tissues leads to sensations that are uncomfortable. For the same reason disease in old age comes insidiously.

Whereas pneumonia, heart disease, stones in the kidney or gall bladder may cause agonizing pain to a young person, they come on so insidiously in older ones they may be unrecognized until they have reached the point where help is difficult. Even cancer comes on insidiously in the aged.

The sensations of taste and smell also become weaker, so that food is not so appetizing. Everyone knows also that sight and hearing are greatly depreciated in the elderly.

One of the most interesting aspects of old age is the change in the mind and ability to sleep. Because the aged sleep less continuously, they frequently estimate the amount of sleep at much less than it really is. However, it is quite certain the aged are able to use much less sleep than vigorous, active people, and it is not desirable to get them into the habit of taking sedative drugs. It is likely, according to Sir Humphry Rolleston, that excessive sleep is more harmful to them than too little.

The mind becomes much more easily fatigued in old age than in middle age. Gradually the power of affection wanes in the old, perhaps because they have become habituated to the loss of relatives and friends. Possibly they are more self-centered; time passes slowly, and their minds are occupied with their own feelings.

DISEASES OF OLD AGE

According to Sir Humphry Rolleston, it cannot be said that any diseases are confined to old age. Even premature senility may occur in youth. Heart disease, atrophy of the brain, and hardening of the arteries may also occur in comparatively young people. However, most of the diseases that occur in the aged are the result of gradual breaking down of the tissues. These include hardening of the arteries, heart failure, hardening of the liver, enlargement of the prostate, cancer, obesity, and indigestion. However, old age does modify any disease, so that it is different from the same condition in youth.

Charcot, the famous French psychologist, called pneumonia the great enemy of old people. Osler, on the other hand, referred to it as the "friend of the aged." Both had in mind the fact that pneumonia in the aged is a short and rarely painful illness which saves old people from the long and gradual decay that is sometimes so distressing.

Measles, scarlet fever, typhoid, and diphtheria occur very rarely in old people, probably because they have been infected in youth and thereby developed immunity from these diseases. The form of sick headache called migraine usually becomes less troublesome as age advances and may disappear with increasing years. A recent conception of this disease indicates that it may be the result of sensitivity to some protein food substance, and perhaps the repeated attacks eventually bring about desensitization.

Even when an aged person is in good health, he must keep a close watch for the diseases to which his age makes him particularly susceptible. Happiness for all elderly persons is principally a matter of health, and so health must be guarded more and more closely as time goes on.

The changes that occur in the skin of the aged are due to gradual loss of activity on the part of the glands and of the tissues responsible for immunity. Because the aged are likely to be a little less scrupulous in the care of the skin, slight infections occur repeatedly. There are also bed sores. Itching is a stimulus to severe scratching and secondary infections take place in the scratches.

The blood vessels may lose their contractile power, and there are occasionally tiny hemorrhages under the skin. One of the most severe conditions that affects the aged is the reaction called herpes zoster. It is a form of shingles which develops along the course of a nerve and which in the aged may be exceedingly painful. Moreover, once the attack has passed, the pains may continue and return at intervals without the eruption. These conditions must be watched closely and treated immediately.

Of course, the aged suffer frequently with dizziness due to many possible causes. Sometimes it is due to accumulated hard wax in the ear, sometimes to changes that have taken place in the internal ear; frequently it is associated with high blood pressure, hardening of the arteries, and changes in the circulation of the blood in the brain. Sometimes the result is a difficulty of coördination between the eye, the ear, and the sense of balance, so that the aged may stagger or fall when the eyes are raised suddenly or under some similar stimulus.

One of the diseases more likely to occur in the aged than in the young is paralysis agitans, or the shaking palsy. Although this disease may occur in youth, the vast majority of cases occur in people between fifty and seventy years of age. The disease occurs twice as often in men as in women. It is marked by tremor of the hands, with a pill-rolling movement, and it tends to progress, running a complete course in from ten to fifteen years.

The aged should be especially careful to consult a good physician when any of the symptoms described in this article occur. While they may be simple results of old age, without more serious implication, they should be checked at frequent intervals by the family doctor.

EXERCISE AND HYGIENE

Old people have particular difficulty in walking, for many reasons. First, there may be weakening in the circulation; sometimes pain in the muscles results from imperfect circulation. Often older persons walk with short steps, because in this way they are better able to control their sense of balance.

While the aged may have high blood pressure, it is not so serious as in youth. Thus Dr. David Riesman described a woman ninety-seven years old who for twenty-five years had a blood pressure over 250. In such cases, because of the hardening of the arteries, high blood pressure may be necessary to maintain life. Such high blood pressure is dangerous only when the blood vessels burst and hemorrhage into the brain results in death.

Of course, old people suffer with disturbances of digestion because of the changes that have taken place in their secretions, and also because they have difficulty in keeping infection away from their teeth and because they do not chew the food properly. The constipation of old age is now largely controlled by the taking of mineral oil which serves the purpose of softening the intestinal mass and making elimination easy. This remedy is practically harmless and adds years of health to many older persons. Hemorrhoids are frequent in the aged and are, of course, associated with constipation.

There was a time when the teeth of the human being gradually fell out as he grew older so that he found himself, by the time he reached old age, able to take only liquid food or food that was soft. Modern dentistry has made it possible for the aged to chew steaks or vegetables of considerable fibrous content. It is for this reason that the aged must frequently resort to laxatives or to mineral oil in order to aid the weakened intestinal muscles in handling the waste material.

The aged are likely to suffer particularly with accumulations of mucous material in the lungs; with diminished power of the lungs to repair themselves, small areas of degenerated tissue break down, and the material accumulates and has to be coughed out of the lung. The continued inhalation and coughing results in disturbances such as bronchopneumonia or similar complaints.

The elderly are particularly prone to varicose veins, to inflammations of the joints, and to fixed joints which follow inflammation.

CANCER IN OLD AGE

Cancer has always been recognized by the medical profession as a disease of old age. More recently it has seemed to occur fairly frequently among younger people, and there are many explanations advanced for this fact. It is recognized that heredity plays a large part in cancer, and that inbreeding may bear some responsibility. The British statistician, Karl Pearson, found that the maximum incidence of cancer occurs at the age of forty-six in women, and of fifty-six in men. The chief cancer period is from forty-six to sixty-four years.

According to Sir Humphry Rolleston, the most recently assembled figures in England indicate that mortality from cancer of the most accessible sites continues to increase up to extreme old age, whereas cancer in less accessible positions does not. Obviously, the reason is that cancer in the stomach, the intestines, and similar inaccessible positions is not easy to discover and in most instances advances so rapidly that the person dies of the cancer. Hence such cancer did not occur in people of advanced years.

It is well established that cancer is associated with long continued irritation of susceptible spots in the tissue. Obviously aged people are more subject to long continued irritation than are the young. Men suffer, of course, much more frequently than do women with cancer of the lips and tongue, perhaps because of their smoking habits. Even though women have begun to smoke cigarettes regularly, it is unlikely that they will suffer as much with cancer of the lips and tongue as do men, because women are much more careful about the state of their mouths and teeth. Men suffer with cancer of the prostate; women with cancer of the organs particularly concerned with childbearing.

There have been many attempts to explain cancer in old age, but all of them are theoretical. In old age the degenerative process in the cells leads to the formation of new tissue, and the repeated demands made on the cells in this way may result in the sudden rapid growth that is called cancer. Warthin, eminent pathologist, considered cancer to be merely a sudden rapid aging of a group of cells.

Whatever the cause may be, older persons should be especially careful to treat all slight infections and to visit a physician if these irritations do not respond readily to treatment.

Index

Abdomen, discomfort, symptom of dyspepsia, 395; massaging, during pregnancy, 159; organs, chart showing, 57; pain, never take a cathartic for, 12; pain, sign of appendicitis, 404.

Abdominal binder, tight, harmful, to puerperal woman, 181; binder used in whooping cough to prevent hernia, 260; support advisable for puerperal woman, 175.

Abnormalities: *See* **"Deformities."**

Abortion, all tissues passed in, should be saved, 166; criminal, 145; danger of, during pregnancy due to exercise, traveling, etc., 160; sexual intercourse during pregnancy may cause, 143; threatened, signs of, and first aid in, 166.

Abscess, in external ear, 715, 717; in teeth, diagram showing effects of, 755; perinephritic, 455.

Absinthe poisoning, symptoms, antidotes and treatment, 47.

Absorption, by skin, 665; in small intestines, 383; in stomach, 382; of food, 774.

Acarus or itch mite, 688.

Accidents, death rate from, in U. S., 19; Fourth of July, and tetanus, 280; industrial defined, 643–644.

Acetanilid, industrial hazard, 645; in headache powders, 13; poisoning, symptoms, antidotes and treatment, 41.

Acetic acid, glacial, for removing warts, 821.

Acetphenetidin poisoning, symptom, antidotes and treatment, 41.

Acetylene: *See* **Oxyacetylene.**

Acetylsalicylic acid, 13.

Achilles tendon, exercise for stretching, 814.

Achlorhydria, 388.

Achylia, 388.

Acid (*see also under names of specific acids as* **Acetylsalicylic, Boric,** *etc.*); -base ratio

of food, 773; burns of eye, 707; burns treatment, 27; in mouth and tooth decay, 751; of gastric juice, 382; -producing food, 773.

Acidified evaporated milk, how to make, 203.

Acidophilus milk in constipation, 410.

Acidosis, 773–774.

Acne, in adolescence, 677; keloid, 701; rosacea, 683–684; rosacea, alcohol and, 684; rosacea, cause, prevention, 684; vulgaris, 681–683; vulgaris, "blood purifiers" harmful in, 682; vulgaris, causes, 681, 682; vulgaris, cold cream harmful in, 682; vulgaris involving back of neck, 701; vulgaris, soap and water benefit, 682; vulgaris, treatment necessary by skilled physician, 682.

Aconite, poisoning, symptoms, antidotes, and treatment, 42.

Acrolein, industrial hazard from putty, 657.

Acromegaly, 545.

ADDISON, 549.

Addison's disease, 548, 549.

Adenoids, cause of laryngitis and croup (diagram), 734; enlargement, cause of chronic sinus disease, 727; infected, or obstructing breathing, should be removed, 367; tonsils and, 733.

Adhesions cause of intestinal obstruction, 414.

Adhesive tape, 15, 16.

Adhesive device for removing foreign body from ear, 716–717.

Adolescence (*see also* **Boys, Girls**), acne vulgaris in, 681–682; care of skin in, 677; changes in, 50; "dates" between young people in, 107, 108; dreams in, 102; goiter during, 556 *ff.*; hobbies valuable in, 101; iodine deficiency during, 52; love affairs in, 103; masturbation in, 102; psychology of, 96; sex education in, 96; thyroid during, 52; value of athletics in, 100.

Adoption of children, 119.

Adrenalin, 547.

Adrenals: *See* **Suprarenals.**

Advertising not ethical for physicians, 3.

Aërophagia, 395–396.

AETIUS noted dropsy with hardened kidneys, 432.

Afterbirth, 80; delivering, 171, 172; in abortion, 166.

Agar, mineral oil with, 17.

Age, blood pressure according to, 609; cancer increases with, 626; distribution of deaths from diphtheria and croup, 243; height and weight according to, 769; number of persons over one hundred years of, 848; of onset of allergy, 508; of onset of menstruation, relation to menopause, 56; old: *see* "Old Age"; relation to albuminuria, 435; sleep requirement according to, 223; susceptible to tuberculosis, 324.

Aged: *See* **Old Age.**

Ague, brass, 648; brass worker's, from zinc, 660.

Air, compressed, caisson disease, 640; fresh, for infant, 221; fresh, what it means, 330; swallowing by adults, 395–396; swallowing by infants, 197, 198.

AKRON, OHIO, prevention of goiter in, 557.

Albumin, healthy urine should be albumin free, 434; in dropsical urine demonstrated by Cruickshank, 431, 432; in urine, demonstration by Dekkers and Cotugno, 431, 432; in urine, work of Richard Bright, 432; nature of, described, 434.

Albuminuria, 421; benign, 436, 437; chemical types, 438; diagnostic significance, 434–435; epidemics in West Point cadets, 435; historical aspects, 431–432; in older persons, 439; in soldiers, 434–435; in students, 435; incidence, 434; incidence in military training camp, 434; modern significance of, 433; nonrenal, 437–438; orthostatic, 437; per cent in 17,000 men, 5; relation of, to age, 435; renal, 435; significance of, 418; transient, in children, 436; types of, 435.

Alcohol, absorbed in the stomach, 382; acne rosacea caused by, 684; amyl, industrial hazard, 646; as an antiseptic, 26; butyl, industrial hazard, 648; effect of, on blood pressure, 614; forbidden for syphilitics, 742; in diet, 787; in mouth washes, 730; not to be used on nipples, 164; nursing

mother should avoid, 174; poisoning, symptoms, antidotes and treatment, 42; to relieve eczema, 679; use of, during pregnancy, 153; wood, industrial hazard, 653.

Alkali, in soap, 669–670; poisoning, symptoms, antidotes and treatment, 42.

Alkaline-producing food, 773.

Alkaline toothpaste, value of, 753.

Alkaptonuria, 461.

Allergy, age of onset of, 508; animal hair, 515; antitoxin, 247; bacteria, 518; blood transfusion, 518; cause of, and removal, 525; cold, 518; colds due to, 314; corn products, 516; cottonseed, 516; definition of, 506; deformities caused by, 520; degree of sensitiveness in, 511; diagnosis, 523–524; drug idiosyncrasies in, 517; dust, 517; effect of environment and climate in, 509; egg, in infant, 506; feathers, 515; fish, 507; food, 515, 763; food, cause of sick headache, 39; fungi, 516; glue, 507, 516; hair, 515; heat, 507, 518, 519; heredity in, 508; history of, 507; ill effects of careless advice in, 514; insects, 516; light, 518, 519; light, Bostock description of, in 1819, 504–505; linseed, 516; menstrual blood, 518; molds, 516; multiple sensitiveness in, 510; natural and acquired, 509; nature of cause, 512; pollen, 504 *ff.*, 506, 515; pollen, described by Dunbar, 505; relationship to general health, 512; scratches, 518; sensitiveness of one individual to another, 518; serum, 518; shock and general illnesses, 524; smoke, 517; specificity of, 511; stunting of growth, 521; sunlight, 518, 519; symptoms, 521 *ff.*; treatment, 524; treatment, nonspecific, 528; treatment, pollen avoidance in, 526; treatment, removal of cause in, 525; treatment, results of, 529; treatment, specific, 527; treatment, specific, use of tourniquet, 527.

Almond meal, soap substitute, 673.

Alopecia: *See* **Baldness.**

Alps, endemic goiter district, 555.

Aluminum chloride solution for perspiring feet, 824.

Aluminum dishes not a cause of cancer, 625.

ALVAREZ, W. C., 392.

Ambulance, call for, in gas poisoning, 31.

Amebiasis, 287, 411; carrier, 288, 412; Chicago outbreak, 287–283, 290; control of outbreak of, by boiling water, 290; 5 per cent of population in U. S. have, 412; flies carriers of, 288, 290; food handlers source of, 288, 290; incubation period,

288; symptoms, 289, 413; treatment, 290; vegetables a source of, 288; water a source of, 287, 288.

AMERICAN COLLEGE OF SURGEONS, 2.

AMERICAN HOSPITAL ASSOCIATIONS, 2.

AMERICAN MEDICAL ASSOCIATION, Committee on Foods, 224; Committee on Foods, charts showing food values, 766, 772, 773, 779, 781, 785; committee suggestions on exercises in infantile paralysis, 269; Council on Medical Education and Hospitals, 2; Council on Pharmacy and Chemistry, 14, 498; Council on Physical Therapy, 310, 311; hospitals approved by, for internship, 2; *Journal*, 613; organization described, 3.

American Review of Tuberculosis, 327.

American sleeping sickness, hiccups in, 37.

AMERICAN SOCIETY FOR THE CONTROL OF CANCER, 636.

Amino-acids, 383; basic components of protein, 770; in proteins, 770.

Ammonia, aromatic spirits of, stimulant in fainting, 14, 18, 33; gas, industrial hazard; 645; manufactured by kidney, 425; poisoning, symptoms, antidotes and treatment, 42; spirits of, for faintness during pregnancy, 167; water in peroxide solution for chloasma, 691; water, iodine stain removed by, 673.

Ammonium chloride for loosening cough, 313.

Amyl alcohol and amyl compounds, industrial hazards, 646.

Amylase, enzyme in pancreatic juice, 383.

Amytal, 13.

Anaphylaxis: *See* Allergy.

Anasarca, defined, 425.

Anatomy, of heart, 348; of kidney, 421; of reproductive system, 76.

ANDERSON, 777.

Anemia, aplastic, 470; causes of, 469; causes scanty menstruation, 54; cessation of menstruation in, 140; eating of liver in, 476; gastric secretion in pernicious, 388; pernicious, 471; prevention, 476; primary, 470; quack remedies for, 472–473, 475; remissions, 475; secondary, 470; symptoms, 474; treatment, 472.

Anesthetics, 13, 14; poisoning, symptoms, antidotes and treatment, 42.

Angina pectoris, 371–372, 373; attacks, what brings on, 374–375; coronary thrombosis compared with, 376; exertion brings on attacks of, 374; fatigue brings on attacks of, 375: Heberden description,

375; pain important symptom in, 374; preventing attacks of, 375; prognosis, 375–376.

Angina, Vincent's, 285; germs causing, 284, 285; treatment, 285.

Aniline dye, methyl violet as industrial poison, 654.

Aniline oil, industrial hazard, 646.

Animal, cancer, 630; hair and feathers, sensitivity to, 515; parasites, allergy, 518; reproduction in, 68.

Ankle, sprained, 817; sprained, contrast bath for, 818; sprained, diathermy treatment, 817; sprained, treatment, 817–818; sprained, X-ray picture in, 817, 818, 819; swelling, during pregnancy, 157, 165.

Anthrax, infections of industry, 642.

Antidotes, list of, 41.

Antigen, Dreyer, in treatment of tuberculosis, 324.

Antipyrin poisoning, symptoms, antidotes and treatment, 41.

Antiseptics, douches, 138, 139; douches, dangers of, 144; in medicine chest, 14; skin, 673; used in first-aid treatment of wounds, 26; used in rinsing diapers, 187.

Antitoxin, defined, 246; diphtheria, 241; diphtheria, dosage, 244; erysipelas, 279; scarlet fever, 258; sensitivity to, 247, 509; tetanus, 281, 282; treatment of diphtheria, 247.

Antrum, infection, 727.

Anus (*see also* Rectum), prolapse in infants, 210.

Aorta, 350.

Apoplexy as cause of death in 1904 compared with 1929, 566.

Appendix, tenderness in region of, per cent in 17,000 men, 5; pus, 405.

Appendicitis, 404; chronic, symptoms, treatment, 405; confused with diabetes coma, 604; danger of using cathartics in, 12; distinguishing, from gall-bladder disease and ulcer, 406; in diabetes, 600; symptoms, 405; X-ray diagnosis, 405.

Appetite, 775; guide to normal diet and nutrition, 761; perversion of, during pregnancy, 153.

Apples, food elements in (diagram), 771.

Apricots in infant feeding, 205.

Arches, fallen, 815; fallen, exercises for, 816; fallen, shoes for, 816; fallen, treatment, 815; fallen, what happens in (diagram), 808; footprints indicate quality of, 811; good (diagram), 811.

Arctic, fat in diet in, 780; use of meat in diet in, 777.

ARDERNE, advice on nephritis, 462.

ARETÆUS, description of diabetes mellitus by, 564.

Argyrosis from silver, industrial hazard, 658.

Army (see also Soldiers, World War), United States, instructions to syphilitics, 742.

Arsenic, hazard in tobacco industry, 659; industrial hazard, 646; in sealing wax, industrial hazard, 657; poisoning, symptoms, antidotes, and treatment, 42.

Arteries, coronary system of, 350 ff.; coronary thrombosis, 371–372; hardening of (see "Arteriosclerosis"); renal, 423; thickening, per cent in 17,000 men, 5.

Arteriosclerosis, chronic renal, 454; found in Egyptian mummies, 614; in diabetes, 597; nosebleed in, 724.

Arthritis (see also Rheumatism), 337 ff.; autohemotherapy, 343; chronic, causes of, 338; diets in, 340–342; differentiated from rheumatism, 337; focal infection rôle in, 339; food faddist on diet for, 340–341; hot paraffin baths for, 343; intestinal causes, 340; massage in, 344; periods in which patient is better then worse again, 339; protein therapy, 343; starch digestion question, 341; stiffness of the joints, 339; symptoms, 338; treatment and care, 340; vaccine therapy, 343.

Asbestosis, industrial, 641, 646.

Aschheim-Zondek test of early pregnancy, based on appearance of sex hormone in urine, 545.

Ascites, defined, 425.

Asexual method of reproduction, 69.

ASHBURN, 435.

Asphalt, industrial hazard, 646.

Asphyxiation, resuscitation after, 27.

Aspirin, 13; to relieve menstrual pain, 53; use in treating colds, 312.

Assimilation of food, 774.

Asthenia, neurocirculatory, 377–378.

Asthma, 504 ff.; deformities caused by, 530; pollen in, 514; pollen avoidance in treatment of, 526.

Athlete's foot, 685.

Athletes, given sugar, 589.

Athletics, for girls should be less strenuous, 100, 101; for women, 801; place in physical training, 800; value in adolescence, 100.

Atomizer, 17.

Atophan poisoning, symptoms, antidotes and treatment, 44.

Atrophy of skin, wrinkles first sign of, 694.

Atropine poisoning, symptoms, antidotes and treatment, 43.

AUBURN, NEW YORK, diphtheria elimination in, 248.

Auricle (of the heart), 350 ff.

Auto-eroticism, 133.

Autohemotherapy in arthritis, 343.

Automobile, driving to be avoided during pregnancy, 160; exhaust-gas poisoning, 30; exhaust-gas poisoning, how to prevent, 30.

AVICENNA, 432.

AVERY, DR., research on scarlet fever, 256.

BABINGTON, 447.

Baby: See Infants.

Baby teeth: See Teeth, first.

Bacillus, colon, cause of kidney disease, 444; Döderlein's, positive value in vagina, 139.

Back, stiffness of, suspicious symptom of infantile paralysis, 266.

Bacteria, 230; allergy, 518; cause of kidney disease, 444–445; cause of syphilis and gonorrhea, 738; fly carries over 6 million on its body, 274; invasion, response of body to, 235; paths by which they invade body, 234; selective localization, 235; skin power to protect against, 665–666; soapsuds kill, 670.

Bactericide power of skin, 665.

Bad breath, 756.

Bakelite, industrial hazard, 646.

Baking soda: See Sodium bicarbonate.

Baldness, alopecia areata, 699; dandruff cause of, 698; may result from seborrheic dermatitis, 681; not due to cutting hair, 696; relation to syphilis, 742; senile alopecia, 699; toxic, 698.

Ballet slippers, 812.

Banana in diabetic diet, 583–584.

Bandages (see also Dressings), 16; gauze, 15.

Bandaging, art of, 22.

Banti's disease, 482.

BANTING, 565, 579.

Barber should sterilize comb and brush, 697.

Barber's itch, 701.

Barbital poisoning, symptoms, antidotes and treatment, 43.

Barbituric acid derivatives in medicine chest, 13; poisoning, symptoms, antidotes and treatment, 43.

Barley water, in infant feeding, 200.

BARLOW, 433.

Basal metabolism: See Metabolism.

Bath (see also Bathing), classified according

to temperature, 668; cold, 668–669; cold, during menstrual period, 53; cold, in conditioning against colds, 310; continuous, for mental disorder, 844; contrast, for feet, 809; contrast, for sprained ankle, 818; cool, 668–669; hot sitz, during pregnancy, 163; hot, to control convulsions in infants, 213; infant's (see "Bathing"); itch, 668; medicated, 669; mud, 669; of potassium permanganate helpful in destroying body odor, 684; Russian, during pregnancy, 163; "salt towel" rub during pregnancy, 162; shower, during pregnancy, 162, 163; sponge, during pregnancy, 162, 163; sulphur, 669; sun, 675; sweat, 669; sweat, during pregnancy, 163; tepid, 668; tub, should be avoided in pregnancy, 162, 163; Turkish, during pregnancy, 163; water, temperature of, during pregnancy, 162.

Bathing, 667; during menopause, 59; during menstrual period, 53; during postnatal period, 175; during pregnancy, 162; effect on skin, 667; feet, 809; frequent, to prevent infectious disease, 239; infant, directions, 186, 226; infant, toilet necessities, 169; infant who is sick, 205; open-air, 669; use of soap in, 668.

Battery, storage, manufacture, litharge poisoning in, 653.

BAUER, WALTER, 340, 341.

Bay rum, spirits of, as mild antiseptic for hair and scalp, 698.

B. C. G. vaccine in tuberculosis, 324.

Beans, growing, as a lesson in sex education, 70.

Bearded region, infection in, and treatment, 701.

BECKMAN, HARRY, on diet in tuberculosis, 331.

Bed, for infant, 185; pans, 15, 16; rest in, normal diet for, 791; -wetting, 445; -wetting, Paulus Ægineta remedy for, 445.

Bee sting, first aid for, 34.

Beef, calories in, 766; intestinal "worms" from, 415–416.

Behavior, adjustment of, 832; childhood patterns of, 832 ff.; difficulties in children may be caused by encephalitis, 302; mental disease and, 828; problems and treatment, 842.

BEHRING, VON, 241.

Belching during pregnancy, 166.

BELL, NEIL, in The Marriage of Simon Harper, describes diphtheria epidemic, 241.

Belladonna poisoning, symptoms, antidotes and treatment, 43.

"Bellyache," 764.

Bence-Jones protein (proteinuria), 438, 460.

Benedict test for sugar in urine, 581.

BENNETT, HUGHES, 464.

Benzene, ethyl, industrial hazard, 647; industrial poison, 651.

Benzine, cause of aplastic anemia, 470; industrial hazard, 647.

Benzoin, use in steam therapy, 15.

Benzol, industrial hazard, 647.

Beriberi, a vitamin B deficiency, 491; derivation of the word, 491; historical aspect, 491; symptoms, 492; treatment, 492.

BERNE, SWITZERLAND, goiter in, 555.

BEST, 579.

Betel nut, chewing, cause of cancer, 625.

Bible, references in, to kidneys, 428; reference in, to reins, 428–429.

Bicarbonate of soda: See Sodium bicarbonate.

Bichloride of mercury: See Mercury.

Bichromates, 647.

Bicycle riding, avoid, during pregnancy, 160.

Bile, action in digestion, 383, 384, 385; aids in digestion of fats, 383, 384; composition, 385; in blood, 403–404.

Bilharzia, irritation from, cause of cancer, 625.

"Bilious," 402.

Birds, reproduction in, 71.

BIRKHAUG, KONRAD, research on erysipelas, 278–279.

Birth, estimating day of, 150.

Birth control, 60–63, 118, 119; dangers of contraceptives, 144; "safe period," 60–63; should be discussed before marriage, 111; young married couple and, 116.

Birthmarks, 690; not due to prenatal influence, 691; superstitions about, 177; vascular, 690.

Biscuit in diabetic diet, 584.

Bismuth formic iodide dusting powder for soft corn, 823–824.

Bismuth treatment of syphilis, 744.

Bisulphide of carbon, industrial hazard, 647.

Bites, dog, and hydrophobia, 282, 283, 284; first aid for, 34.

Black and blue marks, first aid for, 22; tendency to, in purpura, 480.

Black damp, industrial hazard, 659.

Black eye, 22, 705; don't apply beefsteak, knife handle, or strong lotions, 22; eyeball likely to be injured, 22.

Black urine, 461.

Black widow spider, first aid for, 35.

BLACKALL, on albumin in urine, 432.

Blackheads (acne vulgaris), 681–683; don't pick at pimples and, 683; steaming face for, 675; treatment, 682–683.

BLACKLEY, 505, 508.

Bladder, cancer, 633; cancer in the male, 142; habits, training infant in, 226; place in journey through kidney, 427; symptoms of allergy, 522.

Blanching of skin, 663.

Bland diet, 793.

"Bleeder," 479.

Bleeding (see also Hemorrhage), abnormal, 479; after shaving, how to stop, 15; control of, 21; first aid for, 20; from scalp, how to control, 22; from varicose vein, how to control, 21; from wounds, how to stop, 15.

Blindness, caused by cataract can be cured, 712; caused by fireworks, 24, 25; caused by glaucoma, 713; caused by gonorrhea, 745, 746; caused by sinus infection, 726; caused by vitamin A deficiency, 489.

Blisters, chicken pox, 262, 263.

BLOCH, 488.

Blood, 464 ff.; bile in, 403–404; circulation, 351–353; circulation, increasing, in foot by contrast bath, 809; convalescent (see "Convalescent"); count, meaning of, 465; diseases, 464 ff.; first examination with microscope, 464; history of research on, 464; in tears, 710; Kahn test on, 468; laboratory tests, meaning of, 468; "medicines" in anemia, 472; "medicines" in syphilis, 742; platelets, 467; poisoning, 465; poisoning, syphilis not form of, 742; "purifiers" make acne vulgaris worse, 682; quantity of, which flows through kidney, 425; red coloring matter, standard, 466; skin nourished by, 666; sugar, almost normal in treated diabetic, 591; sugar, excess in untreated diabetic, 590; sugar, normal, in healthy person, 569; sugar, regulated by pancreas, 589; supply of heart, 372–373; supply of heart interfered with in angina pectoris, 373; tests in kidney disease, 442; tonics, 475; urea concentration in uremia, 447; urea concentration in, test of kidney function, 442, 443; vomiting in gastric and duodenal ulcer, 400; Wassermann test, 468.

Blood cells, number, increase, decrease, 467; red, 465; red, anemia, 469 ff.; red, development, 466; red, length of survival, 471;

red, number in healthy person, 466; red, too many or polycythemia, 476; white number in normal person, 467; white, too many, 478.

Blood-letting in polycythemia, 477.

Blood pressure, 607 ff.; acute or temporary, 618; definition, 608; diastolic, average by age, 609; diastolic, definition, 610; effect of alcohol on, 614; effect of coffee, etc., on, 613; high, as a symptom, not a disease, 611; high, causes, 611; high, defined, 610; high, diet in, 615; high, importance of, 610; high, in aged, 852–853; high, inflammation of retina in, 713; high, kidney secondary to, 454; high, meatless diet fad, 762; high, nosebleed in, 724; high, per cent in 17,000 men, 5; high, treatment, 614; high, work and, 616; high, worry cause of, 615; increased by adrenalin, 547; low, 617; low, causes, 619–620; low, chronic or persistent, 619; low, defined, 610; low, in various diseases, 619; low, influenza cause of, 617–618; low, per cent in 17,000 men, 5; low, suprarenals cause of, 618; low, symptoms, 618–619; low, treatment, 620; low, treatment, exercise, 620–621; low, what is it? 619; measuring, 608; Nicholson's rule, 610; normal, 610; systolic, 608; systolic, average by age, 609.

Blood transfusion, 473; donor, 473.

Blood vessels tumors of older skin, 691.

Blue moles, 690.

B.O. (body odor), 665, 684.

Boards for certifying specialists, 6.

Body, alkalinity different from stomach acidity, 773; lice, 686; localization of germs in, 235; odor, 665, 684; odor, cause of, 665; paths by which germs invade, 234; response to germ invasion, 235; weight (see "Weight").

Boil, in external ear, 715, 717; in nose, 721.

Bone, broken, first aid for, 19, 20; swallowing, relief for, 23.

BOOERHAAVE, research on urine, 431.

Borax poisoning, symptoms, antidotes and treatment, 43.

BORDET, research on whooping cough, 259.

Boric acid, added to cold cream, 672; antiseptic use, 14, 26, 674; compress, 674, 769; in dusting powder, 671; in gargles, 730; poisoning, symptoms, antidotes and treatment, 43; solution, concentrated, 18; solution for sunburn, 679; solution, how to make, 674; solution, saturated, as antiseptic, 26; solution, saturated, for washing out eye, 24; solution to relieve eczema, 679.

Boron poisoning, symptoms, antidotes and treatment, 43.

Bostock, 433, 504–505, 508.

Bottles, containing old prescriptions should be emptied and washed, 9; in medicine chest should be clearly labeled, 18; nursing, choice and care, 203; shake before measuring medicine, 11.

Bowels (see also Intestines, Stools), care of, during pregnancy, 155; medicines for moving (see "Cathartics and Laxatives"); not necessary to move every day, 408; training infant to develop regular habit, 188, 225.

Bowman's capsule, 422, 423.

Boys, descent of testicles in, 84.

Boy Scout Manual, 101.

Braasch, 462.

Braces for straightening teeth, 751.

Bradford, William L., 735.

Brain, hemorrhage, death rate, 1932 567; hemorrhage death rate compared with heart disease, 347; inflammation of (see "Encephalitis," "Epidemic"); tumor, hiccups with, 36.

Bran, harmful, in smooth diet for indigestion, 393; water as soap substitute, 673.

Brass, industrial hazard, 648.

Brass chills, from zinc, 660.

Brassière to be worn during pregnancy, 158, 163.

Bread, copper and iron in, 772; in diabetic diet, 584; protein yield, 789; rye, Slavic tradition of, 765.

Breakfast, caloric yield of, 789–790; distribution of protein, fat, and carbohydrate, 790.

Breast (see also Nipples), caked, 196; cancer, 142, 632; cancer in men, 629, 633; cancer, life expectancy with, 623–624; care of, in breast feeding, 173; care of, in pregnancy, 163; care of, in weaning baby, 176; feeding of infants, 196; feeding, technic, 197; milk, as preventive of rickets 498; milk, compared to cow's milk, 199; milk in, in infant, 187; supports worn during pregnancy, 158, 163.

Breath, bad, 756; in dyspepsia, 397; odor of, indication in unconsciousness, etc., 32; shortness of, during pregnancy, 165.

Breathing (see also Respiration), through mouth cause of bad formation of teeth, 751.

Bridges, dental, 757.

Bright, Richard, coined the word "uremia," 447; history of kidney before time of, 428; work of, 432.

Bright's disease, 421, 428, 432; acute, 453; causes, 444; chronic, 453; death rate in 1932, 567; gouty, 457.

Britten, 435.

Brodie, Maurice, developed infantile paralysis vaccine, 267.

Bronchitis, unfavorably influenced by removal of tonsils, 737.

Bronchopneumonia, result of vitamin A deficiency, 489.

Bronze powders, industrial poisoning, 648.

Bronze workers, lead poisoning, 648.

Brown moles, 690.

Brown, Lawrason, editor of material on tuberculosis, 333.

Brown-Sequard, 549.

Brucellosis: See Undulant Fever.

Bruises, 22; first aid for, 22; ice-water pads for, 22.

Brunettes, 663.

Brushes, 697; seborrheic dermatitis spread by, 681; shaving, sterilizing, 701; sterilizing in formalin solution, 697; toothbrush, 752.

Brushing the hair, 696.

Bunions, 822; treatment, 822.

Burning sensation on tongue, 719.

Burns, acid, treatment, 27; area, of slight, should be covered with cold water, 27; danger of, in diabetes, 599; electric, treatment, 27; lime or calcium oxide, industrial hazard, 652; of eye, 707; treatment, 26; treatment, liquid or melted petrolatum application, 27; treatment, tannic acid, 27.

Butter, fat in, 585; food value of, 782; fuel value of, compared to sugar, 780.

Buttermilk, protein in, 788.

Buttocks, infant's, should be washed after each stool, 187.

Butyl alcohol, industrial hazard, 648.

Cabbage, calories in, 766.

Cadmium, industrial hazard, 648.

Cæsarean section, 143; superstitions regarding, 179.

Caffeine, cause of high blood pressure, 613.

Caisson disease, 640.

Caked Breast: See Breast.

Calcium, in diet, 773; in relation to tooth decay in adults, 752; in treatment of tuberculosis, 330; metabolism and parathyroids, 543; necessary in formation of good teeth, 750; oxide, industrial poison, 652; value of various foods, 781.

Calculi of kidney, 455.

Calmette vaccination against tuberculosis, 324, 336.

Calories, content of various foods, 585; defined, 189, 765; in diabetic diet based on patient's weight, 587; number needed, calculating, 767; number needed according to type of work done, 767; translating suggested diet in, for diabetic, 587; values of foods by, 766; weight reduction and, 767; yield of breakfast, 790; yield of dinner, 790; yield of luncheon, 790; yield of various foods, 789.

CALVIN, 435, 439.

CAMP, WALTER, "daily dozen" exercises for low blood pressure, 620.

CAMPBELL, C. MACFIE, 837.

Camphor poisoning, symptoms, antidotes and treatment, 44.

Camps, diabetic, 604.

Cancer, 622 ff.; aluminum does not cause, 625; American Society for Control of Cancer, 636; animal, 630; bladder, 633; bladder, in men, 142; breast, 142, 629, 632; breast, in men, 629, 632; causes, 624; causes, heat, 625; causes, irritation, 624; causes, parasites, 625; causes, research on, 622; causes, tobacco, 625; cells, types of, 631; classification, 627; contagion, 630; death from, in 1904 compared with 1929, 566; death from, decrease in women under fifty-five, 624; death in, cause of, 628; death in diabetics due to, 602; death rate according to location in body, 632 ff.; death rate compared with heart disease, 347; death rate, geographic distribution, 626; death rate in 1932, 567; death rate in Switzerland, 626; death rate in United States, 626–627; definition, 624, 627; derivation of word, 627; diagnosis, 634; diet in relation to, 622–623, 625; distribution, 625; education by *Hygeia*, 636; education of the public, 636; esophagus, cause of difficulty in swallowing, 395; gall-bladder, 629; gall-bladder, relation to gallstones, 403; genitals, 141; geographical distribution, 625; heredity, 628; houses, villages, districts, 630; in Negroes, 629; in old age, 853; intestines, 628, 633; kidney, 633; larynx, 632; lip, 629; mouth, 629; nature of, 627; not a disgraceful disease, 627; penis, 629; prevention, 637; prostate, 142, 633; quack never cured any cancer, 637; racial distribution, 629; rec-

tum, 413, 633; rectum, intestinal obstruction first sign, 415; sex distribution, 629; sigmoid, 413; skin, 627, 692; stomach, 407, 628, 629; squamous cell, 631; symptoms, 630; syphilis not cause of, 742; thyroid, 628; transference from animal to animal, 630; treatment, radium, 631 ff., 636; treatment, surgical, 636; treatment, X-ray, 631 ff., 636; uterus (womb), 629, 632; varieties, 630.

Cantharides, as sexual stimulant, 145; poisoning, symptoms, antidotes and treatment, 44.

Capsules, correct way to give, 11.

Carbohydrates (*see also* **Starch, Sugar**), absorption in small intestines, 383; cereals equal a 75 per cent sugar solution, 784; distribution of, according to meal, 790 ff.; food element, 768, 770, 771; in diabetic diet, 582; in diet, 780; in diet during pregnancy, 152; in fruits, 784; in fruits and vegetables per cent, 583; in milk formula for infants, 199; in various foods, 585; journey of, 386–387; metabolism and the pancreas, 588, 589; rôle in nutrition, 189, 190; value in diet, 770.

Carbolic Acid (phenol) in glycerine as eardrops for otitis media, 718; industrial hazard, 648; inks, 652; poisoning, first aid for, 41; poisoning, symptoms, antidotes and treatment, 48; skin antiseptic, 674.

Carbon bisulphide, industrial hazard, 647; industrial hazard in rayon manufacture, 657.

Carbon dioxide, hazard in tobacco industry, 659; in mines, "black damp," 659; in sewer gas, industrial poison, 657; industrial hazard, 649.

Carbon hazard in Portland cement, 656.

Carbon monoxide in mines, "white damp," 659; in sewer gas, industrial poison, 657; industrial poison, 649; poisoning, methylene blue injections for, 31; poisoning, resuscitation, 31; poisoning, symptoms, antidotes and treatment, 45.

Carbon oxychloride, industrial poison, 656.

Carbon tetrachloride, industrial hazard, 649; industrial poison in pyrene, 657.

Carbonyl, nickel, industrial poison, 654.

Cardiospasm, 394–395.

Cardiovascular disease, cause of death of diabetics, 602; symptoms in kidney disease, 443.

Carditis: *See* **Heart, rheumatic inflammation.**

Carotene cause of violet odor of sweat, 665; precursor of vitamin A, 490.

Carriers of disease: *See* **Disease.**

Carrots, food elements in, 771.

Cascara, aromatic, in medicine chest, 12.

Castor oil, 17; disguising, 11; laxative in medicine chest, 12.

Casts in the urine, 440.

Cataract, 711; in diabetics, 597; quack remedies for, 712; surgical treatment only treatment, 712.

Catarrh, vernal, in sensitiveness to light, 519.

Cathartics and laxatives, 11, 17, 417; danger of using, 12; effect of certain articles in infant's diet, 216; for nursing mother, 174; fruits are mild laxatives, 784; habitual use of, cause of constipation, 409; in colds, 311, 314; mineral oil for aged, 853; usually found in medicine chest, 12; use in colds, 311, 314; use in constipation, 409–410; use in pregnancy, 156.

Catheter, ureteral, use in examining kidney function, 442.

Cattle, tuberculosis in, 325.

Caul or veil on new-born child, 181.

Cellulose, in fruits and vegetables, 785; in potato peel, 785.

Cement, Portland, industrial poison, 656.

Centipede, bite of, first aid for, 35.

Cereals, carbohydrates of, 782, 784; food value of, 782; in infant's diet, 205; protein value of, 782–783; protein yield of, 789; 75 per cent carbohydrate, 784; specially prepared for children, 225.

Cerumen or wax of the ear, 716.

Chafing, 678.

Change of life: *See* **Menopause.**

Chaperons, 109.

Chapping, 678.

Charcot, 851.

Charleston, West Virginia, goiter in, 558.

Cheese, calories in, 766; fat in, 585; food value of, 782; protein yield of, 789.

Chemicals, hiccups due to, 36; used in industry, poisoning from, 645.

Chest, cavity, position of heart in, 349; ice bag applied to, in lung hemorrhage, 21; medicine (*see* "Medicine chest").

Chewing betel nut cause of cancer, 625.

Chicago outbreak of amebiasis, 287, 288, 290.

Chicken pox, 261 *ff.;* blisters, 262, 263; cause of, 262; diet in, 263; how spread, 262; in adult may be mistaken for smallpox,

263; incidence, 238; incubation period, 232; quarantine period, 262.

Child, unborn: *See* **Fetus**

Childbirth (*see also* **Confinement, Labor**), afterbirth, 171, 172; Cæsarean section, 179; care of baby as soon as it is born, 171; injuries of cervix, etc., should be repaired to prevent cancer, 637; preventing death after, 148; superstitions about, 177; tying and cutting the cord, 171, 172; what to do if baby born at home, 171; why painful in humans, 75.

Children (*see also* **Adolescence, Boys, Girls, Infants**), adoption of, 119; behavior problems may be result of encephalitis, 302; care and feeding of, 182 *ff.;* care of skin in, 676; diabetic (*see* "Diabetes mellitus"); exposure to tuberculosis, 320; flat-feet in, 810; goiter in, 557; infectious diseases of, 241; love affairs of, 91, 92; maladjustment, treatment, 832–833, 841; mental development of, 229; mental training in, 834; of couple past forty, 122; posture, 797 *ff.;* primary purpose of marriage, 130, 132; protein needed in diet of, 777; psychology, 91 *ff.*, 830 *ff.;* seats for, 797; sex education, 82 *ff.;* sitting posture, 797 *ff.;* susceptible to tuberculosis, 324, 325; taller than their parents and grandparents, 182; training, 833; young married couple and, 116, 118, 119.

Chilling, predisposing factor in catching cold, 309, 310.

Chills, brass, from zinc, 660; in typhoid, 274; zinc or foundrymen's, 648.

Chiropodists great help to diabetics, 599.

Chittenden, 777.

Chloasma, 691; treatment, 691.

Chloral hydrate, poisoning, symptoms, antidotes and treatment, 44.

Chloride of lime, industrial poison, 649.

Chlorination of water in control of amebiasis, 290.

Chlorine, industrial poison, 649–650.

Chloroform, industrial hazard, 649; poisoning, symptoms, antidotes and treatment, 42; to remove insect from ear, 716.

Chlorosis, 471.

Chocolate, 786.

Choking, first aid for, 23.

Cholesterol probable cause of old age, 598.

Chordee, 746.

Chorea (St. Vitus's Dance), manifestation of rheumatic fever, 356, 359; tonsils and, 736.

Christian, Dr.,

Chrome ulcers, 647.

Chromic acid as foot wash for perspiring feet, 824; for removing warts, 821.

Chromium, in green putty, industrial hazard, 657; industrial hazard, 647; plating, industrial hazard, 644.

Chromosomes, rôle in sex determination, 81.

Chrysanthemum buds, industrial poison, 650, 652.

Cicatrix: See Scars.

Cigarettes, smoking, by adolescent girls, 51; smoking, during pregnancy, 153.

Cinchophen poisoning, symptoms, antidotes and treatment, 44.

Circulation, of blood, 351–353; of the heart, 373.

Circulatory system, description and function, 348.

Circumcision, 83, 84, 139; prevents cancer of penis, 629.

Citrate of magnesia, directions for using, 17.

Citric acid milk, preparation of, 203.

Civilization of instinct, 831.

CIVIL WAR, "soldiers' hearts" in the, 378.

CLARKE, J. LYELL, 292, 294.

Cleanliness, and infection, 239; of diabetics, 595.

CLEMENCEAU, diabetes in, 577.

CLENDENING, LOGAN, 611, 616.

CLEVELAND, OHIO, goiter in, 555.

Climacteric: See Menopause.

Climate, effect on allergy, 509; in prevention and treatment of tuberculosis, 325; in relation to rheumatic fever, 364.

Clinical thermometer, 16, 17.

Clothing, for prospective mother to take to hospital, 168; in pregnancy, 157; infant's, avoiding pins and buttons in, 227; infant's, list of, 169; infant's, to be worn home from hospital, 168; infant's, what the infant should wear, 228; odor of genitals and, 138; postural effect of, 802; round shoulders and, 803.

Clubbing of fingers in endocarditis, 370.

Club-foot, 819; statistics, 819–820; treatment, 819–820.

Coal tar, industrial poison, 658.

Cocaine poisoning, symptoms, antidotes and. treatment, 44.

Cocoa, 786.

Coconut oil in hard-water soap, 670.

Cod-liver oil, colds in infants and, 207; dosage in rickets, 219; for pregnant woman to insure good teeth, 748; in infant feeding, 204; rich source of vitamin A, 491; treatment of tuberculosis, 330, 331; use

in rickets, 497; value in rickets, 496; viosterol with, 193; vitamin D in, 192.

Codeine-papaverine preparation for colds, 312.

Coffee, 786; black, in narcotic poisoning, 41; cause of high blood pressure, 613; use by adolescents, 51.

Coitus: See Sexual intercourse.

Cold, chapping due to, 678; industrial conditions due to, 651; industrial hazard, 639; sensitiveness to, 518.

Cold bath, 668–669; during menstrual period, 53, 140; technic in conditioning against colds, 310; temperature of, 668.

Cold cream, 17, 672; as substitute for soap, 668; for sunburn, 678; formula, 673; greaseless, 672; harmful for greasy skin, 672; rancid, 672; should not be used in acne vulgaris, 682.

Cold sores on lips in indigestion, 391.

Cold treatment of allergy, 528.

Cold water, covering of area of slight burns with, 27; sponging with, in heat stroke, 34; swimming during menstrual period, 140; use of, in fainting, 33.

Cold weather brings about colds, 306.

Colds, 304 ff.; aspirin used in treating, 312; bare legs in conditioning against, 310; blowing nose, 314; cathartics in, 311, 314; causes of, 305; chilling as predisposing factor, 309, 310; codeine-papaverine preparation for, 312; conditioning against, 310; dampness as predisposing factor, 309; diet in, 312; different from influenza, 305; effect of removing tonsils on frequency of, 736, 737; fatigue as predisposing factor, 309; frequent, per cent in 17,000 men, 5; gargles (antiseptic) in, 14; heat regulation of body and, 306; heating of homes in relation to, 309; humidity in relation to, 309; in Eskimos, 306; in infants, 206, 207; incidence, 304; incidence, relation to infected tonsils and adenoids, 733–734; laxatives in, 311, 314; lemonade for, 314; living conditions responsible for, 307; loosening the cough, 313; mustard poultice for, 313; nose obstruction in relation to, 307; nose sprays for, 313; orangeade for, 314; prevention of, 308; relation of, to "flare up" in rheumatic fever, 365; remedies for, cause of low blood pressure, 619; rose cold, 314; seasonal incidence, 305; "shots" against, 311; sign of beginning of infectious disease, 232; sign of rheumatic fever, 358; summer, 314; susceptibility to, 304; symptoms, 307, 308;

tonsils in relation to, 307, 736, 737; treatment, 311; ultraviolet rays in conditioning against, 310, 311; vaccines against, 311; ventilation in relation to, 309; vitamin A rôle in preventing, 312, 490; water given every hour for, 313–314; weather changes and, 305, 306.

Cole, Rufus, 318.

Colic in infant, 215.

Colitis, 410 ff.; causes of, 410; spastic, diet in, 792.

Collapse therapy of tuberculosis, 323.

College, medical: See Medical college.

College students, posture of, 800.

Collodion dressings, 674.

Colon, cathartics, laxatives and enemas, 417.

Color, of hair, 695; of skin, 663.

Colored lights, seeing, 705.

Columbian spirits, industrial hazard, 653.

Coma, diabetic: See Diabetes mellitus.

Combs, 697; fine, for loosening nits of head lice, 697; seborrheic dermatitis spread by, 681.

Comedoes or acne vulgaris, 681–683.

Communicable disease (see also Infectious Disease), 272.

Complexes, sexual, 136.

Compress, boric acid, 674, 769.

Compressed air, caisson disease, 640.

Conception (see also Sexual intercourse), possible, in menstrual cycle, 60–63; possible in nursing mother, 180; prevention of (see "Birth Control").

Condensed milk: See Milk.

Condiments, 786.

Condom, contraceptive device, 144.

Confinement (see also Childbirth, Labor, Postnatal Period), clothing packed in suitcase to be taken to hospital, 168; preparation for, 168; when to call the doctor, 170.

Conjunctivitis, 708.

Constipation, 407 ff.; cathartics, laxatives, and enemas, 417; cause of headache, 39; cause of high blood pressure, 613; causes of, 408; diet in, 394, 409, 791–793; effect on skin, 667; habitual use of purgatives cause of, 409; in aged, 853; in infants, 215; in pregnancy, 165; in pregnancy, avoiding, 155; "roughage school" of diet for, 762.

Contagious Disease: See Infectious Disease.

Contagion of cancer, 630.

Continence, 145.

Contraceptives, 116, 144.

Contrast bath for sprained ankle, 818; for tired feet, 809.

Convalescent blood, use of, in scarlet fever, 258; use of, in measles, 252.

Convalescent serum in treatment of infectious disease, 239.

Convulsions in infants, 212.

Cool, how to keep, 33.

Cool baths, effect of, on skin, 667.

Coolants, industrial poison, 650.

Copper, in various foods, 772; industrial poison, 650.

Copper cyanourate-potassium cyanide, use of, in treatment of tuberculosis, 323.

Copper treatment of tuberculosis, 330.

Cord: See Umbilical Cord.

Corn, calories in, 766; products, allergy, 516; protein in, 770; syrup, 783; syrup, tablespoon equivalents of ounce of, 202; syrup, use in infant feeding, 200, 202.

Cornea, 704; infection in tuberculosis, 710; inflammation due to syphilis, 711; ulcers in trachoma, 709.

Corns, 688, 822; cause of, 823; hard, 823; hard, treatment, 824; soft, 823; soft, treatment, 823; treatment, 688.

Coronary arteries: See Arteries.

Coronary thrombosis: See Thrombosis, coronary.

Corpus luteum, 552.

Corset, maternity, 158; to be worn during pregnancy, 158.

Cortin, 550.

Coryza, 307.

Cosmetics, cold cream, 672; dusting powders, 671; face powders, 671; powders, 671; soap, 669–670.

Cotton, must not be applied to burned area, 27.

Cotton packs, use of, during menstruation, 55.

Cottonseed, allergy, 516.

Cotugno, demonstration of albumin in urine, 431, 432.

Cough (see also Whooping Cough), loosening, 313; relieved by inhaling steam medicated with benzoin, 261; sodium citrate to loosen, 313.

Couple, points to be considered by young people in selecting prospective mates, 105–106; right of privacy of, 108, 109; young married, 116.

Court plaster, 674.

Courtship, 104.

Cows, examination of herds of, in epidemic

of septic sore throat, 732; tuberculosis in, 325.

Crab louse, 687.

Crab meat, protein yield of, 788.

Cracking joints, symptom of arthritis, 338.

Cramps, heat, 644; leg, during pregnancy, 167; rhythmic, sign of beginning labor, 170.

Cream, fat in, 585; food value of, 782.

Cream, cold: See Cold cream.

Creeping of infants, 184.

Creosote, in treatment of tuberculosis, 331; industrial poison, 650.

Cresols, poisoning, symptoms, antidotes, and treatment, 48.

Cretins, 539, 555.

Crib, infant's, blankets, sheets, etc., required for, 169.

Crisis in pneumonia, 316.

Croup, in infants, 208; kettle, 209; mortality from, 1910–1914, 243.

Crowding, factor in pneumonia, 316.

CRUICKSHANK, albumin in dropsical urine demonstrated by, 431, 432.

Crying in infants, 187.

Crystal pock: See Chicken pox.

Curd in stools of infants, 195.

Cuticle, cutting, harmful, 702.

Cutting oils, industrial poison, 650.

Cutting the hair, 696.

Cyanides, industrial poisoning, 650; poisoning, symptoms, antidotes and treatment, 44; sodium, industrial poison, 658.

Cycling, avoid, during pregnancy, 160.

Cystoscope in examining kidney function, 442.

Damp, white, black, or stink, 659.

Dampness, industrial hazard, 640; predisposing factor in catching cold, 309.

Dancing during pregnancy, 160; exercises for women, 801.

Dandruff, 698; comb should be washed in formalin if owner suffers from, 697; treatment, 698.

"Dates" between young people, 107, 108.

DAVIS, 485, 488.

Day of birth, estimating, 150.

Death, in cancer, cause of, 628; cause of, 1904 compared with 1929, 566, 567; from childbirth, 148; from diphtheria and croup, 1910–1914, 243; rate, effect of periodical medical examination on, 5; rate, falling total, compared with increasing diabetic death rate, 566, 567; rate from accidents, 19.

Deer fly fever, 290.

Deficiency diseases, 483 ff.

Deformities, bad posture, 799; caused by allergy, 520; of foot, club-foot, 819; of foot, congenital, 806; of foot due to syphilis, 806–807; of nose, 721, 722.

DEKKERS, demonstration by, of albumin in urine, 431.

DELABARRE, FRANK A., 750.

Dementia, symptom of diarrhea, 499.

Dementia paralytica, 741.

Dental hygiene for adults, 751; for children, 749.

Dental plates, 757.

Dental work during pregnancy, 164.

Dentifrice for children, 749.

Dentist should care for child's first teeth, 749.

Dentistry, preventive, in children, 750; will diminish mouth cancer, 637.

Department-store workers, foot trouble in, 815.

DEPEW, CHAUNCEY, 616.

Depilatories, for superfluous hair, 700; thallium poisoning, 49.

Depression, economic, malnutrition in, result seen in next decades, 765; mental, in migraine or sick headache, 38; mental, 844–845.

Dermatitis, from copper in industry, 650; from dyeing hair, 697; from external irritants, 680; from orris root in face powder, 671; from rotogravure ink, 657; from tannic acid, 658; from tincture of iodine, 680; from zinc chloride, 660; seborrheic, 681, 698; symptom of pellagra, 499.

Desserts, protein yield of, 789.

DETROIT, MICHIGAN, goiter in, 555, 559.

DEVINE, MRS., diabetic camps, 605.

Dextrin-maltose mixture, use in infant feeding, 200.

Dextrose in infant feeding, 200.

Dhobie itch, 685.

Diabetes, derivation of the word, 564.

Diabetes insipidus, 460, 545, 570.

Diabetes mellitus, 459, 503 ff.; acidosis in, 774; arteriosclerosis in, 597; best studied in children, 577; blamable, 571; blameless, 572; camps, 604; carbohydrates and fat in, 780; care of feet in, 599–600; cataracts in, 597; children with, 572; children with, and early old age, 578; children with, are taller, 577; children with, have splendid teeth, 578; children with, mentally superior, 577; children with, pathfinders for adults, 576; children with, should have a dog, 579; chiropodists great help in, 599; cleanliness in, 595; coma, cause of death in, 602; coma, confused with appendicitis, 600, 604; coma, danger of, 603; coma, danger of, from too much fat in diet, 585; coma, death rate from, 601; coma, how to avoid and prevent, 601; coma needless, 603: coma, symptoms, 602; coma, what to do for, 603; danger of burns in, 599; danger of using hot applications, 599; death in, cause of, pre-insulin and insulin period compared, 602; death rate, 565, 566; death rate, effect of insulin discovery on, 588, 589; death rate from coma, decrease in, 563–564; death rate increasing according to countries, 568; diet, 581 *ff.;* diet, calories in, 587; diet, calories needed based on patient's weight, 587; diet, carbohydrates in, 582; diet, carbohydrates in, per cent in various foods, 583; diet, cereals 75 per cent carbohydrate, 784; diet, composition, 582; diet, fat in, 585; diet, fat in, danger of, 585; diet, grapefruit the safest, 583; diet, lump of sugar and five-cent piece weigh alike, 582–583; diet, menu, 586; diet, menu, calorie translation, 587; diet, milk in, 584; diet, protein in, 584; diet, sugar *vs.* starches, 770; diet, vegetables in, 584; Drumm (Louisa) and what she did, 576; during pregnancy, 157; education of patient regarding treatment, 580; exercise in, 587–588; gallstone patient susceptible to, 575; gangrene, 598–599; great men who had, 577; half a million in our midst, 605; heredity factor, 572, 577; historical aspect, 564; home treatment, 581; hospital week-end for patients with, 580; if you discover diabetes in a relative, 575; infections in, 600; insulin in, 580, 586, 588, 591; insulin in, administration other than by injection, 595; insulin in, cost per day, 592; insulin in, discovery effect on death rate, 588, 589; insulin in, dosage in infections, 601; insulin in, dosage based on color of Benedict test, 601; insulin in, duration of action, 592; insulin in, hypodermic syringe for, should be kept separate, 14; insulin in, League of Nations standard, 592; insulin in, must not omit doses without testing urine, 603; insulin in, site for injection, 592–593; insulin reaction, 593–594; insulin reactions, symptoms, treatment, 594; insulin shock and coma, 604; lessens resistance of skin, 667;

marriage: should a patient marry?, 574; Massachusetts Board of Health survey, 566; medals given patients, 596–597; menu for, 586; old age and, 597; overeating and obesity likely to cause, 573; overeating in, 582, 592; pancreas "lazy" in, 591; patient adequately treated (diagram), 591; patient should never overeat, 582; patient untreated (diagram), 590; pimples, boils, etc., in, danger of, 600; plan your visit to your doctor, 581; prevention, 571; prevention, wise control of weight, 574–575; raising legs 45 degrees each day in, 600; retinitis in, 713; symptoms, 570; tonsillitis in, 600; treatment (*see also* "Diabetes Mellitus, diet"; "Diabetes Mellitus, insulin in"), 579 *ff.;* treatment, exercise in, 587; treatment, home, 581; treatment, week-end hospital, 580; urine output enormous, 459; usefulness, 595; wandering diabetic nurse, 581; weight of patient basis for number of calories in diet, 587; what is it?, 567; why is it increasing?, 571.

Diabetes, renal, 460.

Dial (drug), 13.

Dials, watch: *See* Watch.

Diapers, antiseptic put in rinsing water in washing, 187; applying square diaper, 225; rash from, 187; washing, 187.

Diaphragm, relation to hiccups, 36.

Diarrhea, 410 *ff.;* acute, symptoms, 411; cause of death in 1904 compared with 1929, 566; causes, 411; chronic, 411; in infants, 187, 216–217; symptom of pellagra, 499.

Diastol, 351.

Diastolic pressure: *See* Blood pressure.

Diathermy treatment of sprained ankle, 818.

Dichloro-difluoromethane, industrial poison, 650.

Dick, George F., research on scarlet fever, 256.

Dick, Gladys Henry, research on scarlet fever, 256.

Dick test, 256, 257.

Diehl, 435.

Diet (*see also* Food, Nutrition, Vitamins, etc.), 759 *ff.;* alcohol in, 787; appetite guide to, 761; bland, 793; building, 776; calcium in, 773; calories needed by individuals, 767; cancer and, 622–623, 625; carbohydrates in, 770, 780; cereals in, 782–783; condiments and seasoning of food, 786; copper sources in (diagram), 772; distribution of protein, fat and carbohydrate according to meal, 790 *ff*.; during menopause, 59; eggs in, 778, 779; elimination, in diagnosis of headache, 39; essentials of normal, 791; extraneous factors in, 764; fads in (*see* "Food fad"); fat in, 771–772, 780, 786; faulty, cause of diarrhea, 410–411; fish in, 778, 779; for hyperacidity, 794–795; for hypoacidity, 795–796; for nursing mother, 174, 196; formulation of perfect diet, 760–761; fruits in, 784; fuel requisite, 787; Gerson, in tuberculosis, 331, 332; heredity factor in, 764, 765; Herrmannsdorfer-Sauerbruch, in tuberculosis, 331, 332; in acne vulgaris, 683; in arthritis, 340–342; in chicken pox, 263; in colds, 312; in constipation, 394, 409, 791–793; in diabetes (*see* "Diabetes mellitus"); in gout, 345; in high blood pressure, 615; in kidney disease, 449–450; in measles, 252; in pneumonia, 318; in pregnancy, 151–154; in pregnancy complicated by vomiting, 153, 154–155; in pregnancy no effect on size of baby, 180; in pregnancy to avoid constipation, 156; in pregnancy to insure good teeth in child, 748; in relation to tooth decay in adults, 752; in scarlet fever, 257–258; in sinus disease, 727; in tuberculosis, 331–332; in ulcer of stomach and duodenum, 401; in whooping cough, 261; infant's (*see* "Infant's Dict"); iodine in, 773; iron in, 773; iron sources in, 772; meat in, 778, 779; meat in, value, 762; meat in, varieties of, 778; meatless, fad, 762; milk in, value, 781; normal, basic considerations, 787; nuts in, 786; phosphorus in, 773; phosphorus in various foods, 785; protein in, 770; protein needed in diet for children, 777; protein requirement, 778, 787; relation to form and color of stools, 384; "roughage habit," 762; salt in, 773; smooth, in indigestion, 392–394; source of food supply as factor in, 764; sugars in, 783; to prevent teeth decaying during pregnancy, 164; tradition factor in, 764, 765; unbalanced, 763; vegetables in, 785; vitamins place in, 787; water in, 772; well-balanced, needed during adolescence, 51; what daily diet should include, 788; "white flour" danger, 762.

Digestion, 380 *ff*., 774; end products of, 384; gastric, 382; intestinal, 382; intestinal, of food, 776; journey of carbohydrate (diagram), 386–387; method of studying, 388; of infants, 194; stools, form and color 384–385.

Digestive diseases, 380 *ff*.

Digestive tract, 380–381.

Digitalis poisoning, symptoms, antidotes and treatment, 45.

Dimples, cause of, 663.

Dinitrobenzene, industrial poison, 650.

Dinner, caloric yield of, 790; distribution of protein, fat and carbohydrate, 791.

Diphtheria, 241 *ff*.; antitoxin defined, 246; antitoxin, discovery of, 241; antitoxin, dosage, 244; bacilli, discovery of, 242; bacilli, recovered from throats weeks and months after child is well, 244; carrier, 242; carrier, infected tonsils in, 735; diet in, 245; distinguishing from tonsillitis, 732; 85 per cent of deaths occur in children under six, 242; elimination of in Auburn, N. Y., and New Haven, Conn., 248; epidemic, described in *The Marriage of Simon Harper*, by Bell, 241; heart strain in, 248; immunization, 239; immunization defined, 246; immunization, elimination by, 248; immunization of infant, 220; immunization with toxin-antitoxin, 246; intubation tubes (O'Dwyer's), 245, 248; laryngeal (croup) in infants, 208; mortality from, 1910–1914, 243; mortality from, twice that of measles, 253; prevention, relation of removal of tonsils to, 735, 736; quarantine, when should child be released, 244; Schick test, 245; smears taken from throat in suspected cases, 242; symptoms of, 244; throat symptoms in, 734; tonsils in or out in relation to, 734–735, 735–736; toxin, defined, 246; toxin-antitoxin defined, 246; toxoid, defined, 246, 247; transmission, 242; treatment, antitoxin, 247.

Dirt: *See* Filth.

Discoveries, new, in medicine, 4.

Disease, caisson, 640.

Disease carriers (*see also under names of specific diseases as* Diphtheria, Typhoid, *etc.*), 233; control of, 237.

Disease, digestive, 380 *ff*.

Disease, infectious: *See* Infectious Disease.

Disease, industrial: *See* Industrial Disease.

Disease of genitals, 141.

Disease of old age, 851.

Disease, respiratory, 304.

Disease, stamping out, 236.

Disease, transmissible, 272.

Disinfecting wounds, 26.

Diuresis, defined, 450.

Diuretics, use in kidney disease, 450.

Dizziness, 32, 33; during pregnancy, 166; headache in cases of, 38; in old age, 852.

DOBSON on sugar in urine, 431.

DOCHEZ, DR., research on scarlet fever, 256.

Doctor: *See* **Physician.**

Döderlein's bacillus, value in vagina, 139.

Dogs, and diabetics, 579; bites of, first aid for, 34, 35; prohibiting stray, to control hydrophobia, 283; should not be killed after biting, 284; superstition of "dog days," 282; transmission of hydrophobia by, 282.

Donor, blood, 473.

Door-stop exercise, 816.

Douches, antiseptic, danger of, 144; antiseptic or cleansing, 138, 139; before and after menstrual period, 55; dangerous, 139; mercury, may injure kidneys, 448.

Dreams, 137; in adolescent period, 102.

Dressings (*see also* **Bandages**), collodion, 674; moist epsom salts, for tired feet, 809.

Dreyer antigen treatment of tuberculosis, 324.

"Drives" or instincts, 829.

Dropsy (*see also* **Edema**), 451; defined, 425; lipoid nephrosis in, 459; mercury preparation for, 451; symptom in various types of nephritis, 453 *ff.;* tapping in, inscription on gravestone of Lady Page, 451 *footnote.*

Drowning, first aid, 27, 28, 29.

Drugs (*see also* **Medicines**), idiosyncrasies, 517; poisoning from, used in industry, 645.

DRUMM, LOUISA, diabetic, what she did, 576.

Dry cleaning, carbon tetrachloride poisoning, 649; hazard of ethylene dichloride, 651.

Dryness of mouth, relieving, 730–731.

DUKE, WILLIAM W., 504.

DUNBAR, 505.

Duodenum, description, 383; examination of function, 390.

Duodenum ulcer, 398; causes, 398–399; diet in, 401; distinguishing between gall bladder disease and appendicitis, 406; pain in, 399–400; perforation of, 400; symptoms, 399; treatment, 400; vomiting blood in, 400; X-ray examination in, 401.

Dust, allergy, 517; as an industrial hazard, 641.

Dusting powder, 671; applied to feet, 809, 824; boric acid in, 671; for heat rash, 681; for infants, dangers to be avoided, 671–672; for perspiring feet, 824; for prickly heat, 681; for soft corns, 823.

Dwarfs, cretins, 539, 555.

Dyeing the hair, 696–697.

Dyes, injecting, to determine excretory function of kidney, 441, 443.

Dynamite head, nitroglycerin responsible for, 655.

Dysentery, 411 *ff.;* amebic (*see* "Amebiasis"); bacillary, 411; chronic, symptoms, 411; in infants, 216.

Dyspepsia, 380; defined, 395; symptoms of, 395.

Dysphagia, 394.

Dystrophy, adiposo-genital, of Froehlich, 546.

Ear, and its disturbances, 714; boil or abscess in external, 715, 717; canal, infection, 715; "cauliflower" or "tin" ear, 715; diagram showing, 734; don't clean out ear with wires, toothpicks, earspoons, etc., 715; erysipelas, 714; foreign body in, 23; foreign body in, adhesive device for removing, 716–717; foreign body in external, how to remove, 716; frost bite of, 715; infant's, cleaning, 186, 282; infected, prevented by spraying nose or throat, 717; infection, symptoms, 717; inflammation of the middle, 718; inflammation of the middle, in infant, 207; insects in, 716; insects in, how to remove, 23, 716; otitis media, 718; protruding or large ear, surgical treatment for, 715; protruding, plastic surgery of, 715; spraying, 23; syringing, method of, 716; "tin ear," 715; washing, of infant, 228; washing out with syringe, 716; wax, 716.

Earache, 717; glycerine advised for, 17; in scarlet fever, 258.

Eardrops, glycerin with phenol, 718.

Eardrum, puncturing, for otitis media and mastoiditis, 718; puncturing, no damage from, 718.

EASTMAN, successful diabetic, 577, 606.

Eating, learning to eat with false teeth, 758.

Eclampsia, 456.

Economic depression, malnutrition in, result in next decades, 765.

Eczema, 504 *ff.,* 679; boric acid solution to relieve, 679; "don't scratch," 679; made chronic by wrong treatment, 680; not a sign of "bad blood," 679; pollen avoidance and pollen disease, 526; promptly cured, 679; rubbing makes eczema worse, 680; soap and water irritate, 680.

Edema (*see also* **Dropsy**), defined, 425; protein, 777.

EDISON, THOMAS A., successful diabetic, 577, 606.

Effort, sensitiveness to, 518, 519.

Egg cells, fertilization process by sperm cell, 80; in humans, 78.

Eggs, albumin source of protein, 770; allergy in infant, 506; food elements, 771; in infant's diet, 224; of lice, 686; protein in, 778, 779, 789; protein value in terms of round steak, 780; whites as first aid in poisoning, 40; whites for washing hair, 696; yolk in infant feeding, 204, 205; yolk necessary for pregnant woman to insure good teeth, 748.

Egyptian mummies, arteriosclerosis found in, 614.

EHRLICH, PAUL, 464, 743.

EIJKMAN, CHRISTIAAN, 485, 491.

Elastic bandage or stocking for varicose veins, 167.

Electric burns, treatment, 27.

Electric needle for removing superfluous hair, 700.

Electric shock, resuscitation after, 28, 29, 30.

Electricity applied to skin, 675.

Elimination diet in diagnosis of migraine, 39.

Embolus, sign of endocarditis, 370.

Embryo (see also Egg cells, Fetus), development of, 80.

EMERSON, KENDALL, 321.

Emotional difficulty, treatment of in adult, 842.

Emotional security, 834.

Emotional strain cause of high blood pressure, 611; cause of high blood pressure, can be controlled, 614.

Encephalitis, epidemic, 300; case of Patricia Maguire, 301; course of, three stages, 301–302; geographic epidemiology, 300; hiccups in, 37; historical aspect, 300; seasonal incidence, 301; treatment, 302–303.

Encephalitis lethargica: See Encephalitis, Epidemic.

Endocardium, 350.

Endocarditis, 368; acute form, 369; acute, symptoms, 369; emboli sign of, 370; Osler's node sign of, 370; petechiæ sign of, 370; subacute, after rheumatic fever, 369; subacute, organism causing, 369; subacute, symptoms, 369–370.

Endocrines, 532.

Endurance test of good posture, 799.

Enemas, 417; in pregnancy, inadvisable, 156.

Energy rate, or basal metabolism, 768.

Energy value of certain foods, 766.

Engagement, prenuptial agreement and arrangements, 110–111.

Entameba histolytica, 287, 288.

Enteritis, cause of death in 1904 compared with 1929, 566.

Environment, effect on allergy, 509.

Enzymes in gastric juice, 381, 382; in pancreatic juice, 383.

Ephedrine solutions for colds in infants, 207.

Epidemic Encephalitis: See Encephalitis.

Epidermis, structure of, 661.

Epilepsy in infants, 213.

Epilating paste for removing superfluous hair, 700.

Epinephrine: See Adrenalin.

Epsom salts, compresses, ice cold, in erysipelas, 278–279; dosage, 17; laxative in medicine chest, 12; moist dressings for tired feet, 809; use in carbolic-acid poisoning, 41.

Ergosterol, irradiated: See Viosterol.

Ergot poisoning, symptoms, antidotes and treatment, 45.

Eruptions in infectious disease, 232.

Erysipelas, 277 ff.; antitoxin, 279; course of disease, 277; history of, 277; incubation period, 232; of ear, 714; recurrence likely, 279; seasonal incidence, 277; transmission of, 277; treatment, 278–279; treatment, antitoxin, 279.

Erythrocytes: See Blood cells, red.

Eskimos, colds in, 306.

Esophagus cancer, difficult swallowing may be due to, 395.

Esophagus, diagram showing, 734; examination by lighted tube, 395; function in digestion, 281; spasm, 394.

Ether poisoning, symptoms, antidotes and treatment, 42.

Ethics, medical, 3.

Ethyl-alcohol poisoning, symptoms, antidotes and treatment, 42.

Ethyl benzene, industrial poison, 651.

Ethyl nitrate, industrial poison, 651.

Ethylene dichloride, industrial poison, 649, 650, 651, 652.

Eugenics, knowledge of, spread by diabetic, 596.

Eunuchs, 553.

Eustachian tube, diagram showing, 734.

Evaporated milk, 199.

Ewald test breakfast in studying digestion. 388.

Exercise, corrective, during higher school

grades, 798; corrective, in kindergarten training, 798; door-stop, 816; during menstrual period, 53, 103, 802; for faulty posture, 804–805; for infant, 188, 220; for nursing mother, 175; for stretching tendon of Achilles, 814; golf-ball exercise, for fallen arches, 817; in aged, 852; in infantile paralysis, American Medical Association committee suggestions on, 269–270; in postnatal period, 172; in treatment of diabetes, 580; in treatment of low blood pressure, 620–621; in water in infantile paralysis, 268; marble, for fallen arches, 817; pencil, for fallen arches, 817; to correct flat-foot, 813; to strengthen foot, 814; towel, for fallen arches, 816; treatment of allergy, 528; value in diabetic treatment, 587; violent, avoid, in pregnancy, 160.

Exertion, angina pectoris attacks brought on by, 374.

Exhaustion, heat, what to do in case of, 34.

Explosions of fireworks, 24.

Eye, boric acid solution for washing out, 24; boric acid solution for washing out, not necessary in infants, 226; camera-like mechanism of, 712; care in industry, 707; cleaning, in infants, 186, 226; conjunctivitis, 708; construction of, 704; diseases of, 704; drops, how to put in, 24; dryness of, symptom in xerophthalmia, 488; effects of abscessed teeth (diagram), 755; foreign bodies in, 23, 706, 707; foreign bodies in, how to remove, 24; glaucoma, 713–714; in measles, care of, 252; inflammation of iris, 711; inflammation of retina, 712; injuries from ultra-violet and infra-red rays, 643; no condition of, should be neglected, 714; penetrating injury, 706; pink eye, 708–709; retina, detachment, 713; seeing colored lights, 705; spots or specks in vision, 705; sympathetic ophthalmia, 706; symptoms in disease unrelated to eye, 711; symptoms of allergy, 521; trachoma, 709; ulcer on, 710.

Eye, black, 705; don't apply beefsteak, knife handle, or strong lotions, 22; first aid for, 22; treatment, 706; X-ray picture, 706.

Eyeball, don't remove foreign body from surface of, 24; likely to be injured in black eye, 22.

Eye dropper, how to use, 24.

Eyelids, rolling back eyelids to remove foreign body, 24; styes, 709.

Eyesight: See Vision.

Eyestrain cause of headache, 38.

Face deformity caused by allergy, 520; lifting for wrinkles, 693; powder, 671; powder for sunburn, 678; powder, lead salts in, 671; powder, orris root in, 671; steaming, for blackheads, 675; superfluous hair on, 700; swelling, during pregnancy, 157, 165; wrinkles, 693.

Faddists: See Food.

Fainting, aromatic spirits of ammonia for, 14, 18; during pregnancy, 166; first aid for, 32, 33; spells during pregnancy, 165; symptoms of oncoming faint, 33; what to do after a person faints, 33.

Fallen arches: See Arches.

Fallopian tubes, 80.

Falls, constitute 40 per cent of accidents in the home, 19; first aid for, 19–20.

False teeth: See Teeth.

FALSTAFF, Shakespeare's, on urine examination, 440.

Family medicine chest: See Medicine chest.

Family physician: See Physician.

Family, size of, 119; union of, necessary in rearing children, 79.

Farmers, number of calories used daily by, 767.

Fat, absorption, 384; content in various foods, 585; danger of, in diabetic diet, 585; deposit tumors or xanthoma, 694; digestion of, aided by bile, 383, 384; distribution of, according to meal, 790 ff.; food element, 768, 770, 771; fuel value of, 786; fuel value of, compared with protein or carbohydrate, 772; glands, description, 662; in cheese, 585; in cream, 585; in diabetic diet, 582, 585; in diet, 770, 780, 786; in diet during pregnancy, 152; in nuts, 585, 786; lessen fat in infant's feeding during acute illness, 213; not digested in stomach, 382; of skin, 663; per cent in butter, 585; rôle in nutrition, 189, 190; source of, 770; source of, in American dietary, 780; type of, in food which, possibly, causes old age, 598.

Father, attitude on male parent in sex education, 73, 74, 88; reproductive power after fifty-five years of age, 531.

Father-and-daughter complex, 136.

"Father and mother" games, 92.

Fatigue, cause of angina pectoris attacks, 375; predisposing factor in catching cold, 309.

Fear, cause of high blood pressure, 612, 615.

Feathers, allergy, 515.

Feces: *See* Stools.

Feeble-mindedness, 838; due to endemic goiter, 561; in endemic goiter districts, 555; symptoms of, 838.

Feeding: *See* Infants.

Feeding, breast: *See* Infants, Nursing mother.

Feeding fevers instead of starving them, 235.

Feet: *See* Foot.

Ferments, digestive, 381, 382.

FERNALD, WALTER, 838.

Fetus (*see also* Embryo, Infants), cord looped around neck, not result of mother reaching, 181; diet in pregnancy and, 151; effect of goiter in pregnancy on, 560, 561; sex determination, 178; sex of, not determined by shape of abdomen, 181; size of, not dependent on diet of mother, 180.

Fever (*see also* Scarlet fever, Typhoid, *etc.*), as defense mechanism, 235–236; feeding instead of starving, 235; in acute indigestion, 391; in infants, reducing, 205; in tuberculosis, 331; metal fume, industrial, 650; result of germ invasion, 235; symptom in distinguishing ulcer, gall-bladder disease, and appendicitis, 406.

Fever, Rabbit: *See* Tularemia.

Fever, Rat-Bite: *See* Rat-Bite Fever.

Fever, Parrot: *See* Psittacosis.

Fever, Undulant: *See* Undulant Fever.

Filth, flies carry, 274.

Financial worry cause of high blood pressure, 615.

Fingernails: *See* Nails.

Fingers, "clubbed" in congenitally defective hearts, 355; clubbing, in endocarditis, 370; sucking, in infant, 188–189.

Fire, how to put out, 27; repellent, zinc chloride hazard, 660.

Firecrackers, first aid for injuries from, 24.

Fireworks, explosion of, 24; injury from, get doctor at once, 25; phosphorus hazard in making, 656.

First aid, 19 *ff.;* accidents, 19; bite wounds, 34; bleeding, 20; bruises, 22, 642; burns, 26; carbon-monoxide poisoning, 30; choking, 23; drowning, 27, 28; electric shock, 28; eye injury, 707; fainting, 32; falls, 19; firearms, 24; fireworks injuries, 24; food poisoning, 40; foreign bodies, 23; gas poisoning, 30; headache, 37; heat stroke, 33; hemorrhage, 20; hiccups, 35; in childbirth case, 171; in threatened abortion or miscarriage, 166; industrial, for cuts, scratches and abrasions necessary, 642; metallic poisoning, 40; migraine, 37; nose-

bleed, 20; poisoning, 40; resuscitation, **27**; sick headache, 37; sprained ankle, 818; supplies in medicine chest, 15; toy firearm injuries, 24; unconsciousness, 32; wounds, 25.

Fish, allergy to, 507; protein in, 778, 779, 788; reproduction in, 71; tradition of, in diet, 765.

Fish tapeworm, 415–416.

FISHBEIN, MORRIS, 1, 9, 19, 50, 230, 241, 272, 304, 337, 704, 738, 748, 848.

Fishhook, how to remove from skin, 26.

Flames, smothering, with blanket, etc., 27.

Flat-foot, 802–803, 810 *ff.;* diagram showing, 808; example (illustration), 816; exercises to correct, 813; in children, 810; result of accidents, 810; rigid, example of, 816; shoes for, 812; walking, correct way, 810.

Flatulence, 396.

Flea bites, first aid for, 35.

Flies carriers of amebic dysentery, 288, 290; carry over 6 million bacteria on body, 274; filth carried by, 274; life cycle, 275; typhoid transmission by, 273.

Floating kidney, 461.

Flour, "white flour" danger fad, 762.

Flue, defective flue fumes, poisoning from, symptoms, antidotes and treatment, 45.

Flukes, 415.

Fluoride poisoning, symptoms, antidotes and treatment, 45.

Flushing of skin, 663.

Fly: *See* Flies.

Fontanel, calcification, 184; failure to close, sign of rickets, 497.

Food (*see also* Diet, Nutrition, Vitamins), absorption, 774; acid-base ratio, 773; acid-producing, 773; alkaline-producing, 773; allergy, 39, 515, 763; assimilation, 774; avoiding certain foods in pregnancy, 155: calcium value, 781; caloric yield, 789; calories, 765; calories in various foods, 766; canned, does not cause cancer, 325; carbohydrates in, per cent, 583; carbohydrates, protein, fat and calories in various foods, 585; cause of diarrhea, 411; classification, 768; condiments, 786; contaminated, source of intestinal "worms," 416; diabetic (*see* "Diabetes mellitus"); digestion, 774; elements, main, 768, 770, 771; facts about (chart), 771; faddist and cancer, 622–623; faddist on proper diet for arthritis, 340–341; fads and fancies, 761; fads, protein fear, 777; fat in, type of, which possibly causes old age, 598; handlers carriers of amebic dysentery.

288, 290; handlers cause of dysentery, 412; infant's (see "Infants"); irradiated, in rickets, 496, 498; mixtures (see under "Infants"); Mosaic laws, 760; need for, 765; phosphorus in various foods, 785; poisoning, 40, 764; preparation, 776; protein yield of various, 788 ff.; seasoning, 786; sensitivity to, 763; sensitivity to, cause of sick headache, 39; skin, 664, 666, 672; stimulating gastric juice secretion, 382; supply, source of, factor in diet, 764; value of alcohol, 787; value of cheese, 782; value of cream, 782; vitamins in, 774, 775.

Foot (see also Ankle, Heels, Toes), 806 ff.; abnormalities, 806; arch of (see "Arches"); athlete's, or ringworm, 685; bathing, 809; blood circulation, 808; bunion, 822; care in diabetes, 599; club-foot, 819; corns, 688, 822; deformities, 806–807, 819; exercise to strengthen, 814; fallen arches, 808, 815, 816; fallen arches, exercises for, 816; flat-foot, 802–803, 810 ff.; flat-foot, correct way to walk, 810; flat-foot, diagram of, 808, 811; flat-foot, exercises to correct, 813; flat-foot, rigid, 816; flat-foot, shoes for, 812; functions of, 807; infant's, should be examined periodically, 810; massage, 809; normal inner side of, 808; odor from feet, 684; painful heels, 818–819; perspiring, 824; postures, right and wrong, 812; print does not indicate real nature of flatness, 810; print indicates quality of arch, 811; sweating, 824; swelling, in pregnancy, 157, 165; trouble in department-store workers, 815; type of, effect on posture, 802; warts on, 821.

Foreign bodies, in body cavities, 23; in ear, 716; in ear, how to remove, 716; in eye, 707; in nose, 723.

Formaldehyde, industrial poison, 651; poisoning, symptoms, antidotes and treatment, 45.

Formalin, industrial poison, 651; industrial poison in insecticides, 652; sterilizing hair brushes in, 697.

Foundrymen's chills, 648.

Fountain syringe, 16.

Fourth of July accidents and tetanus, 280.

Fracastorius, 738.

Fractures, first aid for, 19, 20.

Francis, research on tularemia, 290, 291.

Freckles, precautions to be taken, 677; preventive treatment, 692; protecting skin that freckles, 678; removers, danger of using in chloasma, 691; senile, treatment, 692.

Freckling, a reaction to protect the skin, 663.

French pox, 738.

Fresh Air: See Air.

Freud's theory, 64, 137.

Frigidity, 135; fear of pregnancy cause of, 136.

Froehlich, adiposo-genital dystrophy of, 546.

Frogs, reproduction in, 72.

Frost bite of ear, 715.

Fruit, alkaline producing, 773; carbohydrates in per cent, 583; common source of carbohydrates, 784; copper and iron in, 772; in infant feeding, 205; phosphorus in, 785; protein yield, 789; unripe or over-ripe, cause of diarrhea, 411.

Fuel value, of alcohol, 787; of butter vs. sugar, 780; of fats, 786; of food, or calorie, 765.

Fungi, allergy, 516.

Fungicide, zinc chloride hazard, 660.

Funk, 485.

Fur, allergy, 515.

Galen, on kidney disease, 429, 448.

Gallant's chart showing when menopause will appear, 56.

Gall bladder, effects of abscessed teeth on, diagram showing, 755; ulcer and appendicitis distinguished, 406.

Gall-bladder calculi: See Gallstones.

Gall-bladder cancer, with calculi, 403; sex distribution, 629.

Gall-bladder, disease, 401; symptoms, 402.

Gallstones, cause stomach symptoms, 389–390; patient with, susceptible to diabetes, 575; removal will prevent cancer of gall-bladder, 637; symptoms of, 402; X-ray examination of, 390.

Gambusia affinis, 294.

Games, playing games during menstrual period, 54, 802; for women, 801.

Gangrene, cause of death of diabetics, 602; diabetic, 598–599.

Garage gas poisoning: See Gas poisoning.

Gargles, 730; antiseptic value of, 14; for tonsillitis, 733; hydrogen peroxide solution for, 18; preventive of colds, 14; soda bicarbonate for, 18; use in sore throat, 730.

Garrison, Fielding, on history of urinalysis, 430.

Garrod, 461.

Garters, round, avoid in pregnancy, 157; round, diabetics should not wear, 599.

Gas, acetylene, industrial hazard, 645.

Gas, ammonia, industrial hazard, 645.

Gas company, call up, in case of gas poisoning, 31.

Gas, exhaust, from auto, poisoning by, 31.

Gas, nitrous, industrial poison, 655.

Gas on the stomach, 396.

Gas poisoning, headache sign of, 31; methylene blue poisoning for, 31; predisposes to pneumonia, 315; resuscitation after, 30; symptoms, antidotes and treatment, 45.

Gas, sewer, industrial poison, 657.

Gasoline, tetraethyl lead, industrial poison, 658.

Gastric juice (*see also* Stomach secretion), 381; acid secretion by, 382; enzymes in, 381, 382; hydrochloric acid in, 381; pepsin absent from, 388; pepsin in, 381–382, 388; rennin in, 381, 382; secretion, foods stimulating, 382.

Gastro-intestinal tract, description, 380–381.

Gastroptosis, 397.

Gaucher's disease, 482.

Gauze, bandages, 15, 16; bandaging with, as an art, 22; sterile, application to stop bleeding, 21; strips may be applied to burned area, 27; wide, must not be applied to burned area, 27.

Gelatin, protein yield, 789.

GENGOU, research on whooping cough, 259.

Genitals (*see also* Masturbation, Reproductive system), cancer of, 141, 142; care of, during pregnancy, 164; care of, in infants, 186; cleanliness of, 138; cleansing, to prevent vaginitis in young children, 212; discharges from, consult physician regarding, 140; diseases of, 141; function of pineal gland, 538; hygiene, 137; infant's, cleaning, 186; odor from, 138; pulling at, in children, 93; washing external, 138.

"Geographic tongue," 719.

GEORGIA WARM SPRINGS FOUNDATION, 268.

Germ: *See* Bacillus, Bacteria.

German measles, incubation period, 23, 232, 254; treatment, 254.

Gerson diet in tuberculosis, 331, 332.

Giantism and pituitary gland, 545.

GILBERT, NEWELL C., 346.

Girls, athletics for adolescent, 101; care of genitals in, 84; physical education for, 801; ruptured hymen in, 84, 114.

Glanders, 297 *ff.*; germ causing, 298; incubation period, 298; in horses, 297; symptoms, 298; transmission, 297; treatment, 298.

Glands, 530 *ff.*; fat or sebaceous, 662; lymph,

enlargement, 481; of internal secretion, 38, 532 *ff.*; sex, 76; sweat, 662.

Glandular products, as sexual stimulant, 145; for headaches, 40.

Glass drinking tubes, 15.

Glass Pock: *See* Chicken Pox.

Glass, swallowing, first aid for, 23.

Glasses, to correct cause of headache, 38.

Glaucoma, 713.

Glomeruli: *See* Kidney.

Glomerulonephritis, acute, 453; chronic, 453.

Glossitis or inflammation of tongue, 719.

Glucose, 783.

Glue, allergy, 507, 516.

Glycerine, 17; with phenol, dropping into ear, 718.

Glycogen, manufactured by liver, 388.

Glycosuria, renal, 460.

Goiter, cause and prevention, 554; defined, 541; district, 555; during puberty, 556 *ff.*; endemic, 554; endemic districts, 555; endemic, feeble-mindedness due to, 561; exophthalmic, heart changes in, 371; periods when most likely to occur, 556; prevention, 557; prevention in pregnancy, 168; prevention, iodine added to drinking water, 557; prevention, iodized salt in, 558, 559; results of, 560; simple, 554; simple, during adolescence, 52; zone, 541.

Gold treatment of tuberculosis, 330.

GOLDBERG, DR., on sanatorium care of tuberculosis, 329.

GOLDBERGER, J., 499, 500.

Golf, avoid playing, during pregnancy, 160.

Golf-ball exercise for fallen arches, 817.

Gonads: *See* Sex glands.

Gonococcus, cause of subacute endocarditis, 369; ulcer on eye, 710.

Gonorrhea, advice to those with, 746–747; caused by germs, 738; cause of blindness, 745; drug-store and self-treatment dangerous, 747; historical aspect, 745; in young children, 212; marriage after, 747; prevention, 747; preventive treatment, 747; quack remedies, 742; symptoms, first, 745; transmission, 745; transmission by sexual contact, 745; transmission, nonsexual, 745; treatment, 746.

Gout, 344–345; description, Sydenham's, 344–345; diet in, 345; treatment, 345.

Gouty nephritis, 457.

Grains, cereal, carbohydrates of, 782, 784; food value, 783–784; oils from, 783.

Grain itch, 651.

GRANGE, M., 560.

Granite cause of silicosis, 651.

Granite quarrying, silicosis from, 658.

Grape sugar, 783.

Grapefruit safest fruit for diabetic, 583.

GRASSI, research on malaria, 292.

GREAT LAKES basin, goiter in, 555.

GREENHILL, J. P., 147.

Green soap, 669, 670.

"Grog blossom" or acne rosacea, 683–684.

"Growing" pains, symptom of rheumatic fever, 357–358.

Growth factor of pituitary, 544; function of thymus, 535, 536; of infant, 183; stunting, caused by allergy, 521.

Guaiacol in treatment of tuberculosis, 331.

Gums, coarse foods to harden, 749; infection, cause of, 756; massage of, during pregnancy, 165.

Gymnasium shoes, 812.

Gymnastics, place in physical training, 800.

Habit of masturbation, 93.

Habits, change in life habits in treatment of sick headache, 39.

Habit-training in infant, 188.

Hahn turpentine test of renal function, 457.

Hair (see also Scalp), allergy, 515; bleaching superfluous, 700; brushes, 697; brushes, seborrheic dermatitis spread by, 681; brushes, sterilizing in formalin solution, 697; brushing, 696; care of, 696; care of during pregnancy, 164; color of, 695; combs, 697; combs, seborrheic dermatitis spread by, 681; curling, with hot irons or heat, 696; curly, form of, 695; cutting, 696; description, 694–695; dyeing, 696–697; follicle infection or barber's itch, 701; follicle, muscle joins sebaceous gland to, 662; follicles of nose, infection of, 720; function, 695; graying, 699; graying, sudden, 699; lice infesting, 686; loss of (see "Baldness"); oil application harmful, 696; oiling, 696; permanent wave, 696; pubic, crab louse in, 687; scalp, 695; shaving seems to make hair seem coarser, 696; singeing, 696; straight, form of, 695; superfluous, 700; superfluous, methods of removing, 700; superfluous, treatment, 700; thickness, cutting does not increase, 696; washing, 696; washing, egg white for, 696; washing, in infant, 186; washing, in pregnancy, 164; washing, soap for, 696; wetting, harmful, 696; wigs, 697.

Halibut, source of vitamin A, 491.

Halitosis, 756; causes of, 756.

Hand-to-mouth infection, defined, 307.

Hands (see also Fingers), swelling during pregnancy, 157, 165; washing before eating, to prevent infectious disease, 239.

HARE, H. A., 613.

Harrison's groove in rickets, 497.

HARTMAN, F. H., 550.

Hay fever, 314, 504 ff.; history of, 505; pollen, 514; pollen avoidance in treatment, 526.

Head, "dynamite," caused by nitroglycerin, 655; fontanels or soft spots, closing, 184; lice, treatment with kerosene and sweet oil, 686; misshapen, preventing, in infant, 184; size increase in infant, 183, 184.

Headache, allergic, 504 ff.; as a symptom, 37; at menstrual periods, 39; constipation cause of, 39; eyestrain cause of, 39; food sensitivity cause of, 39; glands of internal secretion may cause, 39; indigestion cause of, 39; nitroglycerin cause of, in industry, 655; nonspecific protein reaction in treatment of, 40; per cent in 17,000 men, 5; persistent, danger signal in pregnancy, 165; pituitary, 546–547; powders, 13; sick, 37; sign of carbon-monoxide poisoning, 31; sinus disease cause of, 39; symptom of allergy, 522; symptom of gallbladder disease, 402; treatment, glandular preparations, 40; treatment, 39; treatment, H. A. Riley on, 39.

Health, examination, periodic, objections to, 612; hints for tuberculous, 334; mental, 832 ff.; of the young married couple, 117; relationship of allergy to general health, 512.

Health shoes, 810.

Hearing, defective in 17,000 men, 5.

Heart, anatomy, 348; aorta, 350; auricle, 350 ff.; beats, 351; beats, number in child and adult, 346; blood supply, 372–373; changes in hyperthyroidism, 371; changes in structure, 354; circulation of blood, 351–353; congenitally defective, 355; construction, 350; coronary system of arteries, 350 ff.; damage in rheumatic fever, 356, 361, 368; defective because of disease, 356; defective (congenital), 355; defective (congenital), prognosis, care, 355; disease, cause of death in 1904, compared with 1926, 566; disease, chorea manifestation of, 356, 359; disease, death rates, 346–347; disease, death rates, 1932, 567; disease, increase, 1900–1929, 347; disordered action, 377; effects of abscessed teeth, diagram showing, 755; function, 351; energy, electrical equivalent, 346;

"leakage" result of rheumatic fever, 362; location of, 533; muscle, or myocardium, 350 *ff.;* muscle, blood supply interference, 372; muscle involved in rheumatic fever, 362; neurosis of, 377–378; organic murmur, per cent in 17,000 men, 5; pacemaker, 346; pericardium, 349; position in chest cavity, 349; rheumatic inflammation, 360; "soldier's," 378; strain in diphtheria, 248; symptoms in kidney disease, 443; syphilis, 371; valves, 350 *ff.;* valves, deformity result of rheumatic fever, 362; vena cava, 351 *ff.;* ventricles, 350, 351 *ff.;* weight in child, 346; work of, never stops, 346; X-ray examination in syphilis of, 371.

Heartburn during pregnancy, 166; symptom of stomach disorder, 396; treatment, 166.

Heat, cause of cancer, 625; cramps, 644; industrial conditions due to, 651; industrial hazard, 639; prickly, 681; production in human body, 189, 190; rash, 681; regulation of the body and colds, 306; sensitiveness, 507, 518, 519; stroke, symptoms of oncoming, 33; stroke, temperature taken by rectum, 34; stroke, treatment, 33; treatment of allergy, 528.

Heating of homes, in relation to colds, 309.

HEBERDEN first described angina pectoris, 375.

HECK, 435.

Heels, exercise for stretching Achilles tendon, 814; painful, 818; painful, causes, 818, 819; painful, result of gonorrhea. 747; painful, spurs cause of, 818, 819; painful, treatment, 819; rubber, value on shoes, 808.

Height, diabetic children are taller, 577; increase in, of present generation, 182; -weight table for various ages, 769.

Hemeralopia: *See* **Night Blindness.**

Hemoglobin, reduction in chlorosis, 471; significance of standard, 466.

Hemophilia, 479; heredity of, 479.

Hemorrhage (*see also* **Bleeding**), cause of anemia, 470; first aid for, 20; in newborn, 480; in ulcer of stomach and duodenum, 400; of brain death rate compared with heart disease, 347; tendency to, 480.

Hemorrhoids in pregnancy, 167; per cent in 17,000 men, 5.

HENCH, PHILIP S., 418.

Henle's loop, 422.

Heredity, cause of high blood pressure, 611 *ff.;* factor in diet, 764; of allergy, 508; of cancer. 628; of diabetes mellitus, 573,

574, 577; of hemophilia ("bleeder"), 479; rôle in causation of mental disorder, 833; rôle in longevity, 848.

Hermaphrodites, 82.

Hernia, at navel, how to control, 206; in infants, 206; in whooping cough, preventing, 260; inguinal, per cent in 17,000 men, 5; intestinal obstruction complicating, 414.

Herpes on lips in indigestion, 391.

Herrmannsdorfer diet in tuberculosis, 331, 332.

HESS, 494; quoted on vitamins, 486.

HEWITT, 450.

HEWLETT, 447.

"Hex," industrial dermatosis, 647; industrial poison, 652.

Hexamethylenetetramine, industrial poison, 652.

Hexylresorcinol, use as antiseptic, 26.

Hiccups, 35; cause of, 36, 397; chemical, 36; in infants, 37; nervous, 36; symptom of considerable importance, 36; treatment, 36.

Hide handlers, tannic-acid poisoning in, 658.

Hides, industrial hazard, 642.

High blood pressure: *See* **Blood pressure, high.**

Hiking crazes, 820.

HILL, A. V., 306.

HILL, L. C., on incidence of albuminuria in training camp, 434.

HIPPOCRATES, on kidney disease, 428; quotation from, on urine, 429.

Hippuric acid manufactured by kidney, 425.

Histamine, to provoke gastric secretion, 389.

Hives, 504 *ff.*

Hobbies, value in adolescence, 101, 102.

Hodgkin's disease, 481.

Honey, carbohydrate value, 784.

Honeymoon, 111; first sexual intercourse, facilitating, 114.

Hookworms, 415.

HOPKINS, 485.

Hordeolum or styes, 709.

Horse, glanders in, transmitted to man, 297; serum-free toxoid, 247; serum, sensitivity to, 247.

Horseback riding during pregnancy, 160.

Horseshoe kidney, 461.

Hosiery: *See* **Stockings.**

Hospital, community, for mental disorder, 846; custodial, for mental disease, 846; for mental disease, 844; recognized for internship, 2; state, for insane. 846; state, for mental disease, 847; week-end treatment of diabetes, 580.

Hot bath, 668–669.

Hot packs for tonsillitis, 733.

Hot sitz baths during pregnancy, 163.

Hot-water bottle, 16.

Hot water to control bleeding, 21; to control bleeding after tooth extraction, 20.

HULL, T. G., 299.

Humidity in relation to colds, 309.

Hunger pains, stimulation, 775–776.

HURD, LEE M., 725, 726.

Husband, points to be considered in selecting, 105–106.

Hyaline casts in the urine, 440.

Hydrochloric acid, in gastric juice, 381, 382, 388; poisoning, symptoms, antidotes and treatment, 45.

Hydrocyanic acid, industrial poison, 650; industrial poison in insecticide, 652; poisoning, symptoms, antidotes and treatment, 44.

Hydrogen, industrial poison, 652.

Hydrogen peroxide should not be applied to fresh wound, 26; solution, 18, 674; solution plus ammonia for chloasma, 691; solution, use as skin antiseptic, 674; solution, use in halitosis, 756; to control bleeding, 21; treatment of Vincent's angina, 285; use as antiseptic, 26.

Hydrogen, phosphureted, industrial poison, 656.

Hydrogen sulphide, industrial hazard in sewer gas, 657; industrial poison, 652; stink damp of mines, 659.

Hydrophobia, danger from bites of animals, 35; diagnosis in dog made by laboratory examination of brain, 284; dog bites source of, 282, 283, 284; dog should be penned up, not killed, after biting, 283–284· historical aspect, 282; incubation period, 283; Pasteur treatment, 284; prevention by prohibiting stray dogs, 283; superstition of "dog days," 282; transmitted by saliva of animal or person, 282; treatment, Pasteur, 284; virus, 282.

Hygeia, cancer education by, 636; sex hygiene material reprinted from, 64.

Hygiene, dental, for adults, 751; dental, for children, 749; mouth, 752–753; of false teeth, 757–758; of hair, 696; of infant, 185, 220; of nails, 702; of nose, 721; of nursing mother, 174; of old age, 852; of reproductive system,137; of skin, 676 *ff.*; of women, 50; personal, to prevent infectious disease 238; rex, 64.

Hymen, ruptured, 84; ruptured *vs.* intact. in virgins, 114.

Hyperacidity, diet for, 794–795.

Hyperhidrosis of feet, 824.

Hypersensitivity: *See* Allergy.

Hypertension: *See* Blood pressure, high.

Hypnotics, cause of low blood pressure, 620.

Hypoacidity, diet for, 795–796.

Hypodermic syringe, giving medicines by, 14.

Hypophysis: *See* Pituitary.

Hypotension: *See* Blood Pressure, low.

Ice, compresses for black eye, 22; compresses for hemorrhoids, 167; rubbing, over body in heat stroke, 34; source of typhoid, 273; water pads for bruises, 82.

Ice bag, 16, 17; applied to chest in lung hemorrhage, 21; for sore throat, 730; for tonsillitis, 733; to relieve painful breasts, 176.

Ice cream, infected, may cause epidemic of septic sore throat, 732; per cent of carbohydrate in, 583; protein yield, 789.

Idiocy, Mongolian, 560.

Idiot, defined, 839.

Imbecile, defined, 839.

Immunization, defined, 246.

IMPERIAL CANCER RESEARCH FUND, 623.

Impetigo, 681; serious condition in infants, 681.

Impotence, 123.

Incubation period (*see also under names of specific diseases as* Measles, Undulant fever, *etc.*) of infectious disease, 231.

Indelible pencil manufacture, methyl-violet poisoning from, 654.

INDIA, life expectancy in, 849.

Indian walking position, correct, 812.

Indigestion, 380 *ff.*; acute, 391; acute, really acute heart attack, 391–392; cause, 391; cause of headache, 39; chronic, due to disease of appendix or gall bladder, 406; diet (smooth) for, 392–394; differentiated from dyspepsia, 395; symptom of condition elsewhere, 391; symptoms, 391; treatment, 392.

Indigo carmine test of kidney excretory ability, 441, 443.

Industrial accident, defined, 643–644.

Industrial cancer, prevention, 637.

Industrial care of eyes, 707.

Industrial disease, defined, 643–644.

Industrial hazards, 639 *ff.*; mercurial nephrosis, 459.

Industrial injury of eye, 707.

878INDEX

Industrial trades, number of calories which various individuals in, need, 767.

Infantile paralysis, 265; artificial respirator in, 268; cause of, not discovered, 265; death rate, 269; exercises in, American Medical Association committee suggestions on, 269; exercise in water, 268; geographical incidence, 266; Georgia Warm Springs Foundation, 268; historical aspect, 265; incidence, 266; infants seldom have, 266; muscular function, restoring, 268; nursing care in, 268; prevention, 266, 267; Roosevelt (Franklin D.) afflicted with, 265, 269; Scott (Sir Walter) afflicted with, 270–271; seasonal incidence, 266; swimming-pool method in, 289; symptoms, 266, 267; transmission, 265; treatment, 268; vaccines developed, 267.

Infants (see also Children, Embryo, Fetus), acute illness, feeding in, 213; air swallowing by, 197, 198; anus prolapse in, 210; artificial feeding, 199; bath, directions for giving, 186; bathing, directions, 226; bed for, 185; birthmarks, 177; bladder habit, control of, 226; bottles and nipples, 203; bowel habit, developing, 188, 225; breast feeding, 196; breast feeding, difficulties, 197; breast feeding, supplementing, 198; breast feeding, technic, 197; breast feeding, when they should not be given, 196; breast of, milk present in, 187; buttocks should be washed after each stool, 187; care of skin in, 676; caul or veil on newborn child, 181; clothing, avoiding pins and buttons, 227; clothing required for, 169; clothing to be taken to hospital for new baby to wear home, 168; clothing, what the infant should wear, 228; colds in, 206, 207; colic in, 215; constipation in, 215; convulsions in, 212; creeping, 184; crib, sheets, blankets required, 169; croup in, 208; crying, 187; defects in, as birthmarks, 177; development, 183; diapers, antiseptic used in rinsing, 187; diapers, applying square kind, 225; diapers, washing, 187; diarrhea in, 187, 216–217.

Infants' diet (see also Infant, feeding), coarse foods strengthen jaws and harden gums, 749; essentials, 224; foods for child teething, 749; iron in, 193; milk in, 224; to insure sound teeth, 749.

Infants, digestion, 194; diphtheria immunization, 220; disease in, 206; dusting powders for, precautions to be taken, 671; dysentery in, 216; ears, cleaning, 186; ears, washing, 228; exercise, 188, 220;

eyes, cleaning, 186; eyesight, development, 185.

Infants, feeding (see also Infants' diet), acidified evaporated milk for, 203; apricots in, 205; bottle, technic, 204; care of bottles and nipples, 203; cereals in, 205; change in, to correct constipation, 216; citric-acid milk, 203; cod-liver oil in, 204; condensed milk in, 200; corn syrup in, 200, 202; dextrin-maltose in, 200; dextrose in, 200; diluents, 200; during acute illness, 213; egg yolk in, 204, 205; formula, corn syrup in, 202; formula for well babies, 201; formula, measurements, 201; formula, milk in, 201, 202; formula, preparation, 203; formula, sugar in, 201; formula, water in, 201, 202; formula with undiluted milk, 202; in acute illness, 213; in diarrhea, 217, 218; iron in, 204; lactic-acid milk, 203; lactose in, 200; laxative effect of certain food elements in, 216; limewater in, 200; milk (evaporated, dried, condensed, etc.), 199; milk diet, additions to, 204; orange juice in, 204; peaches in, 205; schedule, 201; schedule for newborn, 173; sweet milk dilution, 203; synthetic food mixtures, 200; time, relation to emptying of stomach, 194; vegetables (canned sieved) for, 224.

Infants, fever in, reducing, 205; fontanel, closing, 184; fontanel, failure to close, 497; foot of, should be examined periodically, 810; fresh air for, 221; gastro-intestinal symptoms, 198; genitals, care of, 186; goiter in, 557; growth, 183; habit training, 188; hair, washing, 186; head, misshapen, preventing, 184; head size, increase in, 183, 184; heat production in, 189, 190; heat rash, 681; hernia in, 206; hiccups in, 37; hygiene, 220; impetigo in, 681; intussusception in, 210; iron requirement, 193; length of body, increase in, criterion of growth, 183; malnutrition, 218; mastoiditis in, 208; masturbation, 84; mouth, cleaning, 186; newborn, hemorrhage tendency in, 480; newborn, jaundice, 206; newborn, ophthalmia in, due to gonorrhea, 745; nose, cleaning, 186, 228; nutrition of, 189; otitis media in, 207–208; overfeeding, 198; pacifier, infant should not have, 189; physical care and hygiene, 185; pillow not needed, 185; pneumonia in, 209; pneumonia in, convulsions first sign, 212, 213; prickly heat, 681; pyelitis in, 211; rectal prolapse in, 210; rickets in, 218, 494; rumination in, 214; "rupture" in, 206; scalp, care of, 186; scurvy in, 493; seldom have infantile paralysis, 266; seven-month *vs.* eight-month, vitality of, 178; sick, care of, 205; sitting up, 184, 185; size of newborn, depends on heredity and other conditions, 180; sleep, 185; sleep habits in, 188; smallpox vaccination, 220; spasmophilia in, 219; stomach-emptying time, 194; stools, 195; stools, color of, 195; stools, curd in, 195; stools, mucus in, 195; sunshine exposure, 221–223; talking, first to begin, 184, 185; teeth, care of, 748; teeth, cleaning, 186, 228; teething, 184, 749; temperature high in, reducing, 205; temperature of room for waking and sleeping hours, 185; tetany in, 219; thrush in, 210; thumb sucking, 188–189; toilet necessities required, 169; toilet habits, training, 188, 225; training, 188; truss for, 206; tub baths for, 226; underfeeding, 198; urination, teaching control of, 226; vaginitis in, 212; vision, development, 185; vitamins in diet of, 190, 191, 192; vomiting in, 214; walking, first attempts at, 184, 185; water requirement, 193; weaning, 176, 198; weight, normal rate of increase, 183; what to do as soon as baby is born, 171.

Infection, cause of kidney disease, 444; cause of odor during menstruation, 54, 55; cause of painful heels, 818; cleanliness and, 239; convulsions in, in infants, 212, 213; ear, 715; focal, cause of high blood pressure, 613; focal, effects of abscessed teeth, 755; focal, rôle in arthritis and rheumatism, 339; focal, tonsils as source of, 733; hand-to-mouth, defined. 307; in diabetes mellitus, 600; industrial, 641; prevention of, 237; resistance to, and vitamin A, 190, 191, 490; skin power to protect against, 665–666; wound, physician's attention necessary, 26.

Infectious disease (*see also* Communicable disease), carrier, 233; carrier, control, 237; eruptions characteristic in, 232; germs, 230; incidence, 238; incubation period, 231; of childhood, 241; *ff.;* prevention, 230, 237; prevention by cleanliness, 239; prevention by personal hygiene, 238; resistance to, 232; stamping out, 236; tonsillectomy in relation to, 733–737; transmission, 232; treatment, 230, 239.

Inflammation, of cornea due to syphilis, 711; of iris, 711; of retina, 712; of skin, 678; of tongue, 719.

Influenza, bacillus cause of subacute endo-

carditis, 369; baldness after, 698; cause of death of diabetics, 602; cause of low blood pressure, 617–618; death rate, 1932, 567; epidemic and the common cold, 305; incidence, 238; pandemics of, 305.

Infra-red rays, industrial hazard, 643.

Ingrown Toenails: *See* Nails.

Injection of insulin: *See* Insulin.

Ink, industrial poison, 652; rotogravure, industrial poison, 657.

Insane, 836; commitment to hospital, 844; custodial treatment of, 846; general paralysis of, 741; state hospitals for, 846.

Insanity, 825, 836; definition, 836; symptoms, 842.

Insecticides, fluoride poisoning, symptoms, antidotes and treatment, 45; industrial poison, 650, 652.

Insects (*see also* Flies, Mosquitoes), allergy, 516; bites, first aid for, 34; cross pollination by, 71; in ear, 716; in ear, how to remove, 23, 716.

Instincts, civilization of, 831; or "drives," 829.

Instrument for measuring blood pressure, 608.

Insulin (*see also* Diabetes mellitus), origin of, 588.

Insurance (*see also* Metropolitan Life Insurance Company) for the young married couple, 118; policyholders, albuminuria in, 435.

Intestines (*see also* Bowels), absorption in small intestines, 383; cancer, 413, 628, 633; cancer, symptoms, 413; cancer, X-ray diagnosis, 414; digestion of food by, 383, 776; disorders, allergic, 504 *ff.;* disorders, chronic, cause of halitosis, 757; intussusception in infants, 210; obstruction, 414; obstruction, adhesions cause of, 414; obstruction cause of vomiting in infants, 214; obstruction, diagnosis, 415; obstruction, hernia complication, 414; obstruction in rectal cancer, 414–415; obstruction, symptoms, 415; parasites or "worms," 415; parasites, symptoms, 416; parasites, treatment, 416; secretion of large intestines, 384; secretory glands, 383; symptoms of allergy, 522; tumors obstructing, 414, 415.

Intelligence, impaired, or mental defect, 837 *ff.*

Internal glandular system, 532 *ff.*

Internship, 2; hospitals recognized for, 2.

Intussusception in infants, 210.

Invalid, essential of normal diet for, 791.

Iodine, amount needed for average healthy child, 559; amount of iodine in iodized salt, 560; deficiency region, 541; in artesian water, 559; in "blood purifiers" make acne vulgaris worse, 682; in diet, 773; in diet during pregnancy, 152; in prevention of goiter, 168, 557; in sea foods, 559; in thyroid secretion, 557; indispensable to function of thyroid, 540; mercury must not be applied after using iodine, 673; poisoning, symptoms, antidotes and treatment, 45; small doses given weekly to prevent iodine deficiency in adolescent, 52; stain, removal by ammonia water, 673; tincture of, applying, 17; tincture of, as antiseptic, 14, 26, 673; tincture of, care to be taken in applying, 673; tincture of, may cause dermatitis, 680; tincture of, one application enough, 680.

Iodized salt, amount of iodine per year consumed in, 560; history of, 560; in prevention of goiter, 558, 559.

Ipral, 13.

Iris, 704, 705; inflammation, 711.

Iron, in diet, 773; in infant's diet, 193, 204; in various foods, 772; treatment of anemia, 472.

Irritants, dermatitis from external irritants, 680.

Irritation cause of cancer, 624.

Isaacs, 439.

Isaacs, Raphael, 464.

Islands of Langerhans, 564, 565.

Italians, rickets in, 495; tradition of spaghetti and ravioli, 765.

Itch, barber's, 701; bath, 668; grain, 651; mite, treatment, 35; picric, 656; scabies, 687.

Itching of skin, sodium bicarbonate for, 18; of skin not caused by syphilis, 741; symptom of jaundice, 403.

Ivy, poison, cause of dermatitis, 680.

"Jags, naphtha," 647.

Jaundice, 403; caused by poisons, 403; congenital hemolytic, 472; in gall-bladder disease, 402; in newborn, 206; symptoms, 403; symptom of gallstones, 406.

Jaws, coarse foods to strengthen, 749; effect of nasal obstruction on, 722; normal, and nasal cavity, 722.

Jeans, Philip C., 182.

Jews, Mosaic laws of food for, based on sound concepts, 760.

Joffre, diabetes in, 577.

Johnson, Wingate M., 607.

Joints, cracking, symptom of arthritis, 338; inflammation (*see also* "Arthritis"), sign of rheumatic fever, 358; stiffness, in arthritis, 339; symptoms in rheumatic fever, 358.

Jordan, E. O., 306.

Joslin, Elliott P., 563, 565.

Journal of American Medical Association, 613.

Journey, of the blood, 352; of carbohydrate, 386–387; through kidney, 427.

Kaffee Hag in smooth diet for indigestion, 393.

Kahn test, 468, 740; criterion of cure in syphilis, 744; in syphilis of heart, 371.

Kaiser, Albert D., 736.

Kansas, artesian water contains iodine, 559.

Keloids, 690; acne, 701; treatment, X-ray, 690.

Kenneth, J. H., 728.

Kenyon, Josephine H., on menstruation, 53.

Keratoses, senile, 692.

Kerosene, and sweet oil treatment of head lice, 686; industrial poison, 652.

Kettle, Croup: See **Croup.**

Kidney, anatomy, 421; arteriosclerotic, 454; blood vessels, number of, 423; Bowman's capsule, 422–423; calculi, 455; calculi, recognized at time of American Revolution, 428; cancer, 633; care of, in pregnancy, 156; complications in scarlet fever, 258; derivation of the word, 428.

Kidney disease (*see also* **Nephritis**), 418 *ff.*; albuminuria symptom in, 436; and rheumatism confused by quacks, 446; blood tests in, 442; cause of death of diabetics, 602; causes, 444; classification, 452; diet in, 450; diuretics in, 450; from enlarged prostate, 457; germs causing, 444–445; history before time of Richard Bright, 428; no place for self-treatment of, 452; poisons cause of, 444, 445; quack remedies for, 451–452; rest in, 449; secondary to high blood pressure, 454; significance of albuminuria, 418; symptoms and signs, 445–446; treatment, 448; urine color, etc., symptoms in, 446.

Kidney disturbances during pregnancy, 456; effects of abscessed teeth, diagram showing, 755; examining, modern methods of, 440; excretory ability, tested by injecting dyes, 441, 443; failure, treatment, 448; filter chambers, 422–423; filters or glomeruli, 423; floating, 461; function, 419 *ff.*.

424 *ff.;* function, cystoscope in examination of, 442; function, how it carries on, 425; function, salivary index, 442; function, turpentine test of, 457; function, urea concentration in blood in, 442, 443; function, water concentration test, 441, 443; glomeruli, 422, 423; glomeruli, work in shifts, 449; glomerulonephritis (Bright's disease) acute, 453; glomerulonephritis, 453; chronic, 453; Henle's loop, 422; horseshoe, 461; little journey through, 427; location of, 533; malformation, 461; "palpable," 421; pelvis, 422; perinephritic abscess, 455; physiology, 425; polycystic, 462; "pus," 455; pyelonephritis, 455; quantity of blood which flows through, 425; quantity of water eliminated by, 419; quantity of water that passes through, 426; stones (*see* "Kidney calculi"); tests, knowledge derived from, 443; tuberculosis, 457; tubules, 422, 425; weighing about seventeen pounds, 462; X-ray examination of, 441.

KIMBALL, OLIVER P., 554.
Kindergarten training, posture during, 798.
Kissing, transmission of syphilis by, 743.
KITTLESON-VIMTRUP on tubules of kidney, 422.
KLEBS, discovery of diphtheria bacilli, 242.
Knaus method for determining safe period, 61–63.
KOCH, ROBERT, 231.
Koch's tuberculin, 330
KOLMER, JOHN H., developed infantile paralysis vaccine, 267.
Koplik's spots in measles, 251.
Kosher method of killing, 760.

Label, read directions carefully, 10.
Labor (*see also* Childbirth, Confinement), average duration of, 171; estimating day of, 150; signs of beginning labor, 170; why human childbirth so painful, 75.
Laboratory tests, of blood, 468; of urine, 440 *ff.*
Lacquers, amyl alcohol industrial hazard in, 646.
Lacrimal glands (tear ducts), 709–710.
Lactation: *See* Nursing Mother.
Lactic-acid milk, preparation, 203.
Lactose, or milk sugar, 783; ounce-tablespoon equivalents, 202; use in infant feeding, 200.
Larynx, cancer, 632; diagram showing, 734; tuberculosis, ultraviolet ray for, 335.
LAVERAN discovered cause of malaria, 292.

Laxatives: *See* Cathartics and laxatives.
Layette, infant's, 169.
Lead, cause of nephritis, 445; industrial poison, 652; ingot, industrial hazard, 645; oxide, industrial hazard, 653; poisoning in bronze workers, 648; poisoning, symptoms, antidotes and treatment, 45; salts in face powder, 671; tetraethyl, industrial poison, 658; white, 645.
League of Nations fixed standard for strength of insulin, 592.
Lean men compared with fat men as they walk through life, 573.
LEE, 435.
Leg, cramps, during pregnancy, 167; ulcers and syphilis, 741.
Lemon, juice of, eradication of scurvy with, 493; peel, rubbing chloasma with, 691; vitamin C in, 494.
Lemonade for colds, 314.
Lens, crystalline (of eye), 704, 705; cataract, 711.
Leukemia, 478; symptoms and treatment, 478.
Leukocytes: *See* Blood cells, white.
LEWIN, PHILIP, 806.
Lice, body, 686–687; crab, 687; head, 686; infestation, 686; source of tularemia, 291; treatment, 686.
License, state, of physicians, 2.
Life, Change of: *See* Menopause.
Life, cycle of fly, 275; divided into three epochs, 534; duration with low blood pressure, 617; expectancy, 848–849; expectancy with breast cancer, 623–624; habits, change in, in treatment of headache, 39; span of, 848; starts with union of egg and sperm, 81.
LIFE EXTENSION INSTITUTE, 612.
Life insurance (*see also* METROPOLITAN LIFE INSURANCE COMPANY) policyholders, albuminuria in, 434–435.
Light, allergy, 518, 519; blinding flashes of, in headache, 38; colored, seeing, 705; sensitiveness to, 518; sensitivity to, described by Bostock in 1817, 504–505; treatment of allergy, 528; treatment of skin, 676.
Light-headedness, 32.
Lime, burn of eye, 707; chloride of, industrial poisoning, 649; industrial poison, 652.
Limestone hazard in Portland cement, 656.
Limewater, use in infant feeding, 200.
Linseed, allergy, 516.
Linseed oil, in putty, industrial poison, 657.

Lip, cancer, sex distribution, 629; cold sores on, in indigestion, 391.

Lipase, enzyme in gastric juice, 381; enzyme in pancreatic juice, 383.

Liquor: See Alcohol.

Litharge, industrial poison, 653.

Liver, effects of abscessed teeth on, diagram showing, 755; function, 385; function in digestion, 383–384, 385; function, manufacture of glycogen, 388; jaundice, 403; "liver spots" or chloasma, 691; vitamin A storage in, 491.

Liver (beef), calories in, 766; eating, to prevent anemia, 476; extract in anemia, 472.

Lockjaw: See Tetanus.

Locomotor ataxia, 741.

LÖFFLER discovery of diphtheria bacilli, 242.

Longevity, 848.

Lotion, greaseless, for cleansing skin, 673.

Louse, crab, 687.

Lousiness, 686–687.

Love affairs, 110; of adolescents, 103; of children, 91, 92.

LOVETT, 803.

Lozenges, value of, 730.

LUDWIG, 610.

Lugol's solution, use in preventing goiter in pregnancy, 168.

Lumbermen, number of calories used daily by, 767.

Luminal, poisoning, symptoms, antidotes and treatment, 43.

"Lump" in the throat, 394.

Luncheon, caloric yield of, 790; distribution of protein, fat, and carbohydrate, 791.

Lungs, bleeding in tuberculosis, 331; effects of abscessed teeth, diagram showing, 755; hemorrhage in tuberculosis, first aid for, 21; quantity of water eliminated by, 419; symptoms of allergy, 522; X-ray study of, to prevent asbestosis and silicosis, 641.

Lutein, 552.

Lye poisoning, symptoms, antidotes and treatment, 42.

Lymph, glands, enlargement of, 481; glands, "lumps," 482; nodes, enlargement of, 481; skin nourished by, 666.

Lymphatism, status thymico-lymphaticus, 536, 546.

Lysol, douche dangerous, 139, 144; poisoning, symptoms, antidotes and treatment, 48.

Machine-sewing during pregnancy, 161.

MAC: See also Mc.

MACKENZIE, SIR JAMES, 611.

MACLEAN, 435.

MACLEOD, 565.

MAGATH, 435.

Magnesia, citrate of, directions for using, 17.

Magnesia, milk of, 14; as cathartic for infant, 216; for heartburn in pregnancy, 166; in medicine chest, 12; use during pregnancy, 156.

Magnesium silicate, industrial poison, 653, 658.

Magnesium sulphate: See Epsom salts.

MAGUIRE, PATRICIA, case of, 301.

Maladjustment of children, treatment, 832–833, 841.

Malaria, 292 ff.; and the fall of Rome, 236; control by oiling ponds, etc., 294, 295; death rate, 295; decline of, in United States, 292; geographical incidence, 294; historical aspect, 292; minnows feed on mosquito larvæ, 294; mosquito compared to yellow-fever mosquito, 293; plasmochin control, 295; quinine control, 295; therapeutic, in late syphilis, 641; transmitted by bite of mosquito, 292, 293, 294.

Malformation of kidney, 461.

Malnutrition, 485; during economic depression, result in next decades, 764; eye trouble due to, 488; in infants, 218; relation to tuberculosis, 324; relation to tuberculosis death rate, 324.

Malta fever: See Undulant fever.

Maltose, ounce-tablespoon equivalents, 202.

Manganese, industrial poison, 653.

"Mange, Texas," 651.

Manicuring, 702.

Manual method of resuscitation, 28, 29, 31.

Maple syrup, carbohydrate value, 784.

Marble exercise for fallen arches, 817.

Marching as endurance test of good posture, 800.

MARINE, DAVID, 557, 561.

Marriage (see also Love affairs, Sexual intercourse), after gonorrhea, 747; age for, Nature's standard, 110; arrangements and agreements before, 110–111; children primary purpose of, 130, 132; continence, 145; contraceptives, dangers of, 144–145; honeymoon, 111; lack of preparation for, cause of frigidity, 135; legal, advantages of, 132; mating period, 104; points to be considered in selecting a mate, 105–106; purpose of, 128; safe period for preventing conception, 60–63; selection of proper mate, 105; should a diabetic marry?, 574;

state laws forbidding marriage of persons
with syphilis, 744; syphilis and, 743;
syphilis, when people with, may marry,
744; teaching the sanctity of, 99; wife
working after, 116; young married couple,
116.

MASSACHUSETTS BOARD OF HEALTH survey
of diabetics, 566.

Massage, 675; danger of, 675; during pregnancy, 161; foot, 809; harmful in acne
vulgaris, 682; in arthritis, 344; of scalp
by brushing hair, 696.

Mastoiditis, 718; in infants, 208; puncturing
eardrum for, 718; result of chronic sinus
disease, 727.

Mastoids, infection from otitis media, 718;
inflammation, 717.

Masturbation, 133; habit of, 93; in adolescence, 101; in infants, 84; product of
mental deficiency, 134.

Maternal (see also Mother), impressions,
177; mortality in United States, 148.

Maternity corset, 158.

Mating period, 104.

Maxillary sinus or antrum infection, 727.

MAYO, CHARLES W., on causes of hiccups,
36.

Mc: See also MAC.

McCOLLUM, 458, 485, 488.

McCORD, CAREY P., 639.

McKENZIE, R. TAIT, 797.

McKINLAY, 435.

McPHEDRAN, F. M., 328.

Meals, caloric yield of different, 789–791;
distribution of protein, fat, and carbohydrates according to, 790 ff.; test meal
in studying digestion, 388.

Measles, 249; complications always serious,
253, 254; convalescents should be kept
away from other children, 253; danger in
chilling in, 251; danger of lung complications, 251, 252; derivation of the word,
249; diet in, 252; epidemics, 249; epidemic
in Faroe Islands in 1846, 250; eyes in,
care of, 252; germ not isolated, 250;
German (see "German measles"); incidence, 238; incidence in children with
tonsils in or out, 736; incubation period,
232, 251; Koplik's spots in, 251; mortality
from, 253; room need not be darkened,
252; symptoms of, 251; transmission, 250,
253; treatment and care, 239–240, 251,
252; treatment with convalescent blood,
252.

Meat, calcium in, 781; calories in, 766;
elimination fad, 762; in infant's diet, 224;

intestinal "worms" from, 416; iron and
copper in, 772; juice, stimulates gastric
juice, 382; kosher, 760; packers exposed
to undulant fever, 286; phosphorus in,
785; protein, 770; protein yield, 789;
soups, protein yield, 788; spoiled, cause
of diarrhea, 411; value in diet, 762–763;
varieties, in diet, 778.

Medals given diabetic patients, 596–597.

Medical college, class A, 2; number in 1900,
2; recognized, family doctor should be
graduate of, 2; recognized, what it is, 2.

Medical Examination: See Physical examination.

MEDICAL RESEARCH COUNCIL OF GREAT
BRITAIN, 623.

Medical Society, county, aids in selecting
physician, 7; physician should be a member of, 3.

Medicine, discoveries, 4; organized, 3;
scientific advancement, 4.

Medicine chest, 9; antiseptics in, 14; bottles
should be clearly labeled, 18; disorderly,
illustrated, 10; "don'ts" to be remembered, 16; drugs usually found in, 12;
equipment summarized, 16; first aid supplies in, 15; laxatives found in, 12; pain
relievers in, 13; surgical supplies in, 15.

Medicines (see also Drugs), dosage, 10, 11;
dropper necessary in measuring out, 11;
giving medicines to children, 11; hypodermic administration, 14; measuring, 10;
should be clearly labeled, 18; should be
mixed with water, 11; taking, 9, 11.

Mediterranean fever, 285.

Meerschaum, industrial poison, 653.

Melancholia, 38.

MELTZER, 508.

Memory, loss of, from chronic sinus disease,
727.

Men, few past age of fifty-five have power
of reproduction, 531.

MENDEL, 488.

Meninges, 231.

Meningitis, 231; incubation period, 232;
pneumococcus, 235.

Menopause (change of life), 55, 78, 141;
age at onset, relation to age of first
menstruation, 56; age at onset, statistics,
56; bathing during, 59; bleeding during,
may be sign of cancer, 58; bodily changes
during, 58; care of bowels during, 59;
diet during, 59; itching during, ointment
for, 58; mental changes during, 553;
mental symptoms during, 58; pregnancy

possible after, 180; recreation during, necessary, 59.

Menstruation (*see also* Menopause), absence of, 55; after sterilization, 179; age at onset, and when menopause should occur, 56; bathing during period, 53, 140; blood, allergy to, 518; cessation of, 140; cycle, 78; dancing, games, etc., during period, 802; discontinuance, age statistics, 56; disorders, 52; douching before and after, 55; duration of, 30–32 years, 56; estimating day of birth, 150; exercises during period, 53, 103, 802; exercises for young girls, 53; first period, 50, 141; first period, pregnancy possible before, 180; games during period, 53, 802; headache at periodic function, 38; in adolescent period, 102; mechanism, 552; nosebleeds during, 54; odor during, from infection, 54, 55; organs involved in process of, 54; painful, 53, 54; painful, remedies for, 54; period, twenty-one-day to five-week intervals considered normal, 52; return after childbirth, 175; rhythm of, and prevention of conception, 60–63; "safe period," 60–63; sanitary pads used for, 54; scanty, may be due to anemia, 54; should be regular by end of first year, 52; swimming during period, 140.

Mental aspects in tuberculosis, 333; aspects of pregnancy, 165; conflicts, 830, 832; defects, 837; defects, symptoms of, 838; deficiency, product of, not caused by masturbation, 134; depression, 844–845; depression, feeling of, in migraine, 38; development of children, 229.

Mental Disease, 825; causes of, 828; classification of, 826; community hospitals for, 846; continuous bath treatment, 844; hospital treatment best, 844; per cent cured, 845–846; prevention, 840; psychotherapy, 843; recognized as a kind of sickness, 847; recovery, 845–846; symptoms, 843; "total reaction" method in studying, 828; traveling from mental health to, 1–2–3 method, 835; treatment, 841; what constitutes, 837.

Mental health, modern conception of, 832; normal, traveling to mental disease, 1–2–3 method, 835; hygiene, 841; symptoms during menopause, 58; training in childhood, 834.

Menu, diabetic: *See* Diabetes mellitus.

Menus, suggested, 792 *ff*.

Mercurial nephrosis, 458.

Mercurochrome, use as antiseptic, 14, 26.

Mercury, bichloride of, antiseptic put in rinsing water in washing diapers, 187; bichloride of, douche, dangerous, 139, 144; bichloride of, douche may injure kidneys, 448; bichloride of, poisoning, call doctor at once, 41; bichloride of, poisoning, symptoms, antidotes, and treatment, 43; cause of kidney disease, 445; fulminate, manufacture, ethyl nitrite by-product in, 651; industrial hazard, 653; must not be used after applying iodine, 673; ointment, use after direct exposure to syphilis, 739; preparation for use in dropsy, 451.

Mesothorium, industrial poison, 653.

Metabolism of calcium and parathyroids, 543.

Metabolism, basal, defined, 768; how determined, 768; rate as index of thyroid activity, 542.

Metal-fume fever, industrial, 650.

Metal-plating, industrial hazard, 644.

Metal poisoning, 40.

Metaphen, use as antiseptic, 26.

Methanol, industrial poison, 653.

Methyl alcohol (wood alcohol) in shellac, 657; industrial poison, 653.

Methyl chloride, industrial poison, 654.

Methyl violet, industrial poisoning, 654.

Methylene blue test of kidney excretory function, 441, 443.

METROPOLITAN LIFE INSURANCE COMPANY, 567, 624.

Mexicans, tuberculosis rate in, 321.

MEYER, 435, 439.

Mica, industrial poison, 654.

MICHIGAN, goiter incidence in, 557, 559.

Microscope, blood examination with, first, 464.

Middle age, albuminuria in, 439; care of skin in, 677; physical changes in women during, 58, 59; sex in, 121.

Migraine, 37; occurs as frequently in men as women, 38; occurs between eighteen and thirty-five, 38; symptom of allergy, 522.

Military standing and walking position, 812.

Milk, acidified evaporated, how to make, 203; acidophilus, in constipation, 410; antidote in case of poisoning, 40; boiled, in infant feeding, 199; breast, as preventive of rickets, 498; calcium in, 781; calories in, 766; citric acid milk, how to make, 203; condensed, 199; condensed, in infant feeding, 200; cow's and breast milk compared, 199; dried, 199; evaporated, 199; food elements in glass of, 771;

formula for well baby, 201 *ff.*; formula, preparing, for infant feeding, 203; formula, sugars and carbohydrates in, 199; formula, undiluted, for infants, 202; in diabetic diet, 584; in infant's breast, 187; in infant's diet, 189, 201, 224; infected, cause of epidemic septic sore throat, 731; lactic-acid milk, preparation, 203; malted, in infant feeding, 200; mother's, 196; of magnesia (*see* "Magnesia"); pasteurization, 285–286; pasteurization necessary to prevent tuberculosis in children, 325; pasteurization prevents spread of undulant fever, 285; phosphorus in, 785; protein, 190, 770, 779, 781, 788; scarlet fever spread through, 255; sugar, 783; -sugar formula in infant feeding, 202; sweet-milk dilutions, preparation, 203; tuberculous-cattle control and, 325; typhoid transmitted by, 272–273; undulant fever spread through, 285; value in diet, 781.

Milkers, infected, may cause infected sore throat, 731; should wash their hands frequently to prevent contaminating milk, 731.

MILLER, JAMES A., 325, 326, 327.

MILLER JOSEPH W., on treating laryngeal tuberculosis, 335.

Mind: *See* Mental.

Miner's nystagmus, 644.

Mineral oil, 17; use as laxative, 12; use as laxative for aged, 853; use in pregnancy, 156; with agar, 17.

Mineral salts, food elements, 768, 770, 772; in infant's diet, 193; value in diet, 773.

Minerals in diet during pregnancy, 152; in infant's diet, 224; in vegetables, 785.

Mines, white, black, and stink damp in, 659.

MINKOWSKI, research on diabetes mellitus, 579.

Minnows, little top, feed on mosquito larvæ, 294.

MINOR, CHARLES L., health hints for tuberculous, 334–335.

Mirbane, oil of, industrial poison, 655.

Mirrors, use in treating tuberculosis of larynx, 335.

Miscarriage: *See* Abortion.

Mite, Itch: *See* Scabies.

Mitral stenosis result of rheumatic fever, 362.

Modesty, 85, 86; teaching, 91.

Molars, six-year, importance of, 750, 751.

Molasses, 784.

Molds, allergy, 516.

Moles, 666, 690; blue, 690; brown, 690; danger of becoming cancerous, 637.

MÖLLENDORFF, 423.

Mongolian idiocy, 560.

Monthly periods: *See* Menstruation.

MOREL, 554.

Morning sickness: *See* Pregnancy.

Moron, defined, 839.

Morphine, no place in medicine chest, 16; poisoning, symptoms, antidotes and treatment, 46.

Mortality: *See* Deaths.

Mosaic laws of foods, 760.

MOSHER, ELIZA, 799.

Mosquitoes, malarial and yellow fever, compared, 293; rôle in transmission of malaria, 292, 293, 294.

Mother (*see also* Maternal), care before and after childbirth, 147; care of, upon leaving hospital, 173; clothing for prospective, to take to hospital, 168; "father and mother" games, 92; function of, explained in sex education, 74, 75; mother-and-son complex, 136; nursing (*see* "Milk, mother's," "Nursing").

Motherhood as a career, 95.

Mouth (*see also* Gums, Jaws, Lip, Teeth), acid in, and tooth decay, 751; breathing cause of bad formation of teeth, 751; cancer, sex distribution, 629; care of infant's, after teeth appear, 186, 749; care of infant's, before teeth appear, 749; cavity, normal, compared with cavity as result of nasal obstruction, 722; dryness of, relieving, 730–731; first organ of digestion, 381; hygiene, 752–753; symptoms of allergy, 521; transmission of syphilis by, 743; trench, 285; Vincent's angina, 285; wash, 730; wash, alcohol in, 730; wash, commercial, 730; wash, how to make, 730; wash, value of, 753.

Mucin in treatment of ulcer of stomach and duodenum, 401.

Mucous membrane of nose, 720, 721, 725, 728–729; effect of vitamin A deficiency, 725–726.

Mucus in stools of infants, 195.

Mud baths, 669.

Mummies, Egyptian, arteriosclerosis found in, 614.

Mumps, 263 *ff.*; age incidence, 264; complications, sex gland, 264, 265; epidemic in soldiers in U. S. Army in World War, 264, 265; germs causing, 263–264; historical aspect, 263; in Negroes, 264; incidence, 238; quarantine, 264; seasonal incidence, 264, transmission, 264; treatment and care, 264–265.

MURPHY, JOHN B., 405.

MURRAY, J. A., 623.

Muscle joins sebaceous gland to hair follicle, 662.

Muscles, symptoms in infantile paralysis, 266.

Muscular exercise: See Exercise.

Mushroom, poisoning, 40; poisoning, symptoms, antidotes and treatment, 46.

Mustard poultice, how to make, 313.

MYERSON, ABRAHAM, 831.

Myocardium, 350 ff.

Myxoedema and thyroid gland, 539–540.

Nails, cleansing, 702; description, 701; "gift spots," 703; hygiene, 702; ingrowing toenails, 703, 820; longitudinal ridges, 702; loosening, 702; manicuring, 702; pitting, 702; polish for, liquid, 702; ringworm, 703; shedding, 703; splitting, 702; spoon-shaped, 703; thickening, 703; transverse grooves, 702; white spots on, 703.

Naphtha, "jags," 647; wood, industrial poison, 653.

Napkins, Sanitary: See Sanitary pads.

Narcissin, industrial poison, 654.

Narcissus bulbs, industrial poison, 654.

Narcotics, 13, 14; poisoning, first-aid treatment, 41; poisoning, symptoms, antidotes and treatment, 46.

Nasal Sinus: See Sinuses.

NATIONAL TUBERCULOSIS ASSOCIATION, 333.

NAUNYN, 572.

Nausea, during pregnancy, 153, 154, 155; in sick headache, 37.

Navel, hernia at, 206.

Neapolitan disease, 738.

Neck, "big" (see Goiter); stiffness of, suspicious symptom of infantile paralysis, 266, 267.

Negroes, cancer in, 629; mumps in, 264; pneumonia in, 315; pneumonia more serious in, 315; rickets in, 495; Southerners allergic to, 518; tuberculosis rate in, 321.

NEISSER, 745.

Nembutal, 13.

Nephritis, 420; Arderne's advice on, 462; calculosa (stones) recognized at the time of American Revolution, 428; cause, 444; cause of death in 1904 compared with 1929, 566; chief cause of ill health, 453; chronic tubular, with dropsy, 459; classification, 452; death rate compared

with heart disease, 347; glomerulonephritis gouty, 457; of old age, 454; of pregnancy, 157, 456; pyelonephritis, 455; scarlatinal, 458; trench or war, 453; work of Richard Bright, 433.

Nephrosis (see also Kidney disease), 458; lipoid, 459; mercurial, 458.

Nerves, manifestations of allergy, 522; of skin, 665; optic, 705.

Nervous disorder, 825; hiccups, 36; system, syphilis of, 740.

Neurosis, cardiac, 377–378; result of chronic sinus disease, 727.

Neurosyphilis, 740; treatment, 740.

NEW HAVEN, CONN., diphtheria elimination in, 248.

"New skin," collodion dressings, 674.

NEW YORK STATE DEPARTMENT OF LABOR first-aid measures in gas poisoning, 31.

Nicholson's rule, 610.

Nickel, carbonyl, industrial poison, 654; industrial poisoning from plating with, 654.

Nicotine (see also Tobacco), poisoning in tobacco industry, 659; poisoning, symptoms, antidotes and treatment, 46.

Niemann-Pick's disease, 482.

Night blindness, result of vitamin A deficiency, 489.

Night sweats in tuberculosis, 331.

Nipples, care of, during pregnancy, 163; care of, in nursing mother, 197; nursing bottle, 204; nursing bottle, choice and care, 203.

Nitric acid, burns caused by, treatment, 27; poisoning, symptoms, antidotes and treatment, 46; treatment of warts, 689, 821.

Nitrites poisoning, symptoms, antidotes and treatment, 47.

Nitrobenzene, industrial poison, 655.

Nitrocellulose, industrial poison, 655.

Nitrogen in protein, 770.

Nitrogen peroxide, industrial poison, 655.

Nitroglycerin, industrial poison, 655; poisoning, symptoms, antidotes and treatment, 47.

Nitrous chloride, industrial poison, 655; dioxide, industrial poison, 655; gases or oxides, industrial poison, 655; -oxide poisoning, symptoms, antidotes and treatment, 42.

Nits of lice, 686.

Nobel Prize awarded to Banting and MacLeod, 565; awarded to Laveran, 292.

Nodes, Osler's, sign of endocarditis, 370.

Nodules, rheumatic, sign of rheumatic fever, 358.

Nona, 300.

Nose, 720; abnormalities, 721; anatomy, 720; blowing, in colds, 314; boil or pimple in, 721; bridge of, disappearance of, 721; cleaning, in infant, 186, 228; conditions cause of headaches, 39; deformities, 721, 722; deformities, plastic surgery for, 721, 722; diagram showing, 734; discharge from, constant, sign of sinus disease, 726; foreign bodies in, 23, 723; forms of, 722; hemorrhage (see "Nosebleed"); hygiene, 721; infection cause of halitosis, 756; infections of hair follicles, 720; injuries, 721; lining, 720; lining, infection of, 721; mucous membrane, 720, 725, 728–729; mucous membrane, infection of, 721; mucous membrane, vitamin A deficiency effect on, 725–726; normal cavity, 722; obstruction, effect of, 722; obstruction, long-standing, effect, 722; obstruction, relation to colds, 307; picking, squeezing, pulling out hairs, dangerous, 721; plastic surgery, 722; polyps, 723, 728–729; polyps caused by allergy, 520; saddle, 721, 722; sense of smell, 728; sinuses (see "Sinuses"), spraying, 721; spraying for colds, 313; spraying, petrolatum eucalyptus menthol compound, for, 18; spraying, to prevent ear infection, 717; symptoms of allergy, 521; tumors, 723, 728–729; "whisky," 683–684; worms infestation of, 723.

Nosebleed, 724; causes, 724; don't blow nose after, 725; during menstruation, 54; first aid for, 20, 21; lasting longer than ten minutes demands expert care, 725; symptom, not a disease, 725; treatment, 724.

Nostrums: See Quack remedies.

Nourishment: See Malnutrition, Nutrition, Skin.

Nurse, wandering diabetic, 581.

Nursing baby, position for, 175; reasons for not, 196; technic, 197.

Nursing bottle, choice and care, 203; how to give, to baby, 204.

Nursing mother, care of breasts, 173, 174; care of nipples in, 197; diet for, 174, 196; exercise for, 175; hygiene of, 174; may become pregnant, 180; return of menstruation, 175; use of alcohol and tobacco by, 174.

Nutrition (see also Malnutrition), appetite guide to, 761; of infant, 189.

Nuts, calories in, 766; fat in, 585; in diet, 786.

Nux Vomica poisoning, symptoms, antidotes, and treatment, 48.

Nymphomaniac, 134.

Nystagmus, miner's, 644.

Oak, poison, cause of dermatitis, 680.

Oatmeal water substitute for soap, 668, 673.

Obesity, cause of diabetes, 572; how ten fat and ten lean men fare as they walk through life, 573; overeating cause of high blood pressure, 612; reducing weight and calories, 767; wise control of weight to prevent diabetes, 574.

Obstruction, Intestinal: See Intestines.

Occupational: See Industrial.

Odors, bad breath, 756; body, 665, 684; body, cause of, 665; during menstruation sign of infection, 54, 55; of genitals, 138; psychological research on, 728; sense of smell, 727–728.

O'Dwyer devised intubation tubes for use in diphtheria, 245, 248.

Œdipus complex, 136.

Ohio, goiter in, 557.

"Ohio scratches," 651.

Oil, aniline, industrial hazard, 646; coconut, in hard-water soap, 670; from grain, 783; of mirbane, industrial poison, 655; poisoning, symptoms, antidotes and treatment, 47; sweet oil, warmed, to remove insect from ear, 23; sweet-oil-and-kerosene treatment of head lice, 686.

Oilcloth, substitute for rubber sheet, 16.

Oiling, hair, 696; ponds to control malaria, 294, 295.

Ointment, don't use in eczema, 679–680; don't use in poison-ivy dermatitis, etc., 680; for itching during menopause, 58; of rose water or cold cream, 672.

Old age, 125, 126, 848; cancer in, 853; care of skin in, 677; changes in, 850; constipation in, 853; diabetics and, 597; disease of, 851; early, and diabetic child, 578; eggs possible cause of, 598; exercise in, 852; hygiene, 852; nephritis of, 454; number of persons over one hundred years, 848; rejuvenation in, 531–532; senile freckles, 692; sexual stimulation, 145; type of fat in food which possibly causes, 598; Warthin (A. S.) on, 125.

"Old maids," 123.

Oliver, John Rathbone, 615.

Onions, narcissus bulbs mistaken for, deaths from, 654.

Open-air bathing, 669.

Ophthalmia in newborn due to gonorrhea, 745; sympathetic, 706–707.

Ophthalmoscope in diagnosis of headache, 38; instrument to look into eye, 713.

Opium, no place in medicine chest, 16; poisoning, symptoms, antidotes and treatment, 46.

Optic nerve, 705.

Orangeade for colds, 314.

Oranges, in diabetic diet, 583; juice of, in infant's feeding, 204; vitamin C in, 494.

Orris root, allergy, 515, 516, 524; in face powder, 671.

Orthodontia, 750.

OSBORNE, 485, 488.

OSBORNE, OLIVER T., 619.

OSLER, WILLIAM, 304, 741.

Osler's node sign of endocarditis, 370.

Osteomalacia, 494.

"Ostrich step," 813.

Otitis media, 718; glycerine-phenol eardrops for, 718; in infants, 207–208; puncturing eardrum for, 718.

Ounce-tablespoon equivalents, 202.

Ovaries, 551 ff.; function, 76, 77, 78; involved in menstrual process, 54; location of, 533; one-ovary fallacy in regard to sex of unborn child, 178; rôle in mechanism of menstruation, 553.

Overeating cause of high blood pressure, 612, 615.

Overweight (see also Obesity), per cent in 17,000 men, 5.

Overwork cause of high blood pressure, 613.

Oviducts, 80.

Ovulation, 60–63, 78; mechanism of menstruation, 552.

Ovum: See Egg cells.

Oxalic-acid poisoning, symptoms, antidotes and treatment, 47.

Oxyacetylene gas, industrial hazard, 645.

Oxyacetylene welding, phosphureted hydrogen poisoning in, 656.

Oxychloride, carbon, industrial poison, 656.

Oxygen treatment of pneumonia, 318, 319.

Oxytocin, 546.

Oysters, calories in, 766; protein yield, 788; source of typhoid, 273.

Pacifier, no excuse for infant having, 189.

Packing-house workers exposed to undulant fever, 286.

Packs, cotton, used during menstruation, 55.

Pads, sanitary: See Sanitary.

Painful heels: See Heels.

Pains, "false" in pregnancy, 170; "growing," symptom of rheumatic fever, 357–358; in ulcer, gall-bladder disease, and appendicitis compared, 406; in ulcer of stomach and duodenum, 399–400; labor, 170; not always a symptom of kidney disease, 445; relievers, 11, 13; symptom in angina pectoris, 374.

Palate, diagram showing, 731.

Pan: See Bed pans.

Pancreas as seen in a cross section of the body, 570; description, 383; function in sugar metabolism, 569; "lazy" in diabetes, 591; location of, 533; regulates sugar metabolism, 589; source of insulin, 588.

Pancreatic juice, 383; enzymes of, 383.

Papaverine-codeine preparation for colds, 312.

Paper towels and handkerchiefs, 18.

PARACELSUS on goiter, 554.

Paraffin injections for wrinkles, dangerous, 694.

Paragonimus, cause of liver cancer, 625.

Paralysis, general, of insane, 741.

Paralysis agitans in aged, 852.

Paralysis, infantile: See Infantile paralysis.

Paranitranilin, acetanilid hazard in manufacturing, 645.

Paranitranilin red, industrial poison, 657.

Parasites, allergy, 518; intestinal, 415.

Parathryoid glands, location, function, 533, 542.

Paregoric, 14.

Paresis, 741.

Paris Green poisoning, symptoms, antidotes and treatment, 47.

Parotitis: See Mumps.

Parrot disease: See Psittacosis.

PASTEUR, LOUIS, 231, 241, 242, 282.

Pasteur treatment of hydrophobia, 284.

Pasteurization: See Milk.

Patent medicines: See Quack remedies.

Patterns of personality, 833; of personality in mental disorder, 827–828.

PAULUS ÆGINETA cure for bed-wetting, 445.

PEABODY, AMELIA, 596.

Peaches in infant feeding, 205.

PEARSON, KARL, 853.

Peas, calories in, 766.

PECHEY, quoted on treatment of kidney disease, 450.

Pediculoides ventricosus, 651.

Pediculus, three species infesting man, 686–687.

Pellagra, 498; cause, 499; course, 500; derivation of the word, 498; incidence, 499;

symptoms, 499; symptoms, the three D's. 499; treatment, 501.

Pelvic organs, chart showing, 57.

Pelvis, contracted, and childbirth, 143.

Pencil exercise for fallen arches, 817.

Pencil, indelible, methyl-violet poisoning from, 654.

Penis, cancer, circumcision prevents, 629; cleaning, 139; cleaning, in infant, 186; foreskin tight or adherent, 83; function of, 79.

Pennyroyal poisoning, symptoms, antidotes and treatment, 47.

Pepsin, absent from gastric juice, 388; in gastric juice, 381, 382.

Peptic ulcer, 398 ff.

Perfume in soap, 671.

Pericarditis in rheumatic fever, 360–361.

Pericardium, 349.

Perimeter to determine field of vision, 714.

Perinephritic abscess, 455.

Periods, monthly: See Menstruation.

Peritoneum, outer layer of stomach, 382.

Peritonitis, danger of, in taking cathartics in appendicitis, 12; perforation, 398.

Permanent wave, 696.

Pernicious anemia: See Anemia, pernicious.

Peroxide, nitrogen, industrial hazard, 655.

Peroxide of hydrogen: See Hydrogen peroxide.

Persecution, delusion of, 836.

Personal hygiene: See Hygiene.

Personality, of allergy patient, 513; patterns, 833; patterns in mental disease, 827–828.

Perspiration: See Sweat, Sweating.

Pessaries, danger of, 144.

Petechiæ, sign of endocarditis, 370.

PETERSON, BLANCHE, 333.

Petrolatum, -eucalyptus-menthol compound for nasal spray, 18; in cold cream, 672; liquid or melted, applied to burns, 27.

Petroleum, tar from, industrial hazard, 658.

PFIFFNER, J. J., 550.

PHARMACOPEIA, UNITED STATES, 13.

Pharynx, diagrams showing, 731, 734.

Phenacetin in headache powders, 13; poisoning, symptoms, antidotes and treatment, 41.

Phenobarbital poisoning, symptoms, antidotes, and treatment, 43.

Phenol: See Carbolic acid.

Phenolsulphophthalein test of kidney excretory ability. 441, 443.

Phosgene, industrial poison, 656.

Phospho-bronze, industrial poison, 656.

Phosphorus in diet, 773; in relation to tooth

decay in adults, 752; in various foods, 785; necessary in formation of good teeth, 750; poisoning, industrial, 656; poisoning, symptoms, antidotes and treatment, 48.

Phosphureted hydrogen, industrial poison, 656.

Photography, vanadium hazard in, 659.

Photophobia, 711.

Phrenic nerve, treatment in hiccup, 37.

Physical defects, disclosed by periodical medical examination, 5.

Physical education, for women, 801; university course in, 801.

Physical examination, before pregnancy, 147, 148; during pregnancy, 147, 148, 149; periodical, defects disclosed by, 5.

Physical training, 800.

Physician, diabetics should plan visit to, 581; ethical, characteristics, 3; ethics of, 3; family, 1; family, aptitude test for, 1; family, can care for 85 per cent of conditions, 6; family, choice of, 1; family, consult him first, 7; family, graduation from recognized school necessary, 2; family, internship of, 2; family, licensed by state, 2; family, membership in county medical society, 3; family, of former generations, 1; family, picking, 7; family, qualifications, 1; number of physicians in one month who died from circulatory diseases, 613; traveling, not suitable as family doctor, 4; visit to, in pregnancy, 147, 148, 149; when to call him for confinement, 170.

Physiology, of kidney, 425; of reproductive system, 76.

Physique cause of persistent low blood pressure, 620.

Pica or perverted appetite in pregnancy, 153.

Picric acid, industrial poison, 656.

Picric itch, 656.

Pigment, in hair, 695; of skin, 663, 665.

Piles: See Hemorrhoids.

Pills, correct way to give, 11.

Pillow, infant does not need, 185.

Pimples (acne vulgaris), 681–682; don't squeeze, 683; in nose, 721; not result of syphilis, 741; treatment, 682–683.

Pin, swallowing, first aid for, 23.

Pincette for removing superfluous hair, 700.

PINCUS, 572.

Pineal gland, location, function, 533, 538.

Pink eye, 708–709.

Pitocin, 546.

Pitressin, 546.

Pituitary, anterior lobe, 544; anterior, rôle in mechanism of menstruation, 54, 552; headache, 546–547; intermediate part, 544; lobes, function, 544; location, function, 533, 543–545; posterior lobe, 544.

Pituitrin, 546.

Placenta: *See* **Afterbirth.**

Plants, dermatitis from, 680; reproduction in, 68; sensitivity to, 507.

Plasmochin control of malaria, 295.

Plasmodium, 292.

Plaster, court, 674.

Plastic surgery, of nose, 722; of protruding ear, 715.

Plate, dental, 757.

Platelets: *See* **Blood.**

"Pleasure principle," 831.

Pleurisy, symptom of rheumatic fever, 358–359.

Plumbing: *See* **Water supply.**

Pneumococcus, 231; selective localization, 235; types, 315; ulcer on eye, 710.

Pneumoconiosis, 641.

Pneumonia (*see also* **Bronchopneumonia**), 231, 314 *ff.*; age incidence, 315; alcoholics more susceptible to, 316; cause of, 315: complication in measles, 260; convulsions in, in infants, 212, 213; course of, 316, 317; crisis, 316, 317; crowding factor in, 316; death of diabetics due to, 602; death rate compared with heart disease, 347; death rate in 1904 compared with 1929, 566; death rate in 1932, 567; diet in, 318; gas poisoning predisposes to, 31, 315; germs causing: pneumococcus, 315; in infants, 209; in old age, 850, 851; isolation, 317; oxygen treatment, 318, 319; prevention, 317; serum therapy, 319; symptoms in, 316; tonsillectomy, unfavorable effect on, 737; treatment and care, 317, 318; water requirement in, 318.

Poison, cause of diarrhea, 411; cause of jaundice, 404; cause of kidney disease, 444, 445; dangerous, no place in medicine chest, 9.

Poison ivy, cause of dermatitis, 680; treatment, 680.

Poison oak cause of dermatitis, 680.

Poisoning, antidotes, 41–49; cup of salted water every ten minutes to wash out stomach, 40, 41; food, 40; from drugs and chemicals used in industry, 645; gas, resuscitation from, 30; metallic, 40; ptomaine, 764; symptoms of acute, 41; treatment of acute, 41; what to do before the doctor comes, 40.

Poliomyelitis: *See* **Infantile paralysis.**

Pollen, allergy, 504 *ff.*, 506; allergy, described by Dunbar, 505; avoidance and pollen disease, 526; season, 515; sensitivity to, 514.

Pollination, cross, by insects, 71.

Polycystic kidneys, 462.

Polycythemia, 476; blood-letting in, 477.

Polyps, in nasal sinuses, 729; in nose, 723, 728–729; in nose caused by allergy, 520.

Pomade for the hair, harmful, 696.

Pores of skin, 663.

Pork, calories in, 766; intestinal "worms" from, 415–416.

Port wine marks, 690.

PORTIS, MILTON M., 380.

PORTIS, SIDNEY A., 380.

Portland cement, industrial poison, 656.

Position, best resting, for child, 799.

Postnatal period, abdominal binder (tight) harmful, 181; abdominal support advisable, 175; bathing during, 175; care in home after leaving hospital, 173; care in hospital, 172; examination by physician at end of six or eight weeks, 175; menstruation return, 175; mother must avoid steps until after third week, 173.

Postum, in smooth diet for indigestion, 393.

Posture, 797; bad, described, 799; bad, how to estimate, 799; during kindergarten, 798; effect of clothing, 802; exercises for faulty, 804–805; foot and, 802, 807; foot, right and wrong, 812; good, endurance test of, 799; of students of college age, 800; shoes, effect of, on, 802; sitting, correct, 798.

POSTURE LEAGUE design for shoes, 803.

Potassium-cyanide poisoning, symptoms, antidotes and treatment, 44.

Potassium hydrate forms soft soap, 669.

Potassium-hydroxide poisoning, symptoms, antidotes and treatment, 42.

Potassium permanganate baths to overcome body odor, 684.

Potatoes, calories in, 766; carbohydrate in, 785; food elements in, 771; in diabetic diet, 584; peel of, cellulose in, 785.

Poultice, mustard, how to make, 313.

Powder, dusting: *See* **Dusting powder.**

Powder, face: *See* **Face powder.**

Powder, tooth: *See* **Tooth powder.**

Pox, French, 738.

P-P factor of Goldberger, 499.

Prairie itch, 651.

PRATT, GEORGE K., 825.

Pregnancy (*see also* **Abortion, Childbirth,**

Conception, Confinement, Labor, Miscarriage, Postnatal period), 80, 81, 82; after menopause, 180; alcoholic beverages during, 153; amusement places, visiting, during, 161; automobile driving and rides during, 160; bathing during, 162; baths during, kinds to be taken and avoided, 163; before first menstrual period, 180; belching during, 166; bicycle riding during, avoid, 160; bloody or watery discharge sign of threatened miscarriage, 166; breast care during, 163; breast supports during, 158, 163; breath short during, 165; care of bowels during, 155; cathartics in, 156; clothing in, 157; constipation in, 155, 165; corset worn during, 158; craving for certain foods during, 153; dancing during, 160; dental work during, 164; diabetes during, 157; diagnosis, sex hormone test (Aschheim-Zondek) of, 545; diagnostic signs, 149; diet in, 151–154; diet in, does not affect size of baby, 180; diet in, to avoid constipation, 156; diet in, to prevent tooth decay, 164, 748; dizziness during, 166; enemas during, 156; estimating day of birth, 150; exercise in, 159; exercise (violent) should be avoided, 160; failure to feel baby after it has been definitely felt, 166; fainting spells during, 165, 166; fear of, cause of frigidity, 136; foods to avoid, 155; garters to be worn in, 157; genitals, care during, 164; goiter in, effect on offspring, 560, 561; goiter likely to develop in, 556; goiter prevention during, 168; golf during, 160; hair care during, 164; headache persistent in, 165; heartburn during, 166; hemorrhoids or piles in, 167; "high stomach" after, preventing, 158; horseback riding during, 160; house should be aired out during, 160; housework during, 161; in nursing mother possible, 180; in tuberculosis, 143; iodine medication in, 168; kidney disturbances during, 456; kidneys in, care of, 156; leg cramps during, 167; liquor during, use of, 153; "marking" the child, 177, 691; massaging abdomen during, 159, 161; mind during, 165; minor ailments during, 166; miscarriage during, preventing, 160; morning sickness (vomiting in early pregnancy), 153; mother raising arms will not cause lassoing of baby's neck, 181; nephritis during, 157, 456; nipples during, care of, 163; physical examination before, 147, 148; physical examination during, 147, 148, 149; physician should be consulted early in, 148, 149; position of child does not indicate sex, 181; prevention of, utilizing safe period, 60–63; pyelitis during, 157; "salt towel" to stimulate circulation during, 162; serious symptoms, 150; sewing on machine with foot treadle to be avoided, 161; sex determination of unborn child, 178; sexual intercourse in, 143, 164; shoes to be worn, 158; signs of, 149, 545; signs of beginning labor, 170; signs of trouble, 165; skating during, 160; smoking during, 153; swelling of feet, ankles, hands, etc., in, 157, 165; swimming during, 160; teeth care during, 748; teeth decay during, preventing, 151; underclothing to be worn during, 158; urine examination during, 149, 150, 156, 157; urine output diminished during, 165; varicose veins during, 165; vision blurred or doubled during, 165; vitality of seven- vs. eight-month baby, 178; vomiting after fifth month, 165; vomiting during, 148, 153, 154, 165; vomiting during early months, 153; vomiting during, special diets for, 153, 154–155; walking during, 159; Wassermann test in, 149; water in diet, use of, 152, 155; work (housework) during, 161; young married couple, 117.

Prenatal care: *See* Pregnancy.

Prescription, label on, read carefully, 10; measuring out medicine, 10; old, should be destroyed, 9, 10, 16, 18.

Prickly heat, 681.

PRIESEL, RICHARD, 571.

Primrose, cause of dermatitis, 680.

Prize fighter, tin ear of, 715.

Procaine-hydrochloride poisoning, symptoms, antidotes and treatment, 44.

Prone method of resuscitation, 28, 29.

Prostate, 79; cancer, 142, 633; condition in 17,000 men, 5; enlarged, kidney disease from, 457.

Protein (*see also* Albumin), absorption, in intestinal tract, 384; Bence-Jones, 438; common sources of, 770; content in various foods, 585; digestion of, 383, 384; distribution according to meal, 790 *ff.*; edema, 777; fear of, fad, 777; food element, 768, 770, 771; in diabetic diet, 582, 584; in diet during pregnancy, 152; in diet needed by children, 777; in eggs, 778, 779; in fish, 778, 779; in nuts, 785; in various foods, 779; in various kinds of meat, 778; milk, 781; nature of, 770; reaction, nonspecific in treatment of headaches, 40; requirement, 778; rôle in nutrition of in-

fant, 189, 190; sources of, 770; -starch-in-
diet theory in arthritis, 341; value of
cereals, 782; value of cheese, 782; value
of eggs in terms of round steak, 780;
vegetable, 779; yield of various foods, 788.
Proteinuria, Bence-Jones, 460.
PROTOSPATHARIUS on urine, 429.
Psittacosis, course of, 300; death rate high
in parrots, 299; epidemics, 298; historical
aspect, 298, 299; transmission, 299.
Psycho-analysis, 842–843.
Psychology, Freudian, 64; of adolescence,
96; of children, 91 ff., 830–831; research
on odors, 728.
Psychotherapy, 843; in mental disorder, 843.
Ptomaine poisoning, 764.
Ptyalin, action on starches, 382.
Puberty, 78; acne vulgaris in, 681; in girls,
50.
Pubic region, crab louse in, 687.
Puerperium: See Postnatal period.
Pugilist, tin ear of, 715.
Pulse pressure, definition, 610.
Pupil (eye), 705.
Purpura, 479; tendency to black-and-blue
spots, 480.
Pus in wound, treatment, 26.
Putrefaction, 384, 385.
Putty, industrial poison, 657.
Pyelitis, 455; during pregnancy, 157; in
infants, 211.
Pyelonephritis, 455.
Pylorus obstruction cause of vomiting in
infants, 214.
Pyorrhea, 754.
Pyramidon, 13.
Pyrene, industrial hazard, 657.
Pyrethrotoxic acid, industrial poison, 650.

Quack, confuses rheumatism and kidney
disease, 446; distinguishing, from ethical
physician, 3; never cured any cancer, 637;
remedies for anemia, 472–473, 475;
remedies for cataract, 712; remedies for
gonorrhea, 746; remedies for kidney disease, 451–452; remedies for rejuvenation,
531; remedies for syphilis, 742; urine
examination by, 431.
Quarantine, chicken pox, 262; diphtheria,
when should child be released, 244;
mumps, 264; whooping cough, 260, 261.
"Queerness," 835.
Quinidine poisoning, symptoms, antidotes,
and treatment, 48.
Quinine, in control of malaria, 295; indus-

trial hazard, 657; poisoning, symptoms,
antidotes and treatment, 48.

Rabbit Fever: See Tularemia.
Rabies: See Hydrophobia.
Race, distribution of cancer, 629.
Radiant energy diseases, industrial, 642.
Radiation of skin, 664.
Radium, cause of aplastic anemia, 470;
industrial hazard, 642; penetrates skin,
665; treatment of bone sarcoma, 634;
treatment of cancer, 631, ff., 636; treat-
ment of nose tumors, 729.
Ragweed pollen avoidance and pollen dis-
ease, 526.
Rash, diaper, 187; heat, 681.
Rat-bite fever, 295; course of, 295; death
rate, 295; germ, 296; treatment, 296.
Rat poison, thallium, industrial hazard, 658.
Ravioli, Italian tradition of, 765.
Rayon, industrial poison, 657.
Rays (see also Ultraviolet Rays, X-ray),
industrial hazard, 643.
Razor, 15; for removing superfluous hair,
700; shaving, 700–701.
"Reality principle," 831.
REASONER, 670.
Rectum (see also Anus), cancer, 413, 633;
cancer, intestinal obstruction first symp-
tom, 415; cancer preceded by inflamma-
tion, 637; prolapse in infant, 210; temper-
ature taken by, in heat stroke, 34.
Red blood cells: See Blood cells, red.
Red phosphorus, industrial poison, 656.
REES, 433.
Refrigerant, methyl chloride, industrial
poison, 654; sulphur dioxide, industrial
hazard in, 658.
REHBERG, 425.
Reins, reference to, in Bible, 428–429.
Rejuvenation, 531, 532, 551.
Renal, albuminuria, 435; artery, 423;
diabetes, 460; disease (see "Kidney").
Rennin, enzyme in gastric juice, 381, 382.
Repair, self-repair, 537.
Reproduction, asexual method, 69; career
depends on onset of puberty, 56; in beans,
70; in birds, 71; in fish, 71; in frogs, 72;
in plant and animal kingdoms, 68; in
turtle, 72; power of, in men past fifty, 531;
rôle of father in, 73, 74; rôle of mother in,
74, 75; sexual method, 69; vitamin E relation to, 501.
Reproductive system (see also Ovaries,
Penis, Sex, Testicles, Uterus, Vagina,
etc.), anatomy, 76; cleanliness of, 138;

hygiene of, 137; physiology, 76; three functions, 82.

Resin, Indian, in shellac, 657.

Resin-wax method for removing superfluous hair, 700.

Resistance, to disease and vitamin A, 490; to infectious disease, 232.

Respiration (*see also* Breathing), artificial, technic, 28, 29.

Respirator, artificial, use in infantile paralysis, 268.

Respiratory diseases, 304 *ff*.

Rest, bed, normal diet for, 791; in kidney disease, 449; in tuberculosis, 329.

Resting position, best, 799.

Resuscitation, after asphyxiation, 27; after electric shock, 28, 29, 30; method described, 28, 29; Schäfer method described, 28, 29.

Retina, 705; detachment of, 713; inflammation of, 712.

Rheumatic fever, 356 *ff*.; adenoids relation to, 367; attack on, 363; carditis or inflammation of heart sign of, 360; cause of, 363; climate in relation to, 364; colds in relation to "flare up" of, 365; colds sign of, 358; endocarditis result of, 369; geographic incidence, 364; growing pains sign of, 357–358; heart damage from, 368; heart damage from, discovered four to seven years later, 361; heart inflammation, 360; heart "leakage" result of, 362; heart muscle involved in, 362; heart-valve deformity result of, 362; housing, etc., relation to, 364; manifestation of, in childhood, 356; mitral stenosis result of, 362; more frequent in girls, 365; nodules manifestation of, 358; pericarditis in, 360–361; predisposition to, 363, 364; prevention, 367; seasonal incidence, 365; social strata and, 364; streptococcus cause of, 363; symptoms, in childhood, 357; tonsillectomy in relation to, 736; tonsils and, 366; treatment and care, 367–368.

Rheumatism (*see also* Arthritis), 337 *ff*.; confused with kidney disease by quacks, 446; differentiated from arthritis, 337; focal infection rôle in, 339; intestinal causes, 340; periods in which patient is better, then worse, 339.

Rhinitis, acute catarrhal, 307.

Rhus dermatitis, 680.

RICE, THURMAN B., 50, 64.

Rice, calories in, 766.

RICHARDS, 425, 449.

Rickets, a vitamin D deficiency, 494; cause, 495; cod-liver oil for, 219; derivation of the word, 494; effect of sunlight on, 496; history, 494; in infants, 218; incidence, 495; pelvis contracted as result of, 143; prevention and treatment, 498; symptoms, 497; treatment, 496; X-ray examination, 219.

RIESMAN, DAVID, 852.

RILEY, HENRY A., 39.

Ringworm, 684; causes, 684–685; form of sycosis, 701; of nails, 703; treatment, 685.

Roach powders, fluoride poisoning from, 45.

ROBERTS, R. J., 804.

ROCHESTER, NEW YORK, study of effect of tonsillectomy on scarlet fever and diphtheria, 735–736.

ROCKEFELLER INSTITUTE, 319.

Rocky Mountain spotted fever, 296 *ff*.; carried by lice, 687; death rate, 297; diagnosis, 297; incubation period, 296; symptoms, 296; tick source of, 296; vaccine, 297.

Rodent poisons, antidotes, 49.

Roentgen rays: *See* X-ray.

ROGOFF, 550.

ROLLESTON, SIR HUMPHRY, 848, 850, 851, 853.

ROOSEVELT, FRANKLIN D., afflicted with infantile paralysis, 265, 269.

Rose colds, 314.

Rose water, ointment of, or cold cream, 672.

ROSS, RONALD, research on malaria, 292.

ROTH, BERNARD, 803.

Rotogravure inks, industrial poison, 652, 657.

ROUELLE, research on urine, 431.

"Roughage school" of diet, 762.

Round shoulders and clothing, 803.

Roundworms, 415.

ROUX, 241.

ROWE, 522.

ROWNTREE, L. G., 550.

Rubber heels on shoes, value, 808.

Rubber sheet, 16.

Rubella: *See* German measles.

RUFFER, SIR ARMAND MARC, 61₅.

Rumination in infants, 214.

Running, avoid, in pregnancy, 160.

Rupture: *See* Hernia.

Russian bath, avoid during pregnancy, 163.

Rye bread, Slavic tradition of, 765.

"Safe period": *See* Menstruation.

Sailors, scurvy in, 492, 493.

St. Anthony's fire, 277.

St. Vitus's dance, symptom of rheumatic fever, 356; 359; tonsils in or out, 736.

SALICETO, 432.

Salicylic acid (*See also* **Acetylsalicylic acid**), for hard corn, 824; in dusting powder for perspiring feet, 824; in talcum powder to overcome body odor, 684; preparation for treating corns, 688.

Saliva, function in digestion, 381, 774; hydrophobia transmitted by, 282; index of kidney function, 442.

Salt, cleaning infant's teeth with, 749; in diet necessary, 773, 786; iodized, amount of iodine in, 560; iodized, history of, 560; iodized, in prevention of goiter, 558, 559; solution, value as mouth wash, 730; towel to stimulate circulation during pregnancy, 162.

Salvarsan, treatment of rat-bite fever, 296; treatment of syphilis, 744.

SAN FRANCISCO Health Department list of antidotes for poisoning, 41.

Sanatorium care of tuberculosis, 321, 326–327, 329, 330.

Sandstone, industrial poison, 657; quarrying, silicosis from, 658.

Sanitary cotton packs, pads, or tampons for use during menstruation, 54, 55.

Sanocrysin treatment of tuberculosis, 323.

Sanskrit writings, characteristic urine described in, 429.

Santal poisoning, symptoms, antidotes and treatment, 47.

Sarcoma, bone, 634; definition, 627; treatment, 634.

Satyr, 134.

Sauerbruch diet in tuberculosis, 331, 332.

Scabies (the itch), 687–688; treatment, 35.

Scalds, first-aid treatment for, 27.

Scales, greasy or dry, symptoms of seborrheic dermatitis, 681.

Scalp, bleeding from, how to control, 22; crust on, in infant, 186; dandruff, 698; massaging, by brushing hair, 696; seborrheic dermatitis, 681; use of bay rum spirits as antiseptic, 698.

Scar: *See* **Scars.**

Scarlet Fever, 255; antitoxin in treatment, 258; care of throat in, 258; cause of, 255; complications, 258; Dick test, 256, 257; diet in, 257–258; earache in, 258; epidemics, 255; immunity after one attack, 255; incidence, 238; incubation period, 232; kidney complications, 258, 458; mortality, 253; nephritis in, 458; preventive inoculations, 257; scales probably do not spread the disease, 256; spread directly from person to person, 255–256;

spread through milk, 255; strawberry tongue in, 256; symptoms, 256; throat symptoms in, 734; tonsils in or out, 734–735, 735–736; toxin, 256; treatment and care, 257–258; treatment, antitoxin, 258; treatment, convalescent blood in, 258.

Scars, 666; from blackheads, 682–683; keloids are benign tumors which grow in, 690.

Schäfer method of resuscitation, 28, 29, 31.

SCHAMBERG, J. F., 262.

SCHAUDINN, 739.

Schick test in diphtheria, 245, 735.

School child, sex education of, 90.

School grades, corrective exercises during, 798.

School, medical: *See* **Medical college.**

School seats, proper, 797 *ff.*

Scientific advancement of medicine, 4.

Scissors, 15, 16.

Sclera, 704.

Scorpion sting, first aid for, 35.

SCOTT, SIR WALTER, afflicted with infantile paralysis, 270–271.

Scratches, "Ohio," 651; sensitiveness, 518; treatment of allergy by, 528.

Scretagogues, foods as, 382.

Scurvy, 492; course, 493; due to lack of fruits in diet, 784; history, 493; nosebleed in, 724; symptoms, 493; treatment, 494.

Sea foods, iodine in, 559.

Sealing wax, industrial poison, 657.

Seamstress, number of calories used daily by, 767.

Seasoning, 786.

Seat, proper, for child, 797 *ff.*

Seating, proper, need for, 797.

Sebaceous glands, description, 662.

Seborrheic dermatitis, 681, 698.

Seborrheic warts, 689.

Secretin, excitant of intestinal secretion, 383.

Sedatives cause of low blood pressure, 619.

Seidlitz powder, 12.

Self-control, development of, 94.

Self-repair, 537.

Seminal emissions in adolescent boys, 102.

Senile alopecia, 699.

Senile freckles, 692.

Senile keratoses, 692.

Senility: *See* **Old Age.**

Sense of Hearing: *see* **Hearing.**

Sense of smell, 727.

Sense of taste, 720.

Sensitivity: *See* **Allergy.**

Serum, horse-serum-free toxoid, in dipththeria, 247; therapeutic, allergy to, 518; therapy in pneumonia, 319.

Sewer gas, industrial poison, 657.

Sewing, on machine during pregnancy, 161; wound must not be attempted by laymen, 26.

Sex, appeal, 125; changes in girls, 50; desire sometimes increased during menopause, 58; determination of unborn child, 81, 178; determination of unborn child not based on shape of abdomen, 181; distribution of cancer, 629; education, 65; education, function of father, 73, 74; education, function of mother, 74, 75; education, modesty in, teaching, 85, 86, 91; education of adolescent, 96; education of school child, 90; education of young child, 82; education, shame in, 91; education, why human childbirth so painful, 75; Freud's theory, 64; glands, 76; glands, function, 551, 552; glands, infection complication of mumps, 264, 265; glands, relation to suprarenal cortex, 551; glands, relation to suprarenals, 551; hermaphrodite, 82; hormone diagnosis of pregnancy, 545; hygiene, 64; in advanced life, 121; in middle age, 121.

Sexual complexes, 136; frigidity, 135; functions, abnormalities of, 133; intercourse (see also "Marriage," "Reproduction," "Reproductive system"), 82, 88; intercourse, appetite for, control, 121; art of, 115; intercourse, contraceptives, 144; intercourse during honeymoon, 112; intercourse during pregnancy, 143, 164; intercourse, excessive, 134; intercourse, explanation of, by parents, to adolescents, 98; intercourse, first, facilitating, 114; intercourse, foundation of home, 82; intercourse, frequency of, 120; intercourse, function of, reproductive system, 82; intercourse, gonorrhea prohibits, 746, 747; intercourse, gonorrhea spread by, 745; intercourse, gratification, 120; intercourse, complete, 144; intercourse, method of reproduction, 69; intercourse, "safe period" for prevention of conception, 60–63; intercourse, syphilis contagious period, 742; intercourse, syphilis transmitted by, 739; relations, discussed before marriage, 111; stimulant, gland therapy, 145.

SHAKESPEARE on urine examination, 440.

Shaking palsy in aged, 852.

Shale hazard in Portland cement, 656.

Shame in sex education, 91.

Shampoo: See Hair, washing.

Shaving, 700–701; blood crusts removed with hydrogen peroxide, 701; brush, sterilizing, 701; how to stop bleeding, 15, 701; makes hair seem coarser, 696.

SHAW, N. G., 735.

Shedding nails, 703.

Sheep-dip poisoning, symptoms, antidotes and treatment, 48.

Sheep pock: See Chicken Pox.

Sheet, rubber, 16.

Shellac, industrial hazard, 657.

Shellfish, protein yield, 788.

SHERMAN, 487.

Shock, allergic, 524; electric, resuscitation after, 28, 29, 30; resulting from burns, 26.

Shoe-button spider, bite by, first aid for, 35.

Shoes, 807; corns result of improper kind, 823; corns result of pressure from, 688; for fallen arches, 816; for flat-foot, 812; for ingrown toenail, 820; for soft corns, 823; gymnasium, 812; "health," 810; how to care for, 808; ill-fitted, cause of corns, calluses, etc., 817; postural effect, 802; Posture League design of, 803; rubber heels on, value, 808; type to be worn during pregnancy, 158.

"Shots" against colds, 311; in rheumatic disorders, 343.

Shoulders, round, and clothing, 803.

Shower baths, cold, 668–669; during pregnancy, 162, 163.

Shrimp, protein yield, 788.

Sick headache, 37.

Sick infant, care of, 205.

Sickness: See Disease.

Sigmoid cancer, 413.

Silica, industrial poison, 657; in Portland cement, industrial hazard, 656; in sandstone, industrial hazard, 657.

Silicate, magnesium, in talc as industrial hazard, 658.

Silicosis, 641, 644, 646; due to free silica, 657; due to granite, 651; due to meerschaum, 653; due to Portland cement, 656; due to sandstone, 657.

Silk, artificial, industrial poison, 657.

Silver, industrial hazard, 658.

SIMMONDS, 485.

Singeing the hair, 696

Sinuses, nasal, 720; chronic infection, chances for recovery, 726; disease, 725; disease cause of headache, 38; polyps in, 729; X-ray study of, 729

Sitting posture, correct, 798.

Sitting up in infants, 184, 185.
"606" treatment of rat-bite fever, 296; treatment of syphilis, 744.
Sixteenth century, life expectancy in, 849.
Skating, avoid, in pregnancy, 160.
Skeleton growth dependent on thymus, 535.
Skin, 661, *ff.*; abnormalities, 678; absorption by, 665; antiseptics, 673; antiseptics, boric acid, 674; antiseptics, carbolic acid, 674; antiseptics, hydrogen-peroxide solution, 674; antiseptics, iodine, 673; atrophy, wrinkles first sign of, 694; bactericidal power, 665; birthmarks, 690; blackheads (acne vulgaris), 681–683; blanching, 663; blood vessel tumors of, 691; body odor, 684; bronzing, symptom in Addison's disease, 549; cancer, 627, 630, 692; care at various periods of life, 676; care in adolescence, 677; care in children, 676; care in infant, 676; care in middle life, 677; chafing, 678; changes in aged, 851; chapping, 678; cold cream for, 672; color, 663; corns, 688; dry, 664; dry, and soap, 668; dry, soap substitutes for, 668; effect of bathing on, 667; effect of constipation on, 667; elasticity, 662; electricity applied to, dangerous, 675; eliminant of waste products, 664; fat, 663; fishhook in, how to remove, 26; flushing, 663; food, no such thing as, 664, 666, 672; freckles, 663, 678, 692; functions of, 664; greaseless lotions for cleansing, 673; greasy, care of, 668; greasy, cold cream harmful for, 672; infection (chronic) per cent in 17,000 men, 5; inflammation, 678; itching, not caused by syphilis, 741; itching, sodium bicarbonate for, 18; keeping it healthy, 666; keloids, 690; keratoses, 692; light treatment, 676; lousiness, 686–687; massage, 675; moles, 690; nerves of, 665; "new skin" or collodion dressings, 674; nourishment, 663–664; nourishment dependent on blood and lymph, 666; pigment, function, 665; pimples, 681–682; pores of, 663; protection from sunlight, 665; protective function of, 664; radiation one of the chief functions of, 664; ringworm, 684; scabies or the itch, 687–688; soap for, free alkali in, should not exceed one fourth of one per cent, 670; steaming, 675; structure, 661; sunburn, 678; sweating, excessive, 684; sweat production function of, 664; symptoms of allergy, 522; tanning, 663, 677, 678, 692; tests, 666; tests for tuberculosis, 328–329; texture, 663; tumors, xanthoma, 694; ultraviolet rays' effect on, 675; warts, 689; whiteheads (acne vulgaris), 682; wrinkles, 693.
Skyshine, antirachitic effect, 496.
Sleep, extra, needed during adolescence, 51; for baby, 223; habits in infants, 188; -producing medicines, harmful results, 11; requirements for children according to age, 223.
Sleeping sickness: *See* Encephalitis, epidemic.
Slippers, ballet, 812.
Smallpox, incubation period, 232; mistaken for chicken pox in adult, 263; vaccination, 239; vaccination of infants, 220.
Smears, throat, in suspected diphtheria, 242.
Smell, psychological study, 728; sense of, 727.
Smelling salts, inhaling, use in fainting, 33.
Smoke, allergy, 517.
Smoking by adolescent girl, 51; during pregnancy, 153; forbidden for syphilitics, 743; nursing mother should avoid, 174.
Snow fields, sunburn from, 678.
Soap, alkali in, 669–670; cold cream as substitute for, 668; composition of, 669; eczema irritated by soap and water, 680; for washing hair, 696; greaseless cold creams are really soaps, 672; green, 669, 670; hard, 669; hard-water, 670; history of, 669; kind to use in bathing, 668; laundry, 669; oatmeal water substitute for, 668, 673; perfume in, 670; stick, how to make and use, 225; substitutes for, 668, 673; suds, action of, 670; suds kill germs, 670; superfatted, 670; toilet, 669; transparent, 670.
Society, medical: *See* Medical Society.
Soda ash, industrial poison, 650.
Soda, baking: *See* Sodium bicarbonate.
Soda mint tablets for heartburn, 166.
Soda, washing, poisoning, symptoms, antidotes and treatment, 42.
Sodium bicarbonate, 18; for heartburn, 166; gargle, 730; in medicine chest, 14; treatment of burns, 27.
Sodium carbonate poisoning, symptoms, antidotes and treatment, 42.
Sodium chloride: *See* Salt.
Sodium citrate to loosen the cough, 213.
Sodium cyanide, industrial poison, 658; poisoning, symptoms, antidotes, treatment, 44.
Sodium hydrate forms hard soaps, 669.
Sodium hydroxide poisoning, symptoms, antidotes and treatment, 42.

Sodium perborate treatment of Vincent's angina, 285.

Sodium phosphate in medicine chest, 12.

Sodium tetra-iodo phenolphthalein, 390.

Soldiers, albuminuria in, per cent, 434–435; "hearts," 378; measles in, 249; mumps epidemics in, 264, 265; nephritis in, 453; trench mouth in, 285; typhoid in, 276.

Sore, syphilitic: See Syphilis.

Sore throat: See Throat.

Soups, protein in, 788; stimulate gastric juice secretion, 382.

SOUTH CAROLINA, iodine in soil, thus in vegetables, 559.

Spaghetti, Italian tradition of, 765.

Spahlinger vaccine in treatment of tuberculosis, 324.

Spanish fly as sexual stimulant, 145.

Spasm of esophagus, 394–395.

Spasmophilia in infants, 219.

Specialists, boards for certifying, 6; consult family doctor instead of, 7; development of, 6.

Specialties, membership in societies devoted to, 3.

Specific gravity of urine, diagnostic significance, 441.

Specimen of urine, how to prepare, 149–150.

Speech development in infants, 184, 185.

Spermatozoa, 79; fertilization of egg cell, 80; gonads and, 551–552.

Sphygmomanometer for measuring blood pressure, 608.

Spider bites, first aid for, 35.

Spinach, calories in, 766; use in anemia, 473.

Spirochaeta cause of syphilis, 739.

Spleen, enlarged, 482; enlarged in endocarditis, 370.

Splint, how to make, 20.

Splinters, removing, 26.

Sponge baths during pregnancy, 162, 163.

Spoon, measuring medicine with, 11; -shaped Nails (see "Nails"); variations in sizes of, 11.

Sports (see also Athletics), during menstruation period, 53.

Spotted fever, 296.

Sprained ankle: See Ankle, sprained.

Spraying, ear, 23; nose, 721; nose and throat to prevent infected ear, 717; nose for colds, 313; nose, petrolatum-eucalyptus-menthol compound for, 18.

Spurs cause of painful heels, 818, 819.

Squirrels, plague-like disease in, tularemia, 290.

Staphylococcus, cause of impetigo, 681; cause of kidney disease, 444; infection of nose, 720; resist soapsuds, 670.

Starch, action of ptyalin, 382; digestion in arthritis, 341; digestion in duodenum, 383; form of carbohydrates, 770; in diet, source of, 770; -protein in diet theory in arthritis, 341.

State hospital: See Hospital.

State laws forbidding marriage of syphilitics, 744.

State licensing of physicians, 2.

STATE MEDICAL BOARD OF REGISTRATION AND LICENSURE, 2.

Status hypoplasticus, 536, 546.

Status thymico-lymphaticus, 536, 546.

Steam, devices for creating, 15; medication in croup, 209.

Steaming the skin, 675.

STEFÁNSSON, 777.

STEINACH method of rejuvenation, 531.

Sterility, natural monthly, 60–63; syphilis and, 742.

Sterilization essential in treating wounds, 26; sexual, by surgical means, 144; sexual, not deleterious on woman in after life, 179.

STEWART, 550.

STEWART, W. B., 301.

STILLIANS, ARTHUR W., 661.

Stings, of insects, first aid for, 34, 35.

Stink damp, industrial hazard, 659.

Stockings, elastic, for varicose veins, 167; recommended for soft corn, 824.

Stomach acidity, body alkalinity different from, 773; acidity, diet for hyperacidity, 794–795; acidity, diet for hypoacidity, 795–796; cancer, 407, 628, 633; cancer, sex distribution, 629; cancer, treatment, 407; cancer, X-ray examination in, 407; digestion by, 382, 775; disorders, allergic, 504 ff.; disorders (chronic), cause of halitosis, 757; distention cause of vomiting in infants, 214; effects of abscessed teeth, diagram showing, 755; emptying time in infant, 194; emptying time, study of, 389; falling of, or gastroptosis, 397; function in digestion, 381; "gas on the stomach," 396; "high stomach" after pregnancy, 158; location of, 533; preparations in treatment of anemia, 472; secretion (see also "Gastric juice"), histamine given to provoke, 388; secretion, stimulation of, 382; symptoms of allergy, 522; tube, use in studying digestion, 388; ulcer, 398; ulcer, causes, 398–399; ulcer, diet in, 401; ulcer, distinguishing between gall-bladder disease and appendicitis, 406; ulcer, pain in, 399–400;

ulcer, perforation of, 400; ulcer, symptoms, 399; ulcer, treatment, 400; ulcer, vomiting blood in, 400; ulcer, X-ray examination, 401; X-ray examination, 389.

Stone dressing, silicosis from, 658.

Stones: *See* Gall bladder, Kidney.

Stools, 776; analysis, 385; color of, of infants, 195; curd in, of infants, 195; examination of, value, 390; form and color, significance, 384–385; isolate organism from, in dysentery, 412; mucus in, of infants, 195; tarry or black, in ulcer of stomach and duodenum, 400.

Storage-battery manufacture, litharge poisoning, 653.

Store, workers in, per cent having foot trouble, 815.

Stork fable of where babies come from, 86.

Strain, emotional, cause of high blood pressure, 611, 614.

Straitjackets have been abandoned in treating insane, 844.

Strawberry marks, 690.

Streptococcus, cause of impetigo, 681; cause of kidney disease, 444; cause of rheumatic fever, 363; cause of septic sore throat, 731; infection of nose, 720; *viridans* cause of endocarditis, 369.

Striæ gravidarum, 158–159.

Stroke, heat stroke, 33.

STROUSE, SOLOMON, 759.

Strychnine poisoning, symptoms, antidotes and treatment, 48.

Students, albuminuria in, percentage, 435; college, posture of, 800.

Styes, 709.

Styptic for use after shaving, 15.

Subconscious, theory of, 832.

Succus entericus, 383.

Sugar (*see also* Carbohydrates), cereals 75 per cent sugar solution, 784; consumption in United States, 780–781; different kinds, 783–784; digestion, 385, 388; equivalents, ounce-tablespoon, 202; form of carbohydrates, 770; fuel value of, 780; in blood (*see* "Blood"); in diet, 783; in infant feeding, 201; in milk formula for infant, 199; in urine (*see* "Urine"); lump of, and five-cent piece weigh the same, 582–583; metabolism, 569; -milk formula in infant feeding, 202; ounce-tablespoon equivalents, 202; source of, in diet, 770; tooth decay and, 753; types more laxative than others, 216.

Sulphur baths, 669.

Sulphur dioxide, industrial hazard, 658.

Sulphuric acid, burns caused by, treatment, 27.

Sumac, cause of dermatitis, 680.

Summer colds, 314.

Sun baths, 675.

Sunburn, 678; severe, danger of, 669, 677; treatment, 678–679.

Sunlight, effect of, on rickets, 496; sensitiveness to, 518, 519.

Sunshine, exposure of baby to, 221–223.

Sunstroke, unconsciousness from, 32.

Superstitions about childbirth, 177.

Supper: *See* Dinner.

Suppositories, vaginal, as contraceptives, 144.

Suprarenal cortex, 548, 550, 551; extract in use of Addison's disease, 550; interrelationship to other glands, 551; rôle in mechanism of menstruation, 552–553.

Suprarenals, cause of low blood pressure, 618; function, 547 ff.; location, 533, 547 ff.

Surgery, plastic, of large or protruding ears, 715; of nose, 722.

Surgical powder as styptic for use after shaving, 18.

Surgical treatment of cancer, 636.

Swallowing, air, 395–396; air by infants, 197, 198; difficulty in, 394; glass, bone, or pin, 23.

Sweat, bath, 669; bath, avoid, in pregnancy, 163; cause of body odor, 665; glands, 663; glands, description, 662; insensible, 665; odor of, 684; pores, 663; production of, function of skin, 664; quantity of water eliminated by, 419; sugar containing, in diabetics culture medium for bacteria, 667; violet odor of, carotene cause of, 665.

Sweating, excessive, 684; feet, 824; night sweats in tuberculosis, 331.

Swimming, avoid, during pregnancy, 160; during menstrual period, 140; few women able to save themselves in emergency, 27; in cold water during menstrual period, 140; one of the best exercises for women, 802; or open-air bathing, 669; -pool method in infantile paralysis, 269; resuscitation method described, 28, 29; 25 per cent of men do not know how to swim, 27.

SWINGLE, W. W., 550.

SWITZERLAND, cancer death rate in, 626–627.

Syancuprol treatment of tuberculosis, 323.

Sycosis (barber's itch), 701.

SYDENHAM, THOMAS, 249; description of gout, 344–345.

SYDENSTRICKER, 435.

SYMMERS, DOUGLAS, 297.
Sympathetic ophthalmia, 706–707.
Syphilis, "blood medicines" for, 742; cancer and, not related, 742; cause of high blood pressure, 613; cause of mental disease, 827; caused by germs, 738, 739; cornea inflammation due to, 711; cure of, requires long time, 743; facts which should be known, 741; historical aspect, 738; infection from nonsexual sources, 739; Kahn test, 468; marriage of persons who have had, 744; may attack any part of the body, 235; mercury ointment as preventive after direct exposure to, 739; of heart, 371; of nervous system, 741; primary stage, 739–740; quack remedies, 746; secondary stage, 740–741; serodiagnosis, 740; sore, 739–740, 740–741; sore, healing or removing, does not cure, 740; state laws forbidding marriage of persons with, 744; symptoms, first, 739; symptoms, primary, 739–740; symptoms, secondary, 740; symptoms, tertiary, 741; tests for, 740; third stage of, 741; transmission, 739; transmission by mouth, kissing, etc., 743; transmission, nonsexual, 739; treatment, salvarsan ("606"), 744; U. S. Army instructions for those with, 742; Wassermann test, 468.
Syringe, fountain, 16; how to syringe out the ear, 716; hypodermic, 12.
Syrup: See Corn syrup, Maple syrup.
Systolic pressure: See Blood pressure, systolic.

Tabes dorsalis, 741.
Tablespoon-ounce equivalents, 202.
Tailors, number of calories used daily by, 767.
TAKAKI, 784.
Talc, industrial poison, 658.
Talcum powder, 16, 671; containing salicylic acid for body odor, 684.
Talking, age at which infants begin, 184, 185.
Tallness: See Height.
Tampons, use during menstruation, 55.
Tannic acid, applied to burned area, 27; industrial hazard, 658.
Tanning, 663, 677, 678, 692.
Tansy poisoning, symptoms, antidotes and treatment, 47.
Tantrums, 835.
Tape: See Adhesive tape.
Tapeworms, 415.
Tapping in dropsy, inscription on gravestone of Lady Page, 451 footnote.

Tar, industrial poison, 658.
Tartar deposits on teeth, 756.
Taste, loss of sense of, 720; tasting sweet, sour, salt or bitter, 720; tongue responsible for sense of, 720.
Tea, 786; strong, as an antidote, 40; use of, by adolescents, 51.
Tear ducts, 709–710; infection, 710; obstruction, 710.
Tears, bloody, 710; chemical composition, 709.
Teasing children regarding love affairs, 91.
Teaspoon, measuring medicine by, 10.
Teeth (see also Toothbrush, Toothpaste), abscessed, effects of, diagram showing, 755; abscessed, should be extracted in diabetes, 600; baby (see "Teeth, first"); care of, 748; care of, in adult, 751; care of, in infant, 748; care of, in pregnancy, 164; "clean," 751; cleaning, in infant, 186, 228, 749; cleaning, paste, powders, and mouth washes for, 753; cleaning, toothbrush for, 752; cleaning, with salt, 749; crooked, cause of, 751; decay, 751; decay and sugar, 753; decay, causes of, 754; decay during pregnancy, 151; decay, nutrition in relation to, 752; decay, preventing, 752; defective, per cent in 17,000 men, 5; dentist should look over, every six months, 756; enamel, 752, 753; eruption, in infant, 184; extraction, how to control bleeding after, 20; false, 757; false, care of, 757–758; false, cleaning, 758; false, facial expression and, 758; false, hygiene of, 757–758; false, learning to eat with, 758; fillings, cause of gum irritation, 756; first, dentist should care for, 749; first, disappearance, 751; first, infant's diet to insure sound, 749; first, preserving, 749; first, time of appearance, 749; function in digestion, 381; halitosis due to, 756; in diabetic children excellent, 578, 584; permanent, 750; rôle in digestion of food, 774; six-year molars, 750, 751; straight, 750; straightening, braces for, 751.
Teething, 749.
Temper, fits of, cause high blood pressure, 612; tantrums, 835.
Temperature, body, clinical thermometer for taking, 17; body, high (see also "Fever"), in infant, reducing, 205; body, normal: 98.6 degrees F., 236; body, taken by rectum in heat stroke, 34; body, taken regularly in heat stroke, 34; common colds and, 305; of bath water, 668; of bath water for pregnant woman, 162; of in-

fant's room for sleeping and waking hours, 185.

Tendon of Achilles, exercises for stretching, 814.

Tennis, avoid playing, in pregnancy, 160.

Test meal in studying digestion, 388.

Testicles, descent of, 84; eating of animal, as sexual stimulant, pseudoscientific, 145; function, 76, 77, 78; location of, 533.

Tetanus, 279 *ff.*; antitoxin, 281, 282; course of the disease, 280; deaths from, yearly in U. S., 280; from fireworks, 25; germs causing, 279, 280; history, 279; incubation period, 280; industrial hazard, 642; symptoms, 280–281; treatment and care, 281–282; wounds cause of, 280.

Tetany, in infants, 213, 219; relation to parathyroid, 542.

Tetraethyl lead, industrial poison, 658.

"Texas mange," 651.

"Thalgrain" poisoning, symptoms, antidotes and treatment, 49.

Thallium, poison, industrial, 658; poisoning, symptoms, antidotes and treatment, 49.

Thermometer, clinical, 17.

Thinness, how ten fat and ten lean men fare as they walk through life, 573.

Thorium, industrial hazard, 653.

Threshers' itch, 651.

Throat, 729; diphtheria bacilli found in children apparently recovered, 244; foreign body in, 23; in scarlet fever, 258; inflammation, 730; irritation, 729; lozenges, 730–731; "lump" in, 394; smears taken from, in suspected diphtheria, 242; sore, 730; sore, epidemic septic, 731; sore, ice bag for, 730; sore, in beginning of infectious disease, 232; sore, in relation to "flare up" in rheumatic fever, 365; sore, in scarlet fever, 734; sore, incidence after tonsillectomy, 736; sore, may be diphtheria, 242, 244; sore, sign of rheumatic fever, 358; sore, use of gargle in, 730; spraying, to prevent infected ear, 717; swelling and inflammation, 729; symptoms of allergy, 521; symptoms in diphtheria, 734; tickling back of, to induce vomiting, 40.

Thrombosis, coronary, 372; compared with angina pectoris, 376; in diabetics, 597; symptoms, 376; treatment and care, 377.

Thrush in infants, 210.

Thumb sucking, cause of bad formation of teeth, 751; in infant, 188–189.

Thymus, function, 535; location of, 533.

Thyroid (*see also* Goiter), 556; activity, basal-metabolism rate index of, **542;** anatomy, 556; cancer, 628; condition during adolescence, 52; enlargement during pregnancy, 168; function, 539; location of, 533, 539; overactive, 540; rôle in mechanism of menstruation, 553; secretion, chemistry, 557; secretion deficient, tongue abnormally large, 719; secretion, iodine in, 557; toxic, heart changes in, 371.

Ticks, source of Rocky Mountain spotted fever, 296; source of tularemia, **291.**

Timidity, 835.

TIMME, WALTER, 530.

Tin, industrial hazard, 659.

"Tin ear," 715.

TISDALL, FREDERICK F., 182, 220.

Tissue, inner connective layer, of skin, 661; repair by protein, 770.

Tobacco, cause of cancer, 625; effect on blood pressure, 614; forbidden for syphilitics, 742; industrial poison, 659; poisoning, symptoms, antidotes and treatment, 46; smoking by adolescents, 51; smoking by nursing mother, 174; smoking during pregnancy, 153; smoking forbidden for syphilitics, 743; use of, and precancerous lesions on tongue, 637; use of, and Vincent's angina, 285.

Toenails: *See* Nails.

Toes, pinched, diagram showing, 811; turned out, 803.

Toilet habits, training infant in, 188, 225–226.

Toilet necessities required for infant, 169.

Toluene, industrial poison, 659.

Toluol, industrial poison, 659.

Tomato juice, vitamin C in, 494.

Tomatoes, calories in, 766.

Tongue, 718; burning sensation, 719; coated (furred) in acute indigestion, 391; coated (furred), in dyspepsia, 397; diagram showing, 731, 734; "geographic," 719; inflammation, 719; inflammation, causes, 719; painful, 719; place in digestion, 381; responsible for sense of taste, 720; tongue-tie, 719; too large, 719; white spots on, may develop into cancer, 637.

"Tonic" in anemia, 472–473.

Tonics, blood, 475.

Tonsillectomy: *See* Tonsils, removal.

Tonsillitis, 732; chronic, 733; distinguishing between diphtheria and, 732; treatment and care, 732.

Tonsils, cause of halitosis, 756; diagram showing, 731, 734; enlarged, cause of chronic sinus disease, 727; enlarged, relation to colds, 307; enlarged septic or buried, per cent in 17,000 men, 5; infected (*see also* "Tonsillitis"), in diabetes mellitus, 600; infected, may be source of disease elsewhere, 733; infected, relation to diphtheria, 735; infected, should be removed, 366; lingual, diagram showing, 734; normal and enlarged, should not be removed, 366; purpose of, 732; relation to rheumatic fever, 366; removal, 733; removal, indications, advisability, 733–737; removal, relation to various diseases, 733–737; removal, surgical *vs.* electrical, 737.

Tooth: *See* Teeth.

Toothbrush, 752; care of, 752; each person should have two, 753; new, should be put in salt-water solution, 752; when first to use, in child, 749.

Toothpaste, alkaline, value of, 753; child's use of, 749; claims in advertising of, 753–754; value of, 753.

Toothpicks, damage done by, and their substitute, 756.

Tooth powders, value of, 753.

Torus palatinus, 537.

"Total reaction" method in studying mental disease, 827.

"Touchiness," 835.

Tourniquet, how to apply in hemorrhage, 20; may do more harm than good, 22; to stop bleeding, 15; use in specific treatment of allergy, 527.

Towel, as tourniquet, 15; exercise for fallen arches, 816; paper, 18; salt towel to stimulate circulation during pregnancy, 162.

Toxin, cause of kidney disease, 444; defined, 246.

Toxin-antitoxin, defined, 246; diphtheria, 246.

Toxoid, defined, 246; horse-serum-free type, 247.

Toy firearms, blindness from injuries, 25.

Trachoma, 709.

Tradition factor in diet, 764, 765.

Tragacanth in greaseless lotions, 673.

Transfusion: *See* Blood transfusion.

Transmissible diseases, 272 *ff.*

Traut on number of filter chambers in kidney, 422.

Traveling during pregnancy, 160.

Trench mouth, 285.

Trench nephritis, 453.

Treponema, cause of syphilis, 739.

Trichloroethylene, industrial hazard, 649; industrial poison, 659.

Trinitrophenol, industrial poison, 656.

Trional, 13.

Tropics, diseases of, in temperate zones, 236.

Trousseau, 460.

Trudeau, Francis, 327.

Truss for hernia in infants, 206.

Trypsin, enzyme in pancreatic juice, 383.

Tub bath, during pregnancy, 162, 163; for infant, 226.

Tubercle bacillus cause of kidney disease, 444.

Tuberculin, Koch's, treatment of tuberculosis, 330.

Tuberculin test for tuberculosis, 328–329.

Tuberculosis, 319; absent in savage and barbarian races, 321; age susceptible to, 324; B. C. G. vaccine in, 324; beds for patients, increase in number of, 321; calcium in treatment, 330; Calmette inoculation, 324; climate in, changing, ten points to be considered, 327–328; climate in prevention and treatment, 325; cod-liver-oil treatment, 330, 331; collapse therapy, 323; copper cyanourate-potassium cyanide cure, 323; copper treatment, 330; cost of invalid care, 326; creosote treatment, 331; death caused by, in 1904 compared with 1929, 566; death in diabetics due to, 602; death rate, 319, 320; death rate compared with heart disease, 347; death rate in 1932, 567; death rate in, relation to malnutrition, 324; decrease in incidence, 321; detection, 322; diet in, 324; diet in, Herrmannsdorfer-Sauerbruch and Gerson, 331, 332; Dreyer antigen therapy, 324; everyone (practically) has had it by age of fifteen, 321; exposure to, 320; fever in, 331; fresh-air treatment, 330; gold treatment, 323, 330; guaiacol treatment, 331; health hints for patients, 334–335; immunization, Calmette, 336; in cattle, 325; in Mexicans, 321; in Negroes, 321; in young married couple, 117; incidence, 238; infection of cornea in, 710–711; inflammation of retina in, 712; lung hemorrhage in, 331; lung hemorrhage in, first aid for, 21; malnutrition, relation to, 324; may affect any part of body, 235; medical treatment, 323–324; mental aspects in, 333; milk pasteurization to prevent, 325; mother with, should not nurse her baby, 196; National Tuberculosis Association, 333; night sweats in, 331; not caused by cold baths during menstruation, 140; of kidneys, 457; of larynx, ultraviolet ray in, 335; patients must coöperate in treatment, 333; pregnancy in, 143; prevention, 320, 321, 322; research on, 322, 323; rest in, 329; sanatorium care, 321, 326–327, 329, 330; skin test in, 328; Spahlinger vaccine in, 324; syancuprol treatment, 323; treatment, 330 ff.; treatment, coöperation of patient necessary, 333; tuberculin test in, 328–329; tuberculin treatment, 330; X-ray examination in, 328–329.

Tularemia, 290; derivation of name, 290; dressing rabbits source of, 291; Francis's research on, 290, 291; historical aspect, 290; rabbits source of, 291; source, 291; transmitted by deer flies, wood ticks, rabbit ticks, and lice, 291.

Tumors, basal cell, 631; blood vessel tumors of older skin, 691; definition, 627; obstructing intestines, 414, 415; of nose, 723, 728–729; per cent in 17,000 men, 5; yellow, of skin, or xanthoma, 694.

Turkish baths, 669; avoid, during pregnancy, 163.

Turpentine, in sealing wax, industrial hazard, 657; poisoning, symptoms, antidotes and treatment, 47; pure gum spirits of, industrial poison, 659; test of renal function by Hahn, 457; wood, industrial hazard, 659.

Turtle, reproduction in, 72.

Tympanic membrane: See Eardrum.

Typhoid, 231, 272; bacilli, 272; bacilli resist soapsuds, 670; baldness after, 698–699; carriers, 272, 276; carriers, control, 237; death rate declining, 276; death rate, decline since 1890, 272; decline, in U. S. (1900–1923), 273; flies in transmission of, 273; ice source of, 273; in American army in the World War, 276; incidence, 238; incubation period, 232, 273; milk source of, 272–273; oysters source of, 273; stamping out, 236; symptoms, 274; transmission, 272, 273; treatment and care, 275–276; treatment, vaccine, 276; vaccination, 276; vegetables source of, 273; water source of, 272–273; Widal test in, 275.

Typhus carried by body lice, 687.

Ulcer, danger of, becoming cancerous, 637; of leg and syphilis, 741; of stomach and duodenum, 398; on cornea in trachoma, 709; on eye, 710.

Ultraviolet rays, curative effect of, in rickets, 496; effect of, on skin, 675; in conditioning against colds, 310, 311; industrial hazard, 643; treatment of laryngeal tuberculosis, 335; treatment of rickets, 496, 497.

Umbilical cord, cutting and tying, 171–172; function in pregnancy, 151; lassoing child not due to mother reaching, 181.

Umbilicus hernia in infants, 206.

Unconsciousness, first aid for, 32.

Underhill, 501.

Underwear, and odor from genitals, 138; type worn during pregnancy, 158.

Underweight, per cent in 17,000 men, 5.

Undulant fever, 285; incubation period, 286; meat packers exposed to, 286; milk source of, 285; symptoms, 286; treatment and care, 287.

Uneeda biscuit, in diabetic diet, 584, 585.

United States, life expectancy in, 849.

United States Army instructions for syphilitics, 742.

United States Pharmacopeia , 13.

United States Public Health Service, 309.

University: See Medical college.

University of Cincinnati, 733.

Uranium cause of kidney disease, 445.

Urea concentration in blood as test of kidney function, 442, 443.

Uremia, 446–448; blood urea concentration, 447; Bright coined the word, 447; in chronic glomerulonephritis, 454.

Ureter, 422; catheter, use in examining kidney function, 442; place in journey through kidney, 427.

Urinalysis: See Urine examination.

Urination, training infant, 226.

Urine, abnormal but no nephritis present, 459; albumin in (see also "Albuminuria"), demonstration by Dekkers and Cotugno, 431, 432; albumin in dropsical, demonstrated by Cruickshank, 431, 432; albumin in, Wells on, 432; albumin in, work of Richard Bright, 432; Bence-Jones protein, 438; black, 461; Booerhaave research on, 431; casts, 440; characteristic, in twenty different diseases, described in Sanskrit, 429; color, etc., symptoms in kidney disease, 446; curative properties, 429; diminished output, in pregnancy, 165; enormous quantities of, passed in diabetes insipidus, 460; examination, 440; examination, depicted by Dutch painters, 430; examination, diagnosis should not be based only on, 439–440; examination, history of, 430; examination in pregnancy, 149, 150, 156, 157; examination, quacks specialize in, 431; examination, Shakespeare on, 440; healthy, should be albumin free, 434; "honey," reference to, in Sanskrit writings, 429; hyaline casts in, 441;

in pyelitis in infants, 211; incontinence, bed-wetting, 445; manufacture of, by kidney, 424; secretion, increasing with diuretics, 450; specific gravity, diagnostic significance, 441; specimen, how to prepare, 149–150; sugar in, Dobson research on, 431; sugar in, in diabetes mellitus, 459; sugar in, in renal diabetes, 460; sugar in, in untreated diabetic, 590; sugar in, insulin dosage based on color of Benedict test, 601; sugar in, none in healthy person, 569; sugar in, none in treated diabetic, 591; sugar in, per cent in 17,000 men, 5; sweetness of, in diabetes mellitus, 569; therapeutic use, 429–430; weight of, Van Helmont studies on, 431; "white urine," 460.

Uromancy, 430–431.

Uroscopy, 430–431.

Urticaria (hives), 504 ff.

Uterus, 79, 80; cancer, 142, 629, 632; cancer, bleeding during menopause may be sign of, 58; cancer, prevention, 637; involved in process of menstruation, 54; rhythmic contractions sign of beginning labor, 170.

Uvula, diagram showing, 731.

Vaccination, against smallpox, 239; against typhoid, 276.

Vaccines against colds, 311; B. C. G. in tuberculosis, 324, 335; infantile paralysis, 266; Rocky Mountain spotted fever, 297; Spahlinger, in treatment of tuberculosis, 324; typhoid, 276.

Vagina, bacteriology of, 139; bloody discharge or "show" from, sign of beginning labor, 170; bloody or watery discharge from, sign of threatened miscarriage, 166; escape of water from, which is not urine, sign of beginning labor, 170; suppositories for, as contraceptives, 144.

Vaginitis in infants, 212.

Valves of the heart, 350 ff.

Van Helmont, studies on weight of urine, 431.

Vanadium, industrial poison, 659.

Varicella: See Chicken Pox.

Varicose veins, bleeding from, how to control, 21; elastic bandage or stocking for, 167; in pregnancy, 167.

Variola: See Smallpox.

Varnishes, amyl alcohol industrial hazard in, 646.

Vas deferens, tying, to preserve youth, 551.

Vaseline, 17; in cold creams, 672.

Vasopressin, 546.

Vaughan, 522.

Veal, calories in, 766.

Vegetables, 785; calcium in, 781; calories in, 766; canned, sieved, for infant feeding, 224; carbohydrates in, 784; carbohydrates in per cent, 583; copper and iron in, 772; in diabetic diet, 582, 584; in infant's diet, 224; oils from, 783; protein in, 779; raw, source of typhoid, 273; soups, proteins in, 788; source of amebic dysentery, 288.

Veil or caul on newborn child, 181.

Veins, Varicose: See Varicose veins.

Vena cava, 351 ff.

Venereal diseases, 738 ff.

Ventilation, relation to colds, 306, 309.

Ventricles of heart, 350, 351.

Veronal, 13.

Verruca: See Warts.

Vertigo: See Dizziness.

Vimtrup, on number of filter chambers in kidney, 422.

Vincent's angina: See Angina, Vincent's.

Viosterol, fortifying cod-liver oil with, 193; use in rickets, 496, 498.

Virchow, Rudolph, 464.

Virginity, ruptured or intact hymen in, 84, 114–115.

Virility, loss of, 123.

Virus, defined, 282–283; filtrable, cause of warts, 689, 821.

Vision, blurred or doubled, in pregnancy, 165; defective, in 17,000 men, 5; disturbances, headache associated with, 38; in man compared with that of animals, 704; infant's, development, 185; loss of (see "Blindness"); mechanism, 704–705; perimeter to determine field of, 714; seeing colored lights, 705; spots or specks in, 705.

Vital statistics: See Death rate.

Vitamin A, carotene precursor of, 490; deficiency effect on nasal mucous membrane, 725–726; deficiency leads to colds, 207; deficiency and xerophthalmia, 488; described, 190, 191; in relation to colds, 312; resistance to infection and, 490; source, nature and actions, 490; sources, purposes, and deficiencies, 502; stored in liver, 490–491.

Vitamin B, deficiency, beriberi, 491; described, 191; in cereals, 783; sources, purposes, and deficiencies, 502.

Vitamin B₂: See Vitamin G.

Vitamin C, deficiency or scurvy, 492; described, 191; heat detrimental to, 494; sources of, 494; sources, purposes, and deficiencies, 503.

Vitamin D, deficiency, 494; described, 192:

sources, purposes, and deficiencies, 503.

Vitamin-deficiency diseases, 483 *ff*.

Vitamin E, 193, 501; sources, purposes, and deficiencies, 503.

Vitamin G or B₂, 191, 499; deficiency, 486; deficiency cause of pellagra, 499; sources, purposes, and deficiencies, 503.

Vitamins, 774; in diet, 787; in fruits, 784; in infant's diet, 224; in relation to tooth decay in adults, 752; in various foods, 775; necessary for building sound teeth, 748, 750; necessary in diet in chronic sinus disease, 727.

Vocal cords, diagram showing, 734.

Voit, 777.

Volatile oils, poisoning, symptoms, and treatment, 47.

Vomiting, blood in ulcer of stomach and duodenum, 400; how to induce, in case of poisoning, 40, 41; in acute indigestion, 391; in indigestion, 396; in infants, 214; in pregnancy (*see* "Pregnancy"); in sick headache, 37; symptom in differentiating between ulcer and gall-bladder disease and appendicitis, 406.

Von Behring, 241.

Voronoff method of rejuvenation, 531.

Wagner, Richard, 571.

Walking, age when infants begin, 184, 185; during pregnancy, 159; for mother during postnatal period, 175; hiking crazes and the feet, 820; how to walk with flat feet, 810; in old age, 852.

War: *See* World War.

War nephritis, 453.

Warm bath, 668–669.

Warthin, Aldred Scott, 125, 531.

Warts, 689, 821; danger of their becoming cancerous, 637; on sole of foot, 821; removal, 821; seborrheic, 689; treatment, 689; treatment, nitric acid condemned, 689.

Washes, Mouth: *See* Mouth wash.

Washing: *See* Bathing, Diapers, Hair.

Washing soda, poisoning, symptoms, antidotes and treatment, 42.

Washwoman, number of calories used daily by, 767.

Wasp sting, first aid for, 34.

Wassermann test, 740; criterion of cure in syphilis, 744; in syphilis of heart, 371; on blood, 468.

"Waste products," 420.

Watch dials, industrial hazard from painting, 642.

Water, amebiasis transmitted by, 287, 288; bath, temperature of, 668; bath, temperature of, during pregnancy, 162; boiling, safest way to control amebic dysentery, 290; "brash," 396; cause of diarrhea, 411; chlorination, in control of amebic dysentery, 290; cold, cover area of slight burns and scalds with, 27; cold, sponging with, in heat stroke, 34; cold, swimming in, during menstrual period, 140; cold, use in fainting, 33; -concentration tests of kidney function, 441, 443; elimination, by kidney, lungs, and sweat, 419; excretion, 60 per cent by kidney, 424; exercise in, in infantile paralysis, 268; food element, 768, 770, 772; glassful every hour, for colds, 313–314; hard, soap for, 670; hot, to control bleeding, 21; hot, to control bleeding after tooth extraction, 20; in diet during pregnancy, 152, 155; in infant's diet, 193, 201; iodine added to, to prevent goiter, 557; oatmeal, substitute for soap, 668, 673; pock (*see* "Chicken pox"); quantity that passes through kidney, 425; requirement in pneumonia, 318; salted, cup every ten minutes in poisoning, 40, 41; source of typhoid, 272–273; supply, defective, cause of amebiasis in Chicago, 287–288; value in diet, 772; wetting the hair with, 696.

"Water brash," 396.

Waterproofing, danger of nitrocellulose, 655.

Wave, permanent, 696.

Wax, ear, 716; -resin method for removing superfluous hair, 700; sealing, industrial poison, 657.

Weaning, 176, 198; care of breasts in, 176.

Weather changes and colds, 305, 306.

Weight (*see also* Obesity, Overweight, Thinness, Underweight), diabetic estimates number of calories needed according to, 587; diabetic sets example for control in, 595; height-weight table for various ages, 769; increase, at adolescent period, 52; increase, normal rate in infant, 183; increase, too rapid in pregnancy, 165; increasing, cause of diabetes, 571; of heart in child, 346; reduction and calories, 767; wise control of, 574.

Welders, industrial hazard for, 643.

Welding, phosphureted hydrogen hazard in, 656.

Wellcome, 430, 431.

Wells on albumin in urine, 432.

Wendt, Dr., planned a diabetic camp, 605.

West Virginia, goiter in, 558.

Wheat, protein, 770.

"Whisky nose," 683–684.

White blood cells: *See* **Blood cells, white.**

White damp, industrial hazard, 659.

Whiteheads, 682.

White of eggs: *See* Egg whites.

White phosphorus, industrial poison, 656.

WHITE, PRISCILLA, 572, 577, 605.

"White urine," 460.

Whooping cough, 259; blood changes in, 260; complications serious, 260; diet in, 261; epidemics, cause and prevention, 259, 261; germ, 259; hernia or rupture in, prevention, 260; incidence, 238; incubation period, 259; mortality in, 259; prevention of spread of, in neighborhood, 261; quarantine in, 260, 261; relieving the cough, 261; vaccines, 260.

Widal test in typhoid, 275.

Wife, points to be considered in selecting, 105–106; working after marriage, 116.

Wigs, 697.

WILBUR, 425.

WILBUR, DWIGHT L., 483.

WILDBOLZ on surgical recovery in renal tuberculosis, 457.

WILDER, RUSSELL M., 483.

WILLIAMS, LINSLY, 321.

WILLIS, 564.

Winter itch, 668.

WITHERING, WILLIAM, 249.

Womb: *See* Uterus.

Women (*see also* Girls), games for, 801; hygiene of, 50; physical education for, 801.

WOOD, FRANCIS CARTER, 622.

Wood alcohol, industrial poison, 653; in shellac as industrial hazard, 657.

Wood sawers, number of calories used daily by, 767.

Wood tar, industrial poison, 658.

Wood turpentine, industrial hazard, 659.

Work (*see also* Industrial), calories needed based on type of, 767; diet according to kind done, 791; high blood pressure and, 616; housework during pregnancy, 161; overwork, 613; wife working after marriage, 116.

World War, advice to those in, with gonorrhea, 746; epidemic encephalitis during, 300; instructions during, to syphilitics, 742; measles in, 249; mumps epidemic in American soldiers in, 264, 265; "soldier's heart" in, 378; tetanus epidemic during, 280; trench mouth in, 285; trench nephritis in, 453; tuberculosis death rate before and after, 324; typhoid in, 276.

Worms, in intestine, 415; infestation of nose, 723.

Worry, advice on how not to, 615; cause of high blood pressure, 615, 616.

Wounds, 25; antiseptics for, 673 *ff.*; bite, first aid for, 34; bleeding from, how to control, 15, 21; cleanliness necessary in caring for, 25; disinfection, 26; hydrogen peroxide solution for, 18; infected, doctor's care necessary, 26; packing, with gauze, to control hemorrhage, 21; sewing, must not be attempted, 26; tetanus caused from, 280.

Wrinkles, 693; "face lifting" for, 693; paraffin injection in, dangerous, 694; treatment, 693.

Xanthoma, 694.

Xerophthalmia, 488; history, 488.

X-ray, cause of aplastic anemia, 470; diagnosis and treatment of bone sarcoma, 634; diagnosis of appendicitis, 405; diagnosis of cancer, 635; diagnosis of cancer of bowels, 414; diagnosis of gastroptosis or "fallen stomach," 398; diagnosis of headache, 38; examination in rickets, 219; examination in stomach cancer, 407; examination in syphilis of heart, 371; examination in tuberculosis, 328–329; examination in ulcer of stomach and duodenum, 401; examination of child's first teeth, 750; examination of gall bladder, 390; examination of kidney, 441; examination of stomach, 389; in advancement of medicine, 4; industrial hazard, 642; location of foreign bodies by, 23; location of foreign bodies in nose by, 723; penetrates skin, 665; picture in painful heel, 818; picture in sprained ankle, 817, 818; picture of eye injury, 706; study of lungs to prevent asbestosis and silicosis, 641; study of nasal sinuses, 729; treatment of cancer, 631 *ff.*, 636; treatment of keloids, 690; treatment of warts, 821.

Xylene (xylol), industrial hazard, 660.

Yellow fever, 236; mosquito compared to malarial mosquito, 293.

Yellow jacket, first aid for sting of, 35.

Yellow phosphorus, industrial poison, 656.

Zinc, industrial hazard, 660.

Zinc chills, 648.

Zinc chloride, industrial hazard, 660.

Zinc-oxide ointment, 17.

Zinc stearate in dusting powder, 671.

Zinc sulphate, industrial hazard, 660.